GEMS

A Golden Endeavor for Medical Students

AF891979

Celebrating 50 Years

Passion, Quality and Innovation in Healthcare Publishing

System requirements:

Windows:

- Operating System
  - Windows Vista or above.
  - Macintosh OS X or above
- Recommended Web Browser – Google Chrome & Mozilla Firefox
- Essential plugins – Java & Flash player
  - If facing problems in viewing content – enable/re-install Java plugin on your web browser setting.
  - If Videos don't show up – enable/re-install Flash Player or manage Flash setting on your web browser settings.
  - You can test Java and Flash by using the links from the help section of the CD/DVD.

Accompanying CD/DVD Rom is compatible and playable only in Computers and not in DVD player.

CD/DVD has Autorun function (only for Windows based systems). If Autorun feature doesn't works, then follow the steps below to access the contents manually:

Windows:

- Click on My Computer
- Select the CD/DVD drive and click open/explore – this will show list of files in the CD/DVD
- Find and double click file – "launch.html"

Mac:

Double click the file "launch.html" located on the root after inserting the CD/DVD. The Mac OSX operating system does not support an Autorun feature.

For more information about troubleshoot of Autorun click on: http://support.microsoft.com/kb/330135

CD CONTENTS

Contains Specimens, X-rays and Instruments of:

- Medicine
- Surgery and Orthopedics
- Obstetrics
- Pediatrics

GEMS

A Golden Endeavor for Medical Students

THIRD EDITION

Liyakkath Ali M MBBS MD DNB
Government Medical College
Calicut, Kerala, India

Muhammed Noufal Poongadan MBBS MD DNB
Government Medical College
Calicut, Kerala, India

Jafar Niyas P MBBS MD DNB
Government Medical College
Calicut, Kerala, India

Shameej KV MBBS MS MCh
Government Medical College
Calicut, Kerala, India

Muhammed Navas NK MBBS MS MCh
Government Medical College
Calicut, Kerala, India

JAYPEE BROTHERS MEDICAL PUBLISHERS
The Health Sciences Publisher
New Delhi | London | Panama

Jaypee Brothers Medical Publishers (P) Ltd

Headquarters
Jaypee Brothers Medical Publishers (P) Ltd
4838/24, Ansari Road, Daryaganj
New Delhi 110 002, India
Phone: +91-11-43574357
Fax: +91-11-43574314
Email: jaypee@jaypeebrothers.com

Overseas Offices
J.P. Medical Ltd
83 Victoria Street, London
SW1H 0HW (UK)
Phone: +44 20 3170 8910
Fax: +44 (0)20 3008 6180
Email: info@jpmedpub.com

Jaypee-Highlights Medical Publishers Inc
City of Knowledge, Bld. 235, 2nd Floor
Clayton, Panama City, Panama
Phone: +1 507-301-0496
Fax: +1 507-301-0499
Email: cservice@jphmedical.com

Jaypee Brothers Medical Publishers (P) Ltd
Bhotahity, Kathmandu, Nepal
Phone: +977-9741283608
Email: kathmandu@jaypeebrothers.com

Website: www.jaypeebrothers.com
Website: www.jaypeedigital.com

© 2019, Jaypee Brothers Medical Publishers

The views and opinions expressed in this book are solely those of the original contributor(s)/author(s) and do not necessarily represent those of editor(s) of the book.

All rights reserved. No part of this publication and CD-ROM may be reproduced, stored or transmitted in any form or by any means, electronic, mechanical, photocopying, recording or otherwise, without the prior permission in writing of the publishers.

All brand names and product names used in this book are trade names, service marks, trademarks or registered trademarks of their respective owners. The publisher is not associated with any product or vendor mentioned in this book.

Medical knowledge and practice change constantly. This book is designed to provide accurate, authoritative information about the subject matter in question. However, readers are advised to check the most current information available on procedures included and check information from the manufacturer of each product to be administered, to verify the recommended dose, formula, method and duration of administration, adverse effects and contraindications. It is the responsibility of the practitioner to take all appropriate safety precautions. Neither the publisher nor the author(s)/editor(s) assume any liability for any injury and/or damage to persons or property arising from or related to use of material in this book.

This book is sold on the understanding that the publisher is not engaged in providing professional medical services. If such advice or services are required, the services of a competent medical professional should be sought.

Every effort has been made where necessary to contact holders of copyright to obtain permission to reproduce copyright material. If any have been inadvertently overlooked, the publisher will be pleased to make the necessary arrangements at the first opportunity. The **CD/DVD-ROM** (if any) provided in the sealed envelope with this book is complimentary and free of cost. **Not meant for sale**.

Inquiries for bulk sales may be solicited at: jaypee@jaypeebrothers.com

GEMS—A Golden Endeavor for Medical Students

First Edition: 2012
Second Edition: 2013
Third Edition: **2019**

ISBN 978-93-5270-517-7

Printed at Sanat Printers

Dedicated to

Our beloved friend

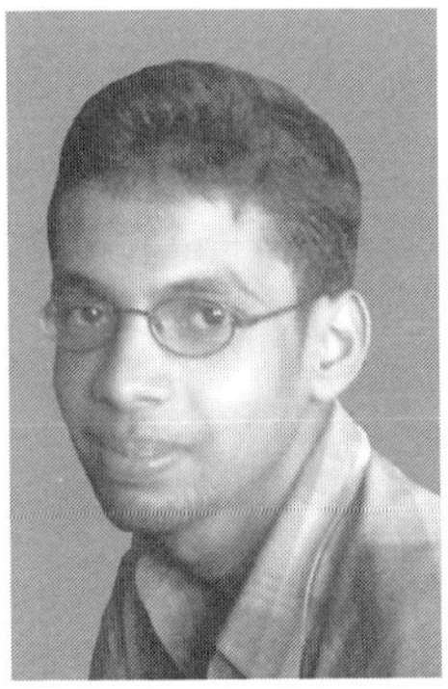

***Late* Shibilu AJ**

It was a day that shook our world...

Our beloved batchmate Shibilu AJ left this world, with lots of unsaid things and dreams...

Our book 'GEMS' is and always will be incomplete without a mention of our brother.

Through this book, we intend to make it an everlasting memory of our brother

who will always and forever remain in our hearts...

Contributors

Ameer VM
Government Medical College
Calicut, Kerala, India

Anilkumar KM
Government Medical College
Calicut, Kerala, India

Mohammed Musthafa PP
Government Medical College
Calicut, Kerala, India

Mohammed Niyaz KV
Government Medical College
Calicut, Kerala, India

Muhammed Basheer KT
Government Medical College
Calicut, Kerala, India

Salal N
Government Medical College
Calicut, Kerala, India

Shamsudheen MP
Government Medical College
Calicut, Kerala, India

Preface to the Third Edition

After the tremendous support and success of its first and second edition, we are immensely happy to bring the next edition of GEMS. A thoroughly revised edition based on the new examination pattern of Kerala University of Health Sciences and readers' suggestions especially the first university batch (54th Calicut Medical College).

The final year, by today terms, has become a hurdle of Darwinian proportions. The fittest survive. The help sought, the classes taken, the books read, all vary. As former aspirants ourselves, we have had to face similar compelling situations. The idea for this book stems from our efforts to perfect a standardized manual handling the vast multitude of topics that the field of medicine holds, concise as required by the undergraduate, keeping in mind the standards set and followed in case handling today.

The correct analysis and evaluation of a situation presented before the candidate is mandatory for every aspirant of the subjects. Hard work has to be put in, without question. But it is the correct analysis of the situation which makes the dart hit the eye.

We have taken every effort to keep the topics to the current scenario, and the cases to the standardized format as prescribed by the latest syllabi of the subjects.

We have put our outmost efforts in bringing out this wonderful book, which is a result of a lot of toil and patience. We sincerely hope that this book will be a guide for those aspirants who are driven to pass the examinations with flying colors.

We have incorporated what we have felt is the need for the aspirants in our age, from our experiences and of those enlightened who have taught us from the very beginning.

It is for the reader to evaluate our work and we sincerely hope our book has the privilege of being the reader companion throughout the journey of the aspirant in being, a doctor of medicine.

Liyakkath Ali M
Muhammed Noufal Poongadan
Jafar Niyas P
Shameej KV
Muhammed Navas NK

Preface to the First Edition

Final year MBBS has become an increasingly tough year with lots of topics, clinical cases and management. So it becomes very important to master the essential cases with correct management to pass this hurdle. It is a need we felt and serves as the driving force to bring up this 'novel' edition of *GEMS—A Golden Endeavor for Medical Students*, a complete manual for overcoming the vast multitude of cases and questions being asked in the practical examinations.

Hard work alone may not suffice to crack this hard nut, but an analytical approach with focused attention on relevant areas.

We have taken every effort to keep this book complete and abreast with all important areas with authentic references. We strongly believe that this manual is bound to invoke a thorough understanding and a holistic approach to the subject.

We have tried our best to bring the best and with our experience feel this book is a must for every aspirant wishing to come out with flying colors in the practical and theory examinations. It is for readers to analyze the truthfulness of our humble work and make it your companion in the eternal journey to be a doctor.

Liyakkath Ali M
Muhammed Noufal Poongadan
Jafar Niyas P
Shameej KV
Muhammed Navas NK

Acknowledgments

To the God, the benevolent, the merciful.

We would like to thank all teachers of Government Medical College, Calicut, Kerala, India, for their blessings and guidance.

Our sincere gratitude to:

Medicine
- Dr Aquil Kalanad, MBBS MD DNB, Government Medical College, Calicut, Kerala, India.
- Dr Nikhil Gladson, MBBS MD (General Medicine) DM, Government Medical College, Calicut, Kerala, India.

Surgery
- Dr Vineeth Rao, MBBS MS (General Surgery), Government Medical College, Calicut, Kerala, India.

Orthopedics
- Dr Sibin Surendran, Assistant Professor, Government Medical College, Calicut, Kerala, India.
- Dr Rejith Valsalan, MBBS MS D Ortho DNB MRCS (Edin), Government Medical College, Calicut, Kerala, India.
- Dr Azhar CM, MBBS MS D Ortho, Government Medical College, Calicut, Kerala, India.

Pediatrics
- Dr Aslam PK, MBBS MD DCH, Government Medical College, Calicut, Kerala, India.

Obstetrics and Gynecology
- Dr Geovin Ranji G, MBBS MS (Obstetrics and Gynecology), Government Medical College, Calicut, Kerala, India.

We would also like to thank all students of our college for their support:

50th Batch
Jithin James, Noufal Yousuf, Nadheem Shah, Shaheera, Lufna, Swetha K, Rubeena Yakoob, Sharmil SK, Bijoy Johnson, Dennis Purackel, Mansoor PM, Abdul Razik T, Swetha B Ram, Sujith Rao V, Jithin K, Jophin John, Mohammed Shafi PK, Rakesh MP, Mohammed Riyas Ali, Muhammed Shameem S, Nizar MMK, Rajeesh S Ravi and Vishnu Sreedath.

51st Batch
Ajmal PM, Ananth Raja, Ishaq TK, Muhsin CH and Praveen MV.

52nd Batch
Adnan Pallikkadan, Fawas Mohammed, Arshad Akram, Roy, Adarsh and Hafeefa.

53rd Batch
Siyad Ahammed PP, Jaseem Sajjad, Ashwin P, Muhammed Mansoof K, Kaleem Ahammed, Ijas and Neethu.

54th Batch
Thomas Kurian, Thejas Lal S and Dileesh AS.

Contents

MEDICINE

SURGERY

MEDICINE

Practical Examinations	**Marks**
Long Case Including Case Sheet	50
Short Cases	
Case 1	20
Case 2	20
OSCE	
Two Stations	5+5
Total	100
Viva	
Four Stations (Charts, Drugs, Instruments, X-rays)	5+5+5+5

CHAPTER 1

General Examination

PALLOR AND ANEMIA

- *Pallor*: Waxy appearance of skin and mucous membrane which depends upon thickness and quality of skin and amount of blood in capillaries.
  - Pallor—clinical term
  - Anemia—biochemical term
- *Anemia*: Decrease in hemoglobin concentration (Hb conc) in blood relation to standard age, sex [2 SD (standard deviation) below the mean for the particular age and sex].
- Sites to be looked—lower palpebral conjunctiva, dorsum of tongue, hard palate, nail bed, palm and soles [palmar crease affected in severe anemia (<8 g%)]
- Pallor but no anemia – Myxedema
  – Nephritic syndrome
  – Vasovagal attack
  – Peripheral circulatory failure.

Red beefy tongue—B_{12} deficiency Balded tongue—Fe deficiency Magenta tongue—B_2 deficiency

- *MCV*: 90 +/– 8 f1.
- *MCH*: 30 +/– 3 pg
- *MCHC*: 33 +/– 2% (Increased in human serum, dehydration)
- *RDW*: 12–16
- *MCV*: Mean corpuscular volume
- *MCH*: Mean corpuscular hemoglobin
- *MCHC*: Mean corpuscular concentration
- *RDW*: Red cell distribution width.

Polycythemia: Defined as Males >18 g% Hb or >52% PCV
Females >16.5 g% Hb or >48% PCV.

Causes of Polycythemia

Primary—Polycythemia rubra vera.
Secondary—
- Due to increased erythropoietin
  - COPD
  - High altitude
  - CCHD
- Inappropriate erythropoietin
  - RCC
  - Hepatoma
  - Fibroid.

- Congenital cyanotic heart disease
- Chronic obstructive pulmonary disease (COPD)
- Polycythemia rubra vera.

Microcytic hypochromic anemia:

- S – Sideroblastic anemia
- I – Fe deficiency anemia
- T – Thalassemia
- A – Anemia of chronic blood loss
- L – Lead poisoning

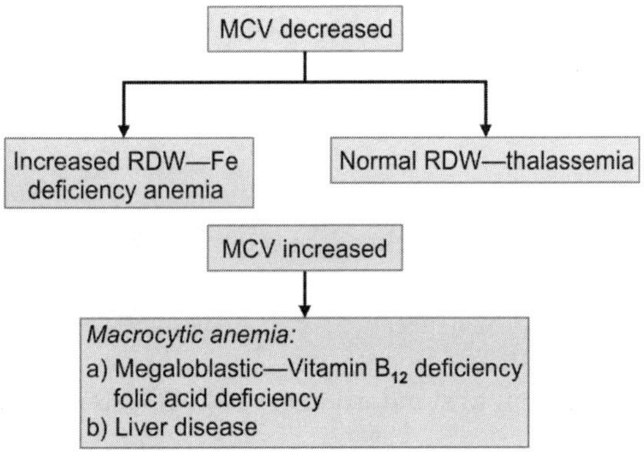

ICTERUS

Yellowish discoloration of skin and mucous membrane.
It is clinical term.
Jaundice—biochemical term
Sites to look for (should be examined in broad daylight):

- Upper bulbar conjunctiva (white background, bilirubin has strong affinity to elastic tissue)
- Under surface of tongue
- Soft palate
- Palms, soles.

DDs of icterus:

- Carotenemia (No yellowish discoloration of sclera)
- Phenol
- Quinacrine.

- Normal serum bilirubin: 0.2–0.8 mg/dL
- Latent jaundice: 1–2 mg/dL
- Evident jaundice: >.3 mg/dL

- Hemolytic (lemon yellow)
- Hepatocellular (orange yellow)
- Obstructive (greenish yellow)

CLUBBING

Bulbous swelling of the terminal part of fingers and toes with an increase in soft tissue mass and increased anteroposterior and transverse diameter of nail with obliteration of onychodermal angle (Lovibond angle).

[Normal angle between nail and nailbed—160°—Lovibond angle]

Index finger of nondominant hand to be used to look for clubbing.

Degree of clubbing:

Grand I — Increased fluctuation
Grand II — Obliteration of onychodermal angle
Grand III — Parrot beak or drumstick appearance
Grand IV — Hypertrophic pulmonary osteoarthropathy
Schamroth sign – obliteration of the normal diamond shaped gap when nails are opposed.

Causes		
Respiratory	*Cardiac*	*Others*
A – Abscess	IE	Endocrine—thyrotoxicosis
B – Bronchiectasis	Congenital cyanotic heart disease	GIT—IBD, CLD
C – Carcinoma	Eisenmenger's syndrome	CNS—syringomyelia
D – Diffuse	ILD atrial myxoma	
E – Empyema		
F – Fibrosing alveolitis		

Acute clubbing—Infective endocarditis, empyema (painful), lung abscess (painful)
Differential clubbing—PDA (clubbing present in legs, absent in hands)
Put Schamroth sign before degrees of clubbing
Pseudoclubbing—Hyperparathyroidism
—Scleroderma
—Laprosy.

CYANOSIS

Bluish discoloration of skin and mucous membrane due to increased amount of reduced Hb (>5 g/dL), PaO_2 <85%. Other causes—sulfhemoglobinemia and methemoglobinemia.

Central
Sites—Tongue and periphery
Clubbing present
Warm limb
Hypoxemic hypoxia
Cause:
CVS — Congenital cyanotic heart disease
Eisenmenger's, pulmonary edema
Lung — Severe asthma, COPD, fibrosing alveolitis, tension pneumothorax.

Peripheral
Sites—Periphery (lip, ear lobule, nose tip, fingers)
Usually not present
Cool limb
Stagnation hypoxia
Cause:
Exposure to cold
Raynaud's phenomenon

Differential cyanosis—PDA (persistent ductus arteriosus) with reversal
Central + peripheral cyanosis—CCF, shock.

Lymphadenopathy

Levels of lymph nodes:

Level 1 – 1a submental nodes, 1b – submandibular nodes
Level 2 – Upper jugular nodes (upper 1/3 of jugular vein, i.e. between base of skull and level of hyoid bone)
Level 3 – Middle jugular nodes (hyoid bone to cricoid cartilage)
Level 4 – Lower jugular nodes (cricoid cartilage to clavicle)
Level 5 – Posterior cervical group—spinal accessory chain, supraclavicular, transverse cervical)
Level 6 – Anterior compartment nodes—prelaryngeal, pretracheal and paratracheal (medial borders of SCM laterally, hyoid bone above and suprasternal notch below)
Level 7 – Nodes of upper mediastinum (below suprasternal notch).

Significant lymphadenopathy:

- Size >2 cm for inguinal, >1.5 cm axillary >1 cm cervical.
- Hard, tender, matted nodes.
- Any supraclavicular and epitrochlear nodes.

Causes:

- Infections—TB, IMN, brucellosis, HIV
- Leukemia—ALL (acute lymphatic leukemia), CLL (chronic lymphatic leukemia)
- Lymphoma—HL (Hodgkin's lymphoma), NHL (non-Hodgkin's lymphoma).

Epitrochlear lymph node (LN) enlargement:
- NHL
- Syphilis
- IMN (infectious mononucleosis)
- Cat scratch disease
- HIV

MEDICINE

[Mention site, size, shape, consistency, tender/nontender, mobile or not, matting (matting in NHL, TB)]

Generalized lymphadenopathy: >3 noncontiguous site.

Virchow's node—Between two heads of sternocleidomastoid (bronchogenic carcinoma) (left supraclavicular LN).

EDEMA

Accumulation of excessive amount of tissue fluid in subcutaneous tissue or serous sac.

Causes:

1. CCF (increase hydrostatic pressure and increase sodium retention)
2. CLD (decrease oncotic pressure)
3. Nephrotic syndrome (decrease oncotic pressure)
4. Cellulitis (inflammation)
5. Angioneurotic edema
6. PEM (in children).

Nonpitting edema:
- Myxedema
- Filariasis

Examination: Press above medial malleolus for 30 seconds.

Dependent edema: CCF (increase toward evening)—edema first appear is limbs {ambulant person—lower limb, bedridden—sacrum}

First appearance of edema on face: Nephrotic syndrome (increase toward morning).

Unilateral pedal edema:

- DVT (deep venous thrombosis)
- Cellulitis
- Filariasis (nonpitting).

VITAL SIGNS

PULSE

Definition: Waves transmitted across the arterial wall produced by the contraction of blood-filled heart into the already blood-filled aorta, travel through the arterial wall.

Characteristics:

Rate, rhythm, volume, character, condition of vessel wall, radiofemoral delay, other peripheral pulsations.

Peripheral pulses to be looked for:

Superficial temporal, brachial, carotid, radial, femoral, popliteal, posterior tibial, dorsalis pedis (*area to be palpated is described in the last of this chapter*).

Radiofemoral delay:

Normally, there is no radiofemoral delay will be present in aortic aneurysm, coarctation of aorta, Takayasu's arteritis.

Rate:

Number of pulses/min.

Tachycardia >100/min

Physiological	Pathological
Anxiety	Atrial fibrillation
Exercise	Thyrotoxicosis
Children	Drugs (e.g. sympathomimetics)
Relative tachycardia:	Myocarditis

Bradycardia <60/min

Physiological	Pathological
Athlete's foot	Hypothyroidism
Sleep	Obstructive jaundice
	Drugs (sympatholytic)

Relative bradycardia:	Leptospirosis	L
	Yellow fever	Y
	Meningitis	M
	Enteric fever	E

For every 1° rise in temperature, pulse increase by 10 bt/min

Respiration increases by 4/min

Relative bradycardia means there is no rise in pulse rate with increase in temperature.

Rhythm:

Regularly irregular — Extrasystole
Ventricular bigeminy

Irregularly irregular — AF
Multiple ventricular ectopics

Volume:

High volume — Anxiety, fever, thyrotoxicosis
AR, PDA, Beri-Beri

Low volume — Stenotic lesion, MS, Aortic stenosis (AS).

THEORY

Normal pulse

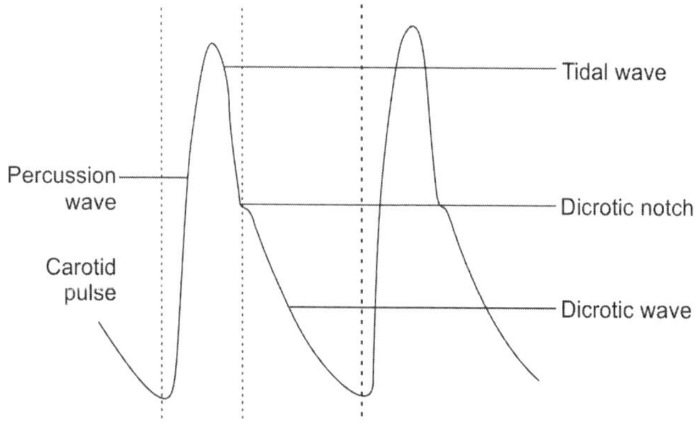

Pulsus parvus – MS—low amplitude slow rising pulse

Parvus et tardus – AS—slow rising, late peaking low amplitude (anacrotic pulse)

Collapsing pulse (Water hammer pulse) – Large volume pulse with rapid upstroke and downstroke
Seen in PDA, AR, AV fistula, rupture sinus of Valsalva

Pulsus bisferiens – Single pulse wave with two peaks in systole
AS and AR
Severe AR
Hypertrophic obstructive cardiomyopathy

Pulsus alternans – Alternating small and large volume pulse in regular rhythm
Seen in severe LV dysfunction

Pulsus bigeminy – Pulse wave with a normal beat followed by a premature beat and a compensatory pause, occurring in rapid succession resulting in alternation of strength of the pulse; it is a sign of digitalis toxicity

Pulsus paradoxus – Exaggerated reduction in the strength of arterial pulse

During normal inspiration or an exaggerated inspiratory fall in systolic pressure of more than 10 mm of Hg during quiet breathing. Causes—cardiac tamponade, constrictive pericarditis, airway obstruction as in acute severe asthma, SVC obstruction.

MEDICINE

Blood Pressure

Definition: The lateral force exerted by the blood column per unit area of the vascular wall that is expressed in mm of Hg.

JNC classification of BP

- Hypertension—140/90 mm of Hg
- Prehypertension—Systolic up to 139; Diastolic up to 89
- Stage 1—Systolic up to 159; Diastolic up to 99
- Stage 2—Systolic >160; Diastolic >100.

Korotkoff sounds:

- Phase 1—Clear tapping
- Phase 2—Soft murmur
- Phase 3—Loud murmur
- Phase 4—Soft muffled
- Phase 5—Disappearance.

Temperature

If febrile, assess temperature using thermometer.

Fever types:

- Continuous fever—Fever does not touch baseline and <1°C variation, e.g. Enteric fiver, infective endocarditis (IE)
- Remittent fever—Fever does not touch baseline and >2°C variation, e.g. Brucellosis
- Intermittent fever—Fever touches the baseline, e.g. malaria, septicemia, pyemia.

Jugular Venous Pulse

It is the reflection of phasic pressure changes in the right atrium observed in right internal jugular vein and consists of 3 positive waves (a, c, v) and two negative troughs (x, y).

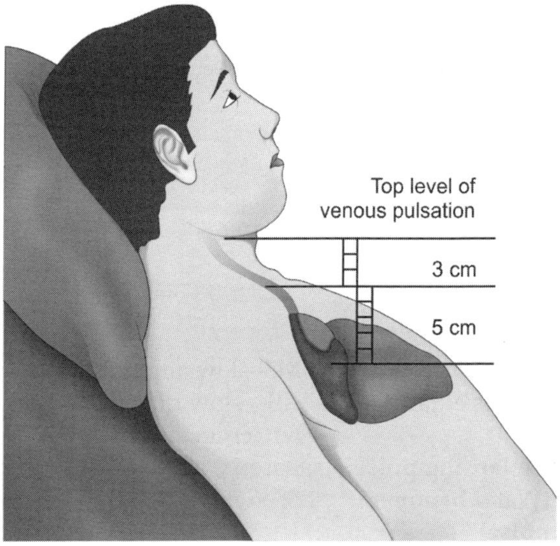

Normal JVP:

A wave — Right atrial systole
C wave — Tricuspid valve closure
V wave — Right atrial filling during ventricular systole or venous return
X descent — Right atrial relaxation with downward descent of tricuspid valve
Y descent — Tricuspid valve opens or emptying of atria.

Giant 'a' wave—Forceful atrial contraction against a stenosed tricuspid valve

TS/PS

Absent 'a' wave—Seen in AF

Cannon 'a' wave—Atrial systole against a closed atrial valve (Seen in systole)

Complete heart block, VT

Giant 'v' wave—Important sign of TR

Prominent 'x' and 'y' descent—Occurs in constrictive pericarditis.

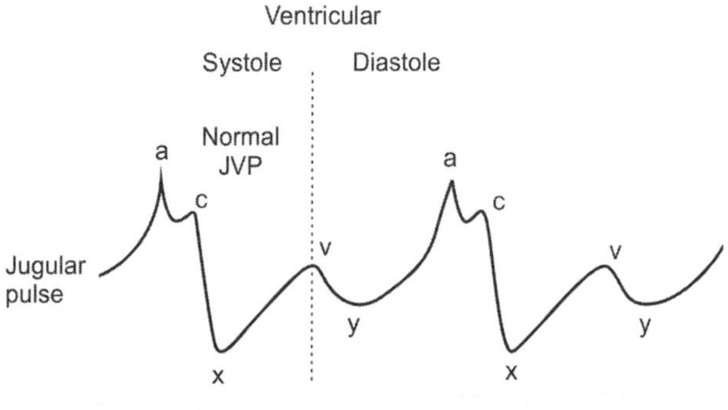

Differentiation from arterial pulse:

- Better seen than felt, definite upper level
- Lateral to SCM
- Upward waves are seen
- Pressure over clavicle, JVP disappears

- Hepatojugular reflex (When pressure applied over right hypochondrium, there is rise in JVP) due to increase in venous return.
- Decrease with inspiration due to decrease in intrathoracic pressure.

Kussmaul's sign—Inspiratory increase in JVP (seen in pericarditis, cardiac tamponade) due to inability to accommodate increased venous return colitis the constrained right side of the heart.

Peripheral Pulsations

Artery	Area to be examined
Radial artey	At the wrist (lower end of radius)
Ulnar artery	At the wrist (lower end of ulna)
Brachial artery	In front of elbow medial to biceps tendon (lower part of humerus)
Axillary artery	Apex of axilla (head of humerus)
Subclavian artery	Middle of supraclavicular fossa (1st rib)
Common carotid artery	At the level of thyroid cartilage, medial to SCM (carotid tubercle—Chassaigne tubercle-C6)
Facial artery	Against body of mandible
Superficial temporal artery	Against temporal bone, in front of tragus
Femoral artery	At midinguinal point
Popliteal artery	Lower part of popliteal fossa (upper end of tibia)
Anterior tibial artery	Midway between 2 malleoli (lower end of tibia)
Posterior tibial artery	Midway between Achilles tendon and medial malleolus (calcaneum)
Dorsalis pedis artery	Proximal part of 1st intermetatarsal space, lateral to tendon of EHL (navicular).

CHAPTER 2

Cardiovascular System

Name: Age: Sex: Address:

PRESENTING ILLNESS

Breathlessness on Exertion

- Onset, duration, progress (class 1–4)
  NYHA classification:
  - Class I—No limitation of physical activity in spite of presence of heart disease
  - Class II—Mild limitation
  - Class III—Moderate limitation but not at rest
  - Class IV—Symptoms at rest
- Aggravating/relieving factors
- Associated symptoms like cough with expectoration, wheeze, chest pain
- History of paroxysmal nocturnal dyspnea, orthopnea, trepopnea, platypnea.

Chest Pain

- Onset, site, duration, radiation, brought on by, lasts for, character
- Aggravating/relieving factors
- Associated symptoms like vomiting, sweating, nausea, heart burns
- Associated with food intake, respiration.

Palpitation

Duration, brought on by, regular/irregular, relieved by, associated symptoms like chest pain, syncope.

Syncope

Duration, number of episodes, brought on by, relieved by, recovery time, associated with convulsions, bladder/bowel disturbances.

Swelling of Feet

Limited to face/legs—unilateral or bilateral/abdomen/generalized, aggravating/relieving factors, duration.

Hemoptysis

Number of episodes, amount, color, sputum present or not.

Sputum

- Duration, quality—frothy/viscid or thick, postural/diurnal variation
- Quantity—copious, foul smelling.

Symptoms of CCF

Anorexia, nausea, vomiting, abdominal distension, decreased urine output, dyspnea on exertion, right hypochondrial pain, nocturia, anasarca.

Symptoms of Rheumatic Fever

Fever with joint pain, sore throat, fleeting joint pain and swelling, involuntary movements, skin rash, nodules.

Symptoms of Infective Endocarditis

Pyrexia, petechial hemorrhages, hematuria.

Pressure Symptoms

Hoarseness of voice (Ortner's syndrome), dysphagia.

Symptoms of Congenital Heart Disease

Cyanotic spells, squatting episodes, recurrent respiratory infections.

PAST HISTORY

Previous similar episodes, history of DM, HT, IHD, TB, STD, RHD, history of obesity, hyperlipidemia, recurrent respiratory infections, neonatal, natal and postnatal history (in case of congenital HD).

PERSONAL HISTORY

Sleep and appetite, bowel and bladder habits, history of addictions (Smoking/Alcohol).

FAMILY HISTORY

Any similar illness in family, any history of DM, IHD, TB, HT, etc. marital history, consanguinity in his parents, sibling history.

DRUG AND TREATMENT HISTORY

General Examination

- Conscious, oriented, cooperative, comfortable/dyspneic at rest, build and nourishment.
- Pallor, cyanosis, jaundice, clubbing, pedal edema, LNE, skin, hair, nail, No thyroid swelling.

Pulse: Rate, rhythm, volume, character, peripheral vessels, thickening, radiofemoral delay, pulse deficit, carotid bruit.

Respiration: Rate, rhythm, character, depth.

Blood pressure: mm Hg in which limb (UL/LL) posture, whether on antihypertensive.

Temperature: Record if febrile, look any features of atherosclerosis (Xanthelasma, Xanthoma, Locomotor brachialis)

Cardiovascular System

Inspection

- JVP—waveform, pressure (cm from sternal angle)
- Chest wall symmetry, precordial bulge, apex, trachea, visible pulsations anywhere, dilated veins, scars.

Palpation

- Apex—site, character, thrill, tracheal position
- Thrill over precordium, palpable sounds, diastolic shock
- Left parasternal heave, palpable pulsations.

Percussion

Right border, left border (apex) 2nd left intercostals space.

Auscultation

Mention each area separately in the order of mitral area, tricuspid area, pulmonary and aortic areas.

Mitral area:
- S1 (soft/N/loud), S2 audible
- Added sounds (S3, S4, OS, non-ejection click, pericardial knock)
- Murmers, pericardial rub.

Tricuspid area:
- S1 (soft/N/loud), S2 audible
- Added sounds, murmers (look for Carvallo's sign), rub.

Pulmonary area:
- S1 audible, S2 (soft/N/loud), S2 splitting (wide, fixed, reverse, narrow)
- Added sounds (ejection clicks)
- Murmers.

Aortic area:
- S1 audible, S2 (soft/N/loud)
- Added sounds (ejection click)
- Murmers.

Examination of other Systems

Respiratory system: Fine basal crepitations, pleural effusion
Gastrointestinal systems: Tender hepatomegaly, splenomegaly, ascites
Central nervous system: Chorea, hemiplegia (embolism).

MITRAL STENOSIS

HEMODYNAMICS

- Mitral stenosis results in obstruction to flow of blood across the mitral valve during left ventricular diastole
- Left atrium compensates for the obstruction by increasing its pressure.
- Hypertrophy of LA (Left atrium).
- As LA is thin walled, capacity for hypertrophy is limited.
- LA pressure transmitted to pulmonary vein (as there is no valve between them).
- There is increase in pulmonary venous pressure.
- Pulmonary capillary engorgement and pulmonary congestion (dyspnea).
- Increase in pulmonary arterial pressure—pulmonary arterial hypertension.
- With mild or moderate MS—forward flow across mitral valve remains normal.
- Severe MS—flow to left ventricle decreases.
- Cardiac output decreases—small volume pulse, cold extremities—peripheral cyanosis.

NATURAL COURSE OF THE DISEASE

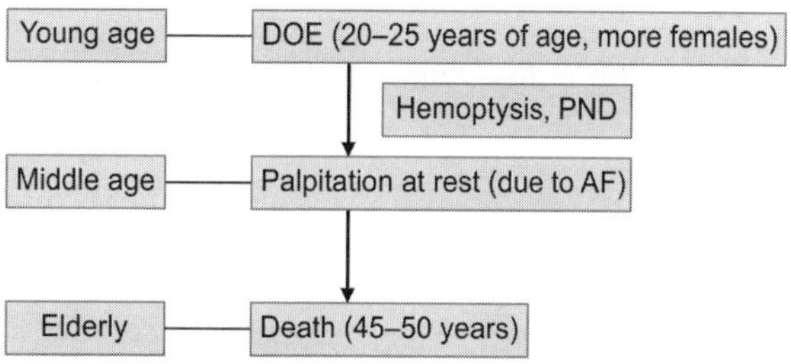

If the initial symptom is

- Dyspnea + angina—MS + AS
- DOE + palpitation—MS + MR.

CAUSES OF HEMOPTYSIS IN MS

- Paroxysmal nocturnal dyspnea
- Pulmonary edema
- Pulmonary apoplexy–rupture of pulmonary-bronchial venous connection due to pulmonary venous HTN
- Pulmonary infarction
- After anticoagulant therapy
- Winter bronchitis.

Why pulmonary infarction—both atria fibrillates in MS

Causes of pulmonary HTN

- Backward transmission of LA pressure
- Second stenosis or reactive pulmonary hypertension due to vasoconstriction
- Interstitial edema
- Organic change in vascular bed (end stage).

Cause of soft S1 in MS

Calcified fibrosed valve
CHF (cardiac heart failure)
Severe PAH (pulmonary arterial hypertension)
Combined mitral valve disease (MS+MR)
AS/AR

COMMON CAUSES

I. Young—rheumatic heart disease (RHD), congenital
II. Middle age—RHD, carcinoid syndrome, connective tissue disorder, mucopolysaccharidosis.
III. Elderly—RHD.

CLINICAL FINDINGS

- Pulse—pulsus parvus (low volume pulse) in severe MS; AF; absent pulse—due to embolism.
- BP—normal/narrow pulse pressure
- Apex—tapping
- Thrill—diastolic thrill at apex
- Left parasternal heave—if PAH, epigastric impulse and palpable P_2.
- S_1 loud (due to widened excursion and forceful closure of mitral valve).
- S_2 loud if PAH present
- Added sounds—Opening snap (Loudest sound is the cardiac cycle due to diastolic buckling of mitral leaflets).
- Murmur—mid-diastolic murmur with presystolic accentuation.

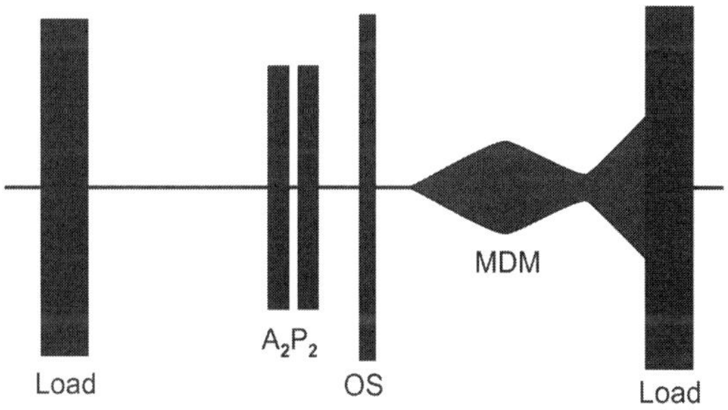

SEVERITY OF MS BASED ON S2-OS INTERVAL

- *Mild MS*: 90–120 ms
- *Moderate MS*: 60–90 ms
- *Severe MS*: 30–60 ms.

Normal area of mitral valve is 4 cm^2; aortic valve—2.5 cm^2
Critical MS <1 cm^2
Critical AS—0.6 cm^2

INVESTIGATIONS

- CXR (chest X-ray)
- ECG (electrocardiogram)
- Echocardiography.

CXR

- *Cardiomegaly*:
  - RVH
  - *LA enlargement*:
    - Double atrial shadow
    - Straightened left heart border
    - Splaying of carina.
- *Pulmonary venous hypertension*:
  - Reverse moustache/antelock sign
  - Perihilar shadow
  - (Batwing sign)—pulmonary edema

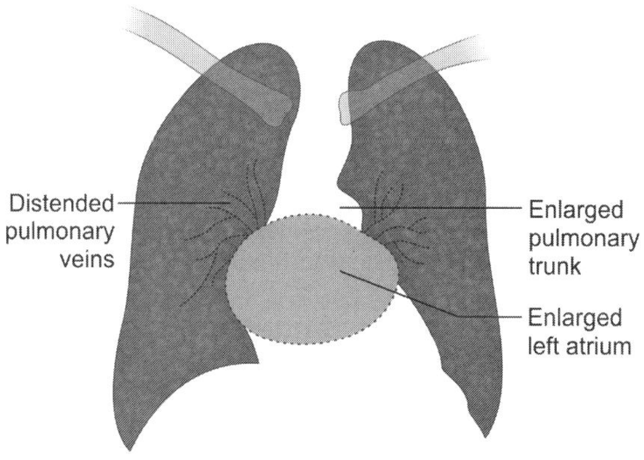

- Kerley B line—interstitial edema
- Ground glass appearance—alveolar edema

- *Pulmonary arterial hypertension*:
  - Peripheral pruning of arteries
  - Pulmonary bay sign
  - Prominence of right descending pulmonary artery
- *Right ventricular hypertrophy*: On lateral CXR—retrosternal translucency will be obliterated.

ECG

- P mitrale—left atrial enlargement
- P pulmonale due to RVH.

Complications of MS

- A/c left atrial failure—pulmonary edema
- PAH
- RVF
- AF
- Embolism
- Hemoptysis
- IE
- Ortner's syndrome.

TREATMENT—MEDICAL

Treatment of left ventricular failure

- Bed rest
- Propped up position
- Oxygen
- Diuretics (frusemide)
- Morphine
- Aminophylline/theophylline
- Antibiotics.

Rheumatic Prophylaxis

Refer rheumatic fever.

Anticoagulant

Aspirin/warfarin (in presence of AF).

SURGERY

- Balloon mitral valvuloplasty (BMV)
- Closed mitral valvulotomy
- Open mitral commissurotomy
- Valve replacement
- Mitral valve replacement
  - Mechanical prosthetic valve
  - Porcine prosthetic valve
- Porcine valves are used in elderly individuals. They last for lesser time than mechanical valves.

Examples of mechanical valves
- Starr-Edward—ball and cage
- Bjork-Shiley—tilting disk
- St Jude—bileaflet

Indications of surgical intervention in a case of MS:

- Critical MS
- Symptomatic MS
- Going for heart failure in pregnancy.

Four requisites for BMV
- No left atrial clot
- No significant MR
- No calcification
- Subvalvular apparatus must be free

MEDICINE

MITRAL REGURGITATION

Hemodynamics—blood in the left ventricle has two options to go:

1. Into the LA
2. Systemic circulation.

   On excertion, the systemic blood flow reduces due to blood flow to left atrium, i.e. in MR, there is fatigue on exertion.

   In **chronic MR**, there is increased blood in LA and LV. So there is volume hypertrophy of LA and LV. Thus, hypertrophied left atrium accommodates regurgitant blood without increasing left atrial pressure and features of LVF are absent.

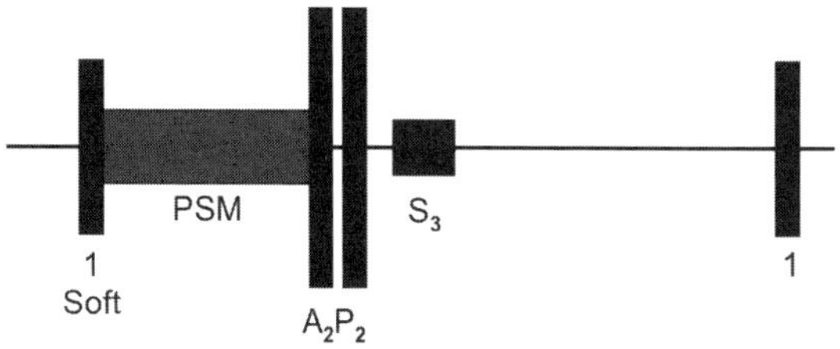

But LVF occurs in:

- Acute MR
- Severe MR
- Failing left ventricular myocardium

In acute MR, left atrial size is normal and the increased volume reaching the LA increases the left atrial pressure and pulmonary venous pressure, resulting in pulmonary venous congestion.

Features of acute MR
- Tachycardia
- Low BP
- Apex—normal
- Loud S1
- Early systolic murmur

Natural Course of MR

Fatigue, palpitation on exertion
↓
DOE
↓
AF—palpitation at rest
↓
Death

Causes of MR
- Rheumatic
- MVP (mitral valve prolapse)
- Bacterial endocarditis
- IHD (ischemic heart disease)
- Blast trauma
- Ostium primum ASD

MR

Ischemic
- Normal S_1
- No PAH
- No much cardiomegaly
- Middle and old age
- Posterior cusp
- Conduction of murmur to left sternal border

Rheumatic
- Soft S_1
- Evidence of MS or PAH
- Cardiomegaly present
- H/o RF in adulthood
- Anterior cusp
- To axilla

Investigations

- CXR
- ECG
- Echocardiography
- *CXR*:
  - LVH
  - LAH (giant left atrium)
  - Signs of pulmonary venous congestion (in acute MR)
  - RVH
  - *ECG*:
    - LAH

Complications of MR
- Acute LVF
- IE
- CCF
- Arrhythmias
- Giant left atrium may produce
- Pressure symptoms—dysphagia, hoarseness of voice (Ortner's syndrome)

- LVH
- AF.

TREATMENT

Medical

- Vasodilators—nitrates, ACE inhibitors—can reduce regurgitation flow and may be helpful in severe cases
- Treatment of LVF
- IE prophylaxis
- Rheumatic prophylaxis
- Anticoagulant prophylaxis (warfarin INR—2–3).

Surgical

Mitral valve replacement/repair.

AORTIC REGURGITATION

There is backward leak from aorta into the left ventricle during diastole → LV hypertrophy
As there is impaired forward flow,

- There is compensatory vasodilation—decrease in diastolic BP
- Increased ejection fraction from LV during early part of systole—increase in systolic BP.

If LV myocardium is failing, the LV diastolic pressure goes up and results in an increase in left atrial pressure and pulmonary congestion.

NATURAL COURSE

Palpitation on exertion (due to large stroke volume)
↓
Dyspnea (due to LVF)

Causes of acute aortic regurgitation (AR)
- IE
- RF
- Trauma
- Dissection of aorta

CAUSES

- Young—RF, congenital, subpulmonic VSD
- Middle age—RHD, anything causing aortic root dilatation (Marfan's syndrome, RA, ankylosing spondylitis).
- Elderly—RHD, aortic root dilatation.

PERIPHERAL SIGNS OF AR

- Corrigan's sign—dancing carotid
- Duroziez's sign—most specific sign of AR—systolic murmur on compression of femoral artery proximally
- Diastolic murmur on compression of femoral artery distally (Duroziez's murmur).
- Hill's sign—used for assessing severity of AR
  - Increase in femoral artery systolic BP >20 mm of Hg above brachial artery systolic BP.
  - Mild AR—20–40 mm Hg
  - Moderate—40–60 mm Hg
  - Severe >70
- De Musset's sign—head nodding
- Traube's sign—booming/pistol shot sound produced after pressing the stethoscope over the femoral artery.
- Quincke's sign—visible capillary pulsations
- Locomotor brachialis
- Water hammer pulse (Corrigan's pulse).

OTHERS

- Pulsation of uvula—Muller's sign
- Liver—Rosenbach's sign

- Spleen—Gerhardt's sign
- Light house sign—alternate flushing and blanching of forehead
- Becker's sign—pulsation of retinal artery.

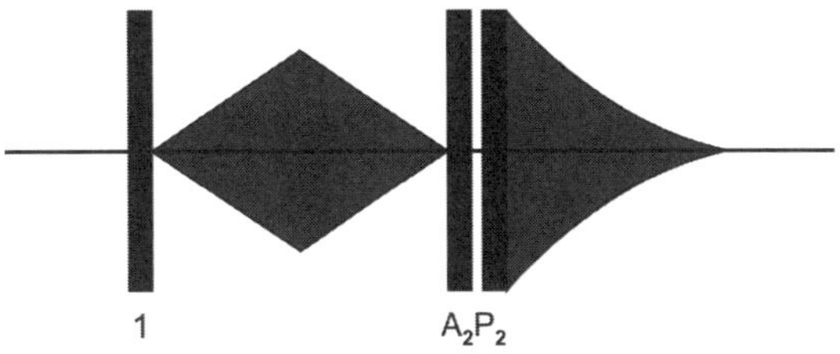

CLINICAL FINDINGS IN AR

- General examination—peripheral signs of AR (Not seen in A/c AR)
- Pulse—high volume collapsing pulse
- BP—wide pulse pressure
- Apex—down and out apex
- Thrill—diastolic thrill
- S1—normal
- S2—soft
- S3.

Murmur—early diastolic murmur.

- In AR of valvular etiology, murmur is best heard in the 3rd left ICS along left sternal edge (new cortic area).
- In AR due to root dilatation, murmur is best heard in the 2nd right ICS along right sternal edge.

> - Austin flint murmur
> - Seen in severe AR
> - Flow murmur—MOM
> - Heard in apex; left lateral position
> - Due to conference of blood flow from LA and aorta

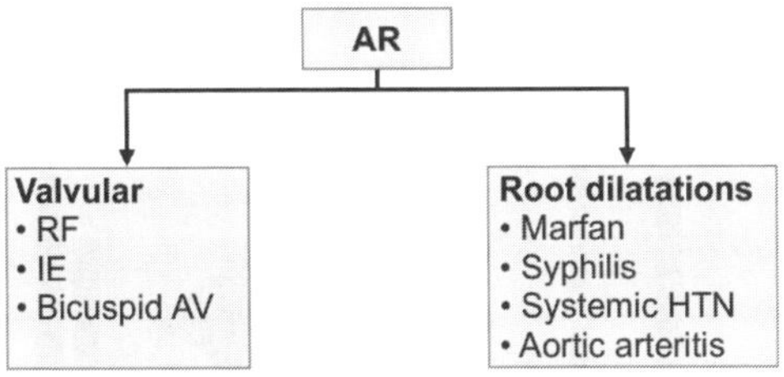

INVESTIGATION—CHEST X-RAY

- Cardiomegaly (LVH)
- Aortic root dilatation (prominent aortic knuckle)
- Pulmonary congestion.

ECG—LVH, conduction defect
Echocardiography.

> **Complication of AR**
> 1. Acute LVF
> 2. IE
> 3. CCF
> 4. Arrhythmias
> 5. Heart block

Treatment

Medical

- Treatment of LVF
- IE, rheumatic, anticoagulant prophylaxis

Surgical—aortic valve replacement.

AORTIC STENOSIS

HEMODYNAMICS

Angina pectoris—imbalance between augmented O_2 requirement and reduced O_2 availability

- Augmented O_2 requirement
  - Increased myocardial mass
  - Increased intraventricular pressure
- Reduced O_2 availability
  - Compression of coronary vessel by hypertrophied myocardium
  - Accompanying CAD.

Syncope on Exertion

Aortic stenosis (AS) is characterized by fixed obstruction cardiac output.

So during exertion, vasodilatation of exercising muscle results in reduced blood supply of brain causing syncope.

Dyspnea

Elevation of the pulmonary capillary pressure caused by elevation of LV diastolic pressure secondary to reduced LV compliance.

Rheumatic AS
- Commissural fusion
- Complete stenosis

Atherosclerotic AS
- Atheromatous deposit as the valve—valve can vibrate

NATURAL COURSE

Exertional angina
↓
Syncope
↓
Dyspnea

CAUSES

- **Young—**congenital valvular stenosis (William's syndrome), Bicuspid aortic valve
- **Middle age***:*
  - RHD
  - Bicuspid aortic valve
  - Connective tissue disorder
- **Elderly**—aortic sclerosis/atherosclerotic AS.

CLINICAL FINDINGS

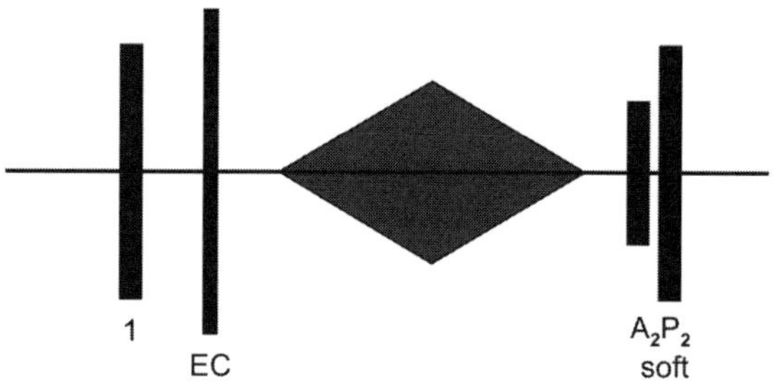

General Examination

- Xanthelasma
- Locomotor brachialis
- Arcus senilis
- Suprasternal pulsations.

Pulse

Pulsus parvus et tardus, carotid shudder (thrill).

BP

- Narrow pulse pressure (low BP—systolic decapitation)
- **Apex**—heaving normal position
  thrill systolic thrill in **aortic area**
- **S1**—normal
- **S2**—soft
- **S4**—may be present
- **Murmur—ESM** conducted to carotid.

- Ejection click—valvular AS
- Gallavardin phenomenon—AS murmur is transmitted to apex

Complications of AS
- Acute LVF
- CCF
- IE
- Angina pectoris, syncope
- Sudden death due to complete heart block or ventricular fibrillation

Investigation

- X-ray
- ECG—LVH with strain pattern
- Echo.

X-ray

- Normal sized heart due to concentric hypertrophy of left ventricle.
- Poststenotic dilatation of ascending aorta.
- Calcification of aortic valve.

Treatment—as in other case.

PULMONARY ARTERIAL HYPERTENSION

PALPATORY FINDINGS

- Palpable P2
- Diastolic shock
- Left parasternal heave
- Epigastric pulsation
- 2nd left intercostal space—dullness
- 'a' wave in JVP.

X-ray findings
- RA, RV enlargement
- Large pulmonary arteries
- Peripheral pruning of arteries

Auscultatory findings—Paulwood's 9 criteria
- loud P2
- narrow spit
- ESM (ejection systolic murmur)
- Pulmonary ejection click
- EDM (early diastolic murmur)
- TR—PSM (pansystolic murmur)
- RV S4
- RV S3
- Flow MDM (mid diastolic murmur)
  *pulmonary hypertension develops earlier in MS, MR.

CONGESTIVE CARDIAC FAILURE

Left heart failure	Right heart failure
• Orthopnea	• Elevated JVP (jugular venous pressure)
• DOE (dyspnea on exertion)	• Tender hepatomegaly
• Bilateral basal crepitation	• Pedal edema
• Pulsus alternans	

ATRIAL FIBRILLATION

FINDINGS

- Irregularly irregular pulse with apex pulse deficit >10/min
- A wave is absent in JVP
- Presystolic accentuation is usually not seen in MS
- Embolic phenomenon.

*in AF, both atria fibrillate
Transient AF is more dangerous than permanent AF.

Causes of artrial fibrillation (AF)—Atrial
- Alcohol
- Thyrotoxicosis
- Rheumatic
- Ischemic
- ASD
- Lone

Differences Between Multiple Ectopics and AF

AF	Multiple ectopics
• Rate >100/minute (but digitalized AF PR <100/min)	• PR <100/min
• Pulse deficit >10 (<10 in digitalized AF)	• Pulse deficit <10
• Following exercise—pulse deficit in digitalized AF >10	• Pulse deficit remains <10 • Following exercise
• Absent a wave in JVP	

MEDICINE

RHEUMATIC FEVER

JONE'S CRITERIA

Major Criteria

- Carditis
- Polyarthritis
- Sydenham chorea
- Erythema marginatum
- Subcutaneous nodules.

Rheumatic prophylaxis
Benzathine penicillin 1–2 million U IM monthly
or
Oral phenoxymethylpenicillin 250 mg 12th hourly.
- With carditis for 10 years or up to 25 years old
- Without carditis for 5 years or up to 18 years old.

Minor Criteria

Clinical

- Fever
- Arthralgia
- Previous rheumatic fever, rheumatic heart disease.

Laboratory

- Acute phase reactants—leukocytosis, elevated ESR and CRP
- Prolonged PR interval on ECG.

Essential Criteria

- Evidence for recent streptococcal infection as indicated by increased antistreptolysin O titer.
- Positive throat culture
- Recent scarlet fever.

Two major or 1 major + 2 minor are required in the presence of essential criteria for diagnosis of acute rheumatic fever.

Rheumatic Reactivation

- Increased ASO titer
- Increased ESR
- RHD, fever with polyarthritis.

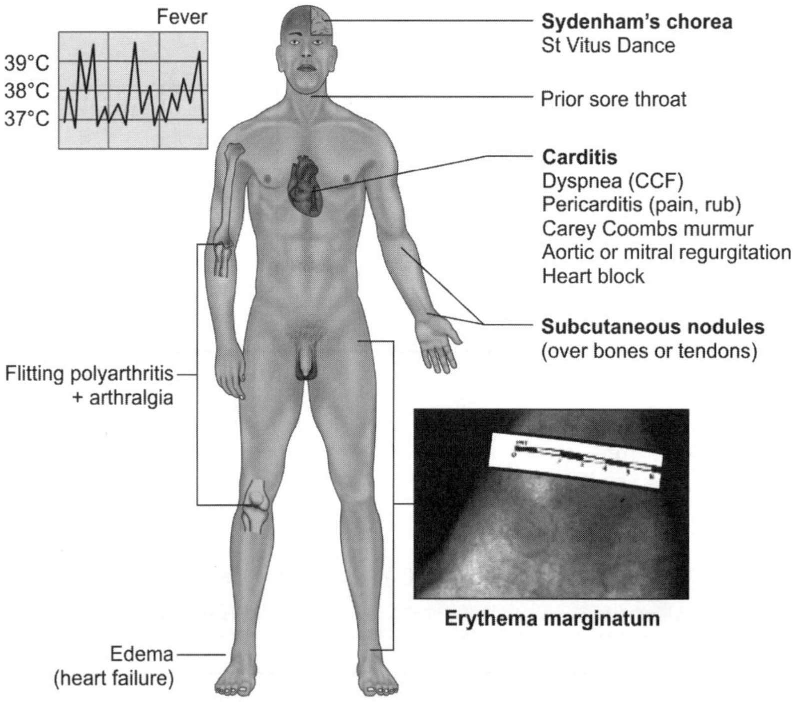

Erythema marginatum

MEDICINE

Duckett Jone's criteria cannot be used in case of:

- Rheumatic reactivation
- Sydenham's chorea.

INFECTIVE ENDOCARDITIS

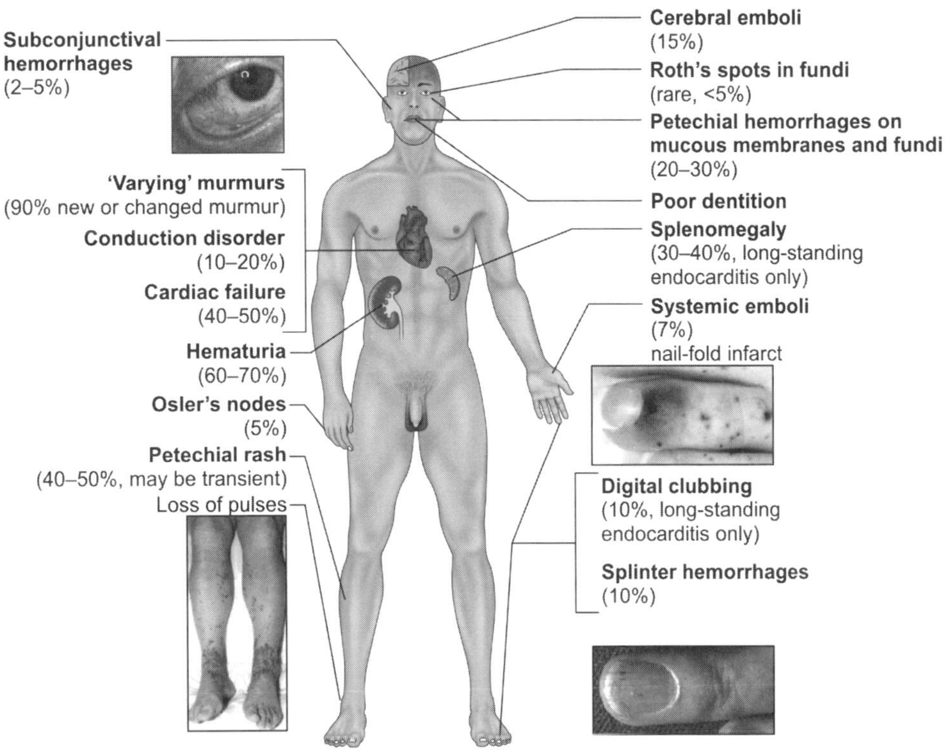

- It is the most dreaded complication of RAD (rheumatic heart disease)
- It is common with MR and AR
- **IE triad pallor, clubbing, splenomegaly.**

Other Features

- Splinter hemorrhage
- Osler's node—tender erythematous nodule over the pulp of finger.
- Roth's spot—seen in retina
- Janeway lesion—nontender erythematous patches on palms and soles.
- Elevated temperature

Diagnosis of infective endocarditis:

- *Modified Duke's criteria*:
  1. *Positive blood culture*:
     - Typical organism from 2 cultures
     - Persistent positive blood cultures taken more than 12 hours apart
     - 3 or more positive cultures taken over >1 hour
  2. *Endocardial involvement*:
     - Positive echocardiographic findings of vegetations
     - New valvular regurgitation.

Minor Criteria

- Predisposing valvular or cardiac abnormality
- IV drug misuse

- Pyrexia >38°C
- Embolic phenomenon
- Vasculitic phenomenon
- Blood culture suggestive—organism grown but not achieving minor criteria.
- Suggestive echocardiographic finding.

Definite endocarditis—two major/one major + 3 minor/5 minor
Possible endocarditis—one major + 1 minor/3 minor.

P's of embolism
- Pallor
- Pain
- Paresthesia
- Paralysis
- Pulselessness
- Persisting cold

Embolic Episodes

Look for all peripheral pulses especially dorsalis pedis.

MARFAN'S SYNDROME

Three out of four criteria should be present

- Autosomal dominant (chromosome 15, fibrillin gene)
- Long tubular bones
- Eye findings—superolateral dislocation of lens
- Root dilatation.

Pulse, BP, JVP—discussed earlier.

Paroxysmal Nocturnal Dyspnea

- During sleep
- Reabsorption of fluid from tissues into plasma
- Increased venous return to the heart
- Elevation of diaphragm
- Decreased sympathetic activity
- As a result of these processes, fluid will reach alveoli stimulating J receptors that in turn stimulate respiratory center.

Apex

- Apex is the lowermost and outermost point where definite cardiac impulse is felt.
- Normal apex—it lasts <1/3rd of systole
- Forceful—>1/3rd of systole, but <2/3rd of systole
- *Diffuse—>2.5 cm²*: Seen in MR, AR, VSD, PDA.
- Heaving apex—lasts >2/3rd of systole
- *Localized*: Seen in AS, systemic hypertension
- *Tapping—palpable S1, seen in MS:* Due to widened excursion, forceful closure.
- Hypokinetic—MI, pericardial effusion, myxedema.

Visible Pulsation

- **Pulmonary area pulsation:**
  - PAH
  - Physiologically
  - ASD, VSD, PDA
- **Visible carotid pulsation:**
  - AR, AS, anemia, thyrotoxicosis, aneurysm of aorta
- **Epigastric pulsation:**
  - RVH
  - Aneurysm of aorta
  - Transmitted pulsation in TR

Causes of right ventricular hypertrophy (RVH)
- Pulmonary hypertension
- PS
- HOCM
- ASD

- **Pulsation over scapula:**
  - Suzman's sign
  - Collateral in coarctation.

Causes of LVH	
Concentric	**Eccentric**
• AS	• AR
• Systemic hypertension	• MR
• Coarctation of aorta	• VSD
	• PDA

Causes of Biventricular Hypertrophy

- DCM
- VSD
- IHD
- Hyperkinetic circulation.

HEART SOUNDS

S1—due to closure of AV valve

Loud S1:
- MS, TS
- Hyperdynamic circulation—anemia, thyrotoxicosis, Beri-beri
- Tachycardia
- MVP+MR
- All short PR interval except WPW syndrome

Soft S1:
- MR, TR
- Prolonged PR interval
- LVF
- Calcified valve
- Obesity
- Thick chest wall
- Emphysema

Varying S1:
- AF
- Extrasystole
- Complete heart block

S2—due to closure of semilunar valve

Loud S2—PAH—due to MS, Eisenmenger's cor pulmonale, primary pulmonary hypertension.

Palpable P2 is called diastolic shock.

SPLITTING OF HEART SOUNDS

Narrow split:
- Late A2
- Left bundle branch block (LBBB)
- AS
- Systemic hypertension.

Wide fixed split
- ASD
- Massive pulmonary embolus
- Total anomalous pulmonary venous connection

Early P2

- Pulmonary hypertension
- RV ectopic.

Paradoxical split
- LBBB
- PDA
- Severe AS

Wide split

- Early A2
- VSD
- MR
- LV ectopic.

Late P2

- Right bundle branch block (RBBB)
- PS

Single S2

- Severe AS—P2 only
- Severe PS—TOF (tetralogy of Fallot)—A2 only.

S3—due to rapid ventricular filling

- Athlete's, young adult, anemia, thyrotoxicosis
- Pregnancy
- Fever
- In LVF, S3 is usually accompanied by tachycardia—gallop rhythm.
- MR, AR.

S_3 after 40 years old—pathological

S4—atrial contraction against a stiff ventricle

- AS
- Hypertrophic obstructive cardiomyopathy (HOCM)
- Systemic hypertension.

Diastolic events

- Opening snap
- S_3, S_4
- Tumor plop
- Pericardial knock

ADDITIONAL SOUNDS

- EC—ejection click
- MVC—mitral valve click
- OS—opening snap.

MURMUR

Heart murmurs are produced by turbulent blood flow across an abnormal valve, septal defect or outflow obstruction or by increased volume or velocity of blood flow through a normal valve.

Levin and Freedman classification of grading of murmurs

Grade 1—Heard by experienced person in a quite surrounding
Grade 2—By careful auscultation
Grade 3—Easily heard
Grade 4—Thrill
Grade 5—Very loud (using part of stethoscope)
Grade 6—Heard with stethoscope off the chest.

Basic mechanism regarding all type of murmurs

Before giong to the topic, you must be thorough with cardiac cycle.

CARDIAC CYCLE

Duration of one cardiac cycle—0.8 s.

Mechanical Event in Cardiac Cycle

- Atrial systole—0.1 s
- Ventricular systole—0.3 s
- Ventricular diastole—0.5 s.

Cardiac Cycle Divided 8 Phases

1. Isovolumetric ventricular contraction
2. Rapid ejection phase
3. Reduced ejection phase
4. Protodiastole
5. Isovolumetric ventricular relaxation
6. First rapid filling phase
7. Reduced filling phase (diastasis)
8. Last rapid filling phase (atrial systole).

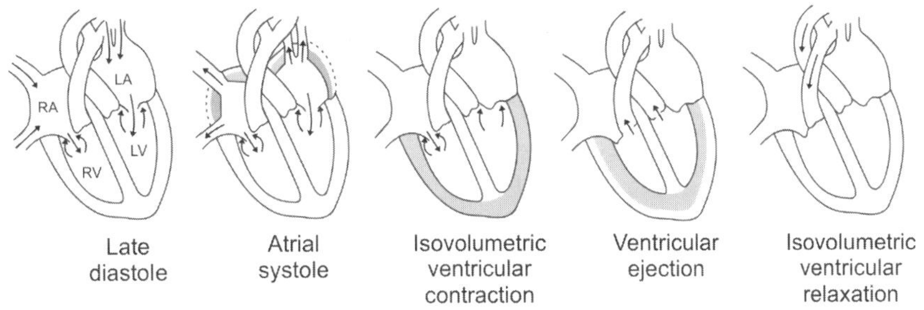

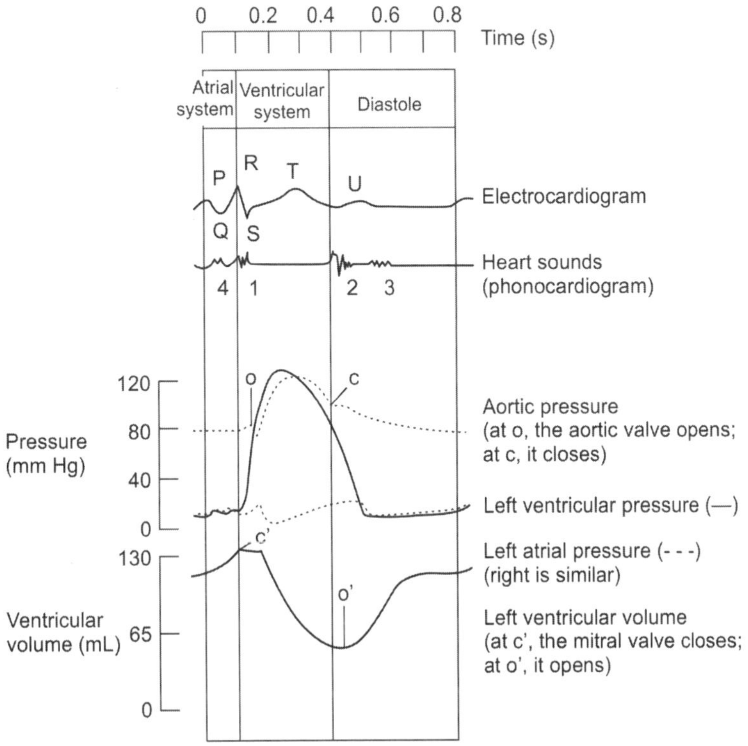

MEDICINE

Pansystolic Murmur

Pansystolic murmur (PSM) is produced when there is flow between the two chambers that have widely different pressure throughout systole. For example, MR, TR, VSD.

Continuous Murmur

This begins in systole, peak near S2 and continue into all or part of diastole results from continuous flow due to a communication between high and low pressure areas that presists through the end of systole and beginning of diastole.

For example: PDA
Systemic AV fistula
Coronary AV fistula.

Carvallo sign–Right-sided murmur–increased during inspiration
Left-sided murmur–increased during expiration.

Graham-Steell Murmur

High-pitched EDM loudest in pulmonary area radiating down left sternal border seen in severe PAH.

MURMURS

Properties	*Mitral stenosis*	*Mitral regurgitation*	*Aortic stenosis*	*Aortic regurgitation*
Grading (Loudness/ Intensity	—	Grade 1–6	Grade 1–6	—
Pitch/Frequency	Low pitch	High pitch	Low pitch	High pitch
Character	Rough rumbling	Soft blowing	Rough rasping	Soft blowing
Timing	Mid-diastolic, presystolic accentuation	Parasystolic	Crescendo-Decrescendo Ejection systolic	Decrescendo Early diastolic
Area best heard	Apex	Apex	Aortic	2nd aortic
Position	Left lateral	Left lateral	Sitting and leaning forward	Sitting and leaning forward
Bell/Diaphragm	Bell	Diaphragm	Diaphragm	Diaphragm
Inspiration/ Expiration	Expiration	Expiration	Expiration	Expiration
Conduction/ Radiation	—	Axilla/Base	Carotid	Left sternal border
Dynamic maneuver	Exercise	Isometric exercise	Decrease on isometric exercise	Isometric exercise

Describe the murmur in a sentence, for example
MS—A low-pitched rough rumbling mid-diastolic murmur with a presystolic accentuation (no grading for diastolic murmur) best heard at the apex with patient in left lateral position with bell of the stethoscope and breath held in expiration.

MEDICINE

CHAPTER 3

Respiratory System

Name: Age: Sex: Address: Occupation:

PRESENTING ILLNESS

Cough

Onset, duration, progress, dry/productive, thick viscid or frothy, how long, diurnal or postural variation, aggravated by dust, pollen, or cold air, associated pain.

Sputum

Thick, viscid, frothy, color, consistency, amount, copious or not, diurnal or postural variation, foul smelling or not.

Hemoptysis

Onset, duration, progress, fresh/altered blood, quantity, purulent sputum or not, any chest pain, hematuria, or any bleeding tendencies.

Breathlessness

- Onset, duration, progress (class 1–4)
- Aggravating/relieving factors
- Associated symptoms like cough with expectoration, wheeze, chest pain.
- History of paroxysmal nocturnal dyspnea, orthopnea, trepopnea, platypnea.

Chest Pain

Onset, site, duration, radiation, brought on by, lasts for, character, aggravating/relieving factors, associated symptoms like vomiting, sweating, nausea, heartburns, associated with food intake, respiration.

Swelling of Feet

- Limited to face/legs—unilateral or bilateral/abdomen, generalized
- Aggravating/relieving factors, duration.

Symptoms of Cor Pulmonale

Anorexia, nausea, vomiting, abdominal distention, decreased urine output, right hypochondrial pain, nocturia, anasarca.

Symptoms of Tuberculosis

Loss of weight, appetite, evening rise of temperature, night sweats.

Symptoms of SVC Syndrome

Facial swelling, radicular pain in arm, hoarseness, dysphagia, dilated veins.

Symptoms of Malignancy

Loss of weight, appetite, chest wall tenderness.

PAST HISTORY

Previous similar episodes, history of DM, HT, IHD, TB, STD, RHD. History of hemoptysis, bronchial asthma or chronic obstructive pulmonary disease (COPD).

PERSONAL HISTORY

- Sleep, appetite, bowel and bladder habits
- Any addictions—smoking, alcohol, IVDA (in detail if one is seen).
- *Smoking*: No. of cigarettes/beedies per day, age at which habit was started, if stopped/reason. History of snuff, tobacco, betel nut chewing.

FAMILY HISTORY

- Any similar illness in the family
- Any history of TB, asthma DM, IHD, HT.

SOCIOECONOMIC HISTORY

Earning member of family, living in what type of house, any overcrowding or not, good sanitary facilities, good well, etc.

GENERAL EXAMINATION

- Conscious, cooperative, comfortable/dyspneic at rest, build and nourishment.
- *Pallor, cyanosis, jaundice, clubbing, pedal edema, LNE*:
  - *Pulse*: Rate, rhythm, volume, character, peripheral vessels, thickening, radiofemoral delay, pulse deficit, carotid bruit.
  - *Respiration*: Rate, rhythm, character, depth
  - *Blood pressure*: mm Hg, in which limb (UL/LL) posture, whether on antihypertensive
  - *Temperature*: Record if febrile
- Look for external markers of TB
- Marfan's syndrome (in pneumothorax).

EXAMINATION OF RESPIRATORY SYSTEM

Upper Respiratory Tract

- *Nose*: Deviated nasal septum, nasal polyps, sinus tenderness, nasal alae.
- *Oral cavity*: Oral hygiene, dental caries, oral thrush, and tonsils.
- *Pharynx*: Postnasal drip and congestion.

RESPIRATORY SYSTEM PROPER

Inspection

- Position of trachea (Trail's sign), apical impulse
- Chest wall deformity—kyphoscoliosis, pectus excavatum (funnel/Cobbler's chest), pectus carinatum (pigeon/keeled chest), flail chest, barrel chest, rickety and scorbutic rosary, Harrison's sulcus, flat chest.
- Chest wall symmetry—look for evidence of volume loss such as drooping, rib crowding, hollowing, decreased spinoscapular distance, kyphoscoliosis, flattening retraction. Any evidence of mass lesion bulging, fullness.
- Movements of chest wall—rate, rhythm, equality, type, intercostals retraction, accessory muscles of respiration.
- Skin over chest wall—dilated veins, pulsations, scar discharging sinus, intercostals swelling, shiny skin.

PALPATION

- Position of trachea, apical impulse may be confirmed.
- Swelling, chest wall, subcutaneous emphysema or intercostal tenderness.
- Movement of chest wall, chest expansion (total, both hemithorax)
- Fremitus (tactile vocal)
- Tracheal tug and inspiratory tracheal descent.

PERCUSSION

- Anteriorly

Right side	*Left side*
Kronig's isthmus	Kronig's isthmus
Clavicular percussion	Clavicular percussion
Infraclavicular area	Infraclavicular area
Mammary area	Mammary area
Liver dullness	Cardiac dullness
Tidal percussion	Traube's space

- *Axilla*: axillary, infra-axillary area on both sides
- *Posteriorly*: subscapular, interscapular, intrascapular area.
- Straight line dullness, shifting dullness (hydropneumothorax)
- Skodaic resonance, crackpot resonance
- Percussion tenderness, percussion myokymia.

AUSCULTATION

- *Breath sound*: Intensity (loud, normal, decreased)
- *Quality*: Vesicular, bronchial (tubular, cavernous, amphoric), bronchovesicular
- *Added sounds*: Crepitations (fine/coarse, early/mid/late inspiratory, post-tussive), bronchi, pleural rub
- *Vocal resonance*: Increased/decreased, bronchophony, egophony, whispering pectoriloquy
- *Other features*: Post-tussive suction, post-tussive creps, coin sound, succession splash, Hạmman's crunch, stridor.

Examination of other systems: CVS/Abdomen/CNS

SPIROMETRY

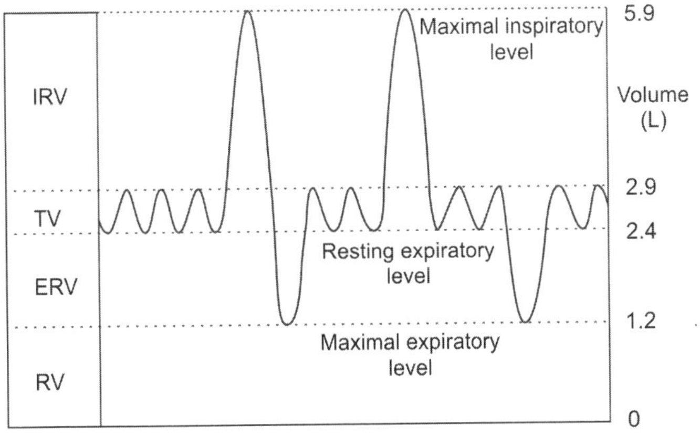

IRV = Inspiratory reserve volume
TV = Tidal volume
ERV = Expiratory reserve volume
RV = Residual volume

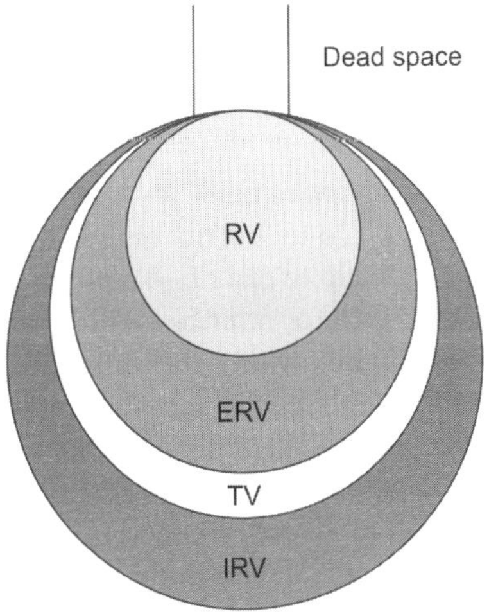

DISCUSSION

ANATOMY

- *Lungs*: 6th, 8th, 10th intercostal space
- *Pleura*: 8th, 10th,12th intercostal space in the midclavicular line, midaxillary line and posterior scapular line, respectively.
- *Major interlobar fissure*: From T2 spine, medial border of scapula (with arm hyperabducted) to 6th costochondral junction.
- *Minor interlobar fissure*: From 4th costochondral junction to major fissure.
- Bronchopulmonary segment:

Right lung:

Upper lobe: Apical
Anterior
Posterior
Middle lobe: Medial
Lateral
Lower lobe: Apical
Anterior basal
Posterior basal
Medial basal
Lateral basal

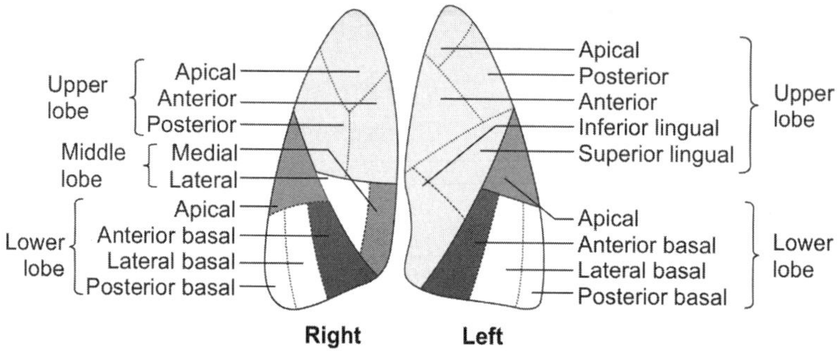

Left lung:

Upper lobe: Apical
Anterior
Posterior
Lingular segment: Superior lingualar
Inferior lingualar
Lower lobe: Apical
Anterior basal
Posterior basal
Medial basal
Lateral basal.

LYMPHATIC DRAINAGE

- *Whole right lung and left lower lobe*: Right supraclavicular lymph node
- *Left upper lobe*: Left supraclavicular lymph node
- *Parietal pleura*: Axillary lymph node.

AREAS

Anteriorly: 1. Above clavicle—supraclavicular area/Kronig's isthmus
2. Up to 3rd rib—infraclavicular area
3. Up to 6th rib—mammary area
Axilla: 4. Up to 6th rib—axillary area
5. Below 6th rib—infra-axillary area
Posteriorly: 6. Above T2—suprascapular area
7. T2–T7—interscapular area
8. Below T7—infrascapular area

Findings of all lobes are obtained in the axilla.
In pleural effusion, patchy dullness beyond the boundaries of a lobe is obtained.

Dull Kronig's isthmus
- Pancoast tumor
- Large lymph node
- Apical fibrosis

Muscles of respiration	Accessory muscles of respiration
Inspiratory: • External intercostal muscle • Internal intercostal muscle • Diaphragm *Expiratory*: Internal intercostal muscle *Hoover's sign*: On inspiration ↓ Negative intrathoracic pressure and positive atmospheric pressure ↓ Intercostal indrawing	**Mnemonic—PASS SALT** • Pectoralis major • Alae nasi • Sternocleidomastoid • Scalenus anterior • Serratus anterior • Abdominal muscle • Latissimus dorsi • Trapezius

CHRONIC OBSTRUCTIVE PULMONARY DISEASE (COPD)

Emphysema-Bronchitis-Bronchiolitis

EMPHYSEMA

Abnormal permanent enlargement of air spaces distal to the terminal bronchiole accompanied by destruction of their wall without obvious fibrosis.

Four Types

1. Centriacinar—smoker
2. Panacinar—alpha-1-antitrypsin deficiency
3. Paraseptal
4. Irregular.

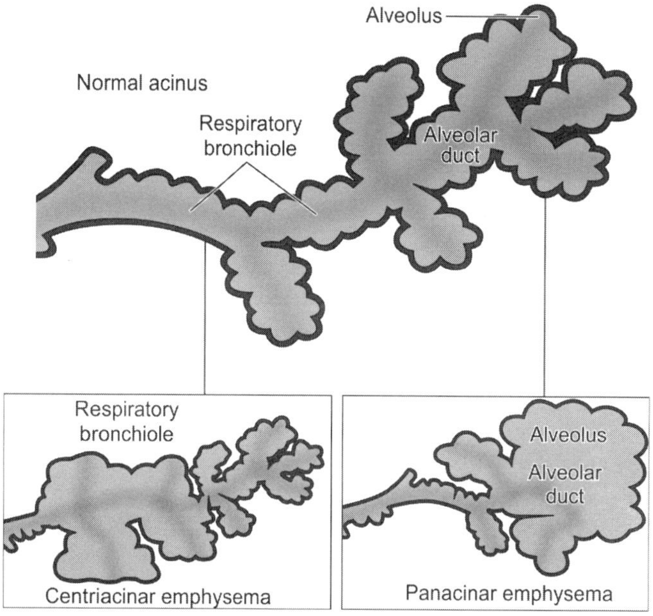

BRONCHITIS

Persistent cough with sputum production for at least 3 months in at least 2 consecutive years in absence of any other identifiable cause.

GOLD CRITERIA FOR COPD

0 – At risk; cough, sputum production
1 – Mild; FEV1/FVC <70%
FEV1 > = 80%
2 – Moderate; FEV1/FVC <70%
FEV1 50%–80%
3 – Severe; FEV1/FVC <70%
FEV1 30–50%
4 – Very severe; FEV1/FVC <70%
FEV1 <30%
OR
FEV1 <50% + respiratory failure/heart failure

CLINICAL FEATURES OF COPD

General Examination

- Tripod posture
- Conjunctival congestion (polycythemia)
- Pedal edema—cor pulmonale
- Respiratory failure
- Flapping tremor
- Warm extremities
- Bounding pulse
- In COPD, do not forget to look for washing.

Respiratory System

- Pursed lip breathing
- Accessory muscles working
- Barrel-shaped chest
- Widened subcostal angle
- Decreased cricosternal distance
- Horizontality of ribs.

Other System

- Cor pulmonale
- Pulsatile JVP
- Tender hepatomegaly.

COR PULMONALE

Right ventricular enlargement with/without right ventricular failure due to problem in lung or ventilatory apparatus with left side being normal.

Etiology of Cor Pulmonale

- COPD
- ILD
- Bronchiectasis
- Ankylosing spondylitis
- Kyphoscoliosis.

Features of Cor Pulmonale

- Bloated up facies
- Pulsatile JVP
- Tender hepatomegaly
- B/L pedal edema
- Most common cause of RVF-LVF
- Most common cause of LVF-IHD
- Acute cor pulmonale—pulmonary thromboembolism.

Respiratory Failure

- Type 1—hypoxia + hypocapnea, e.g. emphysema
- Type 2—hypoxia + hypercapnea
- Type 3—postoperative atelectasis
- Type 4—shock (hypoperfusion of respiratory muscle in shock).

Complications of COPD

- Respiratory failure
- Cor pulmonale

Systemic complications:

- Weight loss, muscular weakness, osteoporosis
- Spontaneous pneumothorax

Type 1 PaO_2 <60 mm Hg, $PaCO_2$ <50 mm Hg

- Alcoholic type
- Irritable
- Emphysema—pink puffer
- Mental confusion

Type 2 PaO_2 <60 mm Hg. $PaCO_2$ <50 mm Hg

- Anesthetic type
- Altered sensorium
- Hypercapnea
- Warm extremities
- Bounding pulse
- Flapping tremor

PNEUMONIA

DEFINITION

Acute respiratory illness characterized radiologically by pulmonary shadowing which may be segmental, lobar or multilobar.

Lobar Pneumonia

Homogenous consolidation of one or more lung lobes often associated with pleural inflammation.

Bronchopneumonia

Patchy alveolar consolidation associated with bronchial and bronchiolar inflammation often affecting both lower lobes.

Types

- *Community-acquired pneumonia (CAP): Pneumococcus, H. Influenzae*
- *Hospital-acquired pneumonia (HAP): E. coli, Staphylococci, Pseudomonas, Klebsiella*
- *Ventilation-associated pneumonia (VAP):*
- *Pneumonia in immunocompromised: Pneumocystis jiroveci.*

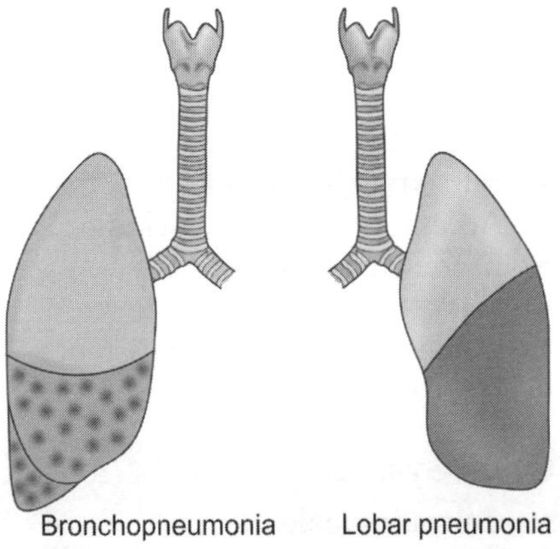

Pneumococcal Pneumonia

- Commonest
- Herpes labialis present
- Rusty sputum
- Rapid onset, high fever, pleuritic pain.

Klebsiella

- Upper lobe
- Red currant jelly sputum
- Bulging fissure sign, pneumatocele
- Seen in: alcoholic, diabetes, leukopenia, thrombocytopenia

Atypical Pneumonia

Dry cough + extrapulmonary manifestation (Diarrhea, hemolytic anemia, erythema nodosum GBS, pericarditis)

- *Legionella*:
  - Diarrhea
  - Neurological manifestations like headache, confusion, malaise
- *Mycoplasma*: Autoimmune hemolytic anemia, GBS
- *Chlamydia Pneumonia*: Perihepatitis (Fitz-Hugh-Curtis syndrome).

DD's of pneumonia

- Pulmonary infarction
- Pulmonary TB
- Pulmonary edema
- Bronchoalveolar carcinoma.

Respiratory defense mechanism

- Cough reflex
- Mucociliary apparatus
- Alveolar macrophage

Any breech in normal respiratory defense mechanism leads to pneumonia

Investigations

- Routine blood (CBC, Hb, ESR)
- X-ray chest—air bronchogram
- Gram staining

S. pneumoniae complications

- Pneumatocele
- Infectious endocarditis associated
- Empyema

MANAGEMENT

Treatment

- Oxygen therapy
  PaO_2 >60 mm Hg and SaO_2 >92% should be maintained
- IV fluids
- Assess CURB-65
- Antibiotics

Gram +ve	— Pencillin/1st generation cephalosporin
Gram –ve	— Aminoglycosides/3rd generation cephalosporin/Fluoroquinolones
Anaerobes	— Metronidazole
Staphylococci	— Cloxacillin/vancomycin/Linezolid/imipenem
Atypical	— Azithromycin
Klebsiella	— Ciprofloxacin + aminoglycoside.

- For pleural pain
  Paracetamol/NSAID
- Physiotherapy — To assist expectorations.

Chest X-ray

- *Air bronchogram*: Air inside terminal bronchiole
- *Hilar adenopathy*: Mycoplasma
- *Cavitation*: Staphylococcal pneumonia
- *Mottled opacity in lower lobe*: Bronchopneumonia

Delayed Resolution

- Sign >2 weeks
- CXR >4 weeks

} Even after antibiotic therapy

Causes

- Incorrect diagnosis
- Inadequate drugs/dose

Complications

- Pleural effusion
- Empyema
- Lung abscess
- Cavity
- Lobar collapse due to retention of sputum
- Pneumothorax—*S.aureus*
- Others:
  Acute respiratory distress syndrome (ARDS), renal failure, multiorgan failure toxic hepatitis, toxic gastric dilatation, metastatic abscess, osteomyelitis, meningioencephalitis

- Complications
- Diabetes or other immunocompromised conditions
- Underlying TB, malignancy
- Drug resistance.

CURB 65

- Confusion
- Urea >7 mmol/L
- Respiratory rate >30/min
- *Blood pressure*:
  - Systolic: <90 mm of Hg
  - Diastolic: <60 mm of Hg
- Age >65 years.

Score: 1 point for each feature present.

Score 0 or 1—likely to be suitable for home treatment
Score 2—short stay inpatient or hospital supervised OP
Score 3 or > manage in hospital as severe pneumonia
ICU admission if score >4

PLEURAL EFFUSION

The accumulation of serous fluid within the pleural space is termed as pleural effusion.

- Clinically—>500 mL
- X-ray–200 mL.

Types

- Exudative: Due to increased microvascular pressure due to disease of the pleural surface or injury in the adjacent lung.
- Transudative: Due to increased hydrostatic pressure or due to decreased oncotic pressure.

Bilateral exudative pleural effusion

- Effusion
- Rheumatoid arthritis
- SLE
- Lymphoma
- Leukemia
- Pulmonary infarction

Predominant left-sided pleural effusion

- Acute pancreatitis
- Esophageal rupture
- Dressler's syndrome (post MI syndrome)
- Aortic dissection

Drug-induced pleural effusion (DAMB)

- Amiodarone
- Bromocriptine
- Dantrolene sodium
- Methysergide

Predominant right-sided pleural effusion

- Amebic liver abscess
- Cirrhosis of liver
- CCF
- Meigs' syndrome

Trachea shifted to same side in pleural effusion

- Same-sided fibrosis
- Same-sided collapse
- Mesothelioma.

Gardland's triangle

Area above the level of pleural effusion
Findings

- Bronchial breath sound
- Increased vocal resonance
- Egophony.

Pleural effusion + trachea in midline

- Mild pleural effusion
- Malignant pleural effusion secondary to bronchogenic carcinoma
- Encysted pleural effusion
- Bilateral pleural effusion
- Pleural effusion associated with mesothelioma

In case of pleural effusion look for 5S

1. Shifting dullness
2. Straight line dullness
3. Succussion splash
4. Sound of coin
5. Shift of mediastinum.

Recurrent pleural effusion even after thoracentesis

- Bronchogenic carcinoma
- Pulmonary TB
- CCF
- Lymphoma

Red flag sign in pleural effusion

- Trachea shifted to same side
- Developing into empyema thoracis.

EXUDATIVE PLEURAL EFFUSION

Causes

- Pneumonia
- Tuberculosis
- Bronchogenic carcinoma
- Pulmonary infarction
- Collagen vascular disease—rheumatoid arthritis, SLE
- Mesothelioma
- Lymphoma
- Meigs' syndrome
- Pancreatitis, subphrenic abscess, liver abscess.

TRANSUDATIVE PLEURAL EFFUSION

Causes

- Nephrotic syndrome
- Congestive cardiac failure
- Cirrhosis of liver
- Myxedema
- Constrictive pericarditis
- Pericardial effusion.

***Remember*: Transudative pleural effusion is usually bilateral (hydrothorax).**

HEMORRHAGIC PLEURAL EFFUSION

- Malignancy
- Tuberculosis
- Bleeding diathesis
- Pulmonary infarction

MANAGEMENT OF PLEURAL EFFUSION

Investigations

- CXR
- Mantoux test
- *Pleural fluid analysis*:
  - Appearance-serous, bloody, pus, milky
  - *Cytology*:
    - Lymphocyte—TB or lymphoma
    - Neutrophils—pneumonia
    - Very high neutrophils—empyema
  - Proteins—high in exudative
  - *Sugar*:
    - Low—all conditions except uncontrolled diabetes
    - Very low—rheumatoid arthritis, empyema
  - Adenosine deaminase (ADA)

    45 IU/L

    ADA –ve not tuberculosis

    (only –ve predictive value
  - AFB in pleural fluid—TB empyema.

Empyema

Presence of pus in pleural space

Etiology

- Pneumonia
- Tuberculosis
- Secondary infection in pleural effusion
- Rupture of subphrenic abscess
- Rupture of lung abscess

MEDICINE

Light's Criteria

Pleural fluid is an exudates if one or more of the following criteria are met:

- *Pleural fluid protein*: Serum protein ratio >0.5
- *Pleural fluid LDH*: Serum LDH ratio >0.6
- Pleural fluid LDH >2/3 of the upper limit of normal serum LDH.

Roth's Criteria

Serum albumin—pleural fluid albumin >1.2

↓

Transudative

Treatment

- ICD tube
- Thrombolysis—to prevent adhesions
- Pleurodesis
- Thoracotomy and decortications
- NSAID-pain

ICD tube in area of maximum dullness

OR

6th, 7th, 8th ICS in MAL

ICD tube removal—< 30 mL/day for 3 consecutive day.

Indication for ICD tube

- Pus
- +ve gram stain
- Very high count
- Very low glucose
- Very low pH
- Encystment of pleural effusion

PNEUMOTHORAX

Pneumothorax is the presence of air in the pleural space.

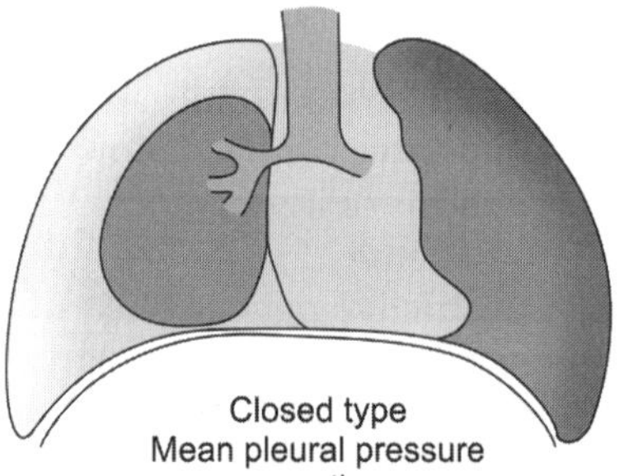

Closed type
Mean pleural pressure negative

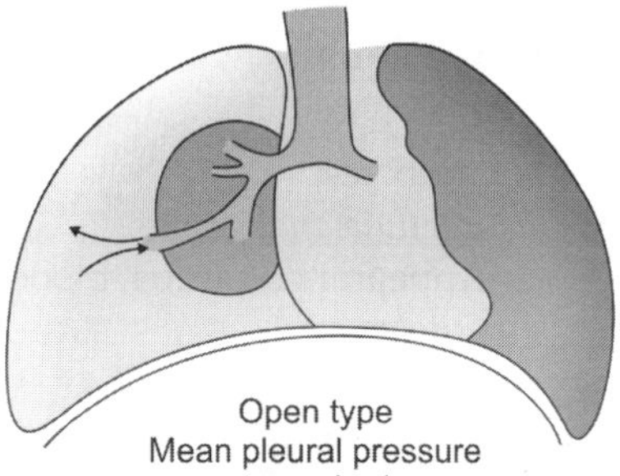

Open type
Mean pleural pressure atmospheric

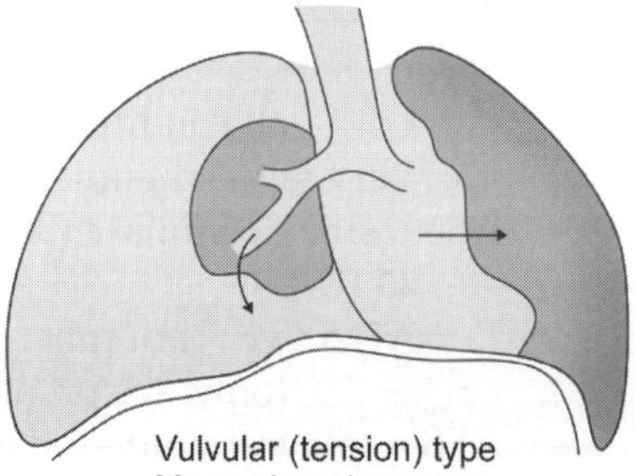

Vulvular (tension) type
Mean pleural pressure positive

Classification

- Spontaneous
- Traumatic

- **Spontaneous pneumothorax**
  - *Primary*
    Affect males aged 15–30 in whom tall stature, smoking and presence of apical subpleural blebs are additional risk factors.
    ↓
    Air escapes from the lung into the pleural space through rupture of a small subpleural emphysematous bulla.
  - *Secondary*
    Underlying lung disease.
    For example, COPD, TB, bronchial asthma, lung abscess, bronchogenic carcinoma, all forms of fibrotic and cystic lung diseases.

- **Traumatic pneumothorax**
  - Non-iatrogenic
  - Iatrogenic.

Types of Pneumothorax

- Closed
- Open
- Tension.

TENSION PNEUMOTHORAX

Communication between the airway and pleura is small. It can act as a one-way valve allowing air to enter the pleural space during inspiration but not to escape on expiration.

CLOSED PNEUMOTHORAX

When the communication between the lung and pleural space seals off as the lung deflates and does not reopen.

OPEN PNEUMOTHORAX (BRONCHOPLEURAL FISTULA)

Communication fails to seal and air continues to transfer freely between the lung and pleural space.

FLOWCHART IN MANAGEMENT OF SPONTANEOUS PNEUMOTHORAX

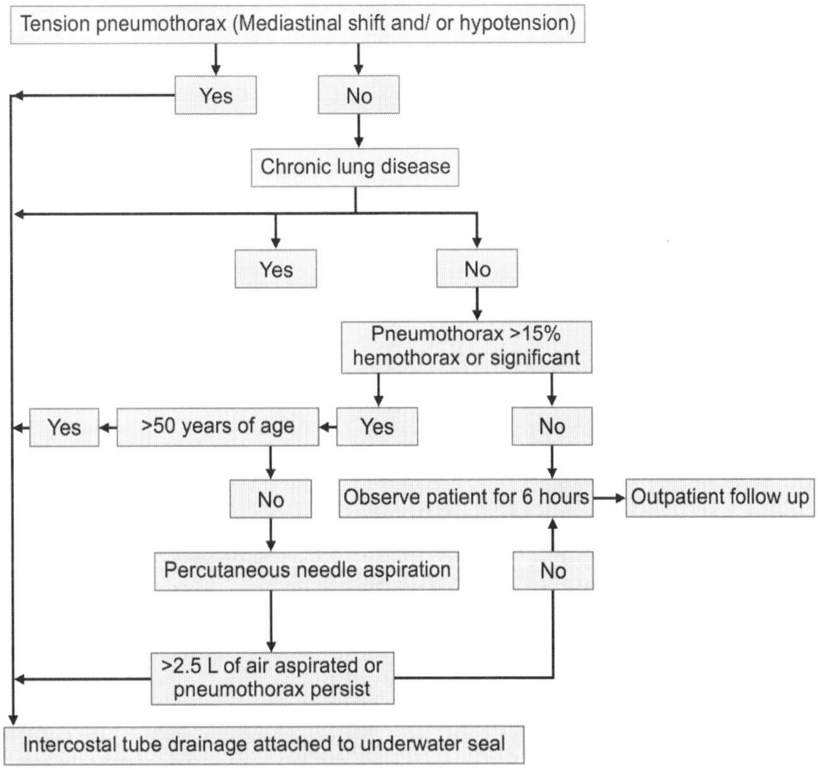

INVESTIGATIONS

- X-ray.

TREATMENT

- In case of tension pneumothorax immediate decompression is required prior to insertion of intercostal drain.
- Aspirate in the 2nd intercostal space anteriorly in the midclavicular line using 16 F cannula.

TUBERCULOSIS

In children: Primary tuberculosis → Ghon focus → Ghon complex → Ranke complex

Primary Tuberculosis

It includes:
- Progressive primary tuberculosis (dissemination within lung)
- Miliary tuberculosis
- Meningitis.

How is miliary tuberculosis spread?

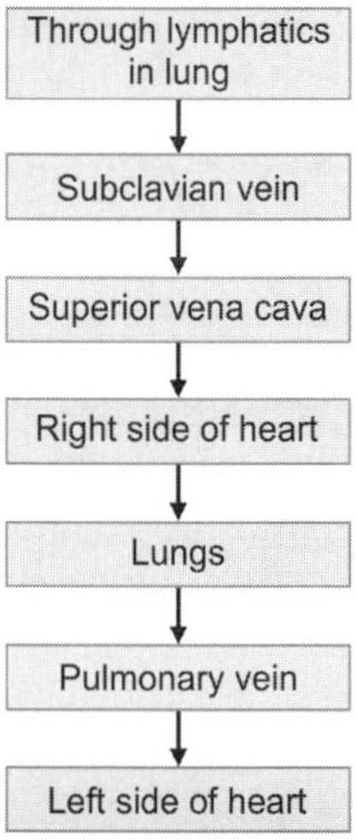

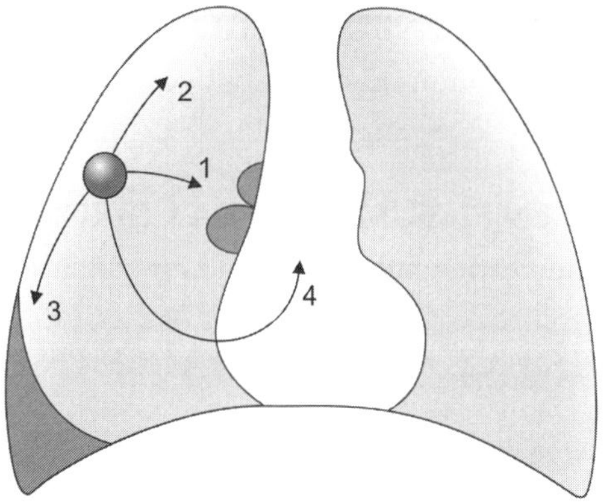

Primary pulmonary tuberculosis. 1. Spread from primary focus to hilar and mediastinal lymph glands to form the primary complex, which in most cases heals spontaneously. 2. Direct extension of the primary focus—progressive pulmonary tuberculosis. 3. Spread to the pleura—tuberculous pleurisy and pleural effusion. 4. Blood-borne spread few bacilli—pulmonary, skeletal, renal, genitourinary infection often months or years later; massive spread—miliary tuberculosis and meningitis.

Secondary Tuberculosis

- Post-primary
- Adult tuberculosis
- Reactivation tuberculosis.

Secondary tuberculosis → Simon's focus in upper lobe
↓
Due to increased ventilation perfusion ratio

- Due to increased ventilation more TB bacilli reaches
- Due to decreased perfusion-reduced antibodies reach.

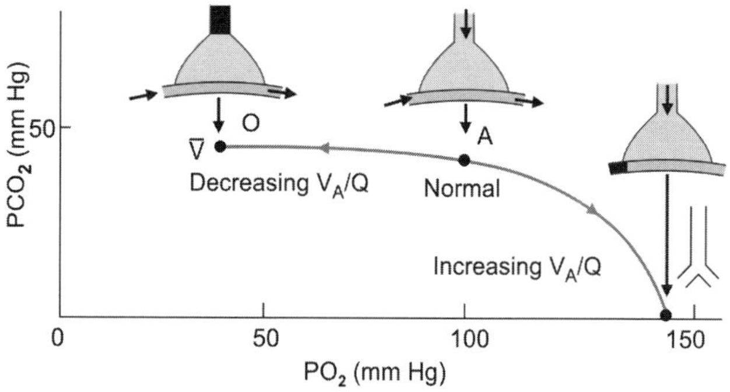

ACTIVE TUBERCULOSIS

Symptoms:

- Fever + evening rise of temperature/night sweats
- Weight loss
- Cough >2 weeks

Signs:

- Signs of cavity
- Post-tussive crepitation.

INVESTIGATIONS

- Increased ESR
- Sputum AFB
- CXR
- Mantoux test.

EMPIRICAL RESPONSE TO ATT

- Do not give rifampicin/fluoroquinolone/aminoglycosides as they are broad-spectrum antibiotics.
- SEATT (Specific Empirical Anti-TB Therapy).

Causes of hemoptysis in tuberculosis

- Bronchiectasis sicca
- TB eroding blood vessel
- Aspergilloma
- Cavitation
- Endobronchial TB
- Rasmussen aneurysm
- Fibrotic scar carcinoma

TREATMENT

- Category I: 2(HRZE)3 + 4(HR)3
- Category II: 2(HRZES)3 + 1(HRZE)3 + 5(HRE)3

Only intracellular acting drug—pyrazinamide
Drugs effective against persisters—rifampicin
In TB:
Exudate → casseation → cavity → fibrosis → bronchiectasis.

BRONCHOGENIC CARCINOMA

Four histological types

1. Squamous cell carcinoma
2. Adenocarcinoma
3. Small cell carcinoma (oat cell Ca)
4. Large cell carcinoma.

Central lung cancers: Squamous and small cell carcinoma.

Diagnosed by bronchoscopy.

Peripheral lung cancers: Large cell carcinoma and adenocarcinoma Diagnosed by CT.

Cavitating cancers: Squamous cell carcinoma and large cell carcinoma.

Paraneoplastic syndrome associated with small cell carcinoma except hypercalcemia (squamous cell carcinoma).

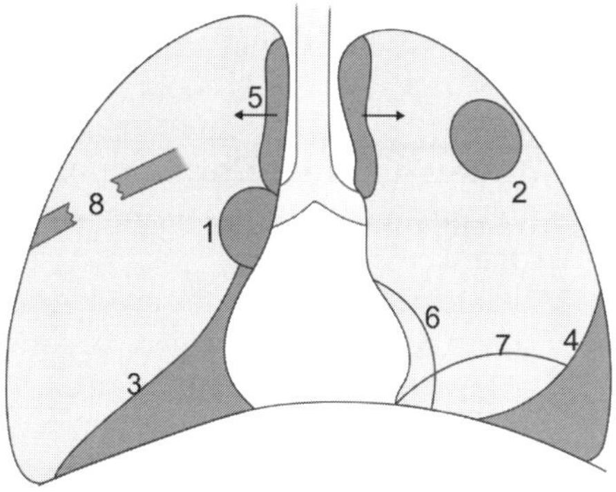

Common radiological presentations of bronchial carcinoma (*See the information box below for details*)

- Unilateral hilar enlargement
- Peripheral pulmonary opacity
- Lung, lobe or segmental collapse
- Pleural effusion
- Broadening of mediastinum, enlarged cardiac shadow, elevation of hemidiaphragm
- Rib destruction

PARANEOPLASTIC SYNDROME

Endocrine

- Syndrome of inappropriate antidiuretic hormone (SIADH)
- Ectopic adrenocorticotropic hormone (ACTH) secretion
- Hypercalcemia due to secretion of PTH-related peptide
- Carcinoid syndrome
- Gynecomastia.

Neurological

- Polyneuropathy
- Myelopathy
- Cerebellar degeneration
- Myasthenia (Lambert-Eaton syndrome).

Others

- Clubbing
- Hypertrophic pulmonary osteoarthropathy
- Nephrotic syndrome
- Polymyositis and dermatomyositis
- Eosinophilia
  - Polycythemia
  - Thrombocytosis

(Eosinophilia, Polycythemia, Thrombocytosis — Hematological)

Clinical features of Pancoast's syndrome

Triad:
1. Pain along inner aspect of arm
2. Small muscle wasting
3. Horner's syndrome

– Seen more often with squamous cell carcinoma of lung. Sometimes with small cell carcinoma

Treatment

- Radiotherapy—for squamous cell carcinoma
- Chemotherapy—cisplatin/carboplatin/paclitaxel

SVC SYNDROME

- Bloated facies
- Non-pulsatile JVP
- Dilated vein with flow from above downward

Treatment

- Propped-up position
- Diuretics
- Corticosteroid
- Radiotherapy.

Causes of SVC syndrome

- Squamous cell carcinoma
- Small cell carcinoma
- NHL
- Secondaries from breast and testes
- Retrosternal thyroid
- Thymoma
- Radiation
- Sarcoma
- SVC thrombosis (due to CVP line)

MEDICINE

GENERAL EXAMINATION IN RESPIRATORY SYSTEM

- *Pallor*:
  - Hemoptysis
  - Any chronic disease
  - INH induced
- *Cyanosis*:
  - Interstitial lung disease
  - Type II respiratory failure
- *Jaundice*:
  - Carcinoma lung with secondaries in liver
  - Pneumonia with sepsis
  - Drug-induced hepatitis
- *Clubbing*:
  - Lung abscess
  - Bronchiectasis
  - Carcinoma lung
  - Diffuse interstitial lung disease
  - Empyema
- *Pedal edema*:
  - Chronic suppurative lung disease—hypoproteinemia
  - Bronchiectasis—amyloidosis.

RESPIRATORY SYSTEM EXAMINATION

- *Position of trachea*: Trail's sign
- *Chest wall deformities*:
  - Kyphosis—exaggerated anterior curvature of the spine
  - Scoliosis—exaggerated lateral curvature of the spine
  - *Kyphoscoliosis may be*:
    - Primary idiopathic
    - *Secondary to childhood poliomyelitis or spinal TB:* Kyphoscoliosis may cause respiratory failure and cor pulmonale.
  - Pectus excavatum—localized depression of lower end of sternum or depression of whole length of body of sternum and of the costal cartilage attached to it (Congenital, Marfan's).
  - Pectus carinatum—localized prominence of sternum and adjacent costal cartilage accompanied by indrawing of ribs to form symmetrical horizontal grooves (Harrison sulcus) above costal margin due to rickets or chronic respiratory disease in childhood (Congenital, Marfan's, Rickets).
- Chest wall symmetry:
  Features of volume loss (seen in fibrosis):
  - Drooping of shoulders
  - Decreased spinoscapular distance
  - Scoliosis (convexity to opposite side)
  - Rib crowding.

Vocal Fremitus

Palpation of laryngeal vibrations on the chest wall when the patient speaks some words repeatedly in a constant tone.

Vocal Resonance

This is the auscultation of laryngeal vibrations transmitted to the chest wall.

Quantitative Change

- *Bronchophony*: Seems to appear from the earpiece of stethoscope.
- *Whispering pectoriloquy*: It seems like spoken right into auscultator's ear.

Qualitative Change

Egophony: This is a qualitative change in vocal resonance with nasal intonation mimicking bleating of a goat.

Breath Sounds

- Vesicular
- Bronchial
- Bronchovesicular

Bronchial Breath Sounds

1. Tubular—high pitch
   For examples: sound—collapse, consolidations, above the level of pleural effusion
2. Cavernous—low pitch sound; heard over large superficial thick walled empty cavity communicating with bronchi.
   For example: TB cavity
3. Amphoric—low pitch sound with high pitch overtone; heard over thin walled cavity.
   For example: Bronchopleural fistula, tension/open pneumothorax.

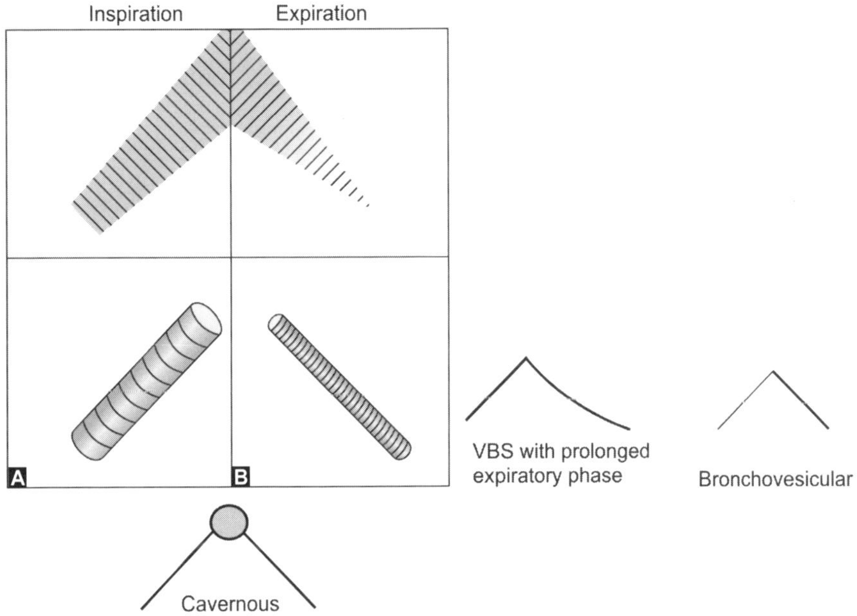

Added Sounds

Wheeze

- Continuous musical sound due to passage of air through narrowed airway.
- Seen in asthma, COPD
- High-pitched wheeze arise from smaller airway and have a whistling quality.
- Low-pitched wheeze arise from larger bronchi.

Crackles

- Interrupted non-musical sound produced by sudden opening of previously closed alveoli or passage of air through fluid filled airway.

Causes of crackles:

- *Early*: Chronic bronchiolitis
- *Middle*: Pulmonary edema
- *Late*: Pulmonary fibrosis
  Pulmonary edema
  Bronchial secretion in COPD, pneumonia, lung abscess, TB lung cavity
- *Biphasic*: Bronchiectasis, COPD.

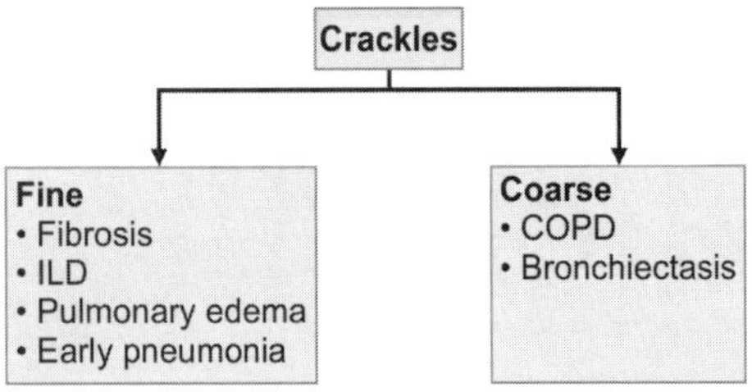

Additional points

- In fibrosis bronchial quality may be obtained due to auscultation over-shifted trachea.
- The sign of fibrosis—post-tussive crepitation.
- Lower lobe fibrosis—fine and inspiratory creps in lung base (Velcro creps in ILD).
- ICD tube is kept under water to prevent air reentry (in pneumothorax).

How to write diagnosis in a case of respiratory system?

1. Anatomy
2. Pathology
3. Etiology
4. Complication
5. Risk factors.

> Right lower lobe pneumonia community acquired, bacterial in etiology, without any complication (respiratory failure, sepsis) with risk factor of smoking and diabetes mellitus

Pathology	*General Examination*	*Trachea*	*Volume Loss*	*Movement*	*Percussion*	*Intensity*	*Quality*	*Adventitious Sounds*	*Vocal Resonance*	*Etiology*
Fibrosis	Emaciated	Shift to same side	++++	↓ed	Impaired	↓ed	NVBS	Crepitations post-tussive	↓ed	Upper lobe fibrosis—TB, Sarcoidosis, Ankyloising SP, Silicosis
Cavity	Emaciated	Central	–	↓ed	Crackpot Resonance (dull if fluid+)	N	Bronchial BS	Post-tussive suction (Absent if surrounding tissue collapsed)	↑ed	TB, Wegner's granuloma, Ca, Lung abscess, Fungal infection
Collapse		Shift to same side	+	↓ed	Dull	Normal-(Partial) or Absent (Total)	BBS (Partial) —(Total)	—	↑ed (Partial) — (Total)	Foreign body (FB)—Child mucous plug—Middle age Ca–old
Bronchiectasis	Clubbing, pedal, edema	Central	—	↓ed B/L	Dull	N	NVBS	MID Insp Coarse leathery crepitations	N	Usually Affects—lower lobe TB—Upper lobe Bronchiectasis (Br. Sicca) Brock's syndrome—Middle lobe bronchiectasis
Consolidation	Febrile, toxic	Central	–	↓ed	Dull	N	BBS (Tubular) Red and Gray heparin—BBS	Creps + Consolidating — Indux Fine Crep Resolution — Redux Coarse creps	Bronch-ophony Whispering Pectoriloquy egophony	Community acquired pneumonia (CAP), hospital-acquired pneumonia (HAP), ventilator-associated pneumonia, pneumonia in immunocom-promised

Contd...

Contd...

Mass lesion	Clubbing, Pancoast Syndrome, SVC Syndrome, para neoplastic Syndrome–Trousseau's Sign, Gynecomastia	Same/ Opposite/ Central	–	↓ed	Dullness, tenderness	N (Depends on Etiology)	N	Fixed, Monomorphic wheeze in obstruction	↓ed/↑ed	
Pleural effusion		Opposite side	bulging	Decreased	Stony dull	Decreased/ increased	—	Pleural rub	Decr/incr	—
Emphysema	Signs of COPD	Central	–	Decreased B/L	Hyper-resonance B/L	Decreased	VBS with prolonged expiration	Rhonchi	Decreased	Smoking, Environmental Pollution
Pneumothorax		Opposite side	—	Decreased	Hyperreso-nance	Decreased/ —	—	—	Decreased —	
Compensatory emphysema		Central	—	N	Hyperreso-nance	N	NVBS	No rhonchi	N	

(BBS: bronchial breath sounds; BS: bronchial sounds; NVBS: normal vesicular breath sound; COPD: chronic obstructive pulmonary disease)

CHAPTER 4

Gastrointestinal System

Name: Age : Sex: Address : Occupation:

PRESENTING ILLNESS

Symptoms of Esophageal Disease

Dysphagia, odynophagia, retching, vomiting, regurgitation, heartburn.

Symptoms of Upper Gastrointestinal Tract

- *Abdominal pain:* Onset, site, duration, radiation, brought on by, lasts for, character aggravating/relieving factors, associated symptoms like vomiting, sweating, nausea, heartburns associated with food intake.
- *Abdominal distension:* Onset, duration, progress, associated leg swelling, facial puffiness, pain, flatulence, dyspeptic symptoms, hiccups.
- *Abdominal lump:* Site, size, shape, onset, duration, progression, pain, weight loss.
- *Vomiting:* Frequency and forcibility, relation to meals, time of day, if preceded by nausea/pain, quantity and nature, ingestion of any drug causing emesis.
- *Hematemesis:* Number of episode, amount and character, color, association with melena, any drug intake, any bleeding tendencies, retching.
- *Jaundice:* Number of episodes, duration, color of urine, stool, drug intake, associated with pain, rigors.

Symptoms of Liver Dysfunction

Nausea, vomiting, jaundice, pruritus, loss of appetite, gynecomastia, loss of hair, loss of libido, loss of weight, reversal of sleep rhythm.

Symptoms of Lower Gastrointestinal Tract

Altered bowel habits, mucus and blood in stool, abdominal pain, lump and distension.

Urinary Symptoms

Oliguria, anuria, dysuria, nocturia, polyuria, hematuria.

Constitutional Symptoms

- *Fever:* Onset, duration, chills or rigors, nature, associated symptoms, any travel outside, similar illness in his house or relatives or friends
- *Weight loss:* Quantify if possible, noticed by relative or himself, loosening of clothes.
- Loss of appetite.

Swelling of Feet

Limited to face/legs—unilateral/bilateral/abdomen/generalized/aggravating/relieving factors duration.

PAST HISTORY

Blood transfusion, jaundice, tuberculosis, drug intake (ATT), travel to outside

PERSONAL HISTORY

Smoking, alcohol (in detail).

FAMILY HISTORY

Similar illness.

SOCIOECONOMIC STATUS

Earning member of family, living in what type of house, any overcrowding or not, good sanitary facilities, *good well*, etc.

GENERAL EXAMINATION

Conscious, cooperative, comfortable/dyspneic at rest, build and nourishment. Pallor, cyanosis, jaundice, clubbing, pedal edema, LNE.

Describe the positive signs of chronic liver disease.

Blood pressure: ....mm Hg, in which limb (UL/LL) posture, whether on antihypertensive.

Temperature: Record if febrile look for signs of liver failure

Pulse: Rate, rhythm, volume, character, peripheral vessels, thickening, radiofemoral delay pulse deficit, carotid bruit.

Respiration: Rate, rhythm, character, depth.

GASTROINTESTINAL SYSTEM

Upper GIT

Teeth, tongue, tonsils, orodental hygiene.

Inspection

- Shape of abdomen (scaphoid/distended), flanks (free/full)
- Umbilicus (position, slit, shape, discoloration, nodules)
- Skin (stretched, shiny, striae, jaundice, scar or sinuses)
- Movements with respiration, visible pulsation or peristalsis
- Dilated veins (around umbilicus, flanks)
- Divarication of recti, surgery marks, pigmentation, hernia orifices.

Palpation

- Local rise of temperature or tenderness, guarding or rigidity
- Organomegaly (site, size, shape, surface border, consistency, tender)
- Dilated veins (direction of flow), fluid thrill, rebound tenderness, shifting tenderness, crossed tenderness, bimanual palpation, dipping palpation, ballotability
- Pulsation (transmitted/expansile)
- Renal angle tenderness.

Percussion

- Liver dullness, liver span, Traube's space
- Shifting dullness, puddle sign, horse-shoe dullness.

Auscultation

Normal bowel sounds, succussion splash, bruit, venous hum, friction rub.

EXAMINATION OF OTHER SYSTEMS

Respiratory system: Percussion, air entry, breath sounds, added sounds.
Cardiovascular system: Loud P2, cardiomegaly, S1, S2, murmur.
Central nervous system: Drowsiness, focal neurological deficit.

A CASE EXAMPLE

Bhagavan Das sixty eight-year-old male, coming from kakkodi mukku.
He worked as office clerk in UP and now doing real estate.
DOA: 2/1/11

Presenting Complaints

Abdominal pain 3 days, abdominal distension 3 days, pedal edema 3 days, fever 2 days.

History of Present Illness

Known case of chronic liver disease, who is on treatment, had abdominal distension since one month. It is gradual in onset, is progressively increased in one month. He noticed severe abdominal distension for 3 days. It is associated with bilateral leg swelling. No history of flatulence, hiccups, it is still persisting abdominal pain is started 3 days back and is associated with abdominal distension.

Diffuse stretching type of pain and is so severe that he is not able to sleep and change his posture frequently. No history of radiating pain not associated with food intake and is relived by rest. Bilateral pedal edema is present. It is associated with abdominal distension, more during the evening. Not associated with facial puffiness. He had history of fever 2 days back, high grade fever with chills and rigor, persistent fever associated with nausea and headache. No history of travel, outside contact. No history of rash, night sweats, evening rise of temperature. He had history of loss of weight. Weight reduced around 6 kg. He had history of constipation since 2 days. He had history of loss of axillary hair, reversal of sleep rhythm, nausea, persistent jaundice, loss of appetite.

No history of hematemesis, cough and expectoration, hemoptysis, palpitation, syncope, chest pain, decreased urine output. No history of weakness of limp and loss of consciousness.

Past History

He had history of fever, jaundice one month back. High grade fever with chills and rigor, persistent in nature. Associated with 2–3 episodes of vomiting/day, nausea. He consulted medical college and adviced to have drug since then. Jaundice is still persisting, but decreased in intensity. No history of pruritis.

Detected to have diabetic since 5 months and is on oral hypoglycemic drug.

No history of TB, BA, COPD, IHD, RHD. No blood transfusion. No history of any surgery.

Personal History

- *Sleep:* Decreased
- *Appetite:* Decreased
- *Bowel:* Constipation since 3 days
- *Bladder:* Normal
- He is a chronic alcoholic sine 40 years using 2–3 pegs per day now stopped since 3 months
- Taking mixed diet
- No other addiction.

Family History

- No history of similar illness in the family
- No TB, IHD, RHD, BA, epilepsy, CAD, liver disease
- Drug or treatment history
- He is on drugs for jaundice.

GENERAL EXAMINATION

Conscious, cooperative and oriented, moderately built and nourished pallor, clubbing, jaundice, pedal edema present.

No lymphadenopathy, cyanosis.

SIGNS OF LIVER FAILURE

Clubbing, jaundice, thick nails, gynecomastia

No palmar erythema and spider nevi

Vital Signs

- Pulse—75, regular in rhythm, normal in volume and character.
  - All peripheral pulsations are normal
  - No radio-radial/radio-femoral delay
- BP—118/76 mm Hg in right upper limp in supine position
- Respiration rate—20
  - Thoracoabdominal
  - Regular
- Temperature—afebrile

EXAMINATION OF GASTROINTESTINAL SYSTEM

- Lips, buccal, mucosa, gums—normal
- Oral cavity—good oral hygiene
- Tongue, teeth, tonsil, tonsilar pillar—normal
- Palate, post-pharyngeal wall—normal.

Inspection

- Shape of abdomen—abdomen grossly distended and flanks full. No dilated veins, scars, visible pulsations.
- Umbilicus central and inverted
- All quadrants move equally and bilaterally with respiration.

Palpation

- Liver—soft, smooth, regular surface, sharp border, non tender, move downward with respiration
- Palpable 5 cm from the costal margin
- Left lobe—liver is palpable
  - Non-tender, soft, regular surface with sharp border, move downward with respiration and 4 cm from xiphisternum
- Fluid thrill—present
- No other mass palpable
- No tenderness, rise in temperature
- No renal angle tenderness.
- External genitalia—normal.

Percussion

- Liver dullness—5th ICS in midclavicular line
- Liver span—15 cm
- Traube's space—dull
- Shifting dullness—present.

Auscultation

- Normal bowel sounds heard
- No hepatic bruit heard.

Examination of CVS System

- Pulse: Mentioned
- BP: Mentioned
- JVP: Not elevated
- Shape of precordium: Normal
- Apex: 5th ICS 1 cm medial to MCL
- Trachea: Central
- S1, S2: Normal
- No murmur and added sounds.

RESPIRATORY SYSTEM

- Trachea—mentioned
- Apex—mentioned
- Shape of chest—normal, bilaterally symmetrical
- Movement of chest wall—equal and symmetrical
- Normal vesicular breath sounds heard
- No adventitious sounds.

CENTRAL NERVOUS SYSTEM

- Higher neural function—WNL
- Cranial nerve examination—WNL
- Sensory and motor system examination within normal limits
- No cerebellar signs
- Skull and spine—normal.

SUMMARY

A 68-year-old male with no significant family history and history of fever and jaundice 1 month back, DM for 3 years, he is a chronic alcoholic, now presented with abdominal distension, abdominal pain, pedal edema for 3 days and fever for 2 days, loss of weight and loss of axillary hair, reversal of sleep rhythm.

On examination found to have pallor, clubbing, jaundice, pedal edema, gynecomastia—present

On examination of GI system, abdomen grossly distented with flanks full and soft nontender, smooth surface with sharp border and liver palpable 5 cm from lower costal margin and liver span is 15 cm. Left lobe of liver is also palpable. On percussion shifting dullness and fluid thrill present and Traube's space is dull.

DIAGNOSIS

Chronic liver disease probably alcoholic liver disease and is decompensated state with spontaneous bacterial peritonitis.

DISCUSSION

* Do not forget past history—history of jaundice, drug intake like ATT, recent blood transfusion.

Definition of some terms:

Melena: Passage of dark, tarry, sticky stool per rectum.

Indicates upper GI bleeding—Min of 60 mL bleeding is required and it remains for at least 8 hours.

with 1 bleed melena may occur up to 7 days

Hematemesis: Vomiting of blood

Hemoptysis: Expectoration of blood

Hematochezia: Passage of red blood per rectum (bleeding distal to ligament of Treitz)

Cirrhosis: Chronic and diffuse involvement of liver of varied etiology characterized by portal hypertension and hepatocellular failure in varying combination and pathologically by irreversible necrosis, extensive fibrosis and nodule formation

Decompensation: When the patient develops jaundice or any of the complications (hepatic encephalopathy, ascites, SBP, hematemesis or hepatorenal syndrome)

Features of Chronic Liver Disease

- Sunken eyes
- Hollowed out temporal fossa
- Frontal balding
- Hollowed out cheek
- Loss of axillary hair
- Gynecomastia in males, breast atrophy in female.
- Spider nevi—seen in superior venacaval drainage area (above umbilicus)

- Palmar erythema (liver, palm, Dawson sign)
- Clubbing
- Terry's nail (Lindsay nail seen in CKD)
- Dupuytren's contracture
- Ascites
- Testicular atrophy—measured by Prader orchidometer
  - Normal testicular volume—15–20 mL/4–6 cm
  - If less than 3 cm—atrophy
- Paper money skin
- Parotid enlargement
- Edema.

Enlarged liver in CLD
- Alcoholic (early stage)
- Wilsons
- Hemochromatosis
- Hepatoma
- Budd-Chiari syndrome

Stigmata of Alcoholic Liver Disease

- Bilateral parotid enlargement
- Gynecomastia
- Dupuytren's contracture
- Testicular atrophy.

Pallor in CLD
- Decreased intake (Fe, B_9, B_{12})
- Decreased absorption
- BM suppression by alcohol
- Increased destruction by
  - Hypersplenism
  - Blood loss.

Spider nevi
- Central dilated alteriolet radiating capillaries
- Blanch central to periphery
- Significant it > 5 – 6 number
- Differential diagnosis
  - Insect bite
  - Telangiectasia

Gynecomastia

Presence of glandular breast tissue in males.

Causes of gynecomastia

- *Physiological:* Newborn, puberty, old age
- *Pathological:* Drugs – digoxin, INH, spironolactone cimetidine
- *Hypogonadism:* Klinefelter
- *Estrogen excess:* Liver failure estrogen secreting tumor of testes.

Etiology of CLD

- Alcoholism
- Non-alcoholic steatohepatitis
- Hepatitis B and C
- Drugs
- Wilson and hemochromatosis (metabolic cause).
- Immune–1° sclerosing cholangitis, autoimmune hepatitis
- C/C venous outflow obstruction.
- Primary biliary cirrhosis.

Alcoholic Cirrhosis

Also called Laennec's cirrhosis

Micronodular pattern (also seen in hemochromatosis, malnutrition, cholestasis)

Micronodular (<3 mm) (macro—Wilson, postnecrotic α_1 antitrypsin deficiency)

Dose of alcohol that cause cirrhosis:
- Males—60–80 mL (consumption for 10 years)
- Females—40 mL (consumption for 10 years)

Stages of alcoholic liver disease

Fatty liver— Alcoholic hepatitis – cirrhosis

Child-Pugh criteria:
- Grade A(good prognosis)
- Grade B
- Grade C

Based on 5 factors
- B—Bilirubin
- A—Albumin
- A—Ascites
- P—PT
- E—Encephalopathy

Treatment

- Stop alcohol
- Nutrition
- Corticosteroids
- Pentoxiphyllin
- Liver transplantation.

Nonalcoholic fatty lever disease (NAFLD)

NAFLD < NAFL / NASH

Mechanism

1st bit

- Increased F-A inflow
- Increased FA synthesis
- Decreased FA oxidation
- Decreased VLDL assembly
- Insulin resistance

} Fatty liver (NAFC)

2nd bit

- TNF-α
- Oxidant stress
- Endotoxin
- Immune factors

} NASH

- NASH $\xrightarrow[\text{Leptin}]{}$ Fibrosis

Investigations

- LFT – Elevated transaminases and GGT
- USG – Fatty Liver
- Liver biopsy – mallory bodies

Treatment

- Weight reduction
- Metformin

Drugs Causing Cirrhosis

A – Arsenic
M – Methotrexate
M – Methysergide
A – Amiodarone
I – Indigenous medicine

HEPATITIS B

History of sexual contact or IV drug abuse, surgeries, blood transfusion, tattooing, vertical transmission

- Manifestations:
  - Rash with arthritis
  - Serum sickness
  - Polyarteritis nodosa
  - AGN and nephrotic syndrome
  - Aplastic anemia.

Hepatitis A virus—Enterovirus
Hepatitis B virus—Hepedine virus
Hepatitis C virus—Flavivirus
Hepatitis D virus—Delta virus
Hepatitis E virus—Calci virus

Investigations

- Serology
  - HbsAg—Active infections
  - HbcAg—Not found in the blood
  - HbcAg—Viral replications
  - Anti-Hbs
  - Anti-Hbc
- Viral load
  HBV – DNA

  R$_x$ – Lamivudin, Alpha-interferon (LAB), entecavir, liver transplantation

Hepatitis C – R$_x$ – Ribavirin, alpha-interferon (CAR)

WILSON'S DISEASE

- To be excluded in young patient with cirrhosis
- Autosomal recessive
- *ATP7B* gene on chromosome 13

Clinical Features

- *KF ring:* In Descemet membrane, disappears with treatment
- Sunflower cataract
- Neuropsychiatric manifestation
- Wing-beating tremor, rigidity, chorea, athetosis, dystonia.

Investigations

- Serum ceruloplasmin < 20 mg/dL
- 24 br urinary copper >38 µg/day
- Liver biopsy – dry weight of copper >250 µg/g
- Rx - D-penicillamine, zinc oxide, trientine
- Liver transplantation in liver failure

HEMOCHROMATOSIS

Autosomal recessive—chromosome 6
Commonly seen in males > 40 years and postmenopausal women.

Manifestations

- Skin pigmentation
- Cardiomyopathy
- Cirrhosis, jaundice
- Diabetes mellitus (Bronze diabetes)
- Hypogonadotrophic hypogonadism
- Arthritis

Other causes of hyper pigmentation
- Addison's disease
- Drugs–clofazimine amiodarone
- Heavy metal–Arsenic
- Kala-azar.

Investigations

- Increased transferrin saturation
- Increased ferritin

Treatment

- Venesection
- Desferrioxamine
- Deferasirox
- Deferiprone.

Primary biliary cirrhosis

- Female
  - Autoimmune disease
  - Features of obstructive jaundice

PORTAL HYERTENSION

- Normal portal pressure—7–10 mm Hg
- If > 12 mm Hg, there is portal hypertension.

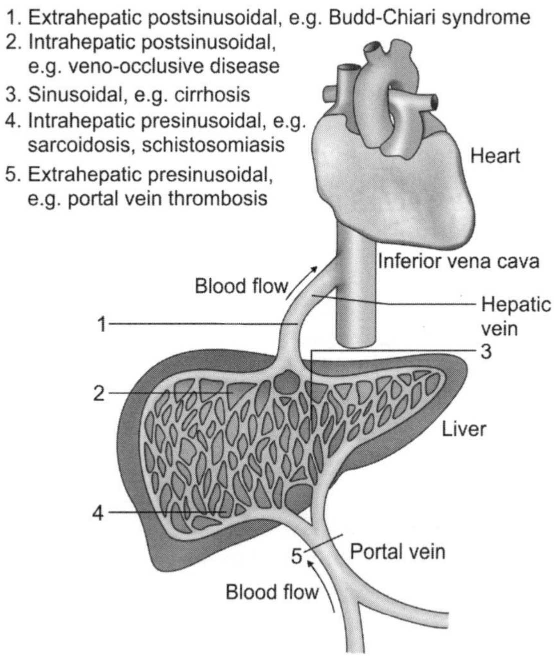

Clinical Features

1. Ascites
2. Splenomegaly
3. Varices [sites of portosystemic anastomoses—esophagus, around umbilicus (caput medusa), rectum (hemorrhoids), bare area of liver, retroperitoneum]

Causes

- *Presinusoidal:*
  - Extrahepatic—Portal vein thrombosis, splenic vein thrombosis
  - Intrahepatic—Schistosomiasis, Banti's syndrome, congenital hepatic fibrosis, sarcoidosis
- Sinusoidal—Cirrhosis due to any cause
- *Postsinusoidal*
  - Intrahepatic—veno-occlusive disorder
  - Extrahepatic—Budd-Chiari syndrome
    —Constrictive pericarditis

Non-cirrhotic Portal Hypertension

- History of umbilical sepsis in neonate
- Normal liver, no ascites (no hypoproteinemia)
- Massive bleed and splenomegaly
- Good prognosis.

Treatment

- Management of variceal bleed
- Primary preventions of variceal bleed—propranolol or Nadolol

HEPATIC ENCEPHALOPATHY

It is the neuropsychiatric manifestation of chronic liver disease.

Flapping tremor causes:
- CLD
- Respiratory failure
- Renal failure
- Phenytoin
- Parietal/thalamic lesion

Clinical Features

- Altered sleep rhythm
- Altered sensorium
- Constructional apraxia
- Fetor hepaticus (due to mercaptans)
- Flapping tremor (asterixis)
  - Inability to maintain posture against gravity.

Grading

I – Poor concentration, slurred speech, slow mentation, altered sleep, constructional apraxia
II – Drowsy but easily arousable, occasional aggressive behavior, lethargic, hyperreflexia, hexor plantar
III – Marked confusion, drowsy, sleepy but responds to pain and voice, gross disorientation, hyporeflexia extensor plantar
IV – Unresponsive to voice, may or may not respond to painful stimuli, unconscious.

Factors Precipitating Hepatic Encephalopathy

- **A**lcohol
- **A**spiration pneumonia (infection)
- **B**leeding
- **C**onstipation
- **D**ehydration, drugs, diuretics
- **E**xcess protein, electrolyte imbalance
- **F**luid paracentesis

Investigations

- EEG—slowing of α wave, delta wave.
- Increased arterial ammonia.

Treatment

- Bowel sterilization – lactulose retention enema
  - Ampicllin, neomycin, metronidazole, rifaximin 400 mg TID × 14 days (gut selective)
- Treat the precipitating factor

MEDICINE

Actions of Lactulose

- Produce acidic diarrhea
- Converts NH_3 to NH_4^+
- Increase in lactose fermenting organisms and suppress NH_4^+ forming bacteria.

ASCITES

Causes

- **A**nasarca
- **S**eptic peritonitis
- **C**irrhosis and cardiac causes
- **I**ntra-abdominal malignancy—Ca ovary, Ca stomach
- **T**B peritonitis
- **E**ndocrine cause—hypothyroidism
- **S**yndromes—Meigs syndrome, Budd-Chiari syndrome

- USG—30 mL
- Puddle sign—150 mL
- Shifting dullness—500–1000 mL
- Fluid thrill—>2 L

Causes of ascites in cirrhosis:
- Hypoalbuminemia
- Portal hypertension
- Lymphatic weep, splanchnic vasodilatation
- Hyperaldosteronism

Treatment

- Salt restriction (<2 g/day)
- Fluid restriction (1–1.5 L/day)
- Diuretics—Spironolactone (100–400 mg/day)
  Frusemide (40–160 mg/day)
- Paracentesis—Usually < 1L of fluid is taken,
  if >1L is taken FFP to be infused.
- Peritoneo—Venous shunt (LeVeen shunt)

Sudden increase in ascites :
- Malignancy
- SBP
- TB.

SPONTANEOUS BACTERIAL PERITONITIS

Clinical Features

- Pain and diffuse tenderness, rebound tenderness
- Local rise of temperature, not much fever
- Sudden increase in ascites.

Investigations

Ascitic cell count > 250 neutrophils

Treatment

- Cefotaxime/Ampicillin + Aminoglycosides
- Low opsonin activity of ascitic fluid—organisms from bowel enter peritoneum causing SBP (commonly *E.coli*, *S.pneumoniae*)

Prevention of SBP

- Norfloxacin (400 mg/day)
- Ciprofloxacin (250 mg 12th hourly)
- Cotrimoxazole.

HEMATEMESIS

- Twenty percent of blood loss—postural hypotension
- Forty percent of blood loss—hypotension

Clinical Features

History of vomiting of blood, history of malena.

Treatment of hematemesis
- Stabilize the patient
- Ryle's tube
- Vasopressin–2 mg 6th hourly Terlipressin up to bleeder stops, this 1 mg 6th hourly for next 29 hour.
- Octreotide (100 microgram IV bolus, 50 microgram IV infusions)
- Endoscopy– sclerotherapy or band ligation
- TIPSS
- Surgery and shunting- lienorenal shunt
- β-blocker or long-acting nitrates

INVESTIGATIONS IN CLD

- CBC
- LFT—SGOT/SGPT > 2:1 (due to pyridoxine deficiency)

- A : G ratio reversal (due to increased Kupffer-cell damage and because of this more antibody produced against antigen)
  Prothrombin time- after LFT
- USG—coarse echotexture of liver, ascites, splenomegaly, portal vein diameter > 10 mm in PHTN
- If Wilson's suspected—serum ceruloplasmin (reduced), serum Cu (increased), urinary Cu (increased), liver Cu (increased)
- Serological markers for hepatitis.
- Paracentesis and ascitic fluid analysis:
  A. Cytology >250 neutrophils = SBP, lymphocyte mainly = TB, malignancy
  B. SAAG > 1.1—indicate ascites due to portal hypertension, transudative
- EEG—slow wave/triphasic wave in hepatic encephalopathy
- Serum ammonia.
- Doppler study in Budd–Chiari syndrome
- OGD scopy

Hepatorenal syndrome

Type I– Progressive oliguria
Rapid increase in creatinine values
No proteinuria
Rx. Albumin infusion + terlipressin

Type II– Common is patients with refractory ascites
Moderate and stable increase in creatinine.
Better prognosis

HEPATOSPLENOMEGALY

LIVER

- Normal liver span is 12–15 cm, if > 15 cm—hepatomegaly, < 8 cm—shrunken
- Tender liver seen in—hepatic abscess, hepatitis, CCF and Budd–Chiarri syndrome
- Pulsatile liver–TR, TS, AR

Consistency

- Soft—CCF, hepatitis
- Firm—Cirrhosis
- Hard—Malignancy.

Function of liver
- Synthetic
- Detoxification
- Storage
- Excretion
- Conjugation

Massive Hepatomegaly

- Hepatocellular carcinoma
- Secondaries
- Amebiasis
- Hydatid cyst.

Function of spleen
- Destruction of RBC—culling
- Removal of pigments in RBC—pitting
- Antibody synthesis and opsonization
- Destruction of foreign body
- Extramedullary hematopoiesis

SPLEEN

Methods of palpation of spleen.
- KIF → Left hypochondriasis
- In right lateral position
- Stand as left side of the patient-Hooking method- Middleton method

Percussions of spleen
- Traube's space—dullness
- Castell's method—If 8th ICS or above dull
- Nixon's method—Is right lateral position, is posterior axillary line, if dullness is greater this 6–7 cm—splenomegaly

MEDICINE

Causes of Massive Splenomegaly

- CML
- *Hairy cell leukemia:*
  - Seen in elderly
  - Clinical features—anemia, massive spleen
  - Invasive PS: Hairy cells with TRAP (tartarate resistant acid phosphatase staining)
  - PAN like picture
  - Treatment—alpha interferon, cladribine, pentostatin
- Myelofibrosis:
  - PS—Dacrocytes/tear drop cells
  - Treatment—Blood transfusion, splenectomy, hydroxyurea, BMT
- Tropical splenomegaly:
  - No malarial parasite in ps
  - Antibodies to malarial parasite present

  Treatment
  - Proguanil 100 mg
- Kala azar:

  Treatment
  - **M**iltifosine
  - **A**mphotericin B
  - **P**entamidine
  - **S**odium stibogluconate

  M A P S
- Storage disorders

PANCYTOPENIA + SPLENOMEGALY

- Myelofibrosis
- Hairy cell leukemia
- Hypersplenism

Hypersplenism
- Splenomegaly
- Pancytopenia
- Bone marrow normal
- Correction with splenectomy

CAUSES OF HEPATOSPLENOMEGALY

I. Infections

a. Bacterial	b. Viral	c. Parasitic
Enteric fever	Hepatitis A	Malaria
Leptospirosis	Hepatitis B	Kala-azar
Brucellosis	IMN	Amebiasis
Miliary TB	HIV infection	

II. Hemolytic anemias—hereditary spherocytosis, thalassemia

III. Malignancies—leukemia, lymphoma, myeloproliferative disorders (CML, PRV)

IV. Immunological—SLE

V. Storage disorders.

VI. *Congestive:* CCF, constrictive pericarditis, cirrhosis with portal HTN, Budd–Chiari syndrome

Fever and hepatomegaly
- Enteric fever
- Leptospirosis
- Malignancy
- Disseminated TB
- HIV infection, viral hepatitis

Pallor and hepatomegaly
- Malaria
- IMN
- Hemolytic anemia
- Malignancy

Jaundice and hepatomegaly
- Viral hepatitis
- Leptospirosis
- Enteric fever
- Hemolytic disorders
- Malignancy

Pallor and splenomegaly
- Infection–IE, malaria, typhoid
- Malignancy
- Cirrhosis
- Hypersplenism

Jaundice and splenomegaly
- Infection
- Cirrhosis
- Hemolytic anemia

Lymphadenopathy and splenomegaly
- IMN
- Brucellosis
- Malignancy—lymphoma

INFECTIONS

Enteric Fever

Clinical features: Fever, headache, pea soup diarrhea, dry coated tongue, rose spots constipation, relative bradycardia, hepatosplenomegaly.

Investigations
- 1st week—Blood culture (bile broth)
- 2nd week—(Antibody) Widal test
- 3rd week—Stool culture
- 4th week—Urine culture
- Later—Bone-marrow culture

B
A
S
U

Treatment: Ciprofloxacin, ceftriaxone, cotrimoxazole, chloramphenicol.

Leptospirosis

- *Clinical features:*
  - Fever
  - Conjunctival congestion
  - Jaundice, HSM
  - Myalgia
  - Anemia
  - Bleeding manifestation
  - Decreased urine output, petechial spots.
- *Four main clinical syndromes:*
  (i) Bacteremia (prodromal)
  (ii) Aseptic meningitis
  (iii) Icteric
  (iv) Pulmonary syndrome
- Triad in Weils's disease—jaundice, renal dysfunction, hemorrhagic manifestation.

Complications
- Myocarditis
- ARDS
- Pancreatitis
- Hepatorenal syndrome

Investigations
- CBC—leukocytosis, thrombocytopenia
- ESR increased
- LFT—conjugated bilirubin increased, RFT elivated
- MAT (diagnostic test)(microagglutination test)
- Culture in EMJH medium.

Treatment
- Crystalline penicillin 1.5 million units qid × 1 week
- Doxycycline 100 mg BD × 1 week.

BRUCELLOSIS

- History of exposure to milk/meat
- Usually seen in Gulf returners
- *Clinical features:* Pallor, fever, arthritis, LNE, HSM.

Investigations: Antibody test.
Treatment: Rifampicin, doxycycline (6 months).

IMN

- Caused by EBV
- *Clinical features:*
  - Anemia, fever

Complications of IMN
- Splenic rupture
- Myocarditis
- Glomerulonephritis
- Pharyngeal edema
- Hemolytic anemia
- Thrombocytopenia

- Jaundice
- LNE—mainly posterior cervical
- Rash–post ampicillin therapy
- Palatal enanthem
- HSM.

Investigations

- Atypical lymphocytes—modified T lymphocyte
- Paul Bunnel test
- Monospot test, IgM, ELISA

Treatment

- Supportive measures
- Pharyngeal edema—corticosteroids

MALIGNANCIES

ALL, AML: Refer Pediatrics

CML

Between 30–60 years
BCR–ABL translocation (9:22)
Clinical features—dragging sensation, massive splenomegaly bruising, tirdness weight loss.
Investigation: Peripheral smear-blast cells
Philadelphia chromosome +
leukocyte alkaline phosphatase—decreased.

Three phases:
- Chronic
- Accelerated (10–19% blasts)
- Blast crisis (>20%)

Leukamoid reaction:
- Toxic featuers present/infections
- Leukocyte alkaline phosphatase—increased
- Toxic granulation present

Differential Diagnosis

Leukemoid reaction.

Treatment

Chronic phase
Imatinib or dasatinib
Allogenic transplantations
Hydroxy urea.
Accelerated phase/blast crisis
Imatinib if not given previously
Hydroxy urea.

CLL

- Seen in elderly
- Most common leukemia
- Investigation—peripheral smear.

Treatment

Chlorambucil + prednisolone

HODGKIN'S LYMPHOMA

- *Clinical features*:
  - Central group of LNE—painless. Usually supraclavicular
  - Contiguous spread
  - Spleen enlarged
  - B symptoms (fever >38°C, night sweats, weight loss)—Bad prognosis
- *Types:*
  - Lymphocyte predominant—popcorn cells
  - Nodular sclerosing—lacunar cells

- Mixed cellularity—typical RS cells
- Lymphocyte depleted
  CBC, ESR, LFT, RFT, LDH, CXR.
- *Investigations*: lymph node biopsy—Reed-Sternberg cells
- *Treatment:* Staging is important for treatment.
- *Staging:*
  I. Single lymph node region (I) or extralymphatic site (1AE)
  II. Two or more lymph node regions (II) or an extralymphatic site and lymph node regions on the same side of (above/below) the diaphragm (IIE)
  III. Lymph node regions on both sides of the diaphragm with (IIIE) or without (III) localized extralymphatic involvement or involvement of spleen (IIIS) or both (IIISE)
  IV. Diffuse involvement of one or more extralymphatic tissues (liver, bone marrow) leukemia/lymphoma

Each stage is subclassified into:
A–No systemic symptoms
B–Weight loss >10%, drenching sweats, fever.
B–symptoms–poor prognosis

Treatment
- Stage I and II—Radiotherapy
- Stage III and IV—ABVD regimen (Adriamycin, bleomycin, vinblastine, dacarbazine)
  MOPP regimen (mechlorethamine, oncovin, prednisolone, procarbazine)

NON-HODGKIN'S LYMPHOMA

- More common than Hodgkin's lymphoma
- Peripheral LNE—tender/matted
- Extralymphatics are more involved
  - Tonsillar enlargement
  - Epitrochlear LNE.

Classification

I. Precursor B-cell neoplasm—precursor B lymphoblastic
II. Peripheral B-cell neoplasm—CLL/SLL
III. Precursor T-cell neoplasm—precursor T lymphoblastic leukemia/lymphoma
IV. Peripheral T-cell and NK-cell neoplasm—T-cell prolymphocytic leukemia.

Treatment
- CHOP regimen (cyclophosphamide, adriamycin, oncovin, prednisolone
- If CD 20 +ve rituximab can be given.

Rituximab given in:
- C—CLL
- H—hemolytic anemia (autoimmune)
- I—ITP
- N—NHL
- A—rheumatoid arthritis

MEDICINE

CHAPTER 5

Central Nervous System

CASE FORMAT

Name: Age: Sex: Occupation: Address:

1. **Presenting complaints:**
2. **History of present illness**: Mode of onset, duration, time of onset, progression

Motor Symptoms

Weakness: Upper limbs, lower limbs, one half of body, all 4 limbs.

Bulk: Noticed any wasting, true or pseudohypertrophy

Power:

UL: Proximal—combing hairs, lifting the arm above head, bringing food to mouth
Distal—difficulty in mixing food, buttoning shirt, sewing, writing

LL: Proximal—getting up from squatting position, climbing stairs up and down, history of buckling of knees
Distal—slippers falling from foot, tripping of toes, dragging of feet

Trunk: Difficulty in turning from side to side, lifting head from pillow

History of muscle twitching or any other involuntary movements.

History of diurnal variation of weakness (s/o myasthenia gravis)

History of pain over muscle, muscle cramps

Higher Function History

History of altered sensorium, loss of consciousness, speech disturbances (difficulty in comprehension, output neologism), dysarthria, convulsions (aura, tonic/clonic, partial/gen, tongue bite, urinary incontinence, postictal state, freq, duration)

History of raised ICT—early morning headache, projectile vomiting, disorientation, memory loss, emotional incontinence.

Cranial Nerve History

1 – History of altered smell sensation
2 – Difficulty in vision/color vision
3,4,6 – Diplopia, squint, drooping of eyelids
5 – Abnormal sensation over face, difficulty in chewing
7 – Facial asymmetry, dribbling saliva, deviation of angle of mouth, stasis of food, taste disturbance over anterior 2/3, hyperacusis
8 – Vertigo, hearing disturbance, tinnitus
9,10 – Nasal regurgitation, nasal twang, dysphagia especially to liquid feeds, hoarseness of voice
11 – Difficulty in shrugging of shoulders, rotate neck
12 – Dysarthria, difficulty to protrude tongue out.

Sensory Symptoms

Loss of sense of temp, loss of touch or absence of pain, tingling, numbness, pins and needle sensation. Posterior column symptoms include history of coordination in dark, symptoms aggravated more in evening, wash basin sign, feeling ground like cotton wool, Lhermitte's sign (electric shock sensation radiating down spine while flexing neck).

Cerebellar Symptoms

History of unsteadiness in standing, walking, tendency to fall or sway towards one side, difficulty in negotiating narrow pathways, tremors while bringing food to mouth (intentional tremor)

Autonomic Nervous System

History of constipation or fecal incontinence, difficulty in feeling bladder fullness, initiation or controlling or complete evacuation of micturation, feeling of residual urine, history of dribbling, retention, overflow of urine, history of catheterizations, postural giddiness, abnormal sweating, salivation, lacrimation, impotency.

After that present status of patient should be described.

3. **Past Histories**
- History of previous similar episodes. TIA? RIND? DM? HT? IHD? TB?
- Exposure to promiscuous sex, fever, trauma, fits, syncope, dog bite, vaccination, ear discharge, sera admin, drug intake, exanthematous fever and diarrhea, LRI.

4. **Personal History**
- Sleep, appetite, bowel and bladder habits
- Any addictions—smoking, alcohol, IVDA
- Diet history—veg/non-veg/mixed
- Exposure to STD, menstrual history
- Educational history

5. **Family History**

   Any similar illness in family, sibling history, consanguinity of parents, parents-age, any diseases, cause of death
6. **Socioeconomic History**

   Earning member of family, type of house, overcrowding or not, sanitary facilities, good well, etc.
7. **Drugs and Treatment History**

   History of drug intake, surgery, any procedures, hospitalization, transfusion

GENERAL EXAMINATION

- Conscious-oriented
- Built, nourishment
- PICCLE, neurocutaneous markers, KF ring, thyroid, vitamin deficiency
- Pulse (Important)
- BP (Important)
- RR

CNS EXAMINATION

- **Higher function**

  Consciousness, orientation to time, place, person, memory, intelligence speech, hallucination, delusion, handedness (COMISH)
- **Cranial nerves**

  1. *Olfactory nerve*: Smell
  2. *Optic nerve*: Visual acuity, field, color vision, fundus

  3,4,6. Ptosis, squint, nystagmus, diplopia, extraocular muscles

  5. *Trigeminal nerve*: Sensory—pain, touch, temp over face
     Motor—opening of jaw, clenching mouth
     Reflex—corneal, conjunctival, jaw jerk, blink reflex
  7. *Facial nerve*: Motor—raise eyebrows, blinking, wrinkling of forehead, tightly closing eyes, blow out cheeks, nasolabial fold, show teeth, purse the mouth, whistle, platysma
     Sensory—taste over ant 2/3
     Secretory—lacrimation, Schirmer's test, salivation
     Reflex—corneal reflex
  8. *Vestibulocochlear nerve*: Positional vertigo, nystagmus, fistula sign, tinnitus, tuning fork test

  9,10. Motor: Palatal contour, movements on saying "aah"
  Reflex: Palatal, gag
  Taste over posterior 1/3, nasal twang, nasal regurgitation

  11. *Accessory nerve*: Shrugging shoulder, move shoulder to opposite side

MEDICINE

12. *Hypoglossal nerve*: Any wasting, fasciculations, tremor of tongue, deviation of tongue, strength of movements

- **Motor System**
  - **Bulk**: Look for wasting, pseudohypertrophy, measure 10 cm above and below olecranon, 10 cm below tibial tuberosity, 18 cm above knee jt, wasting: UL/LL, generalized/partial, proximal/distal
  - **Tone**: UL/LL, normal/hypo/hypertonia—clasp knife, cogwheel, lead pipe, clonus: ankle, patella
  - **Power**: Grade 0–5, UL/LL/trunk muscle
  - **Reflex:**
    - Superficial—corneal and conjunctival, palatal and pharyngeal, abdominal, cremasteric, bulbocavernosus and anal, plantar
    - Deep—jaw jerk, biceps, triceps, supinator, knee, ankle
    - Inverted reflexes—inversion of radial, biceps, knee
    - Primitive reflexes—grasp, groping, avoiding, palmomental, sucting, snout, glabellar tap
    - Reinforcement: UL—ask patient to clench his teeth, LL—Jendrassik's maneuver
    - Any abnormal movements like tremor fasciculations, chorea, seizures, etc.
- **Sensory System**
  - *Primary modalities*: Touch, pain, temp, joint position and vibration, Lhermitte's sign
  - Cortical sensation: Tactile localization, discrimination, stereognosis, graphesthesia, sensory inattention
- **Cerebellar Signs**
  - *Head*: Titubation, nystagmus, scanning or staccato speech
  - *UL*: Finger nose test, tapping in a circle, dysdiadochokinesia, past pointing, rebound phenomenon
  - *LL*: Heel-knee test, pendular knee jerk, hypotonia, tandem walking
  - *Gait*: Wide based ataxic, drunken or reeling gait, swaying towards side of lesion
- **Rhombergs Sign: Specific for Posterior Column**
- **Posture and Gait Disorders**

  Bradykinesia, stooped posture, kyphoscoliosis, lordosis, rigid or tender spine, squatting and standing up (abnormality like Gower's sign), circumduction gait (hemiplegia) scissoring (bipyramidal), ataxic (cerebellar), festinating (parkinsonism), high stepping (foot drop), high stepping and stamping (posterior column), waddling (muscle disease)
- **Autonomic Nervous System**
  - *Skin*: Flushing, cyanosis, temp change, sweating disturbances (horners)
  - *CVS reflexes*: Postural hypotension, deep breath test, hand grip test, heart rate in response to Valsalva, pressure stimuli
  - *Bladder functions*: If catheterized or not, automatic/autonomous type
- **Extrapyramidal System**

  Akinesia, rigidity, abnormal movements (tremors, chorea, etc.)
- **Peripheral Nervous System**

  Nerve thickening, neurofibromatosis, Tinel's sign
- **Signs of Meningeal Irritation**

  Photophobia, neck rigidity, Kernig's sign, Brudzinski's sign
- **Examination of Skull and Spine**

  Spinal deformity such as gibbus, movements of spine, paraspinal spasm, tenderness, vibration sense over spine, look for any deformity of skull or bruit over it
- **Deformities**

  Foot drop, wrist drop, claw hand deformity, straight leg raising test (L5, S1 radicle involvement)
- **Trophic Ulcers:** In UL (syringomyelia) or LL (tabes, peripheral neuropathy)
- **Carotids:** Whether equal on both sides and presence of bruit.
- **Examination of other Systems**
  - *CVS*: RHD, LV dysfunction, cardiomyopathy, infective endocarditis, valvular lesion
  - *RS*: Evidence of malignancy, TB
  - *Abdomen*: Hepatosplenomegaly, ascites, c/c liver disease.

CNS CASE EXAMPLE

Saradha, 48, Wayanad, manual laborer
She is a right handed person

PRESENTING COMPLAINTS

- Deviation of face to right side—4 days
- Weakness of left side—3 days
- Slurring of speech—3 days

HISTORY OF PRESENT ILLNESS

She is known case of sickle cell disease, developed deviation of face to right side and drooling of saliva through left side and weakness of left side 4 days back in the evening around 6 pm after she returned from work. Her daughter noticed that she is about to fall and son supported her. Then she got relieved from weakness. They took her to the hospital immediately. She herself got into the jeep. While she was in the hospital she developed weakness of her left leg initially and she was able to walk but with some instability. But on that day she is not able to get from bed. She had developed complete weakness of left side. She was not able to rise her hand above head, comb her hair, not able to bring food to mouth and she was not able to raise her leg and able to walk. She had difficulty in turning side to side. No history of involuntary movements, twitching of muscles, diurnal variations and cramps over the muscle.

Initially there was no difficulty in speech. On the day she developed facial deviation but later her daughter noticed some slurring of speech, which she cannot understand fully. But now speech is normal. She had history of vomiting episode. No history of altered sensorium, loss of consciousness, convulsions, headache, blurring of vision. Her memory, intelligence are not altered.

She had history of facial deviation to right side. She complains as if food stucks over the left cheek. But she is able to close her eyes. No history of hyperacusis. No history of alteration of smell, diplopia, squint, nystagmus, ptosis, abnormal sensations over the face, difficulty in chewing the food, nasal regurgitation, nasal tone of voice, vertigo, tinnitus, hearing difficulty.

No history of sensory deficit over the left side during the onset of weakness. She is able to appreciate pain, temperature. No history of night worsening of symptoms, incoordination in the dark, electric shock like feeling on the flexing neck.

She had no history of urinary incontinence at the time of onset of weakness. She had no history of rectal incontinence. No history of hypertension, excessive or absent sweating, lacrimation on affected side.

She had no history of swaying to one side during walking, tremors while bringing food to mouth.

She had no history of jaundice for 3 days. They noticed yellow discoloration of urine, eyes, stool is colored normal. No history of pruritis abdominal distension, fever, abdominal pain, drug intake. And it is not relieved.

PAST HISTORY

She is known case of sickle cell disease since 10 years. And she is on treatment. She had no history of crisis after severe dehydration. But no history of neurological problems associated with it.

She had history of palpitation since 3 years. It is gradual in onset, regular in rhythm, more during exertion. And it lasts for 5–10 minutes, relieved by taking rest. No history of chest pain.

She had history of difficulty in breathing for 3 years. It is gradual in onset. Initially she had dyspnea on exertion, and it is relieved on taking rest. And it is progressive, and dyspnea on exertion (grade 3). She had history of orthopnea, paroxysmal nocturnal dyspnea. No history of chest pain, wheeze, cough with expectoration; swelling of feet, anorexia, vomiting, right hypochondriac pain, decreased urine output. No history of fever, petechiae/hemorrhage, hematuria in the past.

She complained of blurring of vision excessive lacrimation 1 week before. And she is relieved from it by 10–15 minutes. No history of headache, convulsions, weakness, aphasia during that time.

No history of diabetes mellitus/hypertension/ischemic heart disease/COPD/TB/epilepsy/trauma/fever chills and rigor.

PERSONAL HISTORY

- Sleep and apetite normal
- Bowel habits normal

- And she is catheterized now
- Taking mixed diet. No addiction.

FAMILY HISTORY

She is born out of nonconsanguineous marriage. No history of similar illness in the family. History of sickle cell disease for her elder brother. No history of diabetes mellitus/hypertension/ischemic heart disease/COPD/TB/epilepsy/bronchial asthma in the family. Her husband died 15 years back due to myocardial infarction.

DRUG HISTORY

She is in treatment for sickle-cell disease. She has not taken other drugs.

GENERAL EXAMINATION

Patient lying supine, with shoulder abduction, elbow extended, flexion of fingers, with extended knee and hip, plantar flexed and externally rotated

- Conscious cooperated oriented
- Moderately built and nourished
- Pallor—present
- No cyanosis, clubbing, lymphadenopathy, pedal edema, icterus,
- Deformed hands
- Locomotor brachialis
- Dilated veins over legs, hands, thigh
- Claw foot

VITALS

- *Pulse*: 72/min, regular in rhythm, character, volume
  - Locomotor brachialis
  - All other peripheral pulsation are palpable equally bilaterally
  - No radio-radial delay
  - No radio-femoral delay
- *BP*: 120/76 mm Hg in right U/L in supine position
- Respiratory rate—28/min, abdominothoracic, regular
- She is afebrile

EXAMINATION OF CENTRAL NERVOUS SYSTEM

Higher Mental Function

She is alert, well oriented in time, place, person with normal memory and intelligence, with good attention, well behavior and is cooperative. She is right handed person. Speech is normal. Her mother tongue is malayalam.

Cranial Nerve Examination

	Right	Left
I . Olfactory nerve	No anosmia, olfactory hallucinations, parosmia	
II. Optic nerve		
• Visual field	Normal	Normal
• Visual acuity	6/6	6/6
• Colour vision	Normal	Normal
• Fundus	Not examined	
III, IV, VI		
• Ptosis, squint, nystagmus, diplopia	Not present	
• Extraocular movements	Full in all direction	
Pupil: Size	Normal	Normal
Shape	Normal	Normal

Reflex

• Direct light reflex	Present	Present
• Indirect light reflex	Present	Present
• Accommodation reflex	Present	Present

V. Trigeminal nerve

Motor part

• Opening of jaw	No deviation	
• Temporalis	Normal	Normal
• Masseter	Normal	Normal
Sensory part (over the face)		
• Touch Present	Present	
• Pain Present	Present	
• Temperature	Not examined	
Reflex		
• Jaw jerk	Absent	
• Corneal reflex	Present	Present
• Conjunctival reflex	Present	Present

VII. Facial nerve

• Wrinkling	Present	Present
• Eye closure	Can close eyes tightly	Can close eyes tightly
• Angle of mouth	Deviated to the right side	
• Nasolabial fold	Prominent on right side	
• Hyperacusis	Not present	Not present
Sensory part		
• Taste over anterior 2/3	Present	Present

VIII. Vestibulocochlear (Nystagmus, tinnitus, vestigo, Rinni's test, Schawback's test, ABC test)

IX, X

• Nasal regurgitation	Not present	Not present
• Palatal contour, position of uvula	Normal	
• Palatal movement	Bilaterally equal	
Sensory		
• Taste over posterior 1/3	Not examined	
• Reflex: 1. Gag reflex	Present	Present
2. Palatal reflex	Present	Present

XI

• Shrugging of shoulder	Present	Present
• Movement of neck against resistance	Present	Present

XII

• Strength of movements	Normal No fasciculation tremor, wasting Deviation of tongue on protrusion of tongue

MOTOR SYSTEM

Bulk	**Right**	**Left**
• Upper limb arm	19	17
• Forearm	19	18
• Lower limb thigh	35	34
• Calf	25	25

There is no wasting

MEDICINE

Tone

• Upper limb	Normal	Hypotonia	
• Lower limb	Normal	Hypotonia	
Power			
• Upper limb shoulder:	Flexion	Grade V	Grade 0
	Extension	Grade V	Grade 0
	Abduction	Grade V	Grade 0
	Adduction	Grade V	Grade 0
• Elbow:	Flexion	Grade V	Grade 0
	Extension	Grade V	Grade 0
• Forearms:	Supinations	Grade V	Grade 0
	Pronation	Grade V	Grade 0
Lower limb:			
• Hip:	Flexion	Grade V	Grade 0
	Extension	Grade V	Grade 0
• Knee:	Flexion	Grade V	Grade 0
	Extension	Grade V	Grade 0
• Ankle:	Dorsiflexion	Grade V	Grade 0
	Plantar flexion	Grade V	Grade 0
	Eversion	Grade V	Grade 0
	Inversion	Grade V	Grade 0
Trunk:	Can raise the head		
	Can turn side to side		

REFLEX

Deep tendon reflex

• Jaw jerk	Absent	
• Biceps jerk	Present	Not present
• Supinator jerk	Present	Not present
• Triceps jerk	Present	Not present
• Knee jerk	Present	Not present
• Ankle jerk	Present	Not present
Superficial reflexes		
• Corneal	Present	Present
• Conjunctival	Present	Present
• Abdominal	Present	Present
• Plantar	Present	Present
• Bulbocavernous reflex (males)	Not done	Not done
• Cremasteric reflex	Present	Present
• Anal reflex	Not done	Not done
Primitive reflexes		
• Snout	Absent	Absent
• Palmo-mental	Absent	Absent
• Grasp	Absent	Absent
• Glabellar tap	Absent	Absent

No involuntary movement

Gait—not examined

SENSORY SYSTEM

Superficial Sensation	**Right**	**Left**
• Pain	Present	Present
• Temperature	Not examined	
• Touch	Present	Present

MEDICINE

Deep sensation		
• Joint sense, fine touch	Normal	Normal
• Vibration sense, position sense	Normal	Normal
Cortical sensation		
• Tactile localization	Present	Present
• Two Point discrimination	Present	Present
• Stereognosis	Present	Present
• Graphesthesia	Present	Present

POSTERIOR COLUMN EXAMINATION

- Romberg sign — Not examined
- No cerebellar signs
- Autonomic nervous system within normal limits
- No signs of extrapyramidal system
- Peripheral nervous system—within normal limits
- Skull and spine—normal
- No trophic ulcer
- No deformities
- Deformity of hand—interphalangeal part
- Fundus examination—not done

EXAMINATION OF OTHER SYSTEMS

Respiratory System
- Trachea—central
- Apex beat—7th ICS lateral to midclavicular line
- Normal vesicular breath sound heard
- No added sounds
- Chest wall moving equally and bilateraly

Cardiovascular system
- Pulse, BP—mentioned above
- JVP—not elevated

Inspection
- Trachea—central
- Apex beat—visible, 7th intercostal
- space lateral to MCL
- Shape of precordium—normal
- No engorged veins
- Suprasternal pulsations seen

Gastrointestinal System

Oral cavity—good oral hygiene
  Lips, tongue, buccal mucosa—normal
  Tonsils and posterior-pharyngeal wall—normal
Shape of abdomen—normal
Umbilicus—central and inverted
No dilated veins, scars, pulsations
No palpable mass
No organomegaly
Bowel sounds—heard normaly

Palpation

Trachea—central
Apex beat—7th ICS 15 cm lateral to midclavicular line
forceful in character
No left parasternal heave, thrill
No palpable heart sounds
No palpable pulsations

Percussion
- Right border of heart within the right sternal margin
- Left heart border corresponds to apex beat
- 2nd ICS—resonant
- Liver dullness in the right 5th ICS

Auscultations
- Mitral area:
  S1 loud
  S2 muffled
  Low pitched rough rumbling mid-diastolic murmur with presystolic accentuation best heard in mitral area in left lateral position,with bell of stethoscope and breath held in expiration
  Opening snap present
- Tricuspid area:
  S1 loud
  S2 muffled
  Systolic murmur of high pitch quality of grade 3 intensity, best heard in expiration with diaphragm of stethoscope

- Aortic area:
  - S1 heard
  - S2 loud with normal split
  - No murmurs
- Pulmonary area:
  - S1 heard
  - S2 heard with normal split
  - No murmurs

SUMMARY

A 48-year-old female with family history of sickle cell disease and past history of rheumatic fever at 10 years of age, and sickle cell disease for 10 years and had a history of palpitation, exertized dyspnea since one month and history of TIA 1 week back, now presented with deviation of face to right, weakness of left side, slurring of speech 4 days back. Initially she developed weakness and deviation of face to one side, but improved after sometimes. After admission she started weakness of leg, which is proposed dense hemiplegia of left side. And history of urinary incontinence.

On examination found to have pallor, deformed hand, locomotor brachialis, pes cavus, dilated veins, over hand and thigh. On examination of nervous system deviation of face to right side, cannot close eye tightly, hypotonia in L/L and in U/L, grade 0 in U/L and L/L, with absent reflexes in both UL and LL. And abnormal plantar response on left and flexor plantar on right.

On examination of CVS, load S1, mid-diastolic murmur with opening snap heard in mitral area and systole murmur of Grade III in tricuspid area.

DIAGNOSIS

Cerebrovascular accident, dense hemiplegia, embolic in pathology, most probably right middle cerebral artery present in neuronal shock, etiology in acquired valvular heart diseases, mitral stenosis, rheumatic in etiology with no featurs of congestive cardiac failure, infective endocarditis, pulmonary hypertension.

NERVOUS SYSTEM DISCUSSION

Diagnosis

- Cerebrovascular accident
- Right sided hemiplegia+right UMN facial palsy
- Broca's aphasia
- Infarct due to emboli/thrombosis
- Left middle cerebral artery territory
- Left internal capsule lesion
- Stage (neuronal shock, recovery)
- Risk factors—systemic hypertension, diabetes, smoking, alcoholism
- Complication-raised ICT
  - Aspiration pneumonia

STROKE

Abrupt onset of focal neurological deficit that is attributable to focal vascular cause (of nonconvulsive origin)

TIA

- Focal neurological deficit lasting <24 hours (usually 5–6 minutes)
- Mainly due to embolism

RIND

- Reversible ischemic neurological deficit
- Resolve within 7 days

PRIND

Progressive reversible ischemic neurological deficit (up to 3 weeks)

ISCHEMIC PENUMBRA

Tissue surrounding core region of infarction which is ischemic but reversibly dysfunctional.
Saving ischemic penumbra is the goal of revascularization.

DIFFERENTIAL DIAGNOSIS OF FOCAL NEUROLOGICAL DEFICIT

- Stroke/TIA
- Seizure with post-ictal Todd's palsy
- Vasculitis
- Metabolic encephalopathy
  - Hyponatremia
  - Hypoglycemia
  - Hypocalcemia
  - Hypoxic ischemic encephalopathy
- Fever/infection
  Tuberculous meningitis
- Trauma related
- Demyelination
- ICSOL
- Hemiplegic migraine.

ETIOLOGY

A. Ischemic (85%)
- *Thrombotic (25%)*: Lacunar (20–25% of thrombosis)
- *Embolic (75%)*: Cardio-embolic (20%)
  Artery-artery (15%)
  Cryptogenic (30%).

B. Hemorrhagic (15%)
1. Hypertensive (Charcot-Bouchard aneurysm)
2. Arteriovenous malformation
3. Amyloid angiopathy (in old)

Most important cause of cardio-embolic stroke—non-rheumatic AF
Site of artery to artery embolism carotid bifurcation.

LACUNAR INFARCTION

Lipohyalinotic/atherothrombotic occlusion of small vessel 30–300 micron diameter (small vessel stroke) producing 2–3 mm sized infarcts (lacunes).

Risk Factors

- Age
- Hypertension

Clinical Features of Lacunar Infarct

- Pure motor hemiparesis lesion in posterior limb of internal capsule, basis pontis
- Pure sensory stroke—thalamus
- Ataxic hemiparesis—ventral pons, internal capsule
- Dysarthria clumsy hand syndrome.

AMAUROSIS FUGAX

Transient monocular blindness—seen in internal carotid artery stenosis.

MEDICINE

INFARCT VS HEMORRHAGE

Infarct	Hemorrhage
• Usually in old age	• Any age
• Risk of atherosclerosis	• Uncontrolled hypertension
• Past history of TIA	• History of headache (due to AV aneurysm)
• During sleeping/early morning	• During daily activities/strain
• Slow onset gradually progressive (stuttering)	• Maximum deficit from the beginning
• Headache after 24 hours (due to development of cerebral edema)	• Headache from the beginning
• Gradual recovery	• Poor recovery
• Presence of seizures without Signs of raised ICT (More common in embolic stroke)	• Seizure in the presence of raised ICT
• Cortical signs present (in embolism)	• Cortical signs absent
• BP-elevated	• Very high BP/coma
• No neck stiffness	• Neck stiffness might be present (due to
	• Intraventricular extension)

Common sites of hemorrhage

- Putamen
- Thalamus **(PTCP)**
- Cerebellum
- Pons

Thrombosis	Embolism
• Elderly	• Any age usually young
• Atherosclerosis	• Risk embolism (AF)
• During sleep/early morning	• During activities
• Slow onset, gradually progressive, slow recovery (stroke in evolution)	• Rapid (stormy) onset, early recovery (due to spontaneous thrombolysis)
• Pulse—regular	• Irregular pulse (AF)
• BP—elevated	• BP—normal
• Cortical signs—absent	• Cortical signs—present
• Seizures—absent	• Seizures—present

Posterior circulation stroke: BP normal/decreased

BRODMANN AREAS: There are total 52 Brodmann's areas.

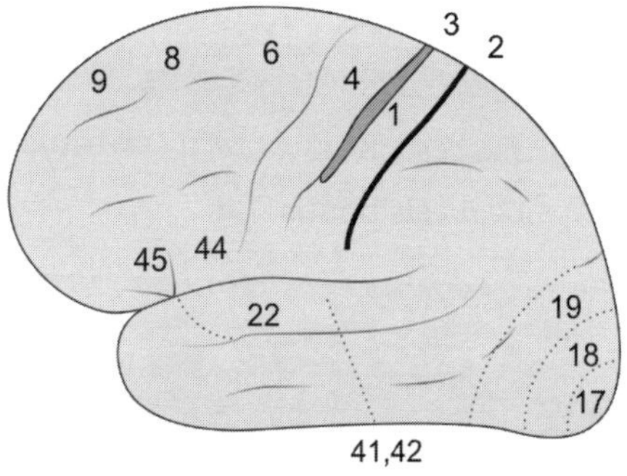

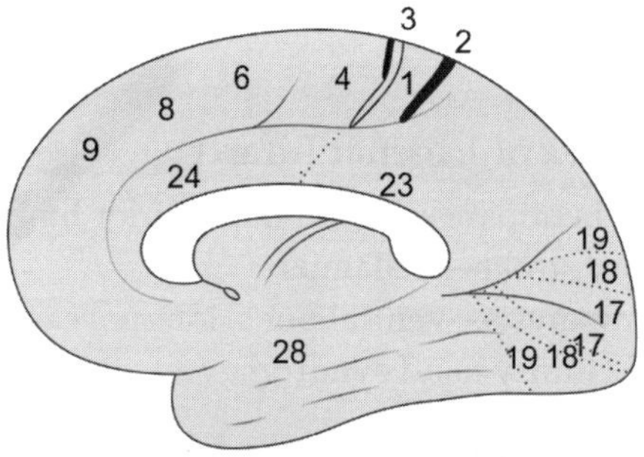

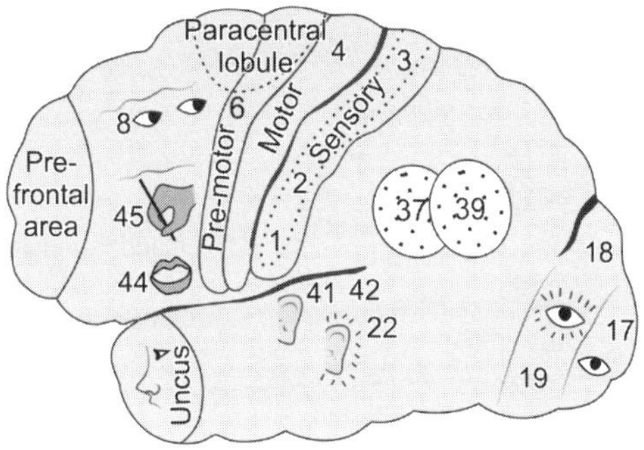

Areas	Functions
1,2,3	Sensory area
4	Motor
6	Premotor area
8	Frontal eye field (saccade)
44	Motor speech area (Broca's area) posterior part of inferior frontal gyrus
45	Exner's area (center for writing)
22	Auditory associative area (Wernicke's area)
41,42	Auditory area
17	Visual area
18,19	Visual associative area (pursuit)
37	Supramarginal gyrus
	Storage and recovery of ideas of speech
	Ideas complex voluntary motor activities
39	Angular gyrus (concerned with reading)

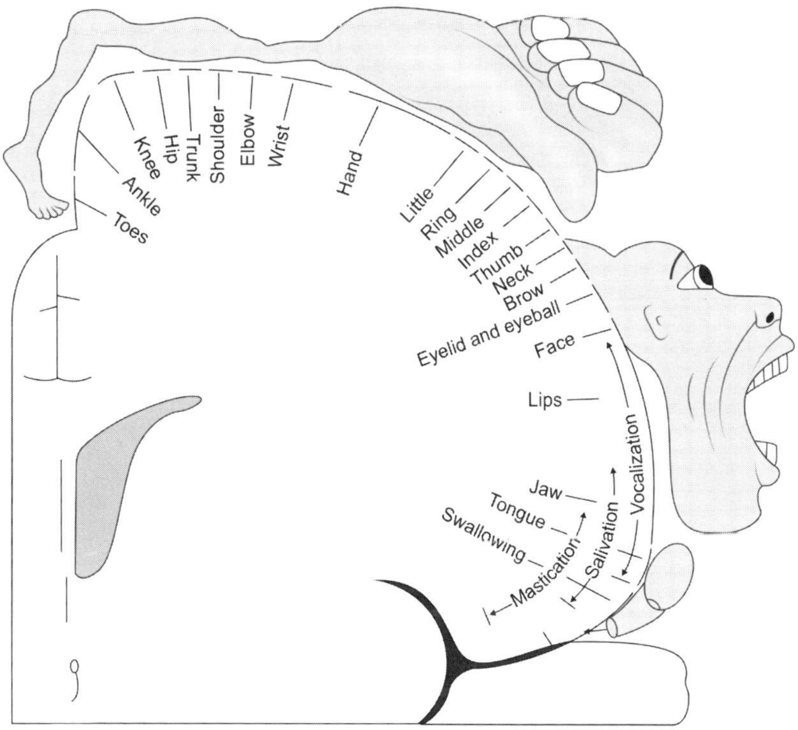

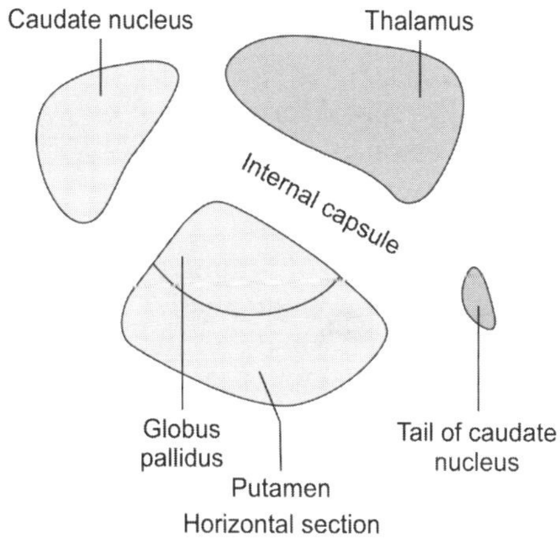

MEDICINE

Pyramidal tract

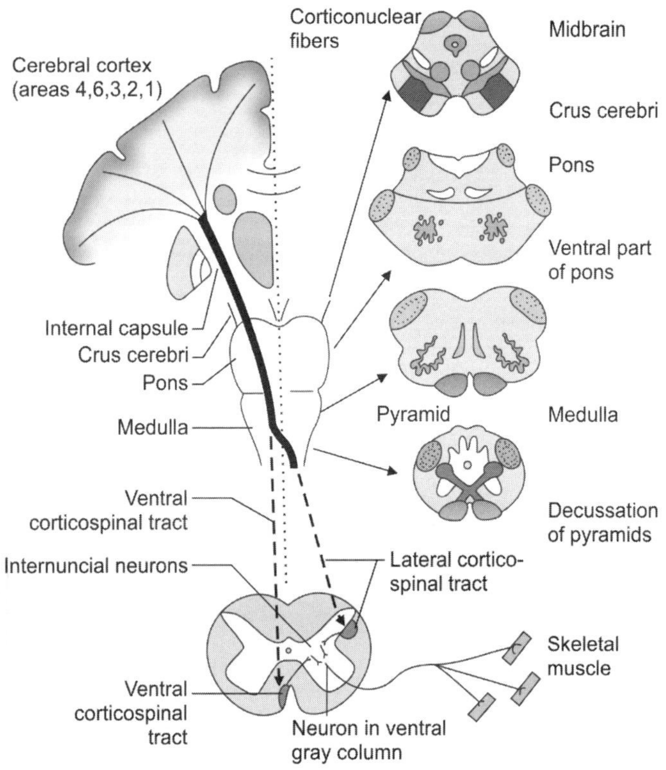

Sensory pathways

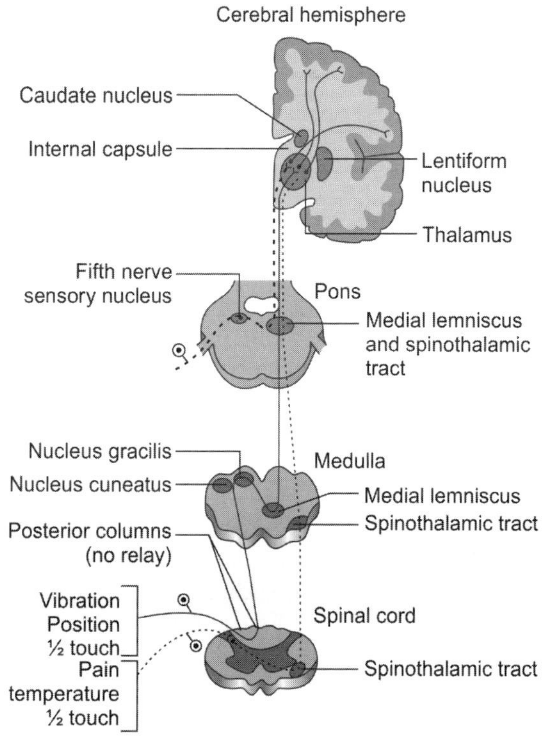

Fibers of pyramidal tract from
30%–1° motor cortex
30%–premotor + supplementary motor cortex
40%–somatosensory cortex

Sensory pathways.

Dorsal column– Fine touch
Beep sensations
Cortical sensations

Anterior spinothalamic tract—crude touch pressure
Lateral spinothalamic tract—pain temperature

CORTICAL LOBAR FUNCTION

LOBE	FUNCTIONS	LESION
Frontal		
1. Prefrontal cortex		
Personality Emotional Social behavior Inhibition of primitive reflex		Personality and behavioral changes, reappearance of primitive reflexes
2. Voluntary motor activity of opposite side of the body		Contralateral hemiparesis
3. Dominant hemisphere—Broca's area		Motor aphasia
4. Paracentral lobule—bowel and bladder control		Involuntary micturition defecation
5. Frontal eye field (voluntary conjugate eye movement to opposite side)		Deviation of eye towards side of lesion
6. Exners area—center of writing		Agraphia

LOBE	FUNCTIONS	LESION
Parietal		
Either lobe		
	• Post-central gyrus Cortical sensation from opposite half	Contralateral hemisensory loss Astereognosis Agraphesthesia
	• Optic radiation	Contralateral homonymous Hemianopia Asymmetry of optokinetic nystagmus
Dominant	• Language • Calculation	**Gerstmann syndrome** • Acalculia • Alexia • Finger agnosia • Right left confusion
Nondominant	• Spatial orientation • Constructional skill	• Neglect of nondominant side • Spatial disorientation • Constructional apraxia • Dressing apraxia

Temporal		
Either lobe	• Optic radiation	Contralateral homonymous—upper Quadranopia
Dominant	• Auditory perception	Receptive aphasia
	• Language	
	• Verbal memory	Impaired verbal memory
	• Smell and balance	
Nondominant	• Auditory perception	Impaired nonverbal memory
	• Melody pitch perception	Impaired musical skill
	• Smell, balance	
Occipital	• Visual processing	Homonymous hemianopia

APRAXIA

Inability to perform complex voluntary motor activities in the absence of paralysis, incoordination or sensory loss

Types:
1. Ideomotor apraxia—inability to translate the idea of complex behavior to action
2. Ideational apraxia
3. Limb kinetic apraxia—dressing apraxia
4. Orofacial apraxia—chewing

Alexia
Inability to read
Agnosia
Inability to interpret sensations correctly although the sense organs and nerves conducting sensations to brain are functionally normal
For example, visual agnosia (can see, but cannot interpret), auditory agnosia and tactile agnosia
Anosognosia–unawareness/denial of any neurological deficit

MEDICINE

BLOOD SUPPLY OF BRAIN

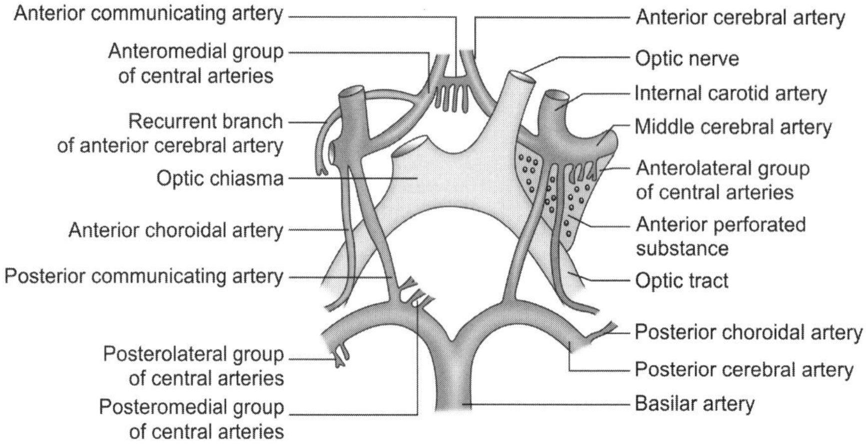

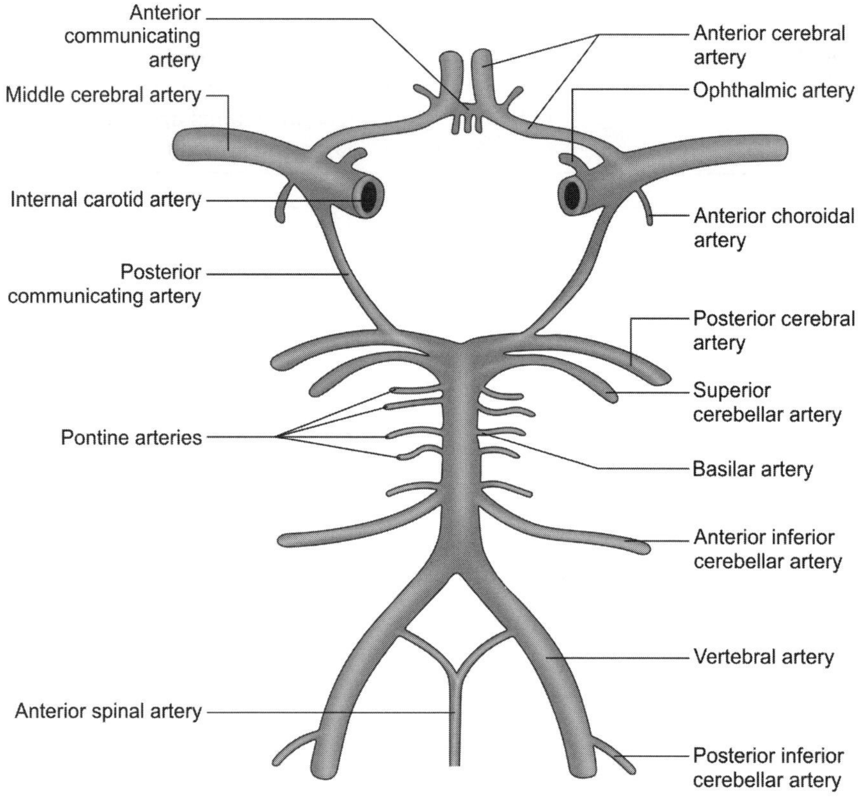

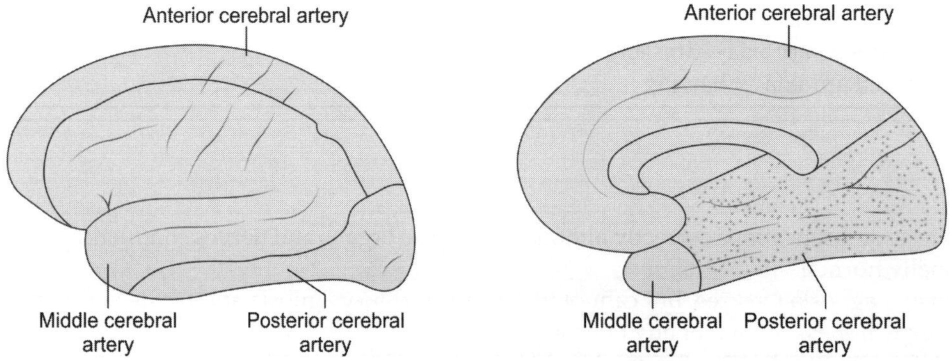

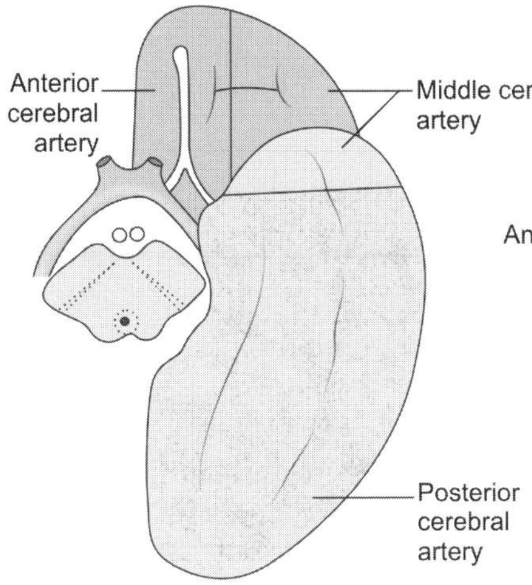

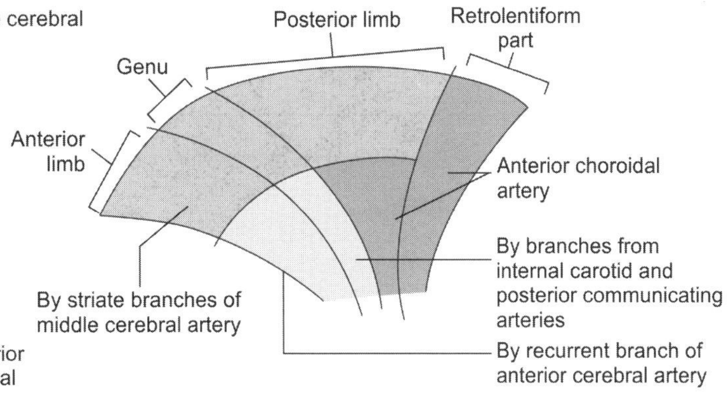

Branches of ICA
- Ophthalmic artery
- Anterior cerebral artery
- Middle cerebral artery
- Posterior communicating artery
- Anterior choroidal artery

Branches of vertebral artery
- Meningeal artery
- Anterior spinal artery
- Posterior spinal artery
- Posterior inferior cerebellar artery (PICA)
- Medullary artery

Branches of basilar artery
- Anterior inferior cerebellar artery
- Labyrinthine artery
- Pontine artery
- Superior cerebellar artery
- Posterior cerebral artery

Artery of cerebral thrombosis—anterior choroidal artery
1. Due to long subarachnoid course
2. Small lumen

Charcots artery of cerebral hemorrhage
Lateral striate artery (branch of MCA)
Recurrent artery of Heubner ***(branch of ACA)***
Faciobrachial monoplegia
Artery of hemiplegia–MCA

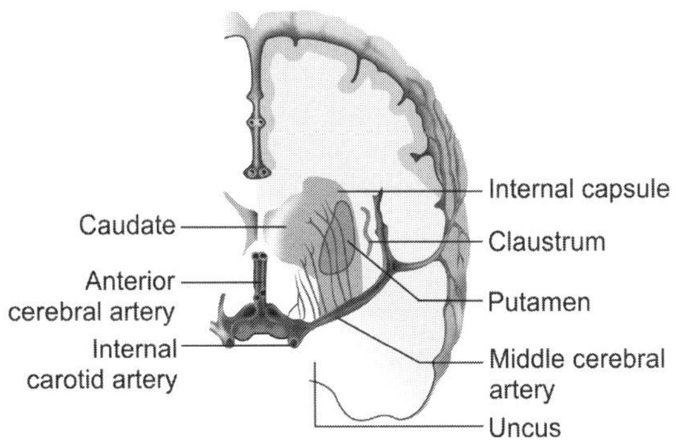

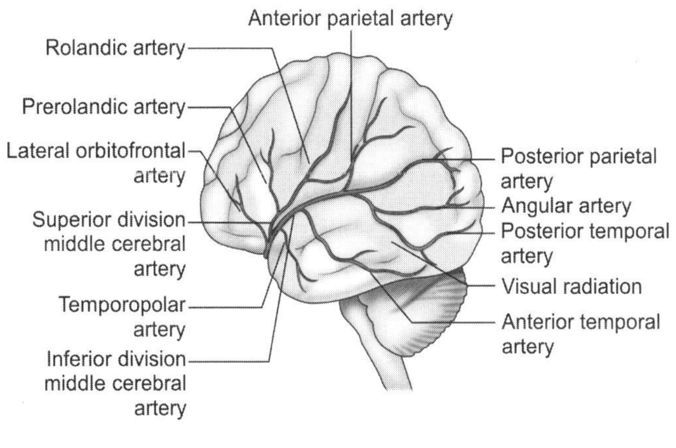

MIDDLE CEREBRAL ARTERY STROKE

M1 segment—lenticulostriate branch supplying putamen, internal capsule, caudate
M2 segment—superior division—frontal and superior parietal branches
Inferior division–temporal and inferior parietal branches

Main artery occlusion

- Contralateral monoplegia—UL > LL
- Contralateral hemianesthesia
- Contralateral homonymous hemianopia
- Coma at the onset
- Cognitive function loss depending on hemisphere

Dominant	*Nondominant*
Speech disturbances	Dressing apraxia
Gerstmann syndrome	Constructional apraxia
	Hemisensory neglect
	Anosognosia

Cortical branches

Superior division
Sensory disturbances
Motor weakness
Motor aphasia

Inferior division
Wernicke's aphasia without weakness
Contralateral homonymous superior
Quadranopia

Branches to internal capsule

Contralateral dense hemiplegia
Contralateral hemianesthesia
Contralateral homonymous hemianopia
No loss of consciousness

Gaze palsy

Frontal lobe—frontal eye field help for conjugate eye movement to opposite side of lesion conjugate deviation of eye to the side of lesion (destructive—infarct)
(weakness of the body is on opposite side of eye deviation)

Pons—for conjugate eye movement to the same side of lesion—eye deviation to opposite side of lesion (destructive)
(i.e. lesion of Pons deviation to Paralysed side...**P FOR P**)

Anterior cerebral artery
A1 segment—precommunal
A2 segment—postcommunal
Symptoms seen only if bilateral involvement
Bilateral weakness
LL>UL
Urinary incontinence
Primitive reflexes
profound aboulia

Internal carotid artery
ACA+MCA+ amaurosis fugax
Posterior cerebral artery
P1 proximal
Midbrain, thalamus, subthalamus
P2 distal to posterior communicating artery
- Occipital and temporal lobe
- Macular sparing present (macular supply is watershed area)

LOCALIZATION IN NERVOUS SYSTEM

1. PURE CORTICAL LESION

Never produce hemiplegia (if dense hemiplegia in cortical lesion—patient comatosed)
Differential limb involvement
Focal seizures/gaze palsy/aphasia
Cortical sensory loss/other cortical signs

2. CORONA RADIATA

One limb more involved than the other
Cortical sensory loss (due to involvement of thalamocortical fibers)
No cortical signs

3. INTERNAL CAPSULE

Dense hemiplegia
Homonymous hemianopia (most important sign)
Hemisensory loss

4. THALAMUS

Anesthesia dolorosa constant burning pain and numbers in an area.
Dejerine–Roussy syndrome—contralateral hemisensory loss associated with agonizing or burning pain

Brainstem syndromes crossed hemiplegia

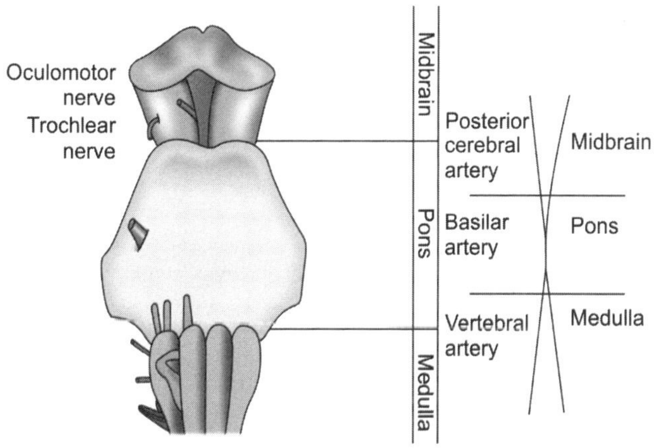

5. MIDBRAIN

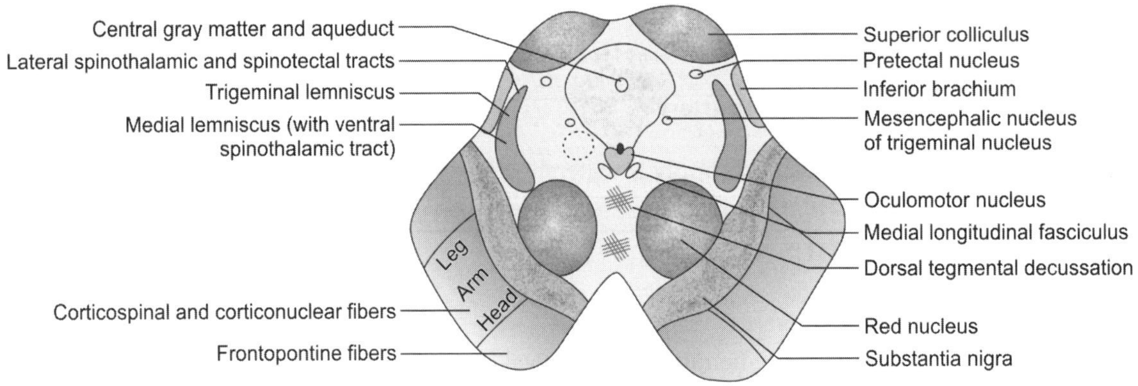

Weber syndrome

Ipsilateral 3rd nerve palsy + contralateral hemiplegia (cerebral peduncle involved)

Claud's syndrome

3rd + contralateral ataxia

6. PONS

Features (4 p's)
Pinpoint pupil
Pyrexia
Paralysis
Gaze palsy
Loss of dolls eye reflex

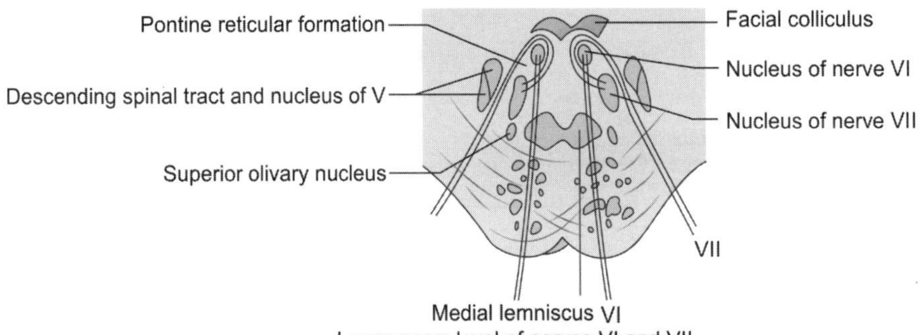

Lower pons; level of nerves VI and VII

Foville's syndrome (Dorsal pons)
- Lateral gaze palsy (6th nerve nucleus + PPRF)
- Ipsilateral facial palsy
- Contralateral hemiparesis

Millard–Gubler (Ventral pons)
- 6th nerve fascicles—lateral gaze palsy
- Facial nerve palsy
- Contralateral hemiparesis

7. MEDULLA

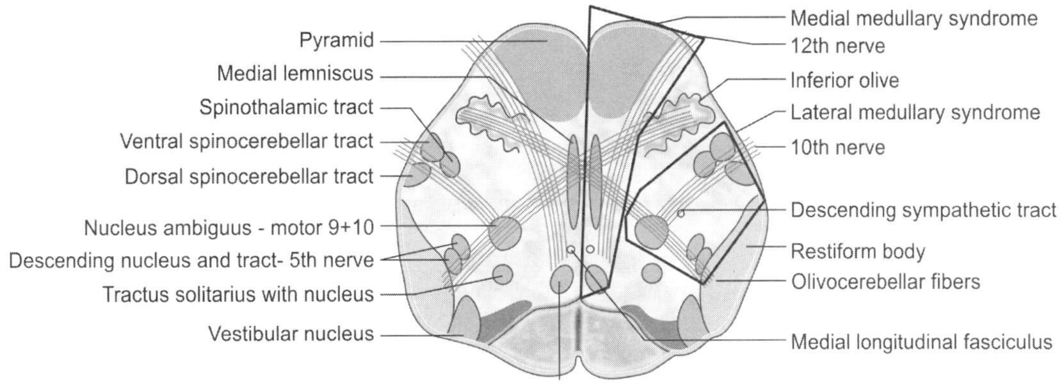

Lateral medullary syndrome/Wallenberg syndrome

Vessels involved

- Vertebral artery
- PICA
- Superior, middle, inferior lateral medullary artery

Ipsilateral side

- Spinal nucleus of trigeminal—(loss of pain and temperature, touch preserved dissociative anesthesia)
- 8th nerve—nystagmus, vertigo
- 10-dysphagia, hoarseness of voice, palatal palsy
- Descending sympathetic tract—Horners syndrome
- Nucleus tractus solitarius—loss of taste
- Restiform body + cerebellar fiber—ataxia

Contralateral side

Spinothalamic tract—loss of pain, temperature of the body.

Medial medullary syndrome

Vertebral artery/lower basilar artery:

- 12th nerve palsy on same side
- Contralateral hemiplegia
- Medial lemniscus—loss of posterior column sensation from opposite side

Avellis syndrome

Ipsilateral 10th nerve palsy + contralateral hemiplegia.

Jackson syndrome

Ipsilateral 10th +12th nerve palsy—contralateral hemiplegia

HIGHER FUNCTIONS (COMISH)

1. CONSCIOUSNESS

It is the state of normal cerebral activities in which the patient is aware of both self and environment and is able to respond to internal and external environment.

Coma

A state of in which patient is unarousable and unresponsive to all internal and external stimulus.

Delirium

Disorientation or dementia occurring in context of drowsiness or clouding of consciousness.

Dementia

Impaired cognitive functions in the setting of normal consciousness.

Drowsy

Patient is unable to sustain consciousness in absence of exteral stimuli.

Stupor

State of disturbed consciousness from which vigorous external stimuli can produce arousal which is brief and incomplete.

GLASGOW COMA SCALE

Eye opening
- 4. Spontaneous
- 3. To speech
- 2. To pain
- 1. Nil

Best motor response
- 6. Obeys commands
- 5. Localizes pain
- 4. Withdraws with pain
- 3. Abnormal flexion
- 2. Extensor response
- 1. Nil

Verbal
- 5. Oriented
- 4. Confused conversation
- 3. Inappropriate words
- 2. Incomprehensible sounds
- 1. Nil

Score = 15- fully conscious
= 3-Deeply comatosed

2. ORIENTATION

In time, place, person

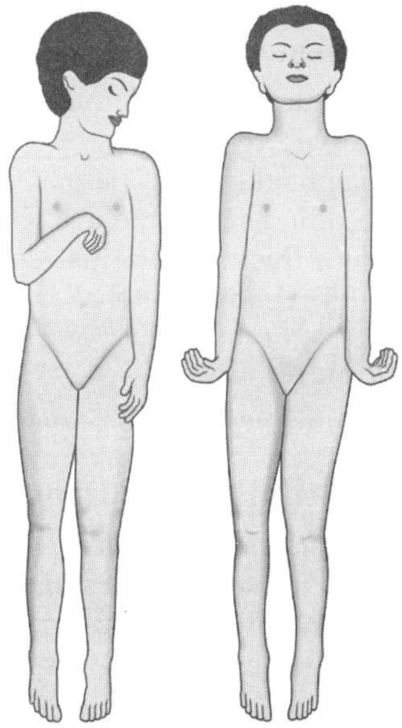

Decorticate	Decerebrate
Internal capsule Thalamus Cerebrum	Pontine stroke

3. MEMORY COMPONENTS

- Registration
- Retention
- Recall
- Reproduction

Types of memory

- Immediate
- Recent
- Remote

4. INTELLIGENCE

Components

- Judgement
- Insight
- Reasoning
- Abstract thinking
- Calculation
- Attention

IQ (Intelligence quotient)
= mental age × 100/ chronological age

Normal range = 90–110
Genius >140
Profound mental retardation <20
Mental retardation < 70

5. SPEECH

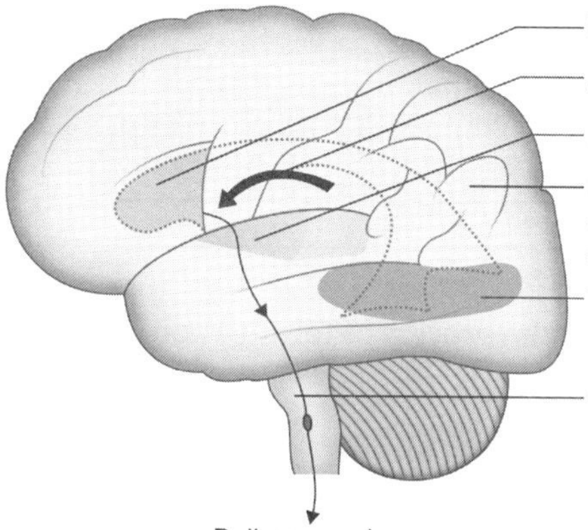

Process of speech involves two stages:

1. Speech formulation
2. Speech articulation

1. Formulation of whether spoken or written is product of three cooperating system:
   A. Sensory system
      - Visual area—17, 18, 19
      - Auditory area—41, 42
   B. Arcuate fasciculus association fibers
   C. Motor system
      - Broca's area—44
      - Exner's area—45
2. Articulation is the function of following:
   a. Pyramidal tract
   b. Cranial nerve nuclei concerned with articulation
   c. Cerebellum for the coordination of muscles of speech
   d. Extrapyramidal system for the speech to be expressive

Components of speech
- Fluency
- Comprehension
- Repetition
- Naming
- Reading
- Writing

Aphasia

It is the loss/impairment of production and or comprehension of written or spoken language due to an acquired lesion of brain

Types

	Fluency	Repetition	Comprehension
1. **Broca's**	Impaired	Impaired	Normal
2. **Wernicke's**	Normal	Impaired	Impaired
3. **Transcortical motor**	Impaired	Normal	Normal
4. **Transcortical sensory**	Normal	Normal	Impaired
5. **Conduction aphasia**	Normal	Impaired	Normal
6. **Global aphasia**	Impaired	Impaired	Impaired
7. **Nominal**	Naming impaired		

Dysarthria

Difficulty in the process of articulation though the process of formulation of speech is normal

Types

a. **Slurred speech** causes:
   1. Central—pseudobulbar palsy—bilateral pyramidal lesion
   2. Nuclear—true bulbar palsy
   3. Nerve—facial nerve
   4. Neuromuscular—myasthenia
   5. Muscle—myopathy

b. **Staccato speech** | **cerebellar**
c. **Scanning speech** | **cerebellar**
d. **Monotonous speech—extrapyramidal lesion**

6. HALLUCINATION

A perception that occurs in the absence of stimuli

Delusion

False unshakable belief which is not amenable to reasoning and is not keeping with patient's sociocultural and educational background

Type of delusions
- Persecutory
- Hypochondriacal
- Grandiose
- Nihilistic

Illusion

A misinterpretation of stimuli arising from external object

For example, Rope seen as snake.

7. HANDEDNESS

MEDICINE

CRANIAL NERVES

1. OLFACTORY NERVE

Unilateral anosmia
- Fractures of cribriform plate
- Basal meningitis
- Foster–Kennedy syndrome

Bilateral anosmia
Common cold
Atrophic rhinitis
Congenital (Kallmann syndrome)
Hysterical

Parosmia post-traumatic

Olfactory hallucination
In temporal lobe epilepsy

2. OPTIC NERVE

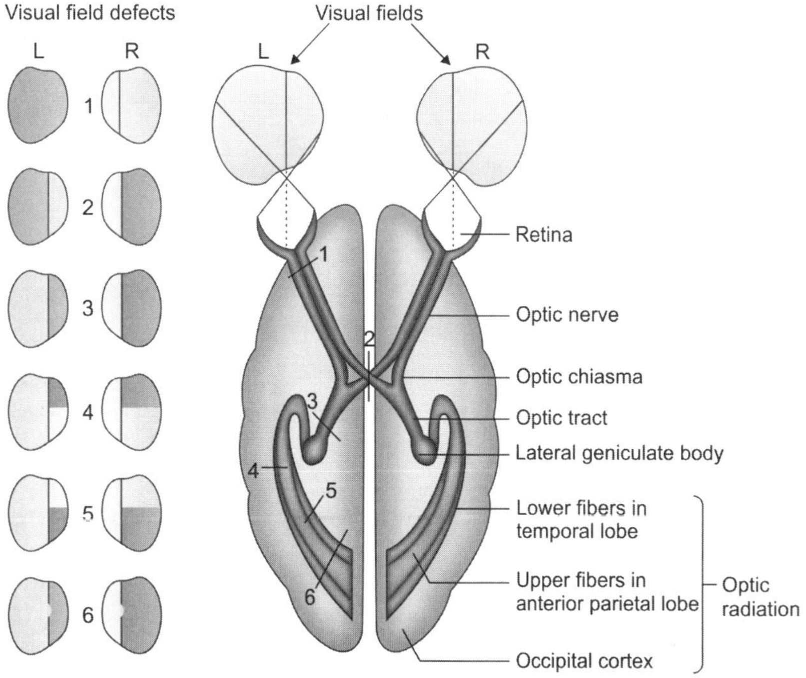

Visual pathways and visual field defects

Blindness
- Visual acuity <6/60
- Visual field
- Confrontation method
- Perimetry
- Color vision—Ishihara's chart

3. OCULOMOTOR NERVE

Nuclei

Motor

Edinger–Westphal—parasympathetic pass between posterior cerebral artery and superior cerebellar artery then through lateral part of cavernous sinus pass via superior orbital fissure

Supplies

Extraocular muscle

Levator palpebrae superioris, all except LR and SO

Intraocular muscles
- Constrictor pupillae
- Ciliary muscles of lens

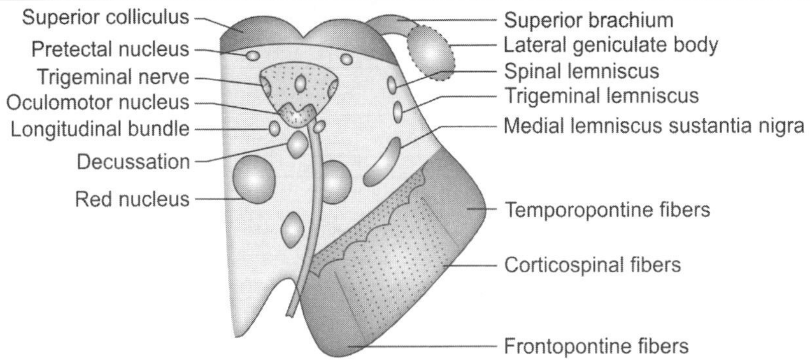
Superior colliculus
Pretectal nucleus
Trigeminal nerve
Oculomotor nucleus
Longitudinal bundle
Decussation
Red nucleus
Superior brachium
Lateral geniculate body
Spinal lemniscus
Trigeminal lemniscus
Medial lemniscus sustantia nigra
Temporopontine fibers
Corticospinal fibers
Frontopontine fibers

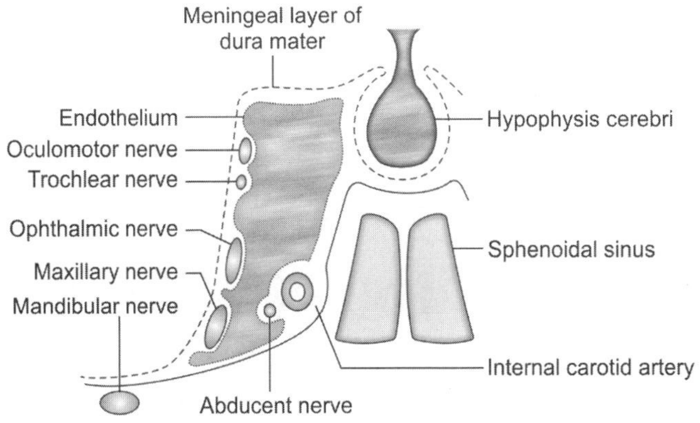
Meningeal layer of dura mater
Endothelium
Oculomotor nerve
Trochlear nerve
Ophthalmic nerve
Maxillary nerve
Mandibular nerve
Abducent nerve
Hypophysis cerebri
Sphenoidal sinus
Internal carotid artery

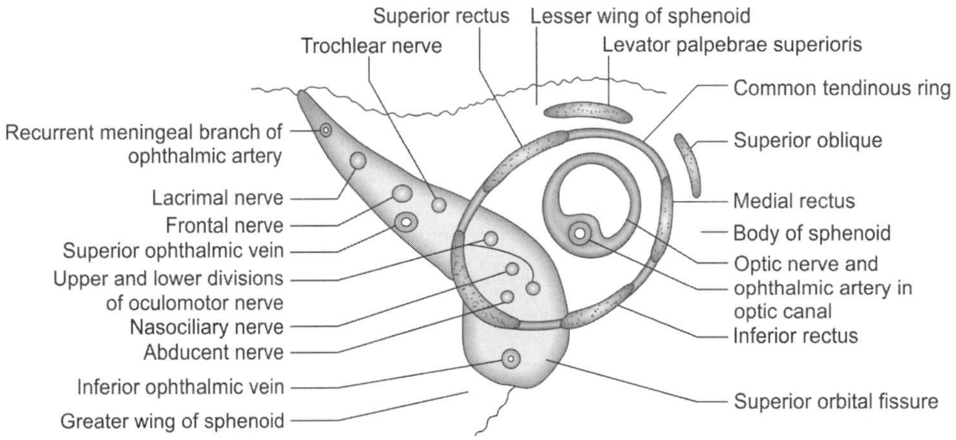
Superior rectus
Lesser wing of sphenoid
Trochlear nerve
Levator palpebrae superioris
Common tendinous ring
Recurrent meningeal branch of ophthalmic artery
Superior oblique
Lacrimal nerve
Medial rectus
Frontal nerve
Body of sphenoid
Superior ophthalmic vein
Optic nerve and ophthalmic artery in optic canal
Upper and lower divisions of oculomotor nerve
Nasociliary nerve
Inferior rectus
Abducent nerve
Inferior ophthalmic vein
Superior orbital fissure
Greater wing of sphenoid

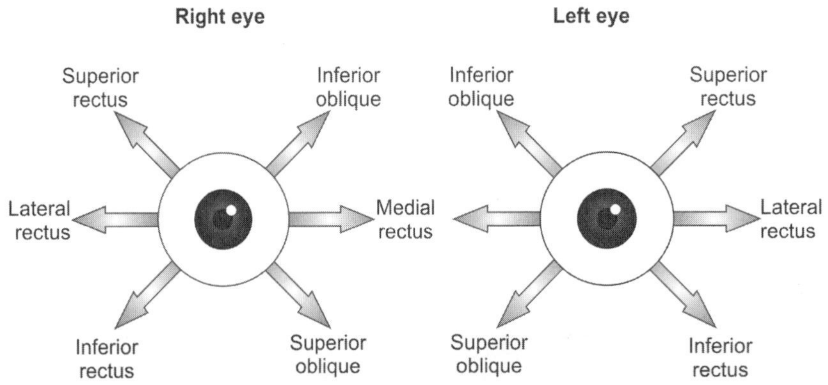
Right eye
Left eye
Superior rectus
Inferior oblique
Lateral rectus
Medial rectus
Inferior rectus
Superior oblique
Inferior oblique
Superior rectus
Lateral rectus
Superior oblique
Inferior rectus

3rd nerve palsy (4D's)

- Drooping of eyelid
- Diplopia
- Down and out deviation of eyeball (these three constitute external ophthalmoplegia)
- Dilated pupil
- Absence of light reflex (last two forms internal ophthalmoplegia)

Light reflex

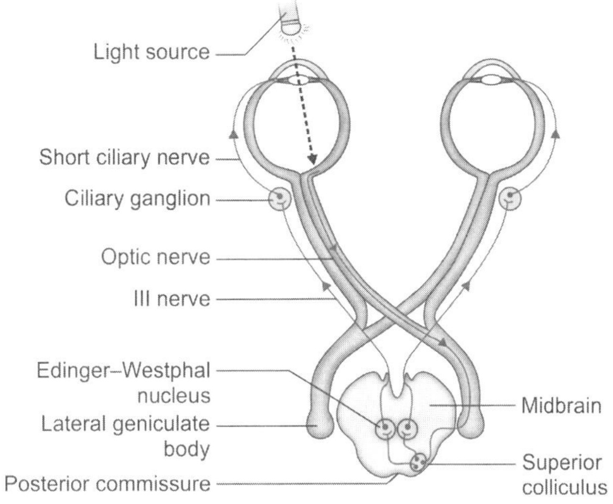

Accommodation reflex

Components: Constriction of pupil
Convergence of eyeball
Increased curvature of lens (contraction of ciliaris muscle)

Argyll-Robertson pupil

(ARP—Accommodation reflex present pupillary reflex absent—lesion of pretectum)

Causes: Syphilis
Diabetes
Alcoholism

- *In oculomotor nerve the autonomous fibers are superficial to motor fibers compression of nerve by tumor results in affection of superficial fibers (mydriasis, loss of light reflex)*
- *While infarction of nerve (ischemic diabetes) results in sparing of superficial fibers*

Causes of ptosis

- 3rd nerve palsy
- Horners syndrome—paralysis of Müller's muscle
- Myasthenia gravis
- Local tumor–neurofibroma of eyelid
- Snake bite
- Muscular dystrophy

NORMAL SIZE OF PUPIL (3–5 mm)	
Causes of miosis (<3 mm) • Horners syndrome • Drugs—organophosphates • Pontine hemorrhage • Opiates • Argyll-Robertson pupil Pinpoint pupil-1 mm-pontine hemorrhage	Causes of mydriasis • 3rd nerve palsy • Drugs—atropine, homatropine • Adie's pupil

4. TROCHLEAR NERVE

Nucleus: In lower midbrain
Supplies: Superior oblique muscles (SO_4)
(function-intorsion and depression of eye in adducted position)
Lesion: Diplopia while looking downward
Limitation of depression in adducted position

6. ABDUCENT NERVE

Nucleus: In lower pons
It is most commonly affected ocular nerve due to its long course and proximity to bony prominence
Supplies lateral rectus (LR6)
Lesion: Diplopia while looking outward towards paralysed side

Longest intracranial course—trochlear
Longest nerve—vagus

INTERNUCLEAR OPHTHALMOPLEGIA (INO)

- Lesion in medial longitudinal fasciculus (MLF)
- Right MLF connected to right 3rd nerve and left 6th nerve
- Lesion of right MLF
- Limitation of adduction in right eye

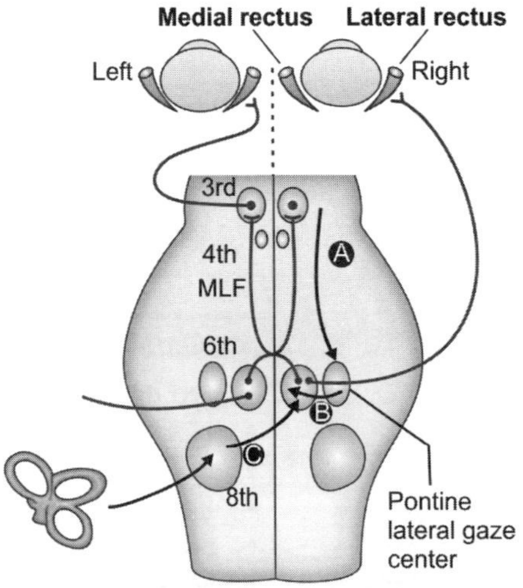

Control of conjugate eye movements

ONE AND HALF SYNDROME

Lesion of MLF and parapontine reticular formation (PPRF) *on same* side due to lesion of right PPRF, there will be limitation in the abduction of right and adduction of left eye

Leison of right MLF

- Limitation of adduction in right eye
- Nystagmus of left eye while abduction

In one and half syndrome only remaining movement is nystagmus in abducting eye

NYSTAGMUS

Rhythmic involuntary and jerky movements of eyeball when they are fixed on an object

Direction of nystagmus is towards fast component

	Peripheral	Central nystagmus
1. Latency	2–20 sec	No latency
2. Duration	<1 min	>1 min
3. Direction of nystagmus	Fixed, towards undermost ear	Changing
4. Fatiguability	Fatiguable	Not fatiguable
5 Accompanying symptoms	Severe vertigo	None/slight

Types

1. Cerebellar—direction towards the side of lesion
2. Labyrinthine—direction opposite to the side of lesion
3. Brainstem lesion—rotatory nystagmus
4. Upper spinal cord lesion—vertical nystagmus

5. TRIGEMINAL NERVE

Nuclei

Mesencephalic – Midbrain
Proprioception, jaw jerk

Main sensory – Pons-touch

Motor nucleus – Pons

Spinal nucleus – Medulla
Pain
Temperature

All receive sensation from same side of face.

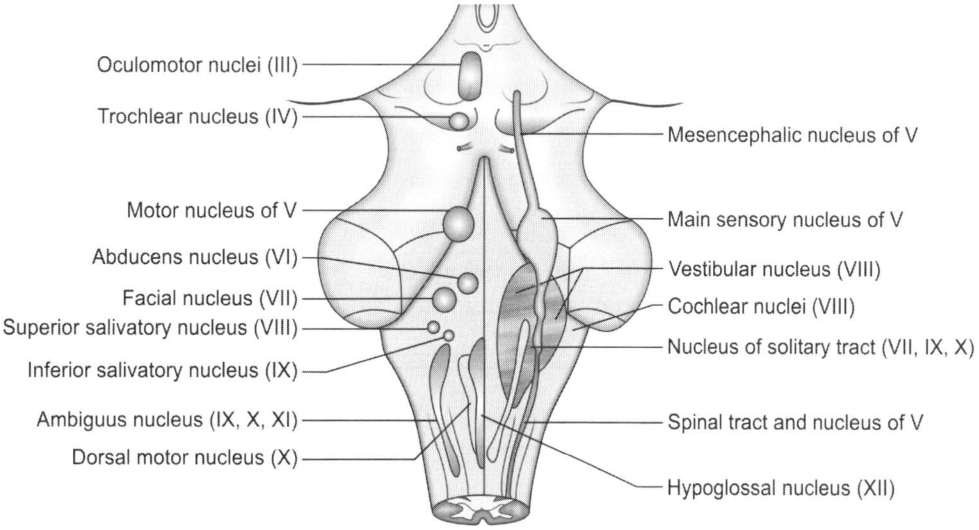

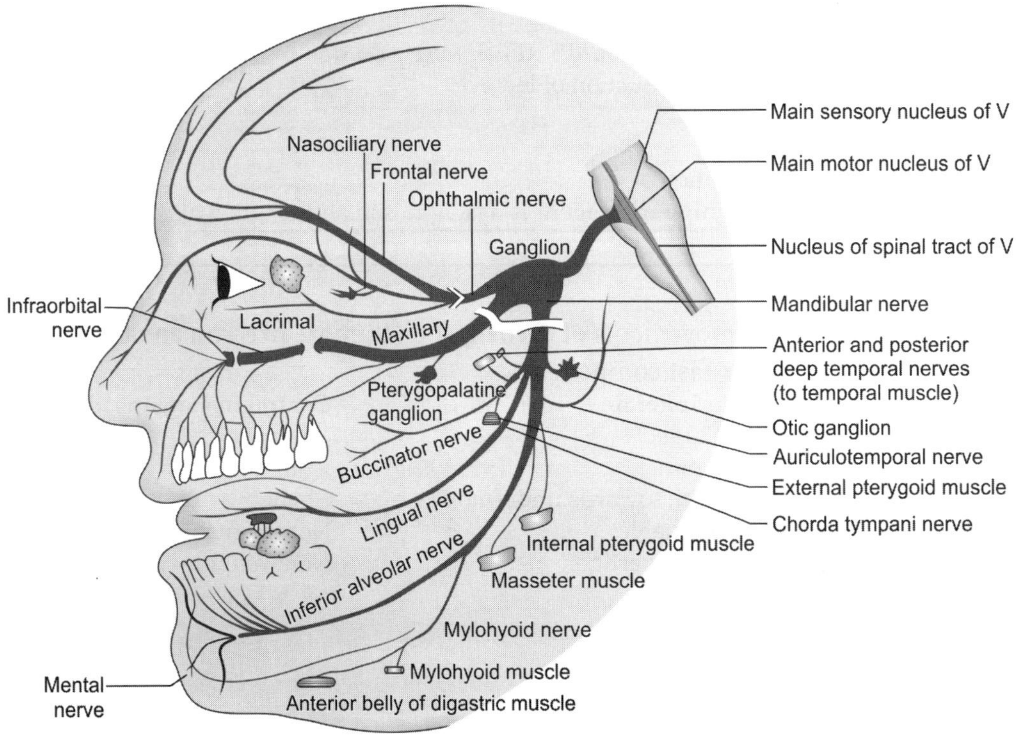

- Ophthalmic nerve—superior orbital fissure
- Maxillary nerve—foramen rotundum
- Mandibular nerve—foramen ovale

- Cavernous sinus—3, 4, 6, ophthalmic, optic, sympathetic chain
- Superior orbital fissure—3, 4, 6 and ophthalmic

Structure passing through foramen ovale
(Male)
- Mandibular nerve
- Accessory meningeal artery
- Lesser petrosal nerve
- Emissary vein

Motor supply
- Muscle of mastication—temporalis, masseter, lateral and medial pterygoids
- Anterior belly of digastric (posterior belly facial nerve)
- Mylohyoid

Lesion
- Loss of sensation on same side of face
- Deviation of jaw to the affected side
- Weakness of muscles of mastication
- Loss of corneal and conjunctival reflex (afferent 5, efferent 7)
- Exaggerated jaw reflex (afferent and efferent 5) (bilateral UMN lesion above pons)

5TH+12TH=17-Deviation to affected side

7TH+10TH=17-Deviation to normal side

FACIAL NERVE

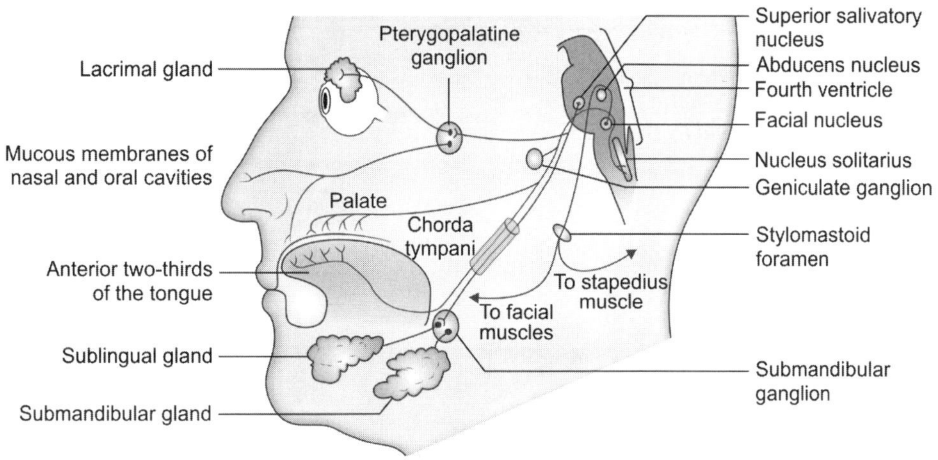

COURSE

Motor nucleus in pons—fibers loop around 6th nerve—emerges at lower part of pons—runs in cerebellopontine angle—enters internal auditory meatus (contain sensory root 8th nerve, labyrinthine artery)—enters facial canal

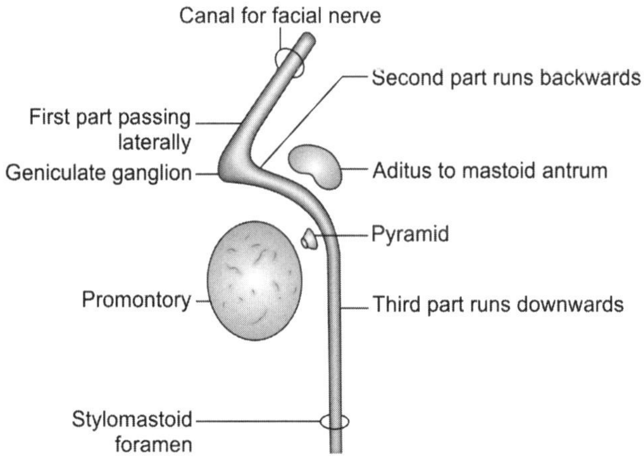

NUCLEI

- Motor nucleus
- Superior salivatory nucleus
- Lacrimatory nucleus
- Nucleus tractus solitarius

BRANCHES

- Greater superficial petrosal nerve—carries secretomotor fibers to lacrimal gland and nasal mucosa
- Nerve to stapedius
- Chorda tympani—*secretomotor fibers to submandibular and sublingual salivary gland, taste from anterior 2/3rd of tongue*

4. Communicating branch—*join with auricular branch of vagus*
5. Posterior auricular nerve—*supplies muscles of pinna, occipital branch of occipitofrontalis*
6. Muscular branch—*to stylohyoid, posterior belly of digastric*
7. Peripheral branches—pes anserinus (goosefoot)
   temporofacial—temporal, zygomatic
   cervicofacial—buccal, mandibular, cervical

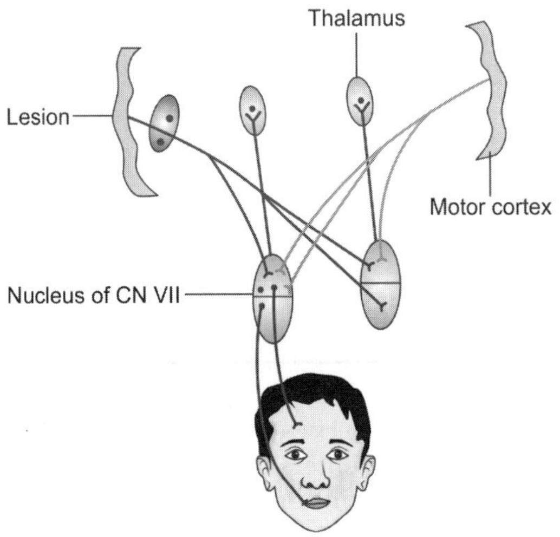

Forehead receives bilateral innervation and is thus saved in supranuclear paralysis. Emotional movements controlled by thalamonuclear fibers are also preserved.

IN UMN—FACIAL PARALYSIS ON AFFECTED SIDE

- Obliteration of nasolabial fold
- Dropping of angle of mouth with drooling of saliva
- Inability to blow the cheek
- Accumulation of food in the vestibule
- Inability to show the teeth properly
- Deviation of angle of mouth to the normal side

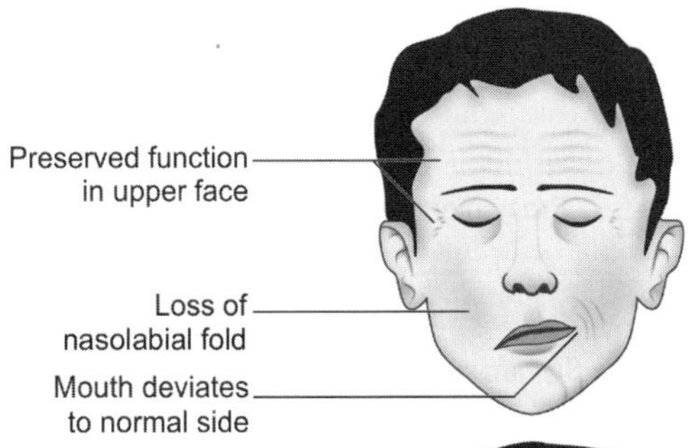

IN LMN—FACIAL PALSY

There are in addition

- Inability raise the eyebrows with absence of wrinkles on forehead
- Inability to close the eye—when the patient attempts to close his eye the eyeball rolls upwards (**Bell's phenomenon**)
- Hyperacusis
- Loss of taste

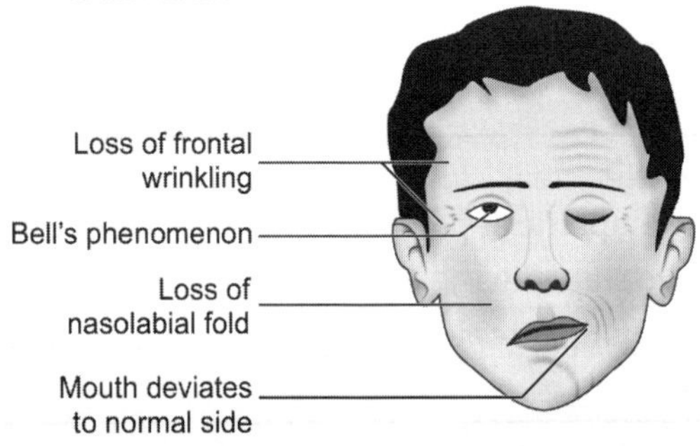

MEDICINE

UMN	LMN
1. Affect pyramidal tract above facial nucleus	Affect facial motor nucleus/nerve
2. Paralysis of muscles of lower part of face of on opposite side of lesion	Paralysis of all muscles of upper part face on the same side of lesion
3. There associated hemiplegia on the same side of facial paralysis	If there is hemiplegia it will be on side opposite to facial palsy
4. It spares emotional and associative movement	Affects emotional and associative movements

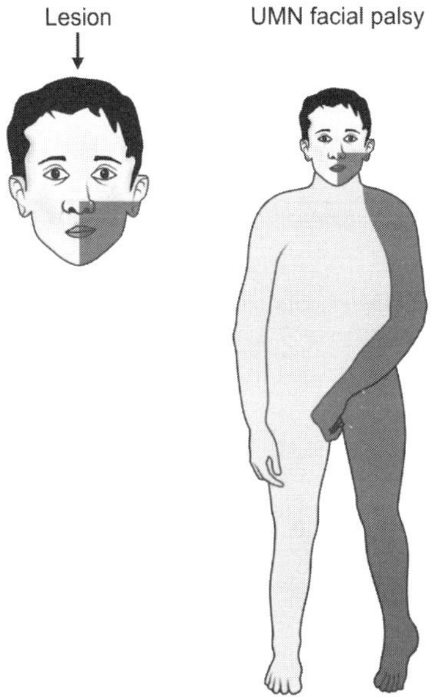

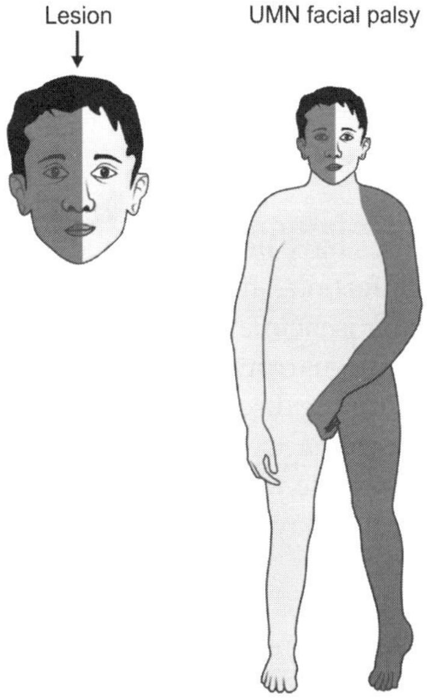

	B/L UMN	VS	B/L LMN
Bell's phenomenon	Absent		Present
Emotional fibers	Spared		Affected
Jaw jerk	Exaggerated		Normal
Corneal reflex	Present		Absent
Pyramidal signs	++		+/−
Taste, stapedial reflex, lacrimation	+		−

CAUSES OF UMN FACIAL PARALYSIS

Lesion causing hemiplegia above pons

(cranial nerve 7 passes very close to pyramidal tract, it has U/L supply lower part of face)

CAUSES OF LMN FACIAL PARALYSIS

A. Nuclear lesion in pons

Vascular—vertebrobasilar insufficiency
Infective—poliomyelitis
Neoplastic—astrocytoma
Demyelinating—multiple sclerosis

B. Cerebellopontine angle

Infective—basal meningitis
Neoplastic—acoustic neuroma

C. Facial canal lesion

Fracture base of skull
Otitis media
Herpes zoster

D. Extracranial lesion

After exit from stylomastoid foramen
Parotid tumor, DM, leprosy

TOPODIAGNOSTIC TESTS IN LMN

1. Schirmer's test—compares lacrimation on both sides
2. Tympanometry—stapedial reflex
3. Taste test
4. Submandibular salivary flow test

CAUSES OF B/L LMN (4 B)

- Basal meningitis
- Bulbar polio
- Guillain-Barré syndrome
- Behcet's disease (sarcoidosis)

BELL'S PALSY

Causes of B/L UMN

- Pseudobulbar palsy
- Diffuse cerebral atherosclerosis

Definition

Idiopathic lower motor neuron paralysis of facial nerve of acute onset

Etiology

Many causes have been suggested

- Viral infection—herpes simplex virus 1 (HSV1)
- Vascular ischemia
- Heredity—narrow facial canal (fallopian canal)
- Autoimmune disease

Clinical features

- Onset is acute with pain behind ear
- One or two days later is complete paralysis of facial muscles on affected side

Treatment

Medical

- Prednisolone 1 mg/kg/day in 2 dose for 5 days, taper over then
- Vitamin B complex, vasodilators
- Protection of exposed cornea with eye ointments during sleep

Physiotherapy: Massage to facial muscles

Surgery

- Decompression of facial nerve
- Facial nerve grafting
- Lateral tarsorrhaphy

Prognosis

Most patients (80%) recovers in 4–6 weeks

Remaining (20%) need surgical interference.

Complications

- Incomplete recovery
- Exposure keratitis—Rx methyl cellulose eye ointment, temporary tarsorrhaphy
- Synkinesis (mass movement) due to cross innervation of fibers
- Contracture
- Crocodile tear (gustatory lacrimation)—tympanic neurectomy
- Frey's syndrome (gustatory sweating)

MEDICINE

8. VESTIBULOCOCHLEAR NERVE

Auditory pathway

E—eight nerve
C—cochlear nucleus
O—olivary nucleus
L—lateral lemniscus
I—inferior colliculus
M—medial geniculate body
A—auditory cortex

Rinne's test

Normally air conduction better than bone conduction in conduction deafness—BC>AC

Weber test

Normally centralized

Localized to one side—conduction deficit on localized side or sensory hearing loss on opposite side

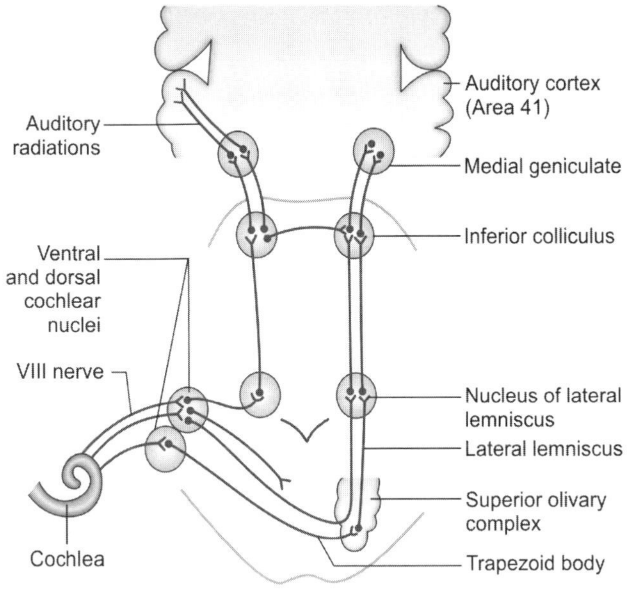

Auditory pathways from the right cochlea. Note bilateral route through brainstrem and bilateral cortical representation.

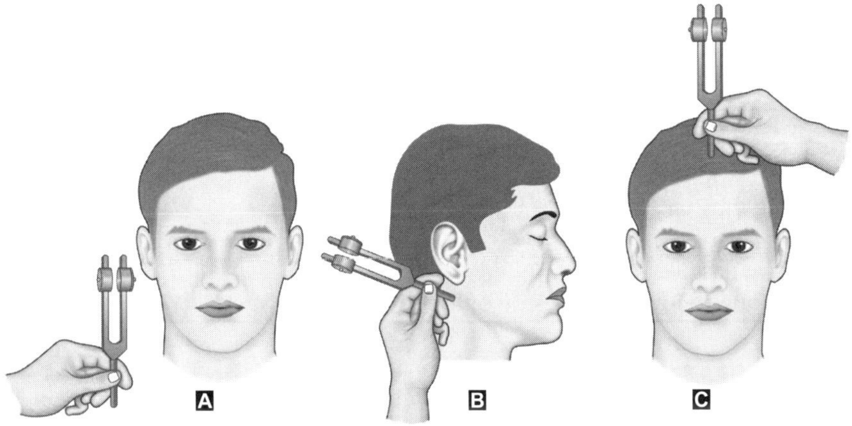

Tuning fork tests: (A) Testing for air conduction; (B) Testing for bone conduction; (C) Water test

9. GLOSSOPHARYNGEAL NERVE

Motor—constriction of pharynx—stylopharyngeus
Sensory—general sensation from posterior 1/3rd of tongue, posterior pharynx, tonsil
Autonomic—parasympathetic to pharynx

10. VAGUS

Motor—soft palate, pharynx, larynx
Sensory—skin over external auditory meatus, thoracic and abdominal viscera
Autonomic—parasympathetic to heart (inhibitory) GIT and bronchial tree (sensory, motor)

Lesions

Dysphagia, dysarthria, nasal regurgitation, hoarseness of voice
Loss of ipsilateral palatal and pharyngeal reflexes.

Pseudobulbar palsy	**True bulbar palsy**
B/L UMN lesion above medulla	LMN lesion medulla
associated with quadriplegia	No quadriplegia
Jaw jerk is exaggerated (if lesion above pons)	Absent jaw jerk
Emotional lability may be present	No emotional lability
Tongue—no wasting or fasciculation	Tongue—flaccid with fasciculation
Causes	
Vascular—B/L stroke	Vertebrobasilar insufficiency
Inflammatory—encephalitis	Diphtheria, bulbar polio, Lyme's disease
Neoplastic—midline brain tumor	Brainstem
Degenerative—motor neuron disease	MND, GBS, snake bite

11. ACCESSORY NERVE

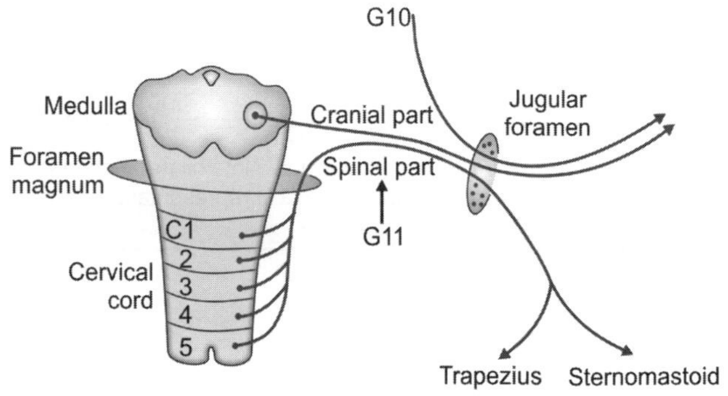

Cranial nerves
Sensory—1,2,8
Motor—3,4,6,11,12
Mixed—5,7,9,10

12. HYPOGLOSSAL NERVE

Motor nerve supplying intrinsic muscles of tongue
Lesion—LMN
Wasting, fasciculation
Deviation of tongue towards the side of lesion

MOTOR SYSTEM

1. **BULK**
   10 cm above and below olecranon
   18 cm above and 10 cm below tibial tuberosity
   Wasting—common with LMN lesion
   Localized cause—disease of joint
   Generalized—cachexia
   (Never miss small muscle wasting in cervical spondylosis)

> 31 pairs of spinal nerves
> 33 vertebral

2. **TONE**
   (It is the state of tension or contraction in healthy muscles resistance offered to passive stretch by a relaxed muscle)
   Inspection—posture
   Palpation—flabby/hard
   Passive movements

Causes of hypertonia
- Pyramidal tract lesion
- Extrapyramidal lesion
- Hysterical
- Tetanus
- Gegenhalten
- Strychnine poisoning

Spasticity

Clasp knife—seen in pyramidal tract lesion
Velocity dependent, stretch sensitive
Antigravity muscle show spasticity
Upper limb: Shoulder adductors
Elbow, wrist flexors
Pronation

Lower limb: Hip extensors
Knee extensors
Plantar flexors and invertors

Causes of hypotonia
- Lower motor neuron lesion
- Shock stage of UMN (due to transient suppression of AHC)
- Cerebellar disease
- Chorea
- Deep sleep

Rigidity

Seen in extrapyramidal involvement
Lead pipe rigidity—there steady increase in resistance
Cog wheel rigidity—resistance is intermittent

	Spasticity	Rigidity
1. Site of lesion	Pyramidal tract	Extrapyramidal tract
2. Velocity	Velocity dependent	Velocity independent
3. Distribution	Distal >proximal Flexors of UL Extensors of LL and trunk (antigravity muscles)	Proximal>distal Flexors of UL, LL,trunk
4. Character	Clasp knife	Lead pipe or cog wheel
5. Deep reflexes	Hyperreflexia	Hyporeflexia

3. **POWER**
It is the force of contraction generated voluntarily by muscle
Grading
0—complete paralysis
1—flicker of contraction
2—movements with elimination of gravity
3—movements against gravity but not against resistance.
4—movement against resistance but not up to normal extent
5—normal power

Hemiplegia

Paralysis of one side of the body involving arm, face, legs due to pyramidal tract lesion anywhere from cerebral cortex to C5 segment of spinal cord.

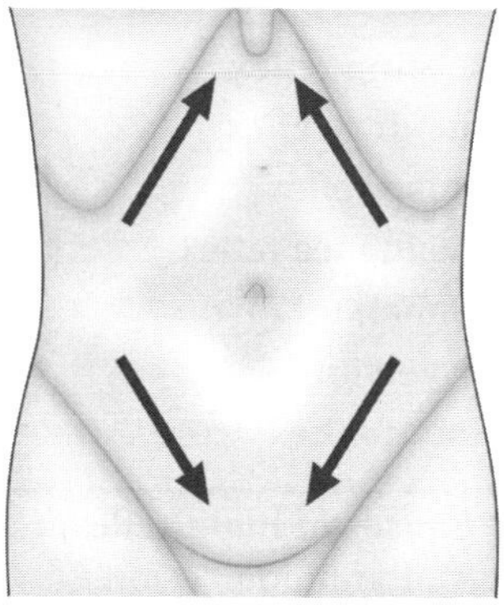

Paraplegia

Weakness of both lower limbs.

Quadriplegia

Weakness of all 4 limbs.

Diplegia

Weakness of all 4 limbs with more weakness on both lower limbs.

4. **REFLEXES**
(Consistent involuntary adaptive response to stimulation of a sense organ)

a. Superficial
1. Plantar reflex—L5, S1
2. Conjunctival and corneal reflex—(afferent 5 efferent 7)
3. Abdominal reflexes—T7–T12
4. Cremasteric reflex—L1
5. Anal—S2, S3, S4
6. Bulbocavernous—S3, S4

b. Deep reflexes
Jaw jerk—(afferent and efferent 5)
Biceps—C5, C6
Triceps—C6, C7
Supinator—C5, C6
Knee—L2, L3, L4
Ankle—S1, S2

(If reflexes are absent do Jendrassiks's maneuver-acts by increasing anterior horn cell excitability by increasing the gamma drive)
Inverted supinator—C5, C6 myeloradiculopathy.

Plantar Reflex

Flexor response
- Slight stimulus—tensor fascia lata contraction, thigh adductors, sartorius contraction.

- Slightly stronger stimulus—flexion of the 4 toes
- Further increase in stimulus—all the toes flexed and drawn together, ankle dorsiflexed and inverted.

Extensor response

- Extension of great toe, fanning of other toes
- Ankle dorsiflexed, knee and hip flexed

Other method to elicit extensor plantar response

In case of wide spread and severe UMN lesion reflexogenic zone is widely enhanced.

Chaddock sign Striking skin around lateral malleolus

Gordon's sign Squeezing calf muscles

Oppenheim's sign Heavy pressure is applied from above downwards on the medial side of anterior surface of tibia

Schaefer's sign Squeezing Achilles tendon firmly

Rossolimo's sign (Homologue of Hoffman sign in upper limb)

Either tap the ball of foot by percussing plantar surface of great toe with hammer or flick the distal phalanges of toes into extension and then allow them to fall back normal position

In pyramidal tract lesion—plantar flexion of all 5 toes

Extensor plantar + Absent ankle reflex.

- SACD
- Taboparesis
- Friedreich's ataxia
- Conus/cauda syndrome
- Combined cervical + lumbar lesions

Upper limb signs of hyperreflexia

1. **Hoffman sign:** Flex tip of middle finger and flick down suddenly, response is brisk flexion and adduction of thumb as well as flexion of tip of other fingers.
2. **Wartenberg's sign**: Interlock the flexed fingers of the patient with your flexed fingers and try to pull apart
   Normally—thumb remains abducted and extended
   In pyramidal lesion—thumb flexes and adducts
3. **Finger flexion response**: Tip of your middle finger and index finger are placed across the palmar surface of the proximal phalanges of the patients relaxed fingers produces flexion of patients finger but a very brisk contraction indicates hyperreflexia
   Root value C7, C8, T1

Primitive Reflexes

Rooting reflex
Sucking reflex
Grasp reflex
Avoidance reflex
Glabellar tap
(Myerson)
Snout reflex

Grading of reflexes
0—absent
1—present-normal as ankle jerk
2—present normal as knee jerk
3—very brisk
4—clonus

Bilateral extensor plantar in hemiplegia patient

- Multi-infarct state—look for release reflex
- Cerebral edema—patient will be drowsy
- Cervical spondylosis—inverted supinator

Causes of hyperreflexia

- Pyramidal lesion
- Anxiety
- Thyrotoxicosis
- Tetanus

Cause of hyporeflexia
LMN
Cerebellar lesion (pendular knee jerk)
Hypothyroidism—*pseudomyotonia*
delayed relaxation of knee jerk

Causes of extensor response

- Pyramidal tract lesion
- Infants
- Deep sleep
- Coma
- Post-ictal
- Post-anesthetic

Nerves involved
Extensor response
Afferent—S1 (tibial nerve)
Efferent—L5 (extensor hallucis longus, deep peroneal nerve)
Flexor
Afferent and efferent S1

5. INVOLUNTARY MOVEMENTS

Chorea—irregular small amplitude semipurposive involuntary jerky movements
Athetosis—slow writhing movements of limbs affecting the distal part
Ballismus—it is more forceful greater amplitude involuntary movement affecting the proximal part of the limb
Chorea—caudate nucleus, Athetosis—putamen, Ballismus—subthalamus

6. CEREBELLAR SIGNS
- Head titubation, nystagmus, staccato speech intention tremor
- Past pointing, dysdiadochokinesia
- Finger nose test (finger nose finger test)
- Rebound phenomenon
- Pendular knee jerk, hypotonia
- Heel-knee test (heel shin ankle test)
- Wide based gate/drunken gate
- Truncal ataxia

7. GAIT
- Pyramidal lesion—circumduction
- Parkinsonism—short step/festinant gait
- Cerebellar—wide based/drunken gait
- Foot drop—high stepping gait
- Posterior column—stamping gait
- Proximal myopathy—waddling gait

SENSORY SYSTEM

Superficial sensation
- Pain
- Touch
- Temperature

Deep sensation
1. Vibration sense
   - 128 Hz
   - Distal to proximal
   - Big toe medial malleolus tibial tuberosity
2. Joint sense
3. Romberg sign*

* Ask the patient to stand with heels together

First with eye opened, then the eye closed
Sways to one side only with eye closed—sensory ataxia
with eye opened—cerebellar ataxia

Cortical sensations
- Tactile localization
- Two point discrimination
- Stereognosis
- Graphesthesia
- Sensory inattention—parietal lobe lesion

Two point discrimination

Lips	2–3 mm
Finger tip	3–5 mm
Dorsum of hand	2–3 cm
Dorsum of foot	3–5 cm

AUTONOMIC NERVOUS SYSTEM

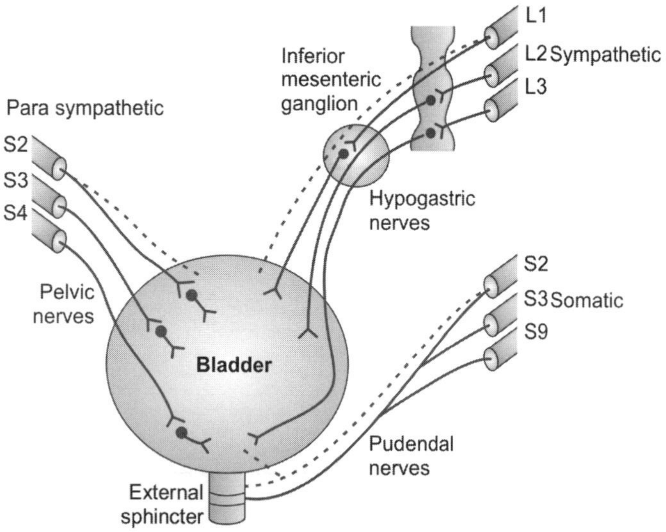

Innervation of bladder. Dashed lines indicate sensory nerves. Parasympathetic innervation is shown at the left, sympathetic at the upper right, and somatic at the lower right.

Micturition reflex
- Afferent—S2 S3 S4
- Center—S2 S3 S4
- Efferent—S2 S3 S4

Higher center
- Facilitatory—pons and posterior hypothalamus
- Inhibitory—cortex and midbrain

LESIONS	
• **Deafferentation**	Tabes dorsalis—bladder distended thin walled and hypotonic
• **Denervation**	Loss of both afferent and efferent fibers *(Autonomus bladder)*, e.g. tumor of cauda equina
• **Spinal transection**	*Automatic bladder* Small spastic with increased frequency, urgency and urge incontinence
• **UMN lesion**	Urge incontinence
• **LMN lesion**	Stress incontinence

PERIPHERAL NERVOUS SYSTEM

Thickening and tenderness of:
- Supraorbital and supratrochlear nerve
- Great auricular nerve—over neck crossing sternocleidomastoid
- Ulnar nerve—palpate behind medial part of olecranon
- Radial nerve—over anatomical snuff box
- Common peroneal nerve—against fibular neck

SIGNS OF MENINGEAL IRRITATION

Neck stiffness

Kernig sign

Flex the knee at 90° then extend the flexed knee. If pain occurs on hamstring it is positive.

Brudzinski's sign

Neck sign—flexion of neck causes hip and knee flexion

Leg sign—flexing one leg other leg will get flexed passively

SKULL AND SPINE

Size, shape, kyphoscoliosis.

CAROTID BRUITS

Auscultate with bell on both sides.

OTHER SYSTEMS

CVS
- Pulse (AF), BP, source of emboli
- Look for bed sores, UTI, pneumonia

Respiratory—TB, malignancy, aspiration pneumonia

DIAGNOSIS

Stages of stroke

a. **Stage of flaccidity**—neuronal shock
   - There is flaccid paralysis, absence of DTR, no plantar response
   - During recovery reflexes appears first followed by tone and power
   - Shorter the duration better prognosis
   - This stage is prolonged by general poor condition of patients health and infection

b. **Stage of spastic paralysis**
   - There is paralysis
   - Hypertonia
   - Exaggerated DTR
   - Positive Babinski's sign

	UMN	LMN
1.	Disuse atrophy	Gross wasting
2.	Groups of muscles affected	Muscles related to nerve is affected
3.	Hypertonia	Hypotonia
4.	DTR brisk	Absent
5.	Plantar extensor	Absent
6.	Flexor spasm may be present	Fasciculation may be present

Syncope—transient loss of consciousness due to decreased cerebral blood flow

Seizure—is any clinical event (motor sensory or autonomic manifestation) due to abnormal electrical activity of brain

Convulsion—*motor component of seizure*

Epilepsy—*it is the tendency to have recurrent seizures*

INVESTIGATIONS

Routine Investigation

- Blood routine
- Urine routine
- RBS, FBS
- RFT
- LFT
- Lipid profile
- Serum electrolytes
- Chest X-ray—look for cardiac lesion, consolidation (complication), TB

Investigation of Choice

- **CT scan**
  For proper evaluation to categorize to ischemic or hemorrhagic stroke
  To decide line of management
  (avoid anticoagulants and antiplatelets in hemorrhagic stroke)
  To rule out condition mimicking stroke
  (MRI—for posterior circulation stroke)
- **ECG, CXR, ECHO**
  To find—cardiac cause

In CT	
Infarct:	*Black*—hypodense area
Hemorrhage	*White*—hyperdense area

MANAGEMENT

- Maintain airway, breathing and circulation
- Control fever, hypoglycemia
- Lower blood pressure, if >186/110 mm Hg (Keep sBP < 160 in intracranial hemorrhage)
  Malignant hypertension
  Concomitant myocardial infarction
- Control seizures

MEDICINE

- Injection 20% mannitol 100–250 mL thrice daily to prevent cerebral edema—other drugs (oral glycerol, IV frusemide, mechanical ventillation).

- **IV THROMBOLYSIS IN ISCHEMIC STROKE**
  Using rtPA (recombinant tissue plasminogen activator)
  alteplase, reteplase, tenecteplase
  Pre-requisites
  - Clinical diagnosis of stroke
  - Onset of symptoms and time of administration <3 hours (from the time patient last seen normal)
  - Age >18 years
  - CT—no hemorrhage or edema over >1/3rd of MCA territory

  Administration
  - 0.9 mg/kg max 90 mg IV alteplase
  - 10% of total dose as bolus
  - Remaining over 1 hour
  - Monitor blood pressure
  - No other antithrombotic treatment for 24 hours
  - Avoid urethral catheterization >2 hours
  - If decline in neurologic status/uncontrolled BP stop and give cryoprecipitate

  Contraindications
  - BP >210/110
  - Treatment with heparin in 48 hours, elevated aPPT elevated INR
  - Stroke/injury in 3 months
  - Surgery in last 14 days
  - Recent MI
  - GI bleed in 21 days
  - Coma, stupor
  - Platelet < 1 lakh, hematocrit < 25%
    Glucose < 50 mg > 400 mg/dL
- **Antiplatelets (in ischemic stroke)**
  - Aspirin 300 mg at once
  - Then 75 mg OD or,
  - Clopidogrel 300 mg at once then 75 mg daily
- **Treatment of atrial fibrillation in valvular heart disease**
- **Indication for surgery:** Life-threatening hematoma in cerebellum
  MERCI (mechanical emboli removal in cerebral ischemia)

GENERAL CARE

- Nasogastric tube feeding: if nasal regurgitation present/in comatosed patient
- Foley catheter in case of retension/incontinence—urinary antiseptics
- Care of skin
  - Frequent changes of patients position and of bedsheets
  - Care of back and pressure points
- Prevent DVT—passive movement of limb or compression stockings
- Care of bowel—daily enema
- Care of respiratory tract—suction of nasal and pharyngeal secretions
- **Physiotherapy**
  - Proper positioning
  - Massage, passive and active exercises after stabilization of neurological condition to minimize the contractures and to strengthen the muscles
  - Rehabilitation, speech and occupational therapy

- **Lifestyle modifications**
  - Cessation of alcoholism and smoking
  - Low salt and fat intake, regular exercise.

YOUNG STROKE (<40 YEARS)

Causes
- Cardiac embolism
- Subarachnoid hemorrhage
  - Saccular (berry aneurysm)
  - AV malformation
  - Vertebral dissection
- Arteritis—TB syphilis collagen vascular disease
- Premature atherosclerosis
- Hyperviscosity syndrome, polycythemia, thrombocytopenia
- Thrombophilia
- APLA
- Homocysteinemia
- Demyelinating disease, intracranial neoplasm
- CADASIL (cerebral autosomal dominant arteriopathy with subcortical infarct and leukoencephalopathy)

Causes
- Cardiovascular
- Hematologic
- Systemic

Corresponding investigations
- ECG, CXR, ECHO
- MRI/angiography
- Mantoux, serology
  ESR, CRP, ANA
- Serum lipids
- CBC
- Protein C, S
  Antithrombin 3, factor 5 leiden
- Anticardiolipin antibody
  Lupus anticoagulant
- Urinary amino acids
- CT/MRI
- MRI brain

EXAMINATION OF UNCONSCIOUS PATIENT

Refer higher mental functions

CRANIAL NERVE

2- Fundus examination, menace reflex

3,4,6- Size and shape of pupil
direct and indirect light reflex

5- Corneal and conjunctival reflex

7-
  a. Look for smoothening or flattening of wrinkles on one side
  b. Uncovering of sclera
  c. Blowing out during expiration and sucking in during inspiration of paralysed side
  d. Apply firm supraorbital pressure which will make patient grimace then look for facial movements while grimacing

8- Oculocephalic reflex or doll's eye reflex
  - If brainstem is normal doll's eye reflex will be present (eyes move in opposite direction to head movement)
  - It is absent in brainstem damage

MEDICINE

MOTOR SYSTEM

- Observe posture
- Bulk, tone examine in normal way
- Power
  - Raise the upper limb and allow it to fall
  - Flex the knees so that soles of feet rest on ground unparalysed limbs slowly extend
  - And paralysed limb fall back to original position
- Reflex examine in normal way

SENSORY SYSTEM AND COORDINATION

It cannot be assessed

LOOK FOR

- **Signs of meningeal irritation**
- **Peripheral nervous system**
- **Skull and spine**
- **Carotid bruit**

PARAPLEGIA

CAUSES OF PARAPLEGIA

1. **Cerebral**
   - Parasagittal meningioma
   - Superior sagittal sinus thrombosis
   - Bilateral anterior cerebral artery occlusion
   - Thrombosis of unpaired ACA
   - Cerebral diplegia
2. **Spinal causes (myelopathy)**
   A. **Compressive**
      1. *Extramedullary*
         A. **Extradural**

Infection:	TB spine, epidural abscess
2°	e.g. breast, prostate, kidney, lymphoma
Trauma	Disc prolapse

         B. **Intradural**

Primary tumors:	neurofibroma, meningioma
AV malformations	
Infections	pachymeningitis/arachnoiditis
Metastasis	leukemia, lymphoma, myeloma

      2. *Intramedullary*

Infections:	Abscess, tuberculoma
Syringomyelia	
Primary tumors:	Astrocytoma, glioma, ependymoma

   B. **Non-compressive myelopathy**
      1. Congenital
      2. Trauma
      3. Vascular, e.g. anterior spinal artery occlusion
      4. Infection—syphilis/epidural abscess/TB
      5. Demyelination
         a. 2°—parainfectious, postvaccinations
         b. 1°—multiple sclerosis/ADEM, neuromyelitis optica
      6. Degenerative—motor neuron disease, Friedreich's ataxia
      7. Nutritional—SCAD, lathyrism, Cu deficiency
      8. Vasculitis—e.g. SLE
3. **LMN type lesion causing paraplegia (flaccid)**
   a. Lesion of anterior horn cell and peripheral nerve—GBS, polio, cauda equina.

5T'S of paraplegia
- Trauma
- Tumor
- TB
- Thrombosis
- Transverse myelitis

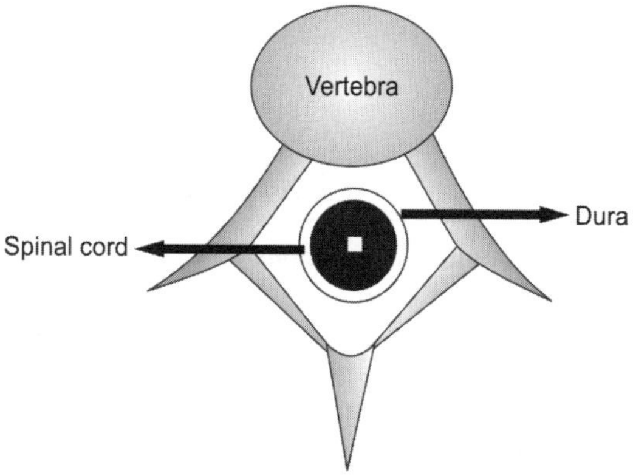

b. Lesion of NMJ—myasthenia
c. Lesion in muscles—myopathy

	Compressive	vs	Non-compressive
1. Bony deformity	+		–
2. Bony tenderness	+		–
3. Girdle like sensation	+		–
4. Upper level of sensory loss	+		–
5. Zone of hyperesthesia	+		–
6. Root pain	+		–
7. Onset and progress	Gradual		May be acute
8. Symmetry	Asymmetrical		Majority are symmetrical
9. Pattern of neurodeficit	U shaped		Bilaterally symmetrical
10. Flexor spasm	Common		Usually absent
11. Bladder and bowel involvement	Early		Late (Early in acute transverse myelitis
12. Classical example	Caries spine		Motor neuron disease

3, 4, 5 often present in acute transverse myelitis
U shaped affection (Elsberg phenomenon): First upper limb (UL) next ipsilateral lower limb (LL) next contralateral LL and finally contralateral UL
In slow cord compression pyramidal tract is affected first followed by posterior column and finally spinothalamic tract

	Extramedullary	vs	Intramedullary
1. Vertebral body tenderness	+		–
2. Root pain	+		–
3. Pyramidal signs	Early and prominent		Late and minimal
4. Pyramidal involvement	Symmetrical		Asymmetrical
5. LMN involvement	Segmental		Wide spread marked atrophy, fasciculations
6. Reflexes	Exaggerated		Late minimal change
7. Dissociative sensory loss	Absent		Present—jacket sensory loss
8. Sacral sensation	Lost		Present till late—sacral sparing
9. Autonomic involvement	Late		Early (bowel and bladder)
10. Trophic changes	Usually not marked		Common
11. Changes in CSF (raised protein)	Frequent		Rare

- Other causes (DM, leprosy, Brown-Sequard syndrome, lateral medullary syndrome, intramedullary compression)
- Pain and temperature sensations lost but touch and deep sensations present
- Jacket sensory loss—hypoesthetic area with normal sensations above and below.

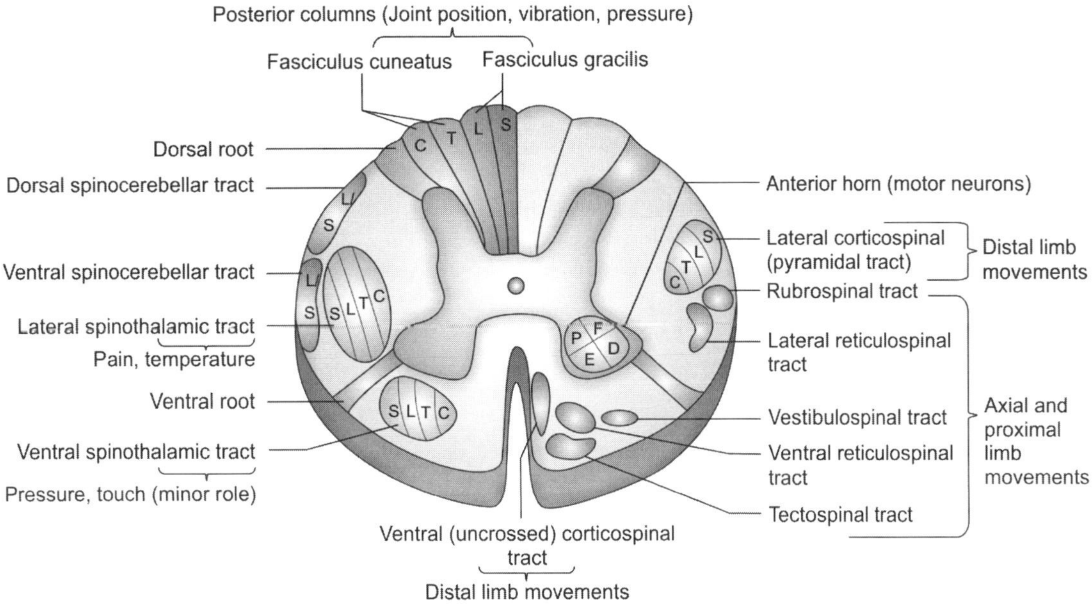

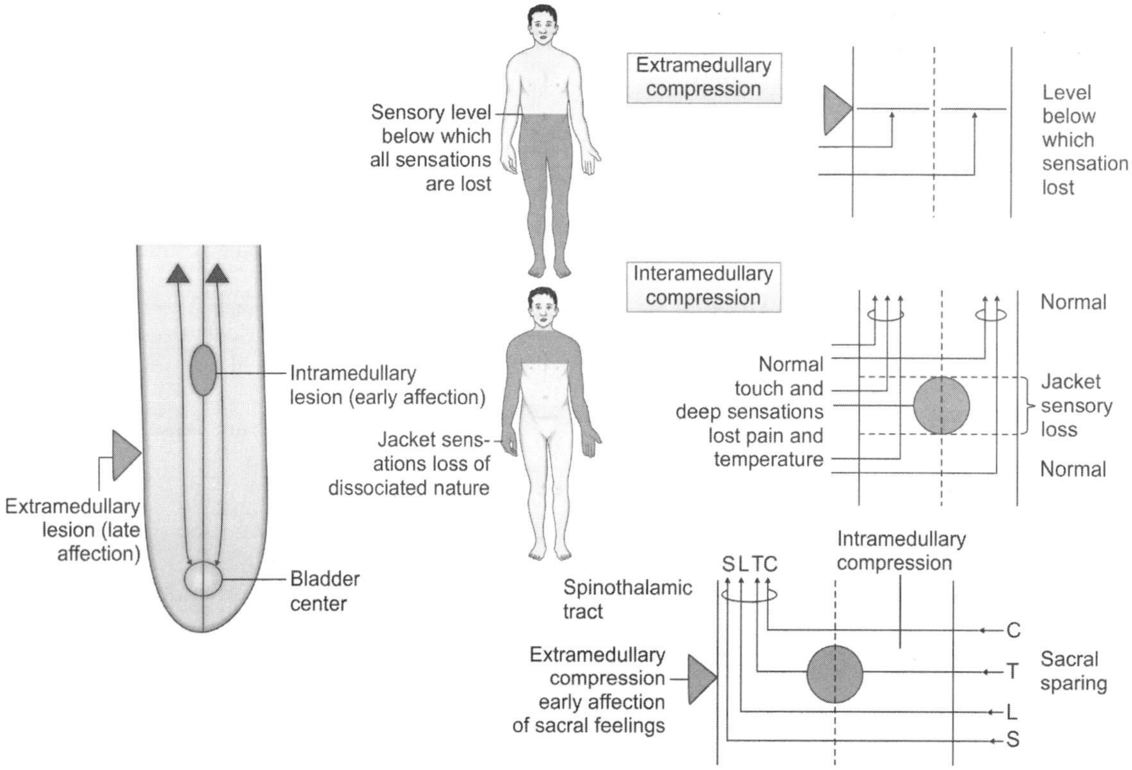

LEVEL OF LESION

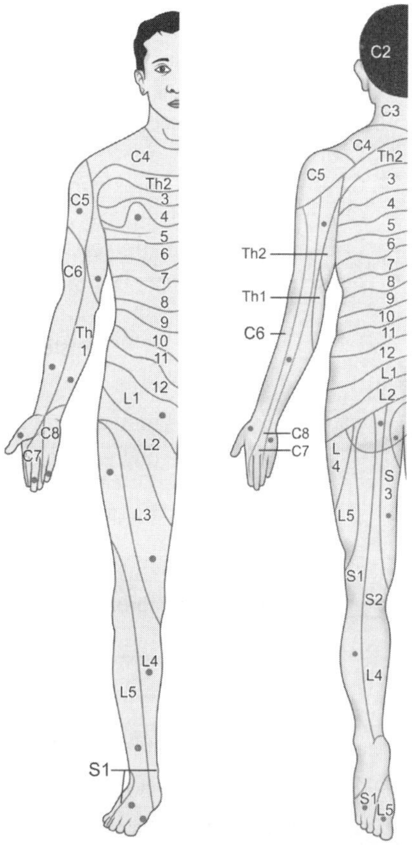

1. Deformity or swelling of vertebra
2. Tenderness in the vertebra
3. **Sensory level**
   a. *Distribution of root pain*: Look for specific dermatomes (due to involvement of posterior nerve root)
   b. Zone of hyperesthesia (due to compression of posterior nerve roots) level of lesion is just below it.
   c. Upper border of sensory loss (due to spinothalamic tract involvement)
   d. Girdle like sensation/sense of constriction at the level of lesion, exaggerated by cough and sneezing (due to involvement of posterior column)

Dermatomes

C1 : No dermatomal supply	T10 : Umbilicus
C5 : Shoulder tip	T12 : Suprapubic
C6 : Thumb	L1 : Inguinal region
C7 : Middle finger	L2 : Medial thigh
C8 : Little finger	L3 : Lateral and lower knee
T1 : Medial upper forearm	L4 : Medial leg and dorsum of foot
T3 : Axilla	Stand on S1
T4 : Nipple	Sit on S2
T8 : Epigastrium	Squat on S3, S4, S5

4. **Motor level**
   - Weakness
   - Fasciculations
   - Neck flexion : C1, C2, C3 Hip flexion L1
   - Shoulder abduction : C5 Hip adduction L2
   - Elbow flexion : C6 Knee extension L3

– Elbow flexion and wrist flexion	: C7	Ankle dorsiflexion	L4
– Finger flexion	: C8	Dorsiflexion of big toe	L5
– Finger abduction	: T1	Plantar flexion	S1
		Knee flexion	S2

5. **Reflex Level**
   Loss of deep reflexes of particular segment is involved
   The reflexes will be brisk below involved segment
   (for level refer reflexes)
   Analysis of Beevor's sign
   In paralysis of lower part of rectus abdominis—umbilicus moves upwards and in paralysis of upper part it moves downwards
6. Determination of spinal segments in relation to vertebrae

Vertebra	Spinal segment
Upper cervical vertebra	equal
Lower cervical vertebra	+1
T1–T6	+2
T7–T9	+3
T10	L1, L2
T11	L3, L4
T12	L5
L1	Sacral and coccygeal segments

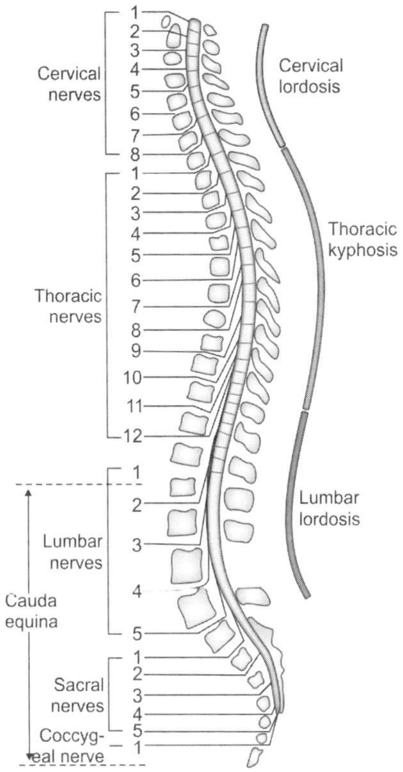

• •

(From motor, sensory, reflex levels find spinal segment, from that find vertebral level)

Paraplegia	**In extension**	**In flexion**
1. Cause	Pyramidal lesion	Pyramidal and extrapyramidal
2. Hypertonia	More in extension	More in flexion
3. Position of lower limbs	Extended	Flexed
4. Deep reflex	Exaggerated	Less exaggerated
5. Clonus	Present	Absent
6. Mass reflex	Absent	May be present

When pyramidal tract alone is at jeopardy, the extrapyramidal system takes the upper hand, resulting in increased tone of antigravity muscles (paraplegia in extension). When extrapyramidal system is also at fault, the spinal arc becomes dominant and there is relative increase in tone of flexors (paraplegia in flexion).

DIAGNOSIS OF PARAPLEGIA

1. Acute or chronic
2. Compressive/noncompressive
3. Flaccid/spastic
4. Paraplegia
5. Extramedullary/intramedullary
6. Spinal cord level
7. Vertebral level
8. Etiology
9. Paraplegia in flexion/paraplegia in extension
10. Complications

	Cauda equina	**Conus medullaris**
1. Onset	Gradually B/L	Sudden B/L
2. Motor deficit	Asymmetric (patchy)	Symmetric
3. DTR	Knee and ankle jerk may be absent	No reflex lose

4. Sensory	Asymmetric U/L All forms affected no dissociation	Symmetric B/L Saddle anesthesia Dissociative sensory loss
5. Bladder and bowel	Late and less marked	Early and marked
6. Sexual functions impaired	Less impaired	Erection and ejaculation

Guillain-Barré Syndrome

It is an acute postinfective polyradiculoneuropathy (inflammatory demyelination involves spinal roots and peripheral nerves)

- It follows viral infections: EBV, *Campylobacter jejuni*, measles, CMV
  Post-vaccines, post-surgical.
- A/c ascending LMN paralysis usually beginning in the leg (proximal muscles are more affected)
- B/L 7th (LMN type) cranial nerve palsy (in 50% cases)
- *Plantar*: Flexor or no response
- Deep reflexes are absent
- There is subjective sensory symptoms (paresthesia) without any objective sensory loss
- Bowel and bladder rarely involved
- Outcome:
  - Complete or near complete recovery : 85%
  - Residual disability : 10%
  - Death : 5%

> Rx—ventilatory support, IV Ig, plasmapheresis

Acute Transverse Myelitis

Though common cause of noncompressive myelopathy clinically behaves like compressive variety (acute onset total transaction of cord)

Follows a viral illness/vaccination:

- Fever may be present before paralysis develops
- Bladder involvement is early
- Absence of root pain, spinal tenderness or spinal deformity
- Back pain and progressive paraparesis are presenting complaints
- Mid thoracic region is the most common site
- Girdle constriction at the level of lesion with zone of hyperesthesia just above
- Partial/complete sensory loss (all modality) with a definite upper level
- Plantar is extensor
- All reflexes are usually lost below level of lesion in stage of neuronal shock (2–3 weeks) thereafter spasticity with brisk reflexes develop.

SUGGESTED READING

1. Davidsons's Principles and Practice of Medicine.
2. Harrison's Principles of Internal Medicine.

NOTES

CHAPTER 6

Viva

CHARTS

JAUNDICE

Liver Function Tests (Normal)

- Serum bilirubin—0.2–0.8 mg%
  - conjugated—0–0.2 mg%
  - unconjugated—0.2–0.6 mg%
- SGPT —10–45 IU/L
- SGOT —10–45 IU/L
- ALP —30–120 IU/L (3–13 KAU)
- Albumin—3.5–5.5 g%
- Globulin—2–3.5 g%

	Hemolytic	**Hepatocellular**	**Obstructive**
Serum bilirubin	10 mg%	10 mg%	10 mg%
Conjugated	0.5 mg%	5.5 mg%	8.5 mg%
Unconjugated	9.5 mg%	4.5 mg%	1.5 mg%
SGPT	26 IU/L	260 IU/L	80 IU/L
SGOT	30 IU/L	290 IU/L	90 IU/L
ALP	8 KAU	20 KAU	40 KAU
URINE			
Bile salts	–	++	++
Bile pigments	–	+	++
Urobilinogen	+++	+	–
Feces			
Stercobilinogen	+++	Normal color	Clay color

CSF STUDY

NORMAL

- *Pressure*: 50–250 mm of H_2O
- *Cells*: 0–5 lymphocytes
- *Protein*: 20–40 mg%
- *Sugar*: 40–80 mg%

	Pyogenic	Tuberculous	Viral
Appearance	Turbid	Clear	Clear
Pressure	++	++	++
Protein	180 mg%	600 mg%	150 mg%
Sugar	12 mg%	30 mg%	65 mg%
Cells	Mainly neutrophil	Lymphocytes	Lymphocytes

URINE ROUTINE

NORMAL

Output: 1.5 L/day
Albumin: Up to 30 mg/dL
RBC: Less than 1/HPF

	AGN	Nephrotic syndrome
Amount	Oliguria (<400)	Normal
Color	Smoky	Clear
Albumin	++	+++
RBC	++	–

GFB—125 mL/mt
Anuria—<50 mL/day
Oliguria—<400 mL/day
Polyuria—>3 L/day

DRUGS

1. **Albendazole**
   Uses:
   - 400 mg single dose for ascaris, hookworm, whipworm, pinworm.
   - Neurocysticercosis

   Advantage over mebendazole:
   - Single administration of drug
   - More active against whipworm

   S/E: Embryotoxicity in animal (so contraindicated in pregnancy)
2. **Azithromycin**
   - Newer macrolide
   - More active than other macrolide against *H. influenzae*
   - *Indications:* Pharyngitis, tonsillitis, sinusitis, otitis media

   Dose: 500 mg daily for 3 days
3. **Beclomethasone dipropionate (Topical steroid)**
   - Anti-inflammatory, immunosuppressive, antiproliferative
   - It is a potent topical steroid

   S/E: Thinning of epidermis, atrophy, delayed wound healing and infections.
4. **Bromocriptine**
   - It inhibits prolactin synthesis
   - It is a selective dopamine D_2 agonist
   - It is an antiparkinsonian drug.
5. **Captopril/Enalapril**
   - ACE inhibitor

   Uses: HTN, MI, diabetic neuropathy and scleroderma crisis
   S/E: Hypotension, hyperkalemia, cough, angioedema, fetal damage.
6. **Cephalosporin**

First generation	Second generation	Third generation	Fourth generation	Next generation
Cephalexin (oral) Cefazolin	Cefuroxime, Cefuroxime axetil (oral), Cefoxitin	Cefotaxime, Ceftriaxone Ceftazidime, Cefixime (oral)	Cefepime	Ceftobiprole Ceftaroline

   Uses:
   1. Alternative to penicillin in patients developing allergic reaction
   2. Penicillinase producing staphylococcal infection
   3. Meningitis, respiratory and urinary tract infections.

   S/E: Nephrotoxicity, diarrhea, bleeding

7. **Cetirizine**
   - Nonsedating anti-allergic (H1 antagonist)

   Dose: 10 mg HS

   Uses: Anti-allergic, common cold, cough, motion sickness.
8. **Chloramphenicol**

   Uses: Enteric fever
   - *H. influenzae* meningitis
   - Intraocular infection
   - UTI.

   S/E: Bone marrow suppression, hypersensitivity reaction, gray baby syndrome.
9. **Cimetidine/Ranitidine**

   Uses:
   - Duodenal ulcer
   - Gastric ulcer
   - Gastritis
   - ZE syndrome

   S/E: Headache, dizziness, gynecomastia (cimetidine)
10. **Cotrimoxazole**

    Trimethoprim + Sulfamethoxazole

    Uses:
    - UTI, respiratory infection
    - Typhoid
    - Bacterial diarrhea/dysentery.

    S/E: Nausea, vomiting, folate deficiency
11. **Finesteride**

    5α reductase inhibitor

    Uses:
    - Prostate cancer
    - Acne
    - Male type of baldness

    S/E: Impotence.
12. **Fluconazole—systemic antifungal**

    Uses:
    - Cryptococcal meningitis
    - Candidiasis
    - Histoplasmosis
    - Sporotrichosis.
13. **Furosemide (Lasix)**

    Diuretic

    Uses:

    Edema

    A/C pulmonary edema, hypertension
14. **Insulin**

Rapid acting	Short acting	Intermediate acting	Long acting
Insulin lispro	Regular (soluble) insulin	Insulin Zn suspension (Lente)	Insulin glargine
Insulin aspart		Neutral protamine hagedorn (NPH) isophane insulin	Insulin detemir
Insulin glulisine			

Reactions to insulin
- Hypoglycemia
- Local reactions
  - Swelling, erythema and stinging
  - Lipodystrophy
- Allergy—Urticaria, angioedema and anaphylaxis
- Edema

15. **Loperamide**

    Antidiarrheal (antimotility) drug

Dose: 4 mg followed by 2 mg after each motion
S/E: abdominal cramps, rashes.

16. **Metoclopramide (Reglan)/Domperidone (Domstal)**
Antiemetic drug (prokinetic drugs)
Dose: 10 mg TDS oral
S/E: Sedation, diarrhea, Parkinsonism, galactorrhea, gynecomastia.

17. **Losartan/telmisartan**
Angiotensin receptor antagonist
Use: Hypertension
S/E: Hypotension, hyperkalemia, fetopathy.

18. **Disease modifying antirheumatic drugs (DMARD)**
   - Gold
   - d-penicillamine
   - Chloroquine
   - Sulfasalazine
   - Immunosuppressants (methotrexate, cyclosporine).

19. **Drugs used in gout**

A/c gout	**C/c gout**
NSAIDs	Uricosurics—probenecid, sulfinpyrazone
Colchicine	Synthesis inhibitor—allopurinol, febuxostat
Corticosteroid	

20. **Atropine**
Anticholinergic drug
Uses:
   - Antisecretory
   - Antispasmodic
   - Bronchial asthma
   - Mydriatic and cycloplegic
   - Cardiac vagolytic
   - Organophosphate poisoning.

   S/E: Dry mouth, dilated pupil, photophobia, palpitation.

21. **Phenytoin**
Antiepileptic drug (prolongation of Na^+ channel inactivation)
S/E:
   - Hirsutism, hypersensitivity
   - Osteomalacia
   - Fetal hydantoin syndrome
   - Megaloblastic anemia
   - Gum hypertrophy.

22. **Propranolol**
Nonselective β blocker
Uses:
   - Antihypertensive
   - Cardiac arrhythmia
   - MI
   - Angina
   - CCF
   - Thyrotoxicosis
   - Glaucoma

   S/E: Bradycardia, exacerbate variant angina, C/I in asthma

23. **Vancomycin**
   - DOC for antibiotic associated pseudomembranous enterocolitis
   - Active against resistant (penicillin) *Staphylococcus aureus*

   S/E: Nephrotoxic, ototoxic, Red man syndrome

24. Rifampicin

First line drug of TB

Uses:
- TB
- Prophylaxis of meningococcal meningitis
- Brucellosis
- Leprosy
- Diphtheroides

S/E:
- Hepatitis
- *Respiratory syndrome*: Breathlessness
- *Cutaneous syndrome*: Flushing, pruritus
- *Flu syndrome*: Fever, chills, rigor
- *Abdominal syndrome*: Nausea, vomiting, cramps

25. Antileprotic drugs

Dapsone, clofazimine, rifampicin

	Dapsone	**Clofazimine**	**Rifampicin**
Paucibacillary (6 months)	100 mg daily	-	600 mg once a month
Multibacillary (12 months)	100 mg daily	300 mg once a month 50 mg daily	600 mg once a month

26. Metronidazole

Tissue amebicides

Uses:
- Amebiasis
- Giardiasis
- Anaerobic infection
- *Helicobacter pylori* infection
- *Trichomonas vaginitis*

S/E: Nausea, anorexia, headache, glossitis

Luminal amebicide—Diloxanide furoate

27. Paracetamol

Analgesics but poor anti-inflammatory

S/E:
- Nausea, rashes
- Analgesic nephropathy
- Hepatotoxic

Treatment of paracetamol poisoning—N acetylcysteine

28. Aspirin

NSAID

Uses:
- Antipyretic
- Analgesic—1 g/day
- Anti-inflammatory—3–5 g/day
- Antiplatelet activity—75–150 mg/day
- Acute rheumatic fever
- Rheumatoid arthritis.

S/E: Nausea, vomiting, epigastric distress

29. Digoxin

Uses:

CCF
- Cardiac arrhythmia
  - AF
  - Atrial flutter
  - PSVT

S/E:
- Extracardiac—nausea, anorexia, abdominal pain, rashes, gynecomastia
- Cardiac-all types of arrhythmia produced by digoxin (pulses bigeminy, ventricular tachycardia).

INSTRUMENTS

1. **Bone marrow aspiration needle**
   SALAH and KLIMA
   SALAH—with guard.
   Indication:
   Hematological malignancies, ITP, storage disorder, infection like kala-azar, PUO, megaloblastic anemia.
   Contraindications:
   Infection, bleeding disorder.
   Sites: Iliac crest/postsuperior iliac spine
   Tibia (childrens)
   Body of sternum.

   Cause of dry tap
   - Myelofibrosis
   - Marrow hypoplasia
   - Metastatic infiltration
   - Faulty technique

2. **Lumbar puncture needle:**
   Sites: Between L_3 and L_4 or L_4 and L_5
   Indications:
   - Therapeutic—to give drugs, (spinal anesthetics, methotrexate)
   - Diagnostic—Meningitis, GBS, convulsions, subarachnoid hemorrhage

   Complications:
   Infections, coning, trauma.
   Contraindications:
   Bleeding disorder, infection, raised ICT.
   Before doing this procedure fundus is examined to r/o papilledema.
3. **Liver biopsy needle:**
   Vim Silverman needle, Menghini needle.
   Indications:
   Cirrhosis, storage disorder, Wilson's disease, hemochromatosis, malignancies.
   Contraindications:
   Prolonged PT, infection at site, thrombocytopenia, biliary obstruction.
   Complications:
   Infection, bleeding, injury to liver.
   Site:
   10th ICS in MAL in the supine position.
4. Laryngoscope
5. Endotracheal tube

   (4, 5) Refer pediatrics instruments
6. Nasogastric tube–refer surgery

X-RAYS

CHEST X-RAY PA VIEW

- For better visualization of lung and anterior structure
- Centering at T5 level
- PA view taken in deep inspiration as maximum air is needed in lung for contrast
- But expiration required when small pneumothorax is suspected (decreased lung contrast on expiration so better visualization of small pneumothorax).

OTHER VIEWS

- Oblique
- Recumbent
- Lateral decubitus

MEDICINE

- Routinely, 6 feet distance between tube and patient
- Time of exposure 1/20th of a second

DESCRIPTION OF CHEST X-RAY

- Soft tissue (muscles, breast, cutaneous tissue)
- Lung hilum, lung field—upper zone (above anterior border of second rib), middle zone (2 to 4th rib), lower zone (below 4th rib)
- Angles—cardiophrenic and costophrenic angles (obliterated in pleural effusion, mass lesion)
- Diaphragm and subdiaphragmatic area (normally right diaphragm is higher)
- Bony shadow (ribs, clavicle, scapula, spine, shoulder joint)
- Heart and mediastinum (heart borders, enlargement, etc.).

Centering

Medial end of the clavicle equidistant from the spinous process.

Penetration

- Whether normal, over or under penetrated
- Normal—vertebral bodies and disc spaces should be just visible down to the T8/T9 level.

On Full Inspiration

- Anterior end of the 6th rib cut the diaphragm
- Posterior end of the 10th rib cut the diaphragm
  - More than this is considered as hyperinflation

1. **Mitral stenosis**
   - Pulmonary venous hypertension—increased prominence of upper lobe veins (Reverse moustache sign)
   - Pulmonary arterial hypertension
     - Central deviation of pulmonary artery
     - Peripheral pruning of pulmonary artery
     - RVH
     - Prominent pulmonary arterial shadow
     - Prominent right descending pulmonary artery
   - Left atrial enlargement—splaying of carina
     - Shadow in shadow sign
     - Straightened left heart border
     - Enlargement of the left atrial appendage
     - Indentation of esophagus in barium swallow.
   - Pulmonary edema—perihilar shadow (Batwing sign)
     - Kerley B lines (horizontal lines at the costodiaphragmatic area)
     - Ground glass appearance (alveolar edema)
2. **Pneumonia**

   X-ray shows an opacity outlining the whole anatomical distribution of a lobe

   As resolution occurs it become irregular and the picture slowly improves to normality

Bulging fissure sign	*Pneumatocele*
Klebsiella pneumoniae due to exudates	*Staphylococcus aureus* and *Klebsiella*
Massive lobar pneumonia	*Air bronchogram*
More than one lobe	Hilar adenopathy

3. **COPD**
   - Horizontality of ribs
   - Hyperinflation
   - Bullae in emphysema
   - Flattened diaphragm (Terracing of diaphragm)
   - Hyperluscent lung field
   - Thickening of bronchial wall due to peribronchial infection (c/c bronchitis)

MEDICINE

4. **Pneumothorax**
   - Increased volume of right hemithorax
   - Hyperlucency on right side
   - Absent lung markings
   - Margin of collapsed lung markings at hilum
   - Mediastinal shift to opposite side
5. **Pleural effusion**
   - Tracheal shift to opposite side
   - Cardiac shift to opposite side
   - Homogeneous opacity, no air bronchogram
   - Obliteration of costophrenic and cardiophrenic angle
   - Ellis S-shaped curve
   - Lateral decubitus film—minimal pleural effusion
6. **Bronchiectasis**
   - Chest X-ray may be normal—increased shadow in the affected area of lung
   - Thickened bronchi—cystic shadows.
7. **Tumors of lung**
   - Primary tumor mass
     - Nodular opacity
     - Rounded lesion in the lung periphery
     - Cavitating lesion
   - Secondary effect or complication
     - Collapse/consolidation
   - Metastatic or local spread
     - Pleural effusion
     - Bony invasion
     - Pathological fracture
     - Elevated hemidiaphragm due to phrenic nerve involvement
     - Secondaries in lung—multiple cannonball appearance.

SURGERY

Practical Examinations	**Marks**
Long Cases Including Case Sheet	50
Short Cases	
Case 1	20
Case 2	20
OSCE	
Five Stations	2+2+2+2+2
Total	100
Viva	
Four Stations	5+5+5+5
(Drugs and Instruments, Operative Procedures, Specimens, X-rays)	

CHAPTER 7

Long Cases

THYROID GLAND

A CASE OF THYROID SWELLING

Anver, 40 years, Malappuram, manual laborer.

Presenting Complaints

Swelling in front of neck—4 months.

History of Present Illness

Patient noticed swelling 4 months back. Initially it was small in size, gradually increased in size and reached present size. There is no associated pain, dyspnea, dysphagia or hoarseness of voice. No history of loss of appetite, heat intolerance, tiredness, palpitation, tremor, diplopia. No history of diarrhea.

No history of lethargy, cold intolerance, loss of memory, weight gain, constipation. No history of dry skin, loss of hair, easy fatigability.

No history of difficulty in get up from squatting position.

Past History

No history of radiation, surgeries in the past. Patient is hypertensive and diabetic and on treatment for last 4 years

Personal History

- He is taking mixed diet
- Sleep and appetite normal
- Bowel and bladder habits not altered
- No addictions.

Family History

There is no similar illness in the family. Father and mother healthy, he has two children.

GENERAL EXAMINATION

- Moderately built and nourished
- PICCLE normal
- Skin, hair and nails normal
- Vitals
  - PR—72/min, regular in rhythm, normal in volume and character
  - BP—128/84 mm of Hg
  - RR—17/min

Signs of Toxicity

Eye Signs

1. Lid retraction—absent
2. Exophthalmos
   a. Von Graefe's sign—lid lag present
   b. Joffroy's sign—wrinkles absent
   c. Stellwag's sign—normal blinking absent
   d. Moebius' sign—failure to converge eyes
   e. Dalrymple's sign—upper sclera visible
3. Ophthalmoplegia—absent
4. No chemosis
   - Tachycardia—absent
   - Tremor—absent
   - Skin—not moist
   - No thyroid bruit

Local Examination of Neck

Inspection

- A diffuse nodular swelling of size 3 × 2 cm, irregular, involving lower part of neck, extending vertically from lower part of thyroid cartilage to 1 cm above suprasternal notch. Horizontally, it extends from anterior border of sternocleidomastoid on both sides.
- Swelling is moving with deglutition, lower border of swelling is visible, plane of the swelling is deep to deep fascia.
- Skin over the swelling is normal with no dilated veins, scar. No visible pulsations, no other visible swelling in neck. Pemberton's sign—negative.

Palpation

- No local rise of temp, tenderness.
- There is a midline oval swelling of size 3 × 2 cm with smooth surface, firm consistency, well-defined borders. Swelling is mobile in horizontal direction. No transmitted pulsations. It is possible to get below the swelling. Plane of the swelling is deep-to-deep fascia. It has got sharp margins.
- No tracheal shift. Carotid pulse palpable in normal site. There are 3 lateral swelling one on anterior aspect of right SCM firm, oval in shape and of size 2 × 1 cm. On making SCM taught, it is becoming less prominent.
- Two other swelling are palpable below angle of mandible of size 1 × 1 cm each present on left side most probably jugulodigastric lymph node. Kocher's test—no stridor.

Percussion

Resonant over manubrium sternum

Auscultation

- No thyroid bruit
- **Skull and spine**—normal
- **CVS**—normal
- **GIT**—normal
- **Respiration**—normal

DIAGNOSIS

Papillary carcinoma thyroid with LN metastasis (in this case)/MNG/SNT/diffuse thyroid.

THYROID GLAND

History Taking

Age

- Teenage: Simple goiter
- Papillary carcinoma: Young girls

SURGERY

- Follicular carcinoma: Middle-aged women
- Anaplastic carcinoma: Old age.

Sex

More common in female.

Swelling

Take history about onset, duration, progression of swelling.

History of Pain

- Usually thyroid is painless
- If pain then it should be:
  - Inflammatory condition—thyroiditis
  - Anaplastic carcinoma
  - Sudden increase in size with pain indicate hemorrhage.

History of Pressure Effect

- May produce dyspnea
- Dysphagia—only in retrosternal extension
- Hoarseness of voice and stridor—involvement of RLN.

Symptoms of Primary Thyrotoxicosis (Mainly CNS Manifestation)

- Loss of weight in spite of good appetite
- Preference to cold, intolerance to heat, excessive sweating
- Nervous excitability, irritability, insomnia, tremor
- Proximal muscle weakness
- Exophthalmos, diplopia, chemosis
- Amenorrhea.

Primary	**Secondary**
1. Diffuse	Bosselated or nodular
2. Abrupt onset	Insidious
3. Severe hyperthyroidism	Mild
5. Cardiac failure rare	Common
6. CNS—common	Rare
7. Eye signs common	Rare
8. Due to thyroid stimulating antibodies	No such antibodies
9. Mx—drugs, radio I_2, surgery	Surgery is choice
10. Entire gland is overactive	Internodular tissue

Symptoms of Secondary Thyrotoxicosis (CVS Manifestation)

- Palpitation
- Tachycardia
- Chest pain
- Dyspnea on exertion.

Symptoms of Secondary Myxedema

- Increase in weight in spite of poor appetite
- Preference to heat, intolerance to cold, dry skin
- Puffiness of face and dull expressions
- Loss of hair and lateral 2/3rd of eyebrow (madarosis)
- Constipation and menorrhagia, oligomenorrhea.

Metastatic Symptoms

- Cough, wheezing, chest pain, hemoptysis
- Bone pain, abdominal distension, jaundice
- History of treatments and investigations (fine needle aspiration cytology).

Past History

- History of radiation to neck—papillary carcinoma
- History of intake of drugs (like Li, sulphonylurea, periodic acid-Schiff (PAS), antithyroid drugs, amiodarone
- History of TB—granulomatous thyroiditis,
- History of any other malignancies
- History of DM (autoimmune), hypertension (HTN) (MEN).

Personal History

About sleep and appetite.

Menstrual History

Menorrhagia, amenorrhea

Family History

- Neoplasm and enzyme deficiency run in family [Pendred syndrome (peroxidase enzyme deficiency)]
- Sometime nonmembers of family affected in endemic goiter.

EXAMINATION OF PATIENT

General Examination

- Built and nourishment:
  - Thin, underweight—thyrotoxicosis
  - Obese, overweight—hypothyroidism
- Facies: Excitement, tension, nervousness, agitation—thyrotoxicosis
- Puddy face without expression (mask like face)—hypothyroidism
- Skin:
  - Moist—thyrotoxicosis
  - Dry and elastic—myxedema
  - Tremor in hands and tongue
- Eyes signs and signs of toxicity
  - Features of Horners syndrome
- Pulse: It is important because thyrotoxicosis, one of the cause of atrial fibrillation (irregularly irregular pulse)
- Sleeping pulse rate is more useful.

Oral cavity examination in thyroid
- Lingual thyroid
- Tremor of tongue
- Mucosal neuroma (MEN II)

CRILE'S grading (Sleeping PR)
- Mild thyrotoxicosis = pulse rate <90
- Moderate thyrotoxicosis pulse rate between 90–110
- Severe thyrotoxicosis pulse rate >110

Local Examination of Neck

Inspection

In short necked person Pizzillo's method is used both hands are placed behind the head and patient is asked to push head backwards against clasped hand.

Describe about:

- Site, shape, size, extent
- Movement with deglutition and protrusion of tongue
- Plane of the swelling—on extending the neck (deep to deep fascia)
- Whether lower border visible or not
- Skin over swelling
- Pemberton's sign: Seen in retrosternal goiter.

Swelling moving on deglutition
- Thyroid
- Thyroglossal cyst
- Subhyoid bursitis
- Pretracheal or prelaryngeal LN

Palpation

Standing behind the patient—classical method/standard

Lahey's method

Criles method

Swelling: Site, size, shape, extend, margin, consistency

- Local rise of temperature and tenderness
- Mobility
- Plane of the swelling, lower border palpable or not

Kocher's test: To rule out obstructed trachea (scabbard trachea)

Position of trachea, carotid pulsation, palpation of cervical LNs.

Consistency
- Soft—colloid goiter
- Hard—Reidels thyroiditis
- Variable—carcinoma

Position of trachea
- Inspection—trail sign
- Palpation—3 finger method
- Auscultation
- Radiological

Percussion

Normally resonant over manubrium sterni

In retrosternal goiter it will be dull.

Auscultation

To look for bruit in superior pole because of increased vascularity.

Why Goiter?
- Butterfly shaped
- Normal anatomical position
- Moves with deglutition
- Plane of the swelling

DISCUSSION

Signs of Toxicity

Eye Signs

- Lid retraction

SURGERY

- Exophthalmos:
  - Von Graefe's sign
  - Joffroy's sign
  - Stellwag's sign
  - Moebius sign
  - Dalrymple's sign
  - Ophthalmoplegia
  - Chemosis
- Tachycardia
- Tremor
- Thyroid bruit
- Moist skin

(described in case format)

- Berry's ligament
- Berry's sign: obliteration of carotid pulsation
- Berry's picking: removal of LNs in papillary carcinoma

- T3—3.5 to 7.5 micromol/L
- T4—10 to 30 nm/L
- TSH—0.3 to 3.3 mIU/L

INVESTIGATION

- Blood routine and urine routine
- Thyroid function test
- FNAC (USG—before FNAC)
- Incision biopsy (anaplastic and Riedel's thyroiditis, lymphoma).
- Thyroid antibody
- Serum calcium: In medullary carcinoma
- Isotope study
- USG neck—features of malignancy
  - Loss of peripheral halo
  - Microcalcification
  - Cervical LNE
  - Irregular margins
  - Central vascularity
  - Hypoechoic lesions

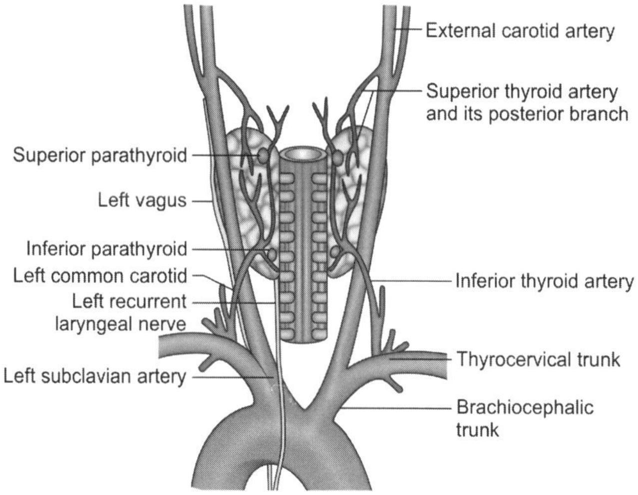

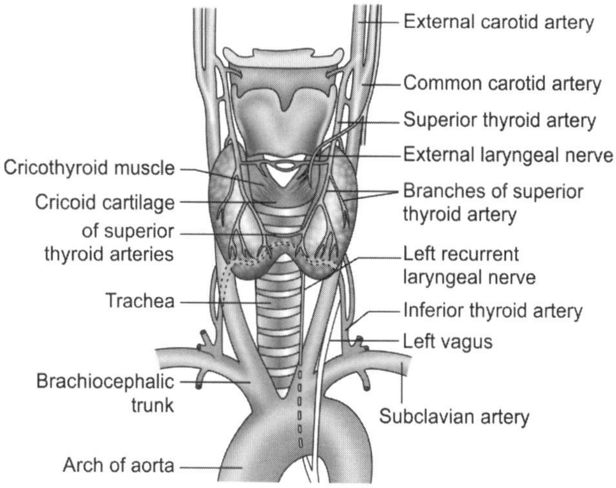

Arterial supply
- Superior thyroid artery—from external cartoid
- Inferior thyroid artery—from thyrocervical trunk
- Thyroidea ima artery—from brachiocephalic/arch of aorta

Venous drainage
- Superior thyroid vein—internal jugular vein (IJV)
- Middle thyroid vein—internal jugular vein (IJV)
- Inferior thyroid vein—left brachiocephalic veins
- Kocher's vein—internal jugular vein (IJV)

Thyrotoxicosis—biochemical and physiological manifestation of excessive thyroid hormone
Hyperthyroidism—over production hormone by thyroid gland
Grave's disease—components
- Diffuse goiter
- Thyrotoxicosis
- Autoimmune—infiltrative ophthalmopathy, dermopathy, myopathy

Signs of Malignancy

- Rapidly growing

SURGERY

- Hard, fixed thyroid
- LN enlargement (papillary carcinoma)
- Hoarseness of voice, and other pressure symptoms
- Pulsatile bony swelling: Mainly in scalp (follicular)
- Berry's sign, Horner's syndrome, chest symptoms

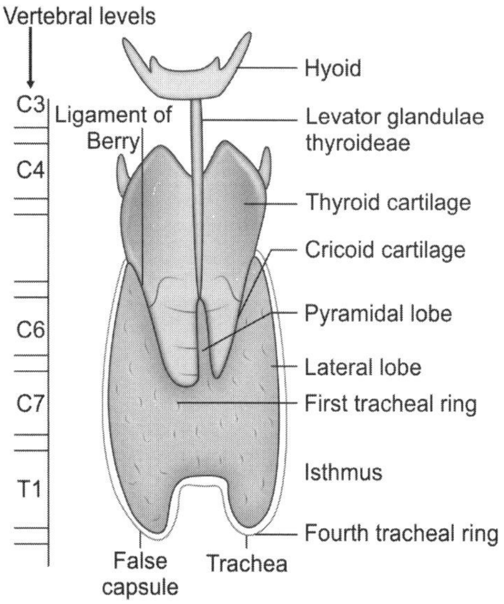

Enlarged thyroid gland may be one of the following
- Benign or malignant
- SNT or MNG
- Dominant nodule (one nodule on one side and other side is palpable)

Stages of MNG

Stage 1—diffuse hypertrophy and hyperplasia of gland
Stage 2—fluctuating levels of TSH
Stage 3—active lobule undergo central necrosis leads to nodular formation.

Complications of MNG

- Acute respiratory obstruction due to hemorrhage
- Secondary thyrotoxicosis
- Calcification
- Carcinomatous changes—follicular carcinoma.

Thyroid moves with deglutition?
Thyropharyngeus and cricopharyngeus (inferior constrictor muscle)
is attached to thyroid and cricoid cartilage respectively. So when patient swallows, inferior constrictor will contract and thyroid and cricoid cartilage moves upwards, thyroid gland is attached to larynx by suspensory ligament of Berry (pretracheal fascia)
- Isthmus at level of 2, 3, 4 tracheal rings

Retrosternal Goiter
Enlargement of lower part of MNG which extends behind the sternum is called retrosternal goiter.
There are three types
1. Substernal—lower border below sternum
2. Intrathoracic—thyroid wholly in the chest
3. Plunging—when intrathoracic pressure raises thyroid plunges out

Cardiac failure, dyspnea, dysphagia, engorgement of neck veins and superior veins of chest.
Treatment of retrosternal goiter
- Resection of thyroid gland followed by sternotomy
- Retrosternal goiter delivered by traction and finger mobilization

Pendred syndrome
- Peroxidase enzyme deficiency
- Goiter + congenital
- Deafness + hypothyroidism

Riedles triangle
- Inferior thyroid artery—above
- Carotid artery—laterally
- Trachea—medially

Pretibial myxedema: Seen in thyrotoxicosis
Thyroid acropatchy: Clubbing and thinning of nail

TREATMENT

- Medical: Antithyroid drugs
  - Propylthiouracil—100 mg TID (given during pregnancy also)
  - Carbimazole
  - Beta blocker propranolol—20 mg TID
- Surgical: Indications for operation
  - Neoplasia (follicular carcinoma)
  - Toxic adenoma
  - Pressure symptoms
  - Cosmetic
  - Patient wishes
  - Recurrent cyst

Operation	Parts of gland removed
• Lobectomy	Now the term obsolete
• Hemithyroidectomy	1 lobe + isthmus
• Bilateral subtotal thyroidectomy	2 g of thyroid kept bilaterally
• Dunhill procedure	Total lobectomy + isthmusectomy on affected side and 4 g remnant kept on other side
• Near total thyroidectomy	1–2 g kept on contralateral side rest PF the gland removed
• Total throidectomy	Entire gland removed
• Isthmusectomy	Removal of isthmus

Antithyroid Drugs—Classification

- Inhibit hormone synthesis—carbimazole, PTU
- Ionic inhibitors—perchlorates, thiocyanate, nitrates
- Inhibit hormone release—iodine, iodides
- Destroy thyroid tissue—radioiodine.

Carbimazole

- Thyroid peroxidase inhibitor
- Dose
  - 40–60 mg daily × 1st 3 weeks
  - 20–40 mg daily × 4–6 weeks
  - Maintenance of 5–20 mg daily for 1.5–2 years (after that surgery should be done)
- Side effects: Agranulocytosis (sore throat: indicates immediate cessation of drug), fever, urticaria, liver disfunction.

Propylthiouracil (PTU)

- Thyroid peroxidase inhibitor + inhibit peripheral conversion of T4 to T3 (100 mg TID)
- Used in pregnant ladies
- Side effects—fever, rash, myopathy, arthralgia, agranulocytosis, hepatotoxicity.

Radioiodine Ablation

- Make the patient euthyroid with drugs
- Discontinue drugs for 5 days, ask the patient not to take iodised salts and compounds
- Administer I131 5–10 mci
- Start antithyroid drugs after 1 week and continue for 6–8 weeks
- After 6 months if no improvement give another dose.

SURGERY

Why in benign thyroid, we go for total thyroidectomy

- Recurrence
- Area of malignant potential
- If we are doing hemithyroidectomy the follow-up cannot be maintained

Strap muscles (supplied by ansa cervicalis)

- Sternothyroid
- Sternohyoid
- Thyrohyoid
- Omohyoid

Preoperative Preparations

- Patient should be in euthyroid state
- Lugol's iodine 10 days before surgery to decrease vascularity [5% I_2 in 10% KI]
- Give propranolol
- Drugs given are antithyroid + Lugols iodine + β-blocker
- Indirect laryngoscopy

Steps in Surgery

- Position: Supine with pillow under the shoulder to extend the neck. Head end with 15 degree elevation to prevent venous engorgement in the head and neck area (Rose's, Fowler's, reverse Trendelenburg position)
- Anesthesia: GA.
- Incision: Kocher's collar incision—transverse incision 2 finger breadth above the suprasternal notch from the anterior border of one SCM muscle to other.

PROCEDURE

- The transverse incision cuts through the skin, subcutaneous tissue and platysma: The two flaps are raised, the superior one up to thyroid cartilage and the lower one up to the suprasternal notch. Hold the flaps with Jolles self-retaining retractor.
- Vertical incision on the investing layer of deep fascia.
- Pull aside the strap muscles.
- Vertical incision on pretracheal fascia.

- Look and ligate and cut the middle thyroid vein. Being a short one it bleeds, when thyroid is pulled.
- Deliver the thyroid, if any difficulty in delivering, cut the strap muscles transversely.
- Ligate and cut the superior thyroid pedicle (artery and vein), close to the gland, as the external laryngeal nerve is away near the gland.
- Ligate and cut inferior thyroid pedicle (vein) as away as possible from the gland, as the RLN (Riedle's triangle) is the near the pedicle when it approaches the gland. Also identify and preserve parathyroid gland.
- Remove the required amount of gland after placing appropriate clamps (2 nos) and cut between them and suture the gland with chromic catgut.
- Close all layers.
- Place suction drainage before closing and bring it out through a separate stab incision, remove drain when the secretions stops (usually 48 hours). Oral feeds can be started next day.

COMPLICATIONS OF THYROIDECTOMY

Peroperative

- Injury to RLN, trachea, carotid, esophagus
- Hemorrhage (primary)
- Thyroid storm

Early Postoperative

Reactionary hemorrhage

Respiratory obstruction due to:

- Tension hemorrhage
- Tracheomalacia
- RLN palsy
- Edema

Late

- Hypoparathyroidism—earliest clinical feature is perioral numbness. Other include carpopedal spasm, Acchoucher's hand, Chovstek sign.
  Treatment: 10% calcium gluconate IV 10 mL for 10 minutes
- Hypothyroidism
- Recurrence
- Wound infection
- Keloid, granuloma
- Flap necrosis.

Postoperative follow-up
- Indirect laryngoscopy
- Side effect or complication after 4–6 hours after surgery
- Withhold thyroxine 1st 6 months as it takes thyroid function to become stable
- Lifelong follow-up for thyrotoxicosis

NEOPLASMS OF THYROID

CLASSIFICATION OF THYROID NEOPLASM

Benign

Follicular adenoma.

Malignant

Primary

- Follicular epithelium—differentiated
  - Follicular
  - Papillary
- Follicular epithelium—undifferentiated
  - Anaplastic
- Parafollicular cells—medullary
- Lymphoid cells—lymphoma

Features of hypoparathyroidism
- Trousseau's sign
- Chvostek-Weiss sign
- Obstetrician's hand (Accoucher's hand)

- **Papillary carcinoma**
  - Psammoma bodies
  - Orphan Annie nuclei
  - Spread through lymphatics
  - Prognostic criteria—AGES, AMES, MACIS
  - Lateral aberrant thyroid
- **Follicular carcinoma**
  - Spread through blood (pulsatile bony swelling)
- **Medullary carcinoma**
  - Amyloid deposition

SURGERY

Secondary
- Metastatic
- Local infiltrations.

1° causing 2° tumor is thyroid
• Breast
• Bronchus
• Kidney

MANAGEMENT

If FNAC report comes as papillary carcinoma after then:
Total thyroidectomy + central compartment dissection (if clinically –ve lymph node) or modified radical neck dissection (for +ve lymph node).

Why total thyroidectomy?
- Intrathyroid lymphatic spread
- Multicentric
- Differentiated carcinomas are TSH dependent
- For follow-up with radioiodine—we have to remove normal thyroid

If FNAC reports comes as follicular neoplasm:
We have to do hemithyroidectomy and specimen sent for HPR.
If reports comes as follicular adenoma do routine follow-up
If report comes as follicular carcinoma we have to do completion thyroidectomy with in 48 hours or after 6 weeks
Why total thyroidectomy?
- Differentiated carcinoma is TSH dependent
- For follow-up with radioiodine 2
- Follow-up in cases of differentiated carcinoma
  - Suppressive dose of thyroxine (300 μg) to keep TSH low
  - Radioiodine scan to look for remnant thyroid tissue
    - Thyroid ablation (30 mci)
    - Whole body iodine scan to look for metastasis
    - Follow-up until 3 scans annually come negative.

Medullary carcinoma—total/near total thyroidectomy + central compartment (clinically –ve LN)/modified radical neck dissection (+ve LN), follow up by calcitonin and CEA
Anaplastic carcinoma—isthmectomy (to reclear compression/for Bx) + radiotherapy + chemotherapy
Lymphoma—radiotherapy + chemotherapy.

THYROIDITIS

AUTOIMMUNE THYROIDITIS (HASHIMOTO'S)

- Clinical features—MNG with hypothyroidism
- Onset—insidious and asymptomatic or sudden and painful initially mild hyper thyroidism—hashitoxicosis
- Later hypothyroidism—due to fibrosis
- Hurthle cells (Askanazky cells)—large granular eosinophilic cells
- Large/small, rubbery or firm consistency
- Common in women at menopause
- Papillary carcinoma and malignant B-cell lymphoma can occur in patients with Hashimoto's disease
- Diagnosis:
  - TFT
  - Thyroid antibodies
  - FNAC
  - ESR (high)
- Treatment:
  - Thyroxine 0.2 mg
  - Steroids—if goiter increases in size and no response to thyroxin
  - Thyroidectomy—if large and cause discomfort.

Causes for hypothyroidism:
• Goitrogens
• Endemic
• Thyroid agenesis
• Autoimmune
• Iatrogenic
• Dyshormonogenesis
• Secondary to pituitary or hypothalamic disease

GRANULOMATOUS THYROIDITIS (DE QUERVAINS OR SUBACUTE)

- Viral etiology
- Clinical features—neck pain fever malaise
- Firm irregular enlarged, self-limiting disease within 6-8 weeks
- Diagnosis
  - ESR—increased
  - Thyroid antibodies—absent
  - FNAC
  - TFT—T_4, high, normal or slightly raised
  - I_{123} —uptake low.
- Treatment
  - Supportive
  - Specific – prednisolone 10–20 mg × 7 days, gradually taper its dose.

RIEDEL'S THYROIDITIS

- Thyroid tissue replaced by dense fibrous tissue, which infiltrates capsule and adjacent nodules, pretracheal connective tissue and carotid sheath
- Reteoperitoneal and mediastinal fibrosis are present.
- Hard and fixed thyroid
- Ureter affected by retroperitoneal fibrosis, hydronephrosis.
- Treatment:
  - Thyroxin—to combat hypothyroidism
  - Isthmusectomy— to relieve compression.

MYXEDEMA

Facial puffiness, supraclavicular puffiness, malar flush, yellow tinge to skin.

Myxedema coma

- Decreased body temperature (100 as 25°C)
- Depressed level of consciousness
- Treatment
  - It is a medical emergency slow warming of body
  - Injection IV hydrocortisone (100 mg)
  - Injection IV T_3 20 mg followed by 20 mg—8th hourly

Thyroxine Doses

- Supplementary—0.1 mg
- Replacement—0.2 mg
- Suppressive—0.3 mg

NO SPECS criteria in toxic goiter

Grade 0 – **N**o signs
Grade 1 – **O**nly signs
Grade 2 – **S**ymptoms (diplopia, periorbital edema)
Grade 3 – **P**roptosis
Grade 4 – **E**xtraocular manifestation
Grade 5 – **C**orneal ulcer
Grade 6 – **S**ight loss.

ANATOMY—RELATIONSHIP

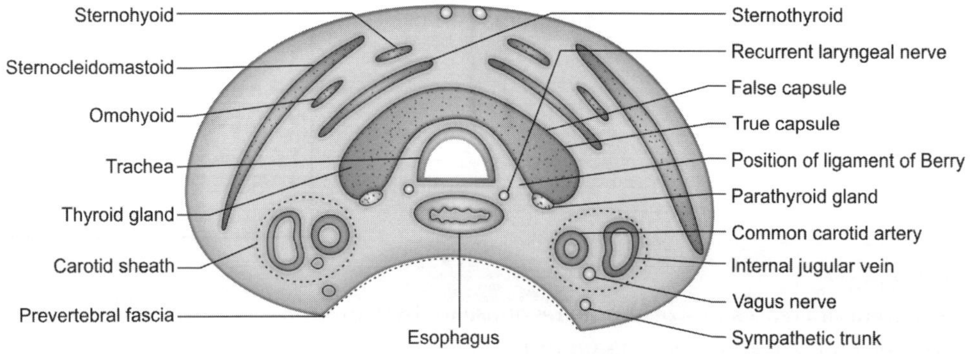

MEN I—Wermer syndrome (3P)
- Pituitary adenoma
- Pancreas—insulinoma, gastrinoma
- Parathyroid—primary hyperparathyroidism

MEN II A (Sipple)
- Thyroid—medullary carcinoma
- Adrenal—pheochromocytoma
- Parathyroid—primary hyperparathyroidism

MEN II B (Most aggressive MEN)
- Medullary carcinoma
- Adrenal—Pheochromocytoma
  Mucosal neuroma of lip, tongue, inner eyelid
- Marfanoid habitus

THYROID STORM

In patients inadequately prepared for thyroidectomy or in thyrotoxicosis patient with infection

Treatment

- General measures
- IV fluids, cooling the patient (Blasket).
- Propranolol 80 mg orally
- Carbimazole 40 – 60 mg
- Sodium ipodate
- Dexamethasone (reduce systemic symptoms)
- Paracetamol (reduce fever)
- Sedations
- Antibiotic

A CASE OF SWELLING IN BREAST

PRESENTING COMPLAINTS

Swelling in the right breast for 6 months duration.

History of Present Illness

Swelling was noticed 6 months back, incidentally while bathing. Initially it was small in size, in the lower part of the right breast. It rapidly increased in size and reached the present size. She consulted a doctor 4 months back and was given three courses of medication. There is no pain, loss of weight or loss of appetite. There is no history of any trauma, nipple discharge, retraction. There is no history of any jaundice, fractures, back pain or abdominal pain. No history of abdominal distention, dyspnea, hemoptysis,

LOCAL EXAMINATION

Inspection (mention the position of patient, e.g. sitting with arms by side)

On inspection, left breast appears to be normal, right breast appears to be elevated than left, with no visible mass, or enlargement, dimpling or ulcer. The nipple of breast partially retracted, no discharge, the right nipple is situated in the 4th intercostals space, in midclavicular line, smooth surface. The left nipple is at 6th intercostals space and is normal. The right breast does not fall forwards on leaning forward.

- Areolas appear to be normal with no cracks, fissures, eczema or discharge.
- Skin over the breasts are normal with no redness, peau d'orange appearance, nodules, engorged veins, ulceration or fungation.
- Arm and thorax are normal.
- Axilla and supraclavicular fossae are normal with no visible swellings.

Palpation

No local rise of temperature, tenderness on both breasts. Left breast appears to be normal. In right breast there is oval swelling of size 14 × 10 cm, extending through all the quadrants of breast, with well-defined margins. The swelling is hard in consistency, with irregular surfaces. There is fixity to skin, but not to the chest wall. The swelling is mobile along with breast tissue, no intrinsic mobility, the plane of swelling appears to be breast tissue (subcutaneous). Nipples, on palpation, there is no discharge, and it is not possible to evert the right nipple.

Examination of lymph nodes: Axillary and supraclavicular lymph nodes not palpable on both sides.

Examination of skeletal system: Normal.

Other systems:

- Abdomen—soft, no mass
- CVS—S1S2 normal, no murmurs
- Respiratory—normal breath sounds, no added sound
- CNS—normal
- PR and PV—not done.

Positions of inspection
- Sitting, arms by side
- Sitting, arms over waist
- Sitting, arms raised
- Sitting, leaning forward

Positions of palpations
- Sitting
- Semirecumbent
- Recumbent

PROVISIONAL DIAGNOSIS

- Carcinoma of right breast
- Stage IIIB T4 N0 M0.

- Pain—acute mastitis
- Throbbing pain—breast abscess
- Cyclical breast pain more during menstruation—fibroadenosis

HISTORY TAKING

- Age:
  - Carcinoma breast—above 40 years
  - Fibrocystic disease—middle age (25–40 years)

SURGERY

- Inflammatory breast abscess—lactating woman
- Fibroadenoma—below 35 years
- Lump: When it noticed, duration, growth, associated with loss of weight, loss of appetite, retraction of nipple
- Pain: Whether associated with pain
- Nipple discharge: Color of discharge
- Symptoms of metastasis—jaundice, bone pain. Hemoptysis, abdominal distension
- Family history—similar illness in the family, less common multipara woman.
- Menstrual history important (whether taken estrogen-containing drugs)
- Past history of breast disease in the same breast or opposite breast.

> - Fresh/altered blood—carcinoma, duct papilloma
> - Serous/greenish—fibroadenosis
> - Pus—mammary abscess
> - Milky—hyperprolactinemia

GENERAL EXAMINATION

Pallor, look for generalized lymphadenopathy.

> **Features of skin involvement**
> - Peau d'orange appearance
> - Ulceration
> - Nodule formation

Local Examination

Mention about normal breast first.

Inspection

- Size, shape, position of breasts
- Dilated veins, ulceration, nodule formation, peau d'orange appearance
- Describe about nipple (present, retracted, destroyed)
- Axilla and supraclavicular fossa—lymph node (LN).

Palpation

Palpation should be made with palmar surface of finger with the hand flat.
Four quadrants should be palpated

a. Local rise of temperature, tenderness
b. Describe about lump: Site, size, shape, surface, margins, mobile/not, hard/cystic/firm (if cystic also look for fluctuation, transillumination)
c. Whether fixed to skin, breast tissue, muscles, chest wall look axillary group of LN, cervical LN
d. Palpation of nipple, areolar complex.

Other System

- GIT—hepatomegaly, ascites, ovaries (Krukenberg's), LN (para-aortic, mesenteric)
- Respiratory—any features of metastasis
- Skull and spine
- PR and PV (important to detect Krukenberg's tumor), if not done, then tell that PR and PV not done.

> **Tethering:**
> Carcinoma spread to Astley Cooper's ligament (lump moved independently of the skin for some distance)
> **Fixity:**
> Cancer infiltrated to the skin (lump cannot moved independent of skin)

> **Fixity**
> - To skin
> - To pectoralis major
> - To latissimus dorsi
> - To serratus anterior
> - To chest wall.

MANAGEMENT OF BREAST LUMP

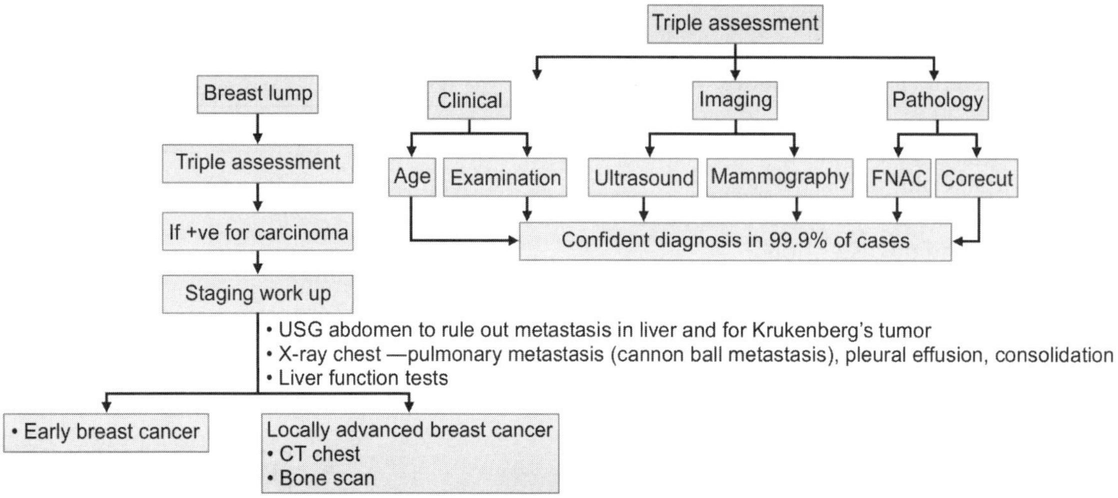

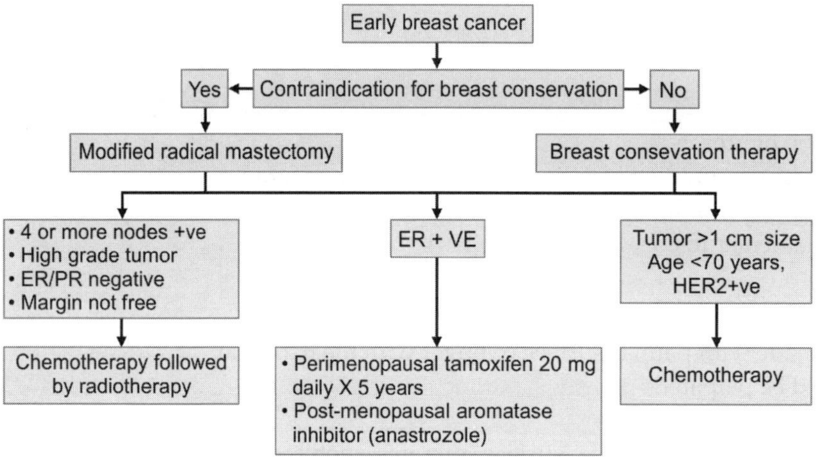

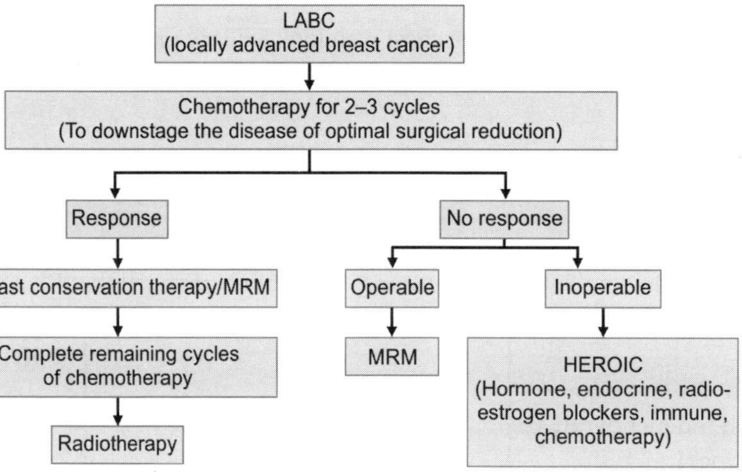

DISCUSSION

Triple Assessment

1. *Clinical Examination*

- Look size, consistency
  - Fixity to skin (present as dimpling)

- Fixity to underlying muscle (make the pectoralis taught and assess mobility along the line of muscle)
- Fixity to chest (ask to lean forward).

- Assess LN status.

Lymphatic Drainage of Breast

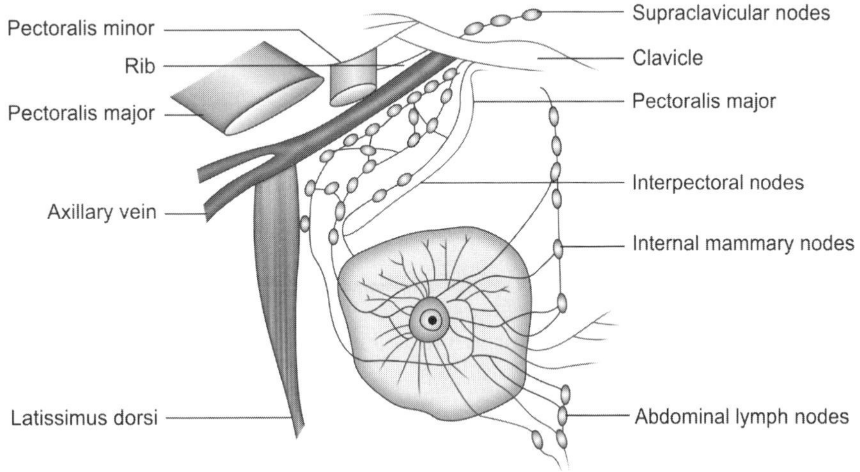

- Lymphatic drainage from subareolar plexus of Sappey and outer quadrant of breast—1st to pectoral then to central and last to apical group of axillary nodes.
- Subscapular and lateral group involved in retrograde way.
- Part of upper quadrant also drain to deltopectoral and apical nodes directly.
- Inner quadrant to internal mammary and to contralateral breast.
- Lower inner-quadrant will transverse through a plexus over the rectus sheath and communicate with subperitoneal lymph plexus.
- Krukenberg's tumor—its transcelomic implantation of malignant cells from the subperitoneal plexus to the surface of the functioning ovaries in premenopausal women.

2. Fine Needle Aspiration Cytology (FNAC)

- Investigation of choice
- Differentiate benign and malignant.

Method:

Using 23 gauge needle with aspiration syringe, lump is held firmly the needle is passed into the lump and with negative pressure continuous aspiration. Needle with syringe is removed with negative pressure (minimum of 6 passes.

FNAC Grading

Grade	*Result*
AC0	No epithelial cells
AC1	Scanty benign cells
AC2	Benign cells
AC3	Atypical cells present
AC4	Highly suspicious of malignancy
AC5	Definitely malignant

If 3 FNAC reports negative do core biopsy (if >2 cm), excision biopsy (if <2 cm)

Core biopsy:

- Helps to differentiate carcinoma in situ from infiltrating
- To assess receptor assay (this is not possible in FNAC)—ER-PR and HER2/neu

If core biopsy fails

- < 4 cm—wide excision
- > 4 cm—incisional biopsy

If FNAC found to be malignant:

- Do staging work up

3. Imaging

- Mammography—preferred if above 35 years
- USG—preferred if below 35 years
- MRI—differentiate scar tissue from tumor recurrence, breast with implant.

Breast image reporting and data system (BIRADS)
0—incomplete assesment
1—negative
2—benign
3—probably benign
4—probably malignant
5—malignant highly suspicious
6—biopsy proven

Indication of mammogram

- Symptoms without mess (palpable)
- Assessment after surgery
- Suspected in opposite breast
- Screening in normal individual.

Mammography findings in Carcinoma (**craniocaudal view, mediolateral view**)

- Mass lesion with clustered microcalcification
- Speckled mass lesion
- Stellate lesion, architectural distortion of breast parenchyma
- Density of lesion will be more than rest of breast

Mammography helps to find multicentricity (tumor foci found in different quadrant) and multifocality (tumor foci found in same quadrant).

STAGING OF CARCINOMA BREAST

TNM

- Tx—primary cannot be assessed
- T0—no evidence of primary
- Tis—carcinoma in situ
- T1—tumor <2 cm
- T2—tumor 2–5 cm
- T3—>5 cm
- T4—any size with direct extension
  - T4a—extension to chest wall (not including pectoralis muscle)
  - T4b—fixed to skin (peau d'orange, nodularity, ulceration)
  - T4c—t4a + t4b
  - T4d—inflammatory carcinoma.

Nx—lymph node cannot be assessed
N0—no regional nodes
N1—mobile, ipsilateral axillary nodes
N2—fixed, ipsilateral axillary or clinically apparent ipsilateral internal mammary
N3—ipsilateral infraclavicular/supraclavicular.

- M0—no mets
- M1—distant mets

Stage Grouping

Stage 0	Tis	N0	M0
Stage I	T1	N0	M0
Stage IIA	T0 T1 T2	N1 N1 N0	M0 M0 M0
Stage IIB	T2 T3	N1 N0	M0 M0
Stage IIIA	Up to T3	Up to N2	M0
Stage IIIB	Any T4	N0/N1/N2	M0
Stage IIIC	Any T	N3	M0
Stage IV	Any T	Any N	M1

Stage I and IIA—**early breast cancer**
Stage IIB, IIIA, IIIB and IIIC—**locally advanced breast cancer (LABC)**
Stage IV—**metastatic breast cancer**

Definite Management

- **Breast conservation therapy (BCR)**
  - Wide excision with 1 cm tumor clearance without excising overlying skin
  - Axillary node dissection through a separate incision in the axilla
  - Radiotherapy to tumor bed to prevent local recurrence

  Contraindications for BCR
  - T3 and T4 tumors, N2, M1
  - Large or central tumor in small breast
  - Multifocal/multicentric disease
  - Collagen vascular disease (CVD)
  - Extensive in situ component
  - Beneath the nipple
  - BRCA1, BRCA2
  - Advanced age >60 years
  - Contraindication for radiotherapy
  - CVD, pregnancy.

Levels of axillary lymph node dissection
- Level I—below and lateral to lateral margin of pectoralis minor
- Level II—behind pectoralis minor (inter pectoral, Rotor's nodes)
- Level III—above and medial to medial border of pectoralis minor

- **Modified radical mastectomy (MRM)**
  - Removal of entire breast nipple and areola
  - Axillary dissection after retracting or dividing the pectoralis minor
  - Preserve pectoralis major, long thoracic nerve, thoracodorsal nerve.

  Types
  - Patey's MRM—where pectoralis minor is removed + level 1, 2, 3
  - Scanlon MRM—where pectoralis minor is divided + level 1, 2, 3
  - Auchinclos MRM—where pectoralis minor is retained + level 1, 2

Other Operative Procedures

Prophylactic mastectomy
- BRCA1 +ve
- Lobular carcinoma (other breast)

- **Halsted complete mastectomy**
  - Entire breast, pectoralis minor + major
  - Regional lymph nodes up to costoclavicular ligament
  - Structures retained—Axillary vein, Bell's nerve, Cephalic vein (ABC)
- **Quart regimen of Veronesi:** Quadrantectomy + axillary dissection + radiotherapy to breast and axilla
- **Lumpectomy—for benign tumors:** Removal of lump with 1 cm margin
- **Simple mastectomy:** Tumor, entire breast, skin over breast, areola, nipple, axillary tail removed.

Steps of Mastectomy

- Put incision (elliptical incision directed obliquely (Kocher's) or transversely enclosing nipple areolar complex)
- Upper and lower flaps are made by electrocautery (minimum flap thickness 5 mm to preserve blood supply)
- Start dissection of breast, elevate the breast of the pectoralis fascia
- Ligate the bleeding vessels, and move laterally, there is clavipectoral fascia
- Cut the clavipectoral fascia and enter the axilla, remove enlarged LNs
- Cut and ligate tributaries of axillary vein
- Put a rubber drain, close the subcutaneous tissue.

To find out axillary vein:
- Trace pectoralis minor insertion
- Trace lattissimus dorsi insertion

Extend of axillary dissections
- Upper Inferior border of axillary vein
- Lower — Angular vein
- Medial — Chest wall
- Lateral — Lateral border of the latissimus dorsi

Complications of Mastectomy

- Psychological trauma
- Bleeding
- Infection
- Flap necrosis
- Lymphedema (later leads to lymphangiosarcoma)
- Injury to axillary vein, thoracodorsal nerve, long thoracic nerve
- Recurrence
- Seroma formation
- Stiffeners of shoulder

Breast reconstruction
- Silicone gel implant under pectoralis muscle
- Latissimus dorsi (LD) flap
- TRAM (transverse abdominis muscle) flap

Systemic Therapy

To tackle micrometastasis

- **Hormone therapy**
  - Indications—estrogen receptor positive, progesterone receptor positive
  - Drugs—tamoxifen (especially in premenopausal), fulvestrant (pure anti-estrogen)
  - Aromatase (postmenopausal) (letrazole)
  - Luteinizing hormone-releasing hormone (LHRH) agonist (buseriline)
- **Chemotherapy**
  - Indication—ER and PR negative
  - Poor prognostic cases
  - To down stage disease
  - Visceral metastasis.

Paclitaxel + adriamycin

Regimen used

- C—cyclophosphamide
- M—methotrexate
- F—fluorouracil.

LOCALLY ADVANCED BREAST CANCER

Treatment

HEROIC

- H—hormone therapy (anastrazole—postmenopausal, tamoxifen—premenopausal)
- E endocrine therapy—growth hormone regulating cytokines
- R—radiotherapy
- O—estrogen blockers—antiprogestrone/antiestrogen)
- I—immune therapy—herceptin if HER2/neu +ve (trastuzumab)
- C—chemotherapy

Theory

Peau d'orange

- Cutaneous lymphatic edema because of blockage of lymphatics draining the skin
- Infiltrated skin is tethered by sweat ducts, it cannot swell.

Pathological Classification

- Ductal
- Lobular

Both have two types:

1. Invasive
2. In situ

Invasive carcinoma (Ca):

- Special types
  - Tubular
  - Mucinous
  - Cribriform
  - Medullary
- Not otherwise specified (NOS)

Common pathological types—infiltrating carcinoma NOS type

Grading (Bloom Richardson):

- **T**—tubule formation
- **N**—nuclear pleomorphism
- **M**—mitotic index

Order of bone metastasis

Lumbar vertebrae > femur > thoracic vertebrae > ribs > sternum (LFT-RS)

Metastasis reach the lumbar vertebrae through
Intercostal vessels→paravertebral of Barton plexus→gravitate and reach the lumbar vertebrae

Van Nuys classification of ductal carcinoma in situ (DCIS)

- Age
- Type of DCIS

- Extent of resection margin
- Size
- Microcalcification

Krukenberg's tumor—occurs in premenopausal women, metastases reach the ovary by gravitating from subperitoneal plexus or blood spread.

Prognostic factors:

- Node metastasis (single most prognostic criteria)
- Tumor size
- Grade
- Lymphovascular invasion
- ER-PR status.

Choudhry Milli's criteria

It is used calling the 2nd tumor a primary are:

- Demonstration of in situ changes in the contralateral tumor
- If it is histologically different from cancer in the first breast
- If the degree of histological differentiation is distinctly greater than the lesion in the first breast
- In the absence of histologic difference, the contralateral is considered as primary, provided there is no evidence of local or distant metastasis from carcinoma (Ca) in the ipsilateral breast.

Paget's disease	vs	Eczema
• Elderly		• Lactating woman
• Itching absent		• Present
• Unilateral		• Bilateral
• Not respond to antibiotics		• Responds
• Nipple may be destroyed		• Intact

Risk factor of Ca breast

- History of Ca in other breast
- BRCA 1 and 2
- Early menarche
- Strong family history
- Age >55 years
- Nulliparity
- Obesity
- Male sex
- Diet rich in phytoestrogens
- Hormone replacement therapy
- Radiation exposure

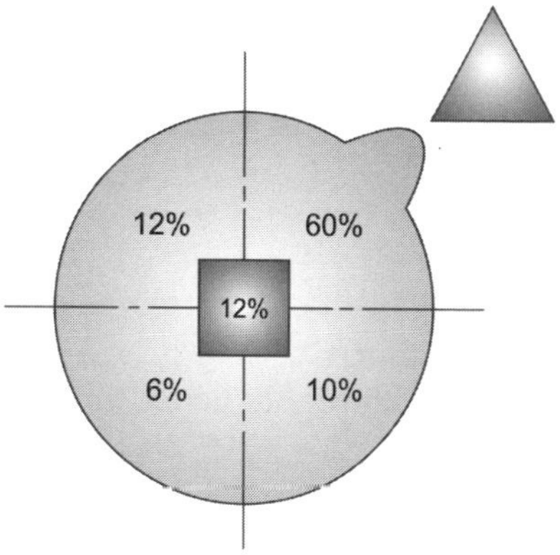

The relationship of carcinoma of the breast to quadrants of breast

Axillary sampling: Before doing wide local excision, 4 palpable nodes are excised through a separate axillary incision

Axillary clearance: Contents of axilla below the axillary vein cleared up to the apex preserving long thoracic nerve, thoracodorsal nerve and vessels.

SURGERY

GYNECOMASTIA

Causes:
- Hyperestrogenism
- Leprosy
- Digoxin, spironolactone, cimetidine
- Paraneoplastic syndrome.

Treatment: Webster's surgery (smiling incision)

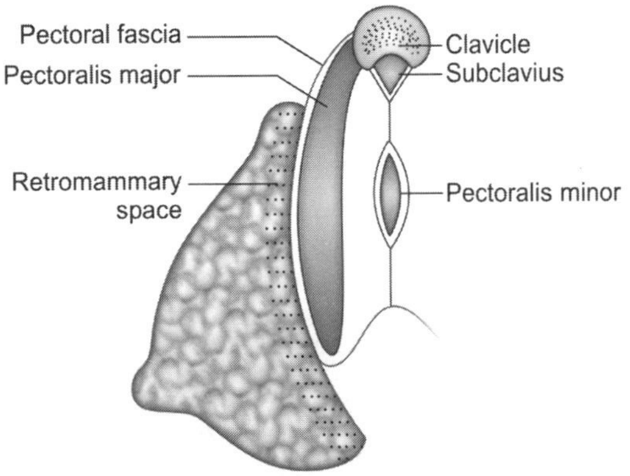

Deep relations of the breast

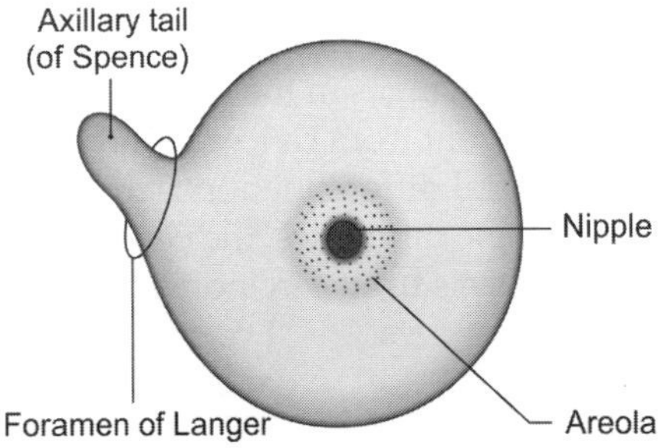

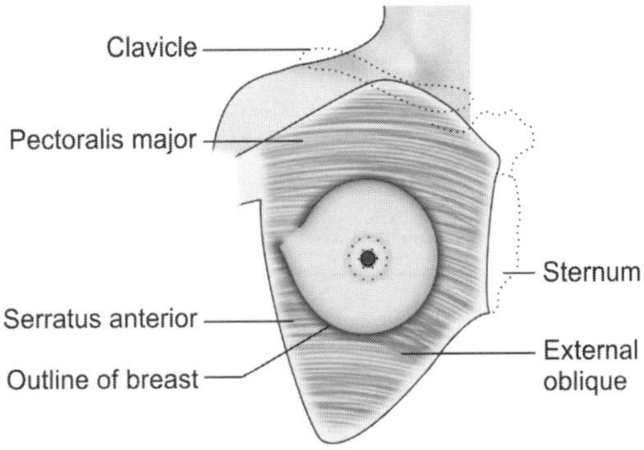

Muscles situated deep of the breast

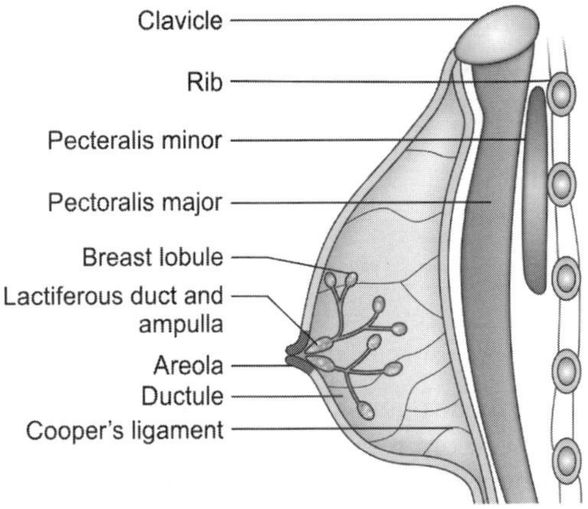

Cross-sectional anatomy of the breast

FIBROADENOMA

a. Pericanalicular
b. Intracanalicular

- Painless lump, slow growing
- It is highly mobile (breast mouse, floating tumor)
- Sometime, it undergo cystic degeneration and form phyllodes tumor.

PHYLLODES TUMOR

- Cystosarcoma phyllodes, serocystic disease of Brodie
- Giant fibroadenoma (>5 cm)
- Huge swelling
- Serous discharge through nipple
- Subcutaneous vein prominent
- It is not a malignant condition.

NOTES

DIFFERENTIAL DIAGNOSIS OF ABDOMINAL LUMP

Abdomen divided into 9 regions, by 2 horizontal and 2 vertical lines.

- Horizontal lines:
  - Upper horizontal—transpyloric line (midway between xiphisternum and umbilicus)—L1
  - Lower horizontal line—transtubercular line (at the level of two tubercle of iliac crest)—L5
- Vertical lines—they are drawn on both sides through the midpoint between anterosuperior iliac spine (ASIS) and pubic symphysis.

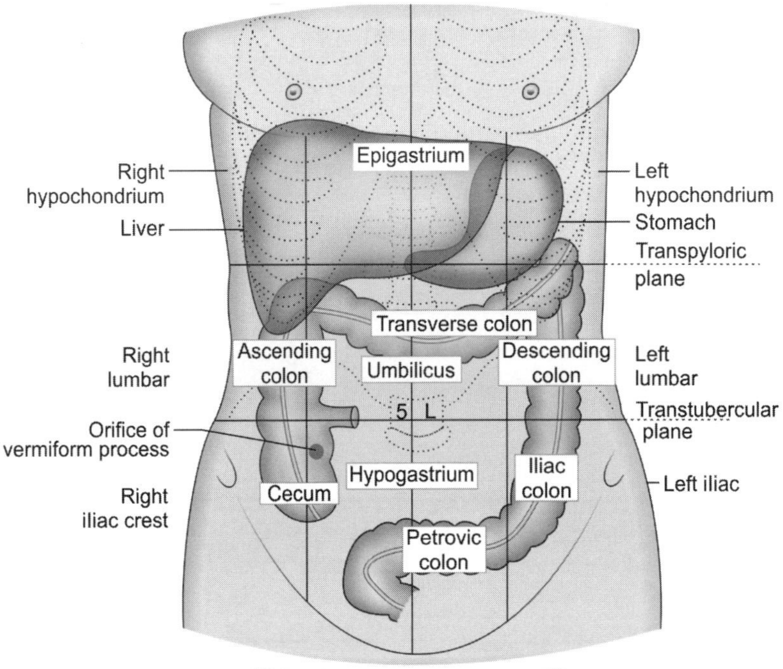

Right hypochondrium
- Liver
- Gallbladder
- Pylorus of stomach and duodenum
- Hepatic flexure of colon
- Right kidney
- Right suprarenal gland

Left hypochondrium
- Spleen
- Stomach
- Left lobe—liver
- Splenic flexure of colon
- Tail of pancreas
- Left kidney
- Left suprarenal gland

Right lumbar
- Liver and gallbladder
- Right kidney
- Ascending colon

Left lumbar
- Left kidney
- Descending colon
- Spleen

Umbilical
- Umbilical hernia
- Stomach and duodenum
- Transverse colon
- Lymph node
- Pancreas
- Aorta
- Retroperitoneal structures

Epigastrium
- Epigastric hernia
- Liver
- Stomach and duodenum
- Transverse colon
- Pancreas
- Lymph node
- Abdominal aorta
- Retroperitoneal structures

Right iliac fossa
- Appendix
- Cecum
- Terminal part of ileum
- Lymph node
- Iliac arteries

Hypogastrium
- Urinary bladder
- Uterus
- Fallopian tube
- Ovary

Left iliac fossa
- Sigmoid colon
- Lymph node
- Desending colon

CARCINOMA STOMACH

PRESENTING COMPLAINT

Abdominal pain—4 years.

History of Present Illness

Complaints started as abdominal pain 4 years back. It was burning type, mainly felt on the upper abdomen radiating to whole abdomen. Initially the pain was intermittent and he was on treatment for dyspepsia. But now the pain is continuous on taking food and the pain is aggravated and there is associated abdominal distension.

Pain get relieved on taking antacids and in sitting position. There was an episode of vomiting two and half years back, which was black in color and contains food particles. He also gives history of black colored stool.

From then onwards he is on treatment. Since then he is having decreased appetite and constipation.

There is loss of weight since 3 months. There is no history of fever or yellowish discoloration of the body. For past 15 days abdominal pain increased in severity and radiates to both axilla. So he was admitted here.

Past history: Peptic ulcer disease, surgery (GJ)

Personal history: Loss of appetite, spicy food, alcohol smoking

Family history: Gastric polyp, atrophic gastritis, pernicious anemia, familial hypogammaglobulinemia.

GENERAL EXAMINATION

Emaciated, pallor +
Loss of skin turgor—due to dehydration (assessment of dehydration important).

Gastrointestinal tract

- Examination of oral cavity
- Oral cavity—normal
- Examination of abdomen.

Inspection

- Abdomen is not distended
- Umbilicus is central and everted
- All regions are moving with respiration
- No dilated veins, scars, sinus or fistula. No visible pulsations
- Visible peristalsis seen in left upper quadrant and moving towards the right side. Hernial orifices are normal. External genitalia—normal.

Palpation

- No local rise of temperature, tenderness
- There is a well-defined mass of 7 × 5 cm with irregular borders in epigastrium and slightly extending to right hypochondrium with irregular surface, hard in consistency, moving with respiration and non-pulsatile. Plane of the swelling is intraperitoneal. The upper border of swelling is palpable. It can insunate fingers between costal margin and the swelling
- No other masses palpable (enlarged liver)
- Renal angle is not tender
- External genitalia and hernial orifices are normal
- No fluid thrill

Percussion

Dullness over the mass, not continuous with liver, no shifting dullness, Traube's space-resonant

Auscultation

- Bowel sounds 3/min, no bruit
- Succussion splash heard
- On **ausculto percussion** stomach is dilated
  - No **left supraclavicular** lymph node enlargement (LNE), axillary LN
  - Skull and spine normal.
  - **PR**—not done.

Other systems: Within normal limits.

CLINICAL FEATURES

• **S**ilent	S
• **T**umor	T
• **O**bstruction	O
• **M**alena	M
• **A**chlorhydria, anemia, asthenia	A
• **C**achexia	C
• **H**ematemesis	H

Why stomach

Symptoms and Signs

- Lump in epigastrium moving up and down with respiration
- Can get above the swelling
- Percussion note impaired
- Ausculto percussion—shows dilated stomach
- Succussion splash is elicited
- Visible gastric peristalsis (VGP)—left to right.

(Ausculto percussion and succussion splash: Suggest gastric outlet obstruction (GOO))

Succussion splash (should not eat or drink within last 3 hours)

Place the bell of the stethoscope in the midepigastrium and fix it with two thumbs and shake the patient's side to side with other fingers of two hands holding the lower end of rib cage. A splashing sound will be heared if it is positive.

Ausculto percussion: Bell of the stethoscope is placed on the midepigastrium. With back of pencil abdominal wall is scratched radially from the edge of bell of stethoscope, starting from below the costal margin up to the left hypochondrium. When scratch is made over the stomach, scratch sound is audible.

GASTRIC OUTLET OBSTRUCTION (GOO)

SYMPTOMS AND SIGNS

- Vomiting
- Visible gastric peristalsis—left to right
- Succussion splash
- Dilation of stomach
- Metabolic abnormalities
- Abdominal distension
- Ball rolling sensation
- Constipation

Causes
- Duodenal ulcer with obstruction
- Distal gastric malignancy
- Acid poisoning with stenosis
- Congenital hypertrophic pyloric stenosis

HYPOCHLOREMIC HYPOKALEMIC METABOLIC ALKALOSIS WITH PARADOXICAL ACIDURIA

Initially the urine has low chlorine and high bicarbonate (reflecting hypochloremia, alkalosis). Bicarbonate is excreted along with sodium and so with time, the patient becomes progressively hyponatremic and more profoundly dehydrated. Because of the dehydration a phase of sodium retention follows and potassium and hydrogen are

SURGERY

excreted in preference. This results in the urine becoming paradoxically acidic and hypokalemia ensues. Alkalosis leads to lowering of circulating ionized calcium and tetani can occur.

JAUNDICE IN CARCINOMA STOMACH

- Infiltration of growth to common bile duct (CBD)
- Secondary lymph nodes in porta hepatis
- Diffuse hepatic metastasis.

Pathway of umbilical nodule formation (Sister Mary Joseph—Nurse to Sir William Mayo)

Growth in lesser curvature
↓
Involvement of lesser omentum
↓
Involvement of ligamentum teres
↓
Umbilicus

VIRCHOW'S NODE

Spread occurs by permeation and embolization through lymphatics to subpyloric, gastric, pancreaticoduodenal, splenic, celiac, aortic and later to left supraclavicular lymph nodes.

CARCINOMA STOMACH—CASE DISCUSSION

INVESTIGATIONS

To Confirm the Diagnosis

- Esophagogastroduodenoscopy (OGDScopy)
  - Can visualize lesion
  - Identify the extent
  - Take biopsy (minimum six samples)
- Barium meal examination.
  - Shows persistent irregular filling defect
  - Shows persistent mucosal irregularity
  - Shows persistent loss of peristalsis

It is superior to OGDScopy
- In linitus plastica
- Lesions in cardia
- Lesions with obstruction

Staging investigation/to know the extent of diseases:

- **USG abdomen tumor thickness**
  - To rule out liver metastasis, ovary
  - To assess regional lymph node
  - Ascites

If LN enlargement FNAC from LN

- **Contrast enhanced computed tomography (CECT)**
  - To determine operability
  - To know mural thickness
  - Invasion to adjacent structures.
- **Endoluminal USG:** Assess tumor thickness and lymph node, local infiltration
- **Diagnostic laparoscopy**
  - To stage the disease
  - Can eliminate need for laparotomy.
- Chest X-ray to rule out pulmonary metastasis
- **PET scan.**

BASELINE INVESTIGATIONS

Management

Preoperative Preparation

- Correct anemia, nutrition, albumin
- Correct fluid and electrolyte distribution

- Arrange blood
- Prophylactic antibiotics.

SURGERY

Principle

- 5 cm proximal and 2 cm distal clearance
- For lesions involving pylorus:
  - Lower partial gastrectomy (<3/4th of stomach removal)
- More proximal lesions involving body:
  - Subtotal gastrectomy (>3/4th removal)
- For lesions involving cardia: Total gastrectomy.

Types of Resection

- **R0**—Resect margin free of gross and microscopic malignancy
- **R1**—Resect margin with microscopic malignancy
- **R2**—Resect margin gross and microscopic malignancy.

Complication of Gastrectomy

Early

- Esophagojejunostomy
- Duodenal stump leak, duodenal blow out
- Biliary peritonitis
- Hemorrhage, sepsis
- Acute pancreatitis

Late

- Due to resection
  - Dumping syndrome, B_{12} deficiency
- Due to anastomosis
  - Leak loop obstruction
  - Alkaline reflex gastritis
  - Retained antrum syndrome
  - Carcinoma of stump

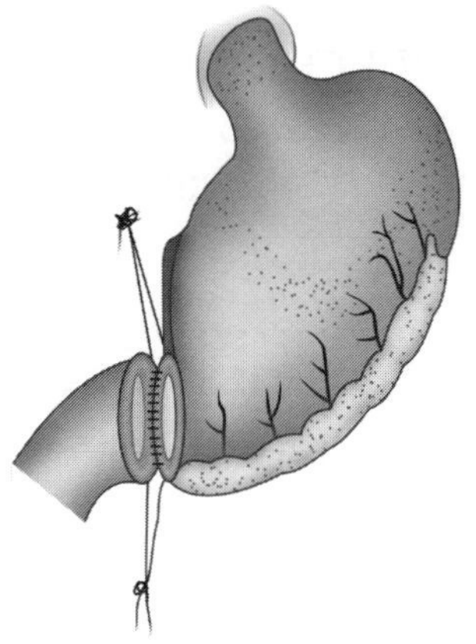

Billroth I gastrectomy. The lower half of the stomach is removed and the cut stomach anastomosed to see first part of the jejunum

Features of early and late dumping syndrome

	Early	*Late*
Incidence	5–10%	5%
Relation to meals	Almost immediate	Second hour after meal
Duration of attack	30–40 minutes	30–40 minutes
Relief	Lying down	Food
Aggravated by	More food	Exercise
Precipitating factor	Food, especially carbohydrate rich and wet	Same
Major symptoms	Epigastric fullness, sweating, light headedness, tachycardia, colic and sometimes diarrhea	Tremor, faintness, prostration

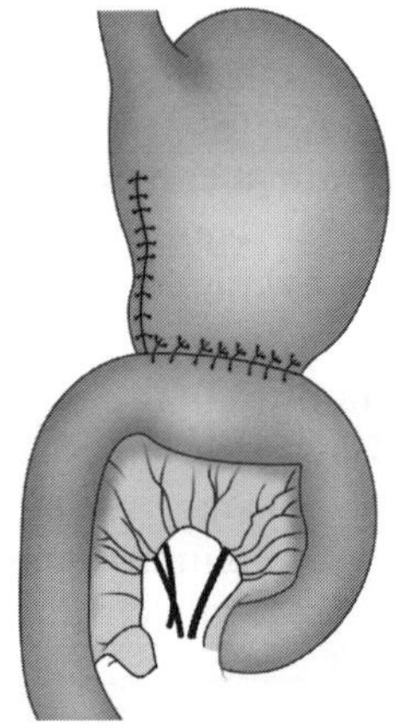

Billroth II. Two-thirds of the stomach are removed, the duodenal stump is closed and the stomach is anastomosed to the jejunum

Signs of inoperability:

- Metastatic liver, presence of jaundice
- Ascites
- Supraclavicular lymph node (Virchow's node/Troisier's sign)
- Irish nodule (enlarged axillary LNE)
- Presence of Blumer's shelf

SURGERY

- Presence of a cutaneous nodule in umbilicus (Sister Mary Joseph's nodule)
- Krukenberg's tumor (enlarged ovaries in pelvic examination)
- Pleural effusion

After resection anastomosis

- **Bilroth II**—side to side gastrojejunostomy
  (Isoperistaltic, retrocolic)
- Polya—End to side anastomosis

After total gastrectomy

- **Roux-en-Y** esophagojejunostomy

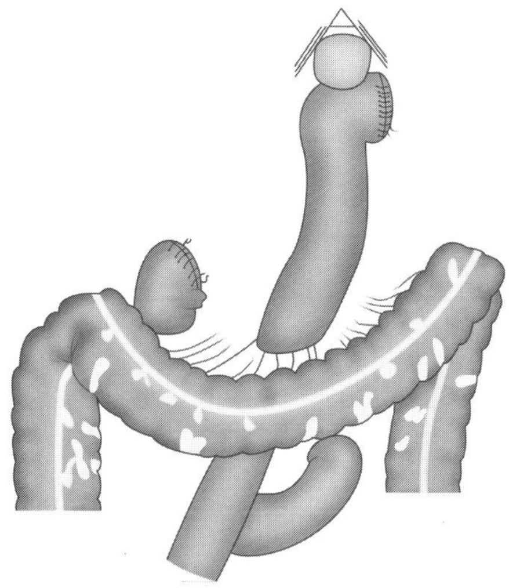

Esophagojejunostomy Roux-en-Y

D2 gastrectomy

Structures removed are:

- Stomach with growth
- Omental bursa
- Entire greater omentum
- Lesser omentum
- Anterior layer of mesocolon
- Anterior pancreatic capsule
- Lymphadenectomy up to N2 nodes

(In general a **D1 resection** involves the removal of perigastric nodes. **D2 resection** involves the clearance of major arterial trunks)

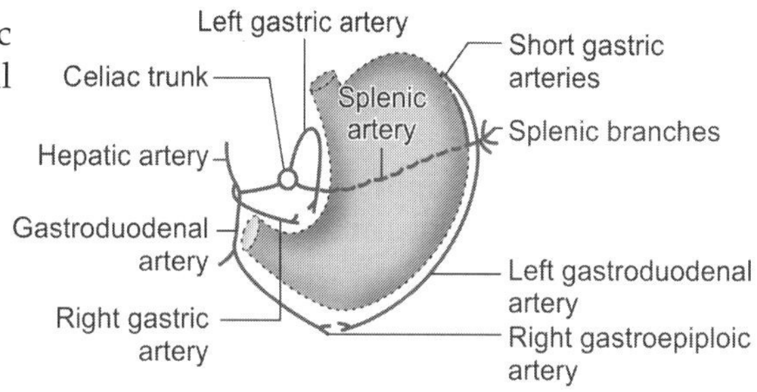

Management of inoperable cases:

- Without complication—chemotherapy
- With complications—palliative surgery and chemotherapy.

Palliative Surgery

- Palliative bypass
  Gastrojejunosotomy + jejunojejunostomy
  Or
  Esophagojejunostomy + jejunojejunostomy
- Stenting
- Laser
- Photodynamic therapy

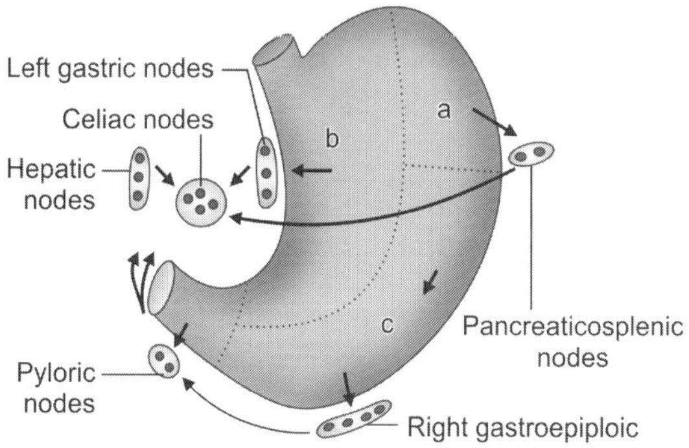

Chemotherapy

- **F**: 5 fluorouracil (5FU)
- **A** : adriamycin
- **M**: mitomycin
- **FOLFOX**: Folinic acid, 5FU, oxaliplatin

Radiotherapy—in bony metastasis

Most common site of recurrence—stomach bed.

Stomach bed

- Diaphragm
- Left adrenal
- Left kidney
- Transverse mesocolon
- Pancreas
- Splenic flexure of colon
- Splenic artery
- Spleen (sometimes)

Treatment: Self-expandable metal stents

Anatomy

- Parts of stomach
- Blood supply
- Lymphatic drain

(i) Early Gastric Cancer: Confined to Mucosa and Submucosa

Japanese classification
- **Type I:** Protruding
- **Type II:** Superficial
  - Elevated
  - Flat
  - Depressed
- **Type III:** Excavated

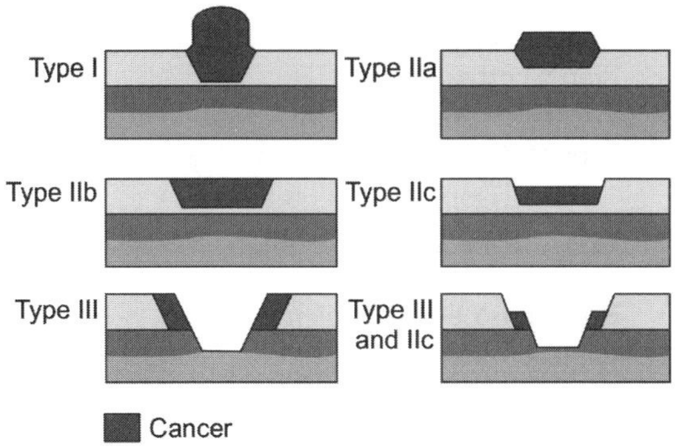

Japanese classification of early gastric cancer

Minimally invasive procedure for early gastric cancer
- Endoscopic mucosal resection
- Laparoscopic wedge resection
- Pylorus preserving gastrectomy
- Photodynamic therapy

(ii) Advanced Gastric Cancer (Involvement of Muscularis)

Borrmann classification of advanced gastric cancer
- **Type I:** Polypoidal
- **Type II:** Ulcerative
- **Type III:** Ulcerative and polypoidal
- **Type IV:** Diffuse—linitis plastica

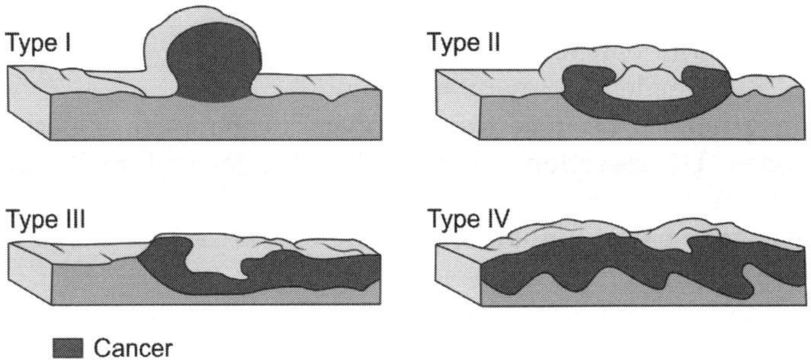

Borrmann classification of advanced gastric cancer

Linitis plastica (leather-bottle stomach)

It is an aggressive diffuse type of carcinoma stomach wherein there is enormous proliferation of tissue involving submucosa of stomach which is thickened mucosa looks and feel normal.

Investigation: Small sized stomach in barium meal study.

Treatment: Poor prognosis.

AJCC staging	
T	**T1**: Involving mucosa and submucosa **T2**: Involving muscularis **T3**: Involving serosa **T4**: Extend beyond serosa
N	**N0**: No nodes **N1**: Involvement of 1–2 nodes **N2**: Involvement of 3–6 nodes **N3**: Involvement of >6 nodes **N3a:** –7–15 nodes **N3b:** – >15 nodes.
M	**M0**: No distal mets **M1**: Distant mets

Japanese Research Society LN Station
- 1-6 nodes: N1 nodes perigastric
- 7-11 nodes: N2 nodes along named vessels
- 12-14 nodes: N3 intraperitoneal
- 15-16 nodes: N4

Stage		Code
0	Tis N_0 M_0	0
IA	T_1 N_0 M_0	1
IB	T_1 N_1 M_0 T_2 N_0 M_0	2
IIA	T_1 N_2 M_0 T_2 N_1 M_0 T_3 N_0 M_0	3
IIB	T_1 N_3 M_0 T_2 N_2 M_0 T_3 N_1 M_0 T_{4a} N_0 M_0	4
IIIA	T_2 N_2 M_0 T_3 N_2 M_0 $T4_a$ N_1 M_0	5
IIIB	T_3 N_3 M_0 T_{4a} N_2 M_0 T_{4b} N_1 M_0	6
IIIC	T_{4a} N_3 M_0 T_{4b} N_2–N_3 M_0	7
IV	Any T, Any N, M_1	

Nodal stations:

1. Right cardiac
2. Left cardiac
3. Lesser curvature
4. Greater curvature
5. Suprapyloric
6. Infrapyloric
7. Nodes along left gastric artery
8. Common hepatic artery
9. Celiac
10. Splenic hilar
11. Splenic artery
12. Hepatic pedicle
13. Retropancreatic
14. Mesenteric
15. Middle colic
16. Para-arortic
17. Infradiaphragmatic
18. Esophageal hiatal
19. Lower esophageal
20. Supradiaphragmatic

Risk factors for Carcinoma stomach

- Diet—smoked fish, excessive salt intake, chilly, deficiency of antioxidants, exposure to nitroso compounds
- Smoking, obesity
- Gastritis, *H. pylori* (direct causation)
- Gastric atrophy
- Gastric polyps
- Pernicious anemia, Menetrier's disease, blood group A
- Postgastrectomy patients.

Lauren's classification (DIO)

- Diffuse—infiltrate deep to stomach
  - Localized
  - Generalized (linitis plastica)
- Intestinal—in cases of intestinal metaplasia better prognosis
- Others.

Correa cycle

H. pylori - gastritis - gastric atrophy - metaplasia - dysplasia - carcinoma in situ - carcinoma

Distal gastric cancer vs proximal gastric cancer

Distal	*Proximal*
Diet and environment related	Not
Instestinal histology	Diffuse
Better prognosis	Bad
Need distal subtotal gastrectomy	Need total gastrectomy

	Diffuse *Vs*	*Intestinal*
Histology:	Normal gastric mucosa	Areas of intestinal metaplasia
Infiltration:	Diffuse	Localized
Metastasis:	Frequent	Infrequent
Sex:	Female>male	Male>female
Prognosis:	Worse	Better

5 modes of spread:

1. Horizontal spread—along the stomach wall
2. Vertical—invasion of stomach wall and to adjacent structures like colon and pancreas, etc.
3. Lymphatic spread
4. Peritoneal dissemination
5. Blood stream spread—to liver, lung, bone (LLB)

Sievert classification for proximal gastric cancer

- **Type I**: Esophageal Ca involving OG junction
- **Type II**: Primary OG junction growth
- **Type III**: Stomach lesion involving junction.

Gastrointestinal stromal tumor (GIST)
Previously called leiomyoma/leiomyosarcoma
- Anywhere in GIT, 50% in stomach
- Tyrosine kinase C kit oncogene
- Treatment—imatinib

Treatment (surgical) duodenal ulcer
- GJ + TV (gastrojejunostomy + truncal vagotomy)

NOTES

COLORECTAL CARCINOMA

INVESTIGATIONS

General:
- Blood routine
- Occult blood
- Carcinoembryonic antigen (CEA)

Diagnostic:
- Colonoscopy
- Virtual colonoscopy CT
- Double contrast barium enema

Staging:
- Chest X-ray
- USG abdomen
- CECT abdomen thorax

Right colon
- Ulcerative growth
- No obstructive features
- Stools are liquid
- Altered blood through rectum
- No history of tenesmus

Left colon
- Cicatrizing
- Obstructive features present
- More solid stools
- Fresh blood through rectum
- Tenesmus

DISCUSSIONS

Etiology of Colorectal Carcinoma

- Dietary factors, red meet, decreased fiber, increased animal fat, refined carbohydrate
- Alcohol, smoking
- Inflammatory bowel disease
- Familial adenomatous polyposis
- Hereditary nonpolyposis colorectal cancer (HNPCC)
- Cholecystectomy.

Blood Supply

- Marginal artery of Drummond: It is a single arterial trunk along the large intestine from ileocecal junction to rectosigmoid junction.
- Arc of Riolan: Collaterals connecting middle colic to left colic artery
- Griffiths point: It is the weak point in the anastomosis between middle colic and left colic artery.

Lymphatic Drainage

There are four groups
a. Epicolic—located on bowel wall
b. Paracolic—along marginal artery
c. Intermediate—located along colic vessels
d. Apical—located along superior mesenteric artery (SMA) and inferior mesenteric artery (IMA).

Dukes staging
A. Tumors confined to the wall
B. Penetrating through bowel wall
C. LN involvement
D. Distant metastasis (in modified Duke's staging)

TNM staging:
T1: Tumor involving submucosa
T2: Involving muscularis propria
T3: Invasion through the muscularis propria, but not through serosa
T4: Directly invades other organs

TREATMENT

- T1—surgery, no chemotherapy
- T2—surgery
  - +/– chemotherapy
  - + if perforation, high levels of CEA, ascites
- T3, T4—surgery + chemotherapy

SURGERY

No touch technique of Turnbull. Here dividing vascular pedicle at the beginning of surgery will reduce tumor embolization.

For operability look for:
- Liver for secondaries
- Peritoneum and omentum for secondaries
- LN palpated

- Look for tumor mobility and adjacent structures involved
  - Carcinoma of right colon and cecum = right hemicolectomy
  - Carcinoma of transverse colon = extended hemicolectomy or V resection
  - Carcinoma left colon= left colectomy
  - Carcinoma of sigmoid colon= sigmoid resection

Prognostic Factors

- Staging
- CEA levels high
- Bowel obstruction, ascitis.

Synchronous carcinoma: In the case of colon cancer look for the presence of second malignancy in colon at different area. This is called synchronous carcinoma.

Metachronous:
- If it develops after the resection of malignancy
- It is called metachronous.

Chemotherapy

FOLFOX regimen

Follow-Up

- CEA level
- Chest X-ray
- Colonoscopy

Pathological types of carcinoma colon
- Ulcerative lesion
- Cauliflower like lesion
- Structure—annular and tubular

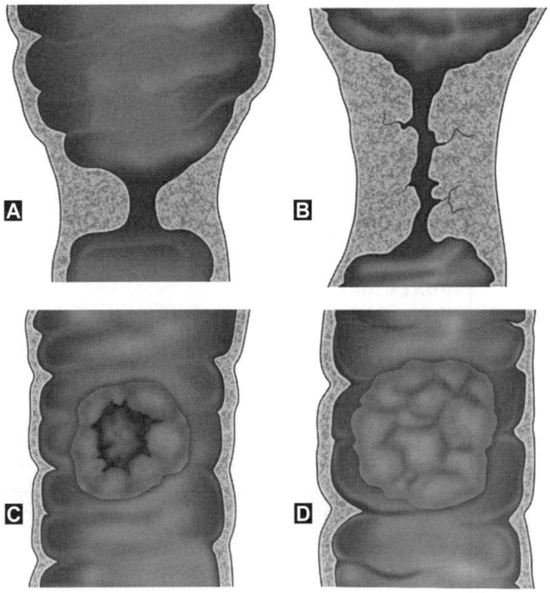

The four common macroscopic varieties of carcinoma of the colon (A) Annular; (B) Tubular; (C) Ulcer and (D) Cauliflower

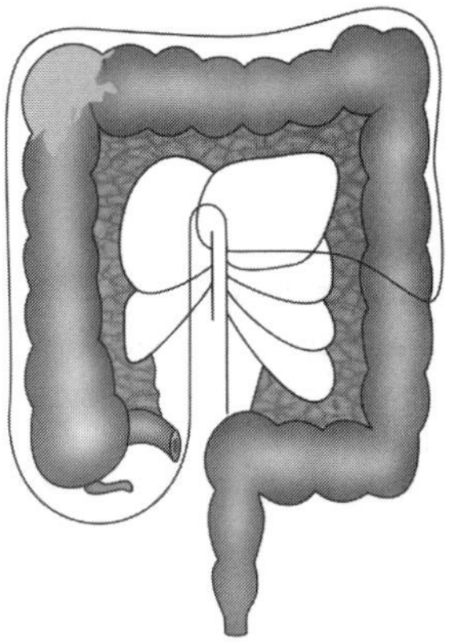

Area to be resected when the growth is situated at the hepatic flexure

RIGHT ILIAC FOSSA MASS

DIFFERENTIAL DIAGNOSIS

Any structure in right iliac fossa (RIF), commonly:
- Carcinoma of cecum
- Appendicular mass
- Ileocecal TB

Others
- Lymph node
- Retroperitoneal mass
- Hydronephrosis, ovarian mass.

CARCINOMA OF CECUM—DISCUSSED EARLIER (CA COLON)

Appendicular Mass

- Short duration
- History of Murphy's triad (fever, pain, vomiting)
- Patient ill looking
- Tender mass in the right iliac fossa

It is the complication of appendicitis (as a result of small perforation in the appendix, omentum try to seal the perforation and leading to mass).

Treatment: Patient treated conservatively (patient is not operated).

Oshner-Sherren regimen
- A—aspiration with Ryle's tube to give rest to gut
- B—bowel care—purgative not used (may cause perforation)
- C—charts—temperature, pulse, respiration, diameter of mass
- D—drugs to cover all organism (antibiotics)
- E—exploratory laparotomy should not done
- F—fluids

During the course of conservative treatment appendicular mass, one should suspect appendicular abscess

Features of Appendicular Abscess

- Rising pulse rate
- Increasing abdominal pain
- Increasing in size of mass
- Patient looking ill

	Carcinoma cecum	Appendicular mass	Ileocecal tuberculosis
Age	Above 50 years	Younger	Middle age
Onset	Insidious/asymptomatic	Acute—3 days after initial symptom attacks	Subacute—recurrent
Symptoms	Lump abdomen	Murphy's triad	Recurrent attacks of abdominal pain, diarrhea, evening raise of temperature
Nature of mass	Hard	Irregular, firm, tender	Irregular, doughy
Intrinsic movement	Fixed	Fixed	Fixed
Response to antibiotics	No response	Become smaller and then disappears	No response
Radiological signs	Irregular filling defect in cecum which is in normal position	No specific signs	Pulled up cecum, obtuse ileocecal angle, Fleischner's sign, Sterlin's sign

RETROPERITONEAL TUMOR

INVESTIGATIONS

- Blood
  - Alpha fetoprotein
  - Human chorionic gonadotropin (hCG)
  - Liver function test (LFT)
  - Renal function test (RFT)
- Contrast enhanced computed tomography (CECT)
- Magnetic resonance imaging (MRI)
- Retroperitoneal core needle biopsy under USG guidance only if inoperable by CECT.

DISCUSSION

- Features of retroperitoneal tumor
  - It would not cross the midline
  - No movement with respiration
  - Tumor fixed
  - Knee elbow position—mass does not fall forward
  - Carnet test—mass is intra-abdominal
- Retroperitoneal structures—kidney, adrenals, pancreas, ureter, duodenum, ascending colon, descending colon.
- Most common retroperitoneal tumor—liposarcoma
- Tumor arise from fat, fascia, lymphatics.

CLASSIFICATION

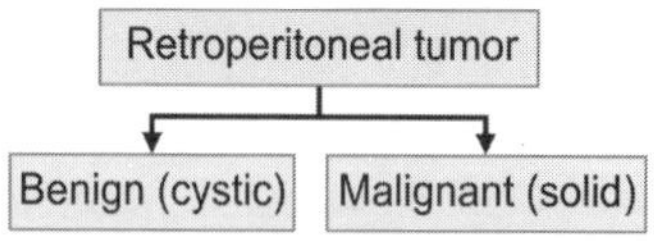

TREATMENT

- Complete en block surgical excision
- Chemotherapy
  - adriamycin, iphosphamide, mesna (AIM)
  - MAID (AIM + dacarbazine).

OBSTRUCTIVE JAUNDICE

CLINICAL EXAMINATION

History

- Duration of jaundice, progress, intermittent or continuous
- Clay-colored stools
- Itching
- Loss of weight and appetite, fever
- Previous history of jaundice (stones). History of abdominal pain
- Drug history [Antituberculous treatment (ATT), oral contraceptive pill, anabolic steroids like testosterone produce cholestatic jaundice]
- Any symptoms of liver failure (bleeding, edema, encephalopathy)
- History of previous abdominal surgery, blood transfusion, travel to outside
- Stools—silvery stools—periampullary carcinoma
- Family history—hemolytic jaundice runs in family are sickle cell anemia, storage disease
- Personal history—addictions.

INVESTIGATION

- Urine
- Blood
- X-ray
- Ultrasonography (USG)
- Contrast enhanced computed tomography (CECT)
- Endoscopic retrograde cholangiopancreatography (ERCP)
- Magnetic resonance cholangiopancreatography (MRCP)
- Endoscopic ultrasound (EUS)
- Diagnostic laparoscopy
- Tumor marker CA 19-9.

Urine

- Bile salt—Hay's test
- Bile pigment—modified Fouchet's test
- Urobilinogen—Ehrlich's test.

Blood

Liver Function Test

- Albumin—if <3 g/dL—give albumin to prevent anastomotic leakage
- Bilirubin—conjugated and unconjugated
- Enzyme—alkaline phosphatase (ALP) and gamma-glutamyl transferase (GGT)
- Prothrombin time/International Normalized Ratio (PT/INR) (give vitamin K 10 mg IM for 5 days/FFP 6–10 units).

X-ray

Bile stone—Seagull/Mercedes-Benz sign (90% renal stone—opaque; 10% gallstone—opaque).

USG

- Intrahepatic biliary radical dilation
- CBD dilatation >10 mm
- Number and size of stone
- If malignant—lymph node, ascites.

CECT : To find site, extent, other structures involved in a case of carcinoma head of pancreas, operability

ERCP :

- Diagnostic—cytology, biopsy
- Therapeutic—stenting, sphincterotomy, stone removal from distal CBD
- Adverse effect—sepsis, pancreatitis.

MRCP: noninvasive, high specificity, sensitivity, diagnostic

EUS: Ca head of pancreas, periampullary carcinoma to know the extent of tumor, lymph node status.

Diagnostic laparoscopy

CA 19-9

TREATMENT FOR CARCINOMA HEAD OF PANCREAS

- Preoperative preparation
- Rehydration 10% or 5% dextrose
- Adequate nutrition
- Maintenance of urine output
- Vitamin K if necessary 10 mg for 5 days
- Procedure – Whipple surgery under GA
  - Roof top/Chevron incision
  - Open—look for ascites, liver, peritoneum
  - Kocherization—mobilization of duodenum

- Look for involvement of superior mesenteric vein, portal vein
- Then remove:
  - Pancreas at the junction of head and neck
  - Distal (40%) of stomach
  - C- loop of duodenum
  - 15 cm proximal jejunum
  - Gallbladder and lower CBD
- Then anastomose
  - Pancreaticojejunostomy
  - Choledochojejunostomy
  - Gastrojejunostomy

COMPLICATION

- Biliary leakage
- Sepsis
- Hepatorenal syndrome.

Why pylorus and C-loop of duodenum is removing along with head of pancreas?
Ans – Because of common blood supply.

Why gallbladder is removing?
Ans – Physiology of gallbladder filling is retrograde filling which depends on sphincter of CBD.
Other optional procedure

- PPPD (pylorus preserving pancreato-duodenostomy)
- Palliative surgery—for inoperable tumor, for pain, GOO, jaundice
- Jaundice—surgical biliary bypass (cholecystojejunostomy
- ERCP stent
- PTC stent
- GOO—gastrojejunostomy
- Duodenal stent.

Pain

- Stepwise escalation of analgesia
- Transthoracic splanchnicectomy
- Celiac plexus block.

BILE DUCT STONE—CHOLEDOCHOLITHIASIS

Treatment

Cholecystectomy

- It may be open or laparoscopic
- After cholecystectomy the indication for CBD exploration
  - Palpable stone in CBD
  - Stone in CBD by radiology
  - CBD dilatation
  - Recurrent attack of jaundice.
- After CBD is longitudinally incised, remove stone and put a T tube and suture over it, then long end of T tube is taken out.
- After 10 days do a T tube cholangiogram
  - If no residual stone:
    - Clip T tube for 48 hours and if no problem is there remove the T tube
  - If there is residual stone:
    - Remove the T tube after 6 weeks until track is matured
    - Then remove the stone by a choledochoscope (Burhene technique) or Fogarty catheter or Dormia basket.

Complication of cholecystectomy
- Hemorrhage from hepatic artery
- Injury to liver
- Stricture CBD
- Post-cholecystectomy syndrome

SURGERY

Difference between choledocholithiasis and Ca head of pancreas

Disease	*Symptom*	*Pain*	*Jaundice*
Choledocholithiasis	Episodes of flatulent dyspepsia	Intermittent severe	Sudden onset, fades
	Pain		Slowly in days
Ca head of pancreas	Loss of weight loss of appetite	Backache	Progressive jaundice

Difference between periampullary Ca and Ca head of pancreas

Features	*Ca head of pancreas*	*Periampullary carcinoma*
Pain and weight loss	Early features	Late features
Jaundice	Persistent and progressive	Intermittent
Occult blood in stool	Absent	Present, stools are silvery
Endoscopic examination growth	Not visible	Growth visible
Prognosis	Not good	Good

BARIUM MEAL

- Reverse 3 sign—periampullary carcinoma
- Pad sign—widened C loop of duodenum in carcinoma head of pancreas.

CHOLEDOCHOLITHIASIS

It is the stone in the CBD and biliary tree.

Clinical Features

- Pain, jaundice, fever with chills and rigors
- Charcot's triad of ascending cholangitis
  - Intermittent pain
  - Intermittent fever
  - Intermittent jaundice

Reynolds pentad of acute obstructive cholangitis—pain, fever, jaundice, shock, altered mental status.

GALLSTONE

Common in fat fertile forty female

Types:
- Cholesterol stones—Solitary, stones soft
- Pigment stones—Multiple
- Mixed stones

PIGMENT STONE

It may be:
- Black—insoluble bilirubin pigment mixed with calcium phosphate and calcium bicarbonate
- Brown pigment—contains calcium bilirubinate, calcium palmitate and calcium stearate.

FACTORS ASSOCIATED WITH GALLSTONE FORMATION

- Altered GB function:
  - Stasis
  - Poor emptying
  - Poor absorption
  - Infection
- Supersaturated bile:
  - Sex—female
  - Age—40
  - Obesity—fat
  - Diet—high calories
- Cholesterol nucleating factors:
  - Glycoprotein
  - Mucus
  - Infection

Renal stone
- Oxalate
- Phosphate— Struvite (ammonium, magnesium phosphate)
- Uric acid, urate calculi
- Cystine calculi
- Xanthine calculi

Only uric acid stone is radiolucent

- Altered enterohepatic circulation:
  - Ileal resection
  - Ileal disease
  - Altered bowel transit time
  - Altered bowel flora
  - Cholestyramine
  - Deoxycholate

Complications of gallstone

In gallbladder	*In bile duct*	*In intestine*
Silent stone	Cholangitis	Obstruction
Cholecystitis	Obstructive jaundice	
Empyema	Pancreatitis	
Gangrene		
Perforation		
Mucocele		
Carcinoma		

Clinical Features

- Right upper quadrant or epigastric pain which may radiate to back
- Dyspepsia, flatulence, food intolerance
- On examination Murphy sign—in acute inflammation, tenderness at right upper quadrant and it is exacerbated during inspiration.

Theories of gallstone
- Indection
- Hemolysis
- Stasis
- Metabolic

Investigation

USG abdomen, X-ray.

Treatment

Conservative treatment followed by cholecystectomy.

Conservative treatment
- NPO and IV fluid
- Analgesic
- Antibiotics—cefazolin, cefuroxime
- Cholestyramine for pruritus.

COURVOISIER'S LAW

In a jaundiced person, if gallbladder is palpable, it is unlikely due to stones because previous inflammation will have made gallbladder thick and nondistensible.

Exceptions

- Mucocele or empyema Gallbladder
- Double impaction of stones occluding cystic duct and CBD
- Oriental cholangiohepatitis (clonorchis sinensis)
- Pancreatic calculi obstructing ampulla.

CAUSES OF OBSTRUCTIVE JAUNDICE

In the lumen	*In the wall*	*Outside the wall*
• Gallstone • Parasite • Foreign	• Strictures • Atresia • Body choledochal cyst • Caroli's disease • Klatskin's tumor • Cholangiocarcinoma	• Ca head of pancreas • Periampullary Ca • Porta hepatis metastasis • Pancreatitis

MIRIZZI SYNDROME

Gallstones impact in the gallbladder and compress it causing pressure necrosis and get adherent to CBD wall and causes compression of CBD:
- Type I: Compression of CBD without lumen narrowing
- Type II: Compression causing CBD lumen narrowing
- Type III: Compression causing CBD wall necrosis
- Type IV: Cholecysto-choledochal fistula.

NOTES

VARICOSE VEIN

CASE FORMAT

- Name
- Biodata

PRESENTING COMPLAINTS

Dilated veins over the left lower limb—4 years.

History of Present Illness

He noticed dilated veins over left lower limb 4 years back. It was extending to thigh also. It was associated with dull aching pain more towards evening and pain was relieved on lying down. He also complaints of ankle swelling towards the end of the day.

About 3 years back he noticed itchy skin lesions over the left leg which later blackened.

There is no history of ulceration, bleeding, painful swelling of leg (DVT), no history of abdominal distension, constipation, micturition problems.

Past History

No history of major surgery, immobilization, drug intake, long air travel, chest pain, breathlessness, hemoptysis (pulmonary thromboembolism).

Personal History

Female—history of OCP.

Family History

No similar illness in family.

LOCAL EXAMINATION

Inspection

There are dilated veins involving the medial aspect of the left lower limb extending from just below the medial malleolus to middle of thigh.

There is loss of hair and skin is shiny. There is no redness, congestion, ulceration or scar. There is no brittleness of nails.

There is no impulse on coughing at saphenous opening (Morrissey's test)—saphena varix.

Palpation

There is no local rise of temperature or tenderness. There is no edema or skin thickening.

- Trendelenburg test 1 and 2 positive
- Tourniquet test +ve in all perforator sites
- Modified Perthe's test—negative
- Schwartz test is positive
- Fegan's test shows multiple defect in deep fascia
  - Signs of DVT [Mose's sign, Homan's sign—usually not done (risk of pulmonary embolism)]

Percussion

Schwartz test is positive.

Auscultation

No venous hum, bruit

- There is no regional lymph node enlargement
- No nerve lesions
- All peripheral pulses felt equally on both sides

Other limb—normal.

SURGERY

Examination of Abdomen

- No mass palpable
- No shifting dullness or fluid thrill.

VARICOSE VEINS—DISCUSSION

Diagnosis

Varicose veins of left lower limb involving long saphenous system with multiple perforator incompetence and saphenofemoral junction incompetence without complication.

CEAP Classification

- C – Clinical classification
- E – Etiological
- A – Anatomical
- P – Pathophysiological

C – Clinical

0 – no visible or palpable sign of venous diseases
1 – telangiectasias/reticular veins
2 – varicose veins
3 – edema
4 – skin changes (eczema, lipodermatosclerosis)
5 – + healed ulceration
6 – + active ulceration

E – Etiological

Ec – congenital
Ep – primary (undetermined cause)
Es – secondary (post-thrombotic, post-traumatic)

A – Anatomical

As – superficial
Ad – deep veins
Ap – perforating veins

P – Pathophysiological classification

Pr – reflux
Po – obstruction
Pro– reflux and obstruction

Investigations for Varicose Veins

- Doppler ultrasound imaging
- Duplex ultrasound imaging
- USG abdomen
- Others
  - Photoplethismography
  - Venography (phlebography)—invasive
  - Ambulatory venous pressure studies
  - Raju's test—arm foot venous pressure studies

- **Doppler USG**: A bidirectional flow probe will identify venous reflux
- **Duplex ultrasound imaging:**
  - It is a combination of Doppler ultrasound and B-mode imaging
  - Gives anatomical, physiological and functional details
  - Can visualize lumen, flow, direction and reflux of blood
- USG abdomen: To rule out abdominal pathology in suspected cases of secondary varicose veins
- Venography—invasive, not used nowadays
  - Indication—recurrent varicose veins, complex anatomy
  - Here dye is injected into femoral veins with patient standing

- Normally the foot pressure is equal to or slightly higher (by 5 mm of Hg) than hand pressure: In venous obstruction this pressure is more (10–15 mm of Hg)—Raju's test.

Management

- Reassurance
- Elastic compression stockings
- Injection selerotherapy
- Surgery
- Laser therapy

Indication for treatment
- Varicose veins that cause discomfort
- Cosmetic
- Complications

Compression stockings

Available in three grades—class 1, 2, 3
- Class I: 14–17 mm Hg
- Class II: 18–24 mm Hg
- Class III: 25–35 mm Hg

Injection sclerotherapy (Fegans method)
- Indications: In the treatment of VV in the absence of junctional incompetence of major perforating veins
- For smaller veins <3 mm in size.
- Agents used
  - STD—sodium tetradecyl sulphate
  - Polidocanol
  - Ethanolamine oleate

Technique: Sclerosant is injected into an empty vein and vein is compressed. Endothelial lining is destroyed (aseptic inflammation—thrombosis and fibrosis).

Foam Sclerotherapy (Tessari technique)

Using a 3 way rapid to and fro movements of the piston of syringe, the foam is produced. The foam is then injected into the vein, the air is absorbed, the vein collapses and the endothelial lining is destroyed. Much large volume can be injected into the vein with a small quantity of sclerosant

Echoscleortherapy: Done under duplex ultrasound

Microsclerotherapy: Using a 30 G needle.

Complications of Sclerotherapy

- Skin pigmentation—due to extravasation of dye
- Injury to skin and ulceration
- Allergic reaction
- Thrombophlebitis
- Deep vein thrombosis.

Surgery

Deep vein thrombosis is a contraindication to surgery, since it may be the only route of venous drainage in lower limb.

- **Trendelenberg's operation**
  - Identification, isolation and ligation of named tributaries: Superficial external pudendal, superficial inferior epigastric and superficial circumflex iliac vein
  - Juxtafemoral flush ligation of saphenous vein with femoral vein
  - Excision of 5–10 cm segment of long saphenous vein
- **Multiple perforator ligation**
  - Extrafacial—identify T junction, ligate and divide branches of T
  - Subfacial—Linton operation (long incision along the medial part of tibia, divide and elevate deep facia and ligate and divide perforator)
- **Stripping**
  - The saphenous trunk is retrogradely stripped to knee using a Myer's stripper or Babcock's or rigid metal pin stripper. Stripping not done below to knee to avoid injury to saphenous nerve

- Stripping of short saphenous vein is done from ankle below upwards after passing stripper from above downwards. There is chance of injury to sural nerve.
- Inverting or invaginating stripping using rigid Oesch pin stripper is better (less postoperative pain hematoma)

- **Hook phlebotomy:** Residual veins after stripping can be managed by small hooks, that is inserted through incisions of 1–2 mm in size
- **VNUS closure:** This is the intraluminal destruction of long and short saphenous vein using ablation catheter under USG guidance.
- **TRIVEX**: Removing of superficial vein by suction followed by injection of large amount of fluids
- **Radiofrequency ablation (RFA)**
- **Endovenous laser ablation**
- **Subfacial endoscopic perforator ligation surgery (SEPS).**

Postoperative Management

- Foot end elevation, analgesia
- Compression bandaging is applied to the limb, after 2 days the bandage may be replaced with compression stockings.

Complication of Varicose Vein Surgery

- Pain, discomfort, bruising
- Nerve injury
  - Saphenous nerve for long saphenous surgery
  - Sural nerve for short saphenous surgery
- Venous thrombosis in residual varices
- Deep vein thrombosis (DVT)
- Recurrence.

Complications of Varicose Veins

- Hemorrhage
- Superficial thrombhophlebitis
- Eczema
- Pigmentation
- Lipodermatosclerosis
- Venous ulcer
- Deep vein thrombosis (rarely)
- Marjolin's ulcer (squamous cell carcinoma)
- Calcification
- Periostitis
- Talipes equinus.

Deep vein thrombosis (DVT)
- Homan's sign
- Moses' sign
- Treatment-May Husni operation, Palma's operation

Varicose ulcer Vs	**Venous ulcer**
• Due to pure superficial insufficiency (long standing SFJ incompetence) • History of long standing superficial varicosity • Painless • Does not penetrate deep fascia • Ankle edema may not be there • Respond to surgical treatment of the	• Due to incompetence of perforator and deep venous incompetence. It may be post-thrombotic venous damage • History of DVT followed by lower limb edema • Painful • Penetrate • Ankle edema • Does not respond to treatment

Features of Venous Ulcer

- Seen at gaiter area—on medial side lower third of leg
- Any shape
- Sloping edge
- Floor with granulation tissue/slough/white fibrous tissue
- Surrounding tissue shows features of chronic venous hypertension—pigmentation, eczema, lipodermatosclerosis
- Movements of ankle joint may be limited by scarring of ulcer—equinus deformity

Pathophysiology of Venous Ulcer

White cell trapping theory:
↓
Venous hypertension
↓
Blood slows down in capillaries
↓
WBC marginate and are trapped
↓
Leukocyte sequestration
↓
Activation of trapped WBC
↓
Release of proteolytic enzymes
↓
Damage to capillary endothelium
↓
Leg ulcer

Fibrin cuff theory:
↓
Persistently raised venous pressure
↓
Increased capillary leakage
↓
Perivascular cuff of fibrin, collagen around capillaries
↓
Fibrotic process affecting the skin and subcutaneous fat
↓
Barrier to diffusion preventing nutrient exchange
↓
Anoxia
↓
Ulcer

Champagne bottle leg (inverted beer bottle appearance)
Lipodermatosclerosis will present as palpable induration in gaiter area contraction of skin and subcutaneous result in narrowing of the ankle area.

The combination of narrow ankle and prominent calf is known as the champagne bottle

Atrophic blanche: Superficial vein are lost from skin and white patches develops (skin damage due to venous valvular incompetence)

Management: Rule out PVD and sensory loss

Investigations
- RBS
- Culture and sensitivity
- Biopsy—if nonhealing.

Treatment of Bisgaard's regime
- Elevation of limb
- Elastocrepe bandage
- Exercise
- Education

Drug Treatment for Venous Ulcer

Aspirin, prostaglandin E analog, calcium dobesilate

ANATOMY

- Superficial veins
  - Long saphenous system
  - Short saphenous system with branches
- Deep veins
  - Three pairs below knee—anterior tibial, posterior tibial, peroneal

- Popliteal vein
- Superficial femoral vein

- Perforating veins—in long saphenous vein:
  - Hunters perforator in thigh
  - Dodd's perforator in above knee
  - Boyd's perforator below knee
  - Cockett's perforator above ankle (5, 10, 15 cm above malleolus)
  - Ankle perforators of May or Kuster.

  For all practical purposes there is no perforator in short saphenous system.

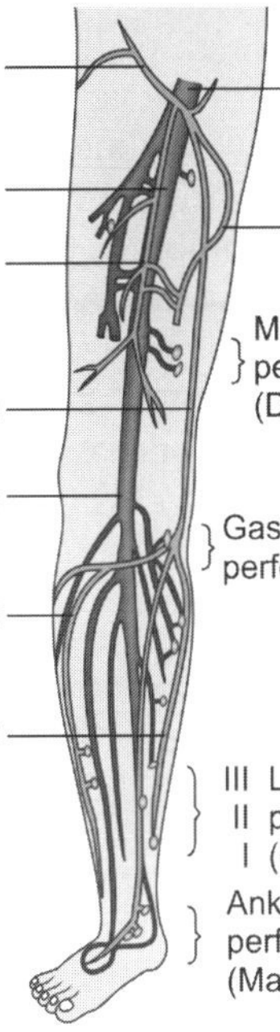

Anatomy of Long Saphenous System

- Biggest vein in body
- Arise in front of medial malleolus
- Ascends behind medial femoral condyle along the medial aspect of thigh and terminate in the common femoral vein through the saphenous opening in groin.

Tributaries

- Posterior arch vein (Leonardo's vein)
- Anterior superficial tibial vein
- Medial and lateral accessory saphenous vein

At saphenofemoral junction

- Superficial inferior epigastric
- Superficial circumflex iliac
- Superficial external pudendal

Short saphenous system

Vein starts behind the lateral malleolus and ascend superficially through posterior aspect of calf to terminate in the popliteal vein after piercing deep fascia.

Physiology

- Normally the venous blood flow (superficial via perforators to deep veins)
- Normal pressure in superficial vein of foot and ankle is around 80–100 mm of Hg
- The venous blood is pumped to the heart from limbs by series of muscle pumps—foot pump, calf pump, thigh pump also called peripheral heart. During walking the pressure within the calf rises to 200–300 mm of Hg and the blood is pushed from the deep system.
- During relaxation of calf muscles the pressure within the calf falls to a low level and the blood from superficial veins flow through the perforators to deep veins and the pressure within superficial system will then automatically fall to about 20 mm of Hg
- Failure of superficial venous pressure fall during exercise is called ambulatory venous hypertension and is the main cause of venous leg ulceration.

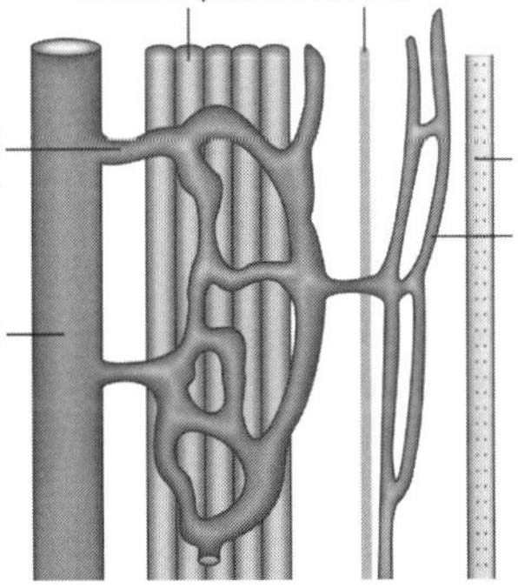

Indirect perforating vein

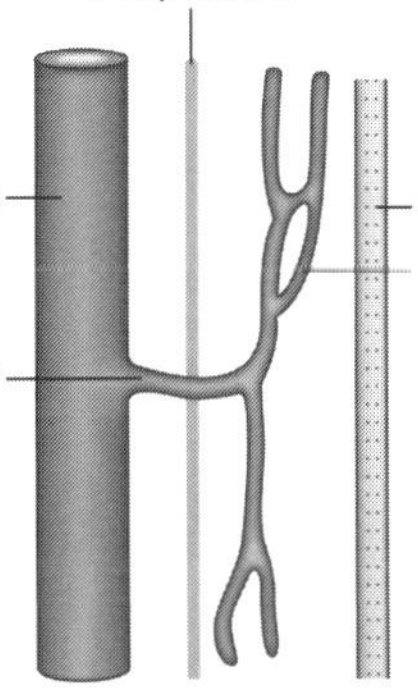

Direct perforating vein

Varicose Veins

- Thin walled tortuous, dilated and elongated veins with incompetence of contained valves:
  - Thread veins (dermal flares)
  - Smaller veins of 0.5 mm diameter seen in the skin in varicosity
- Reticular veins—veins of 1–3 mm in diameter.

SURGERY

Causes of Varicose Veins

- Congenital—rare, due to congenital absence of valves
- Primary varicose vein (cause not known often familial)
  Wall theory (weakness of wall) and valve theory
- Secondary varicose veins (VV)
  - Post-thrombotic, post-traumatic
  - Pregnancy, fibroid, ovarian cyst
  - Pelvic tumors, ascites
  - Retroperitoneal fibrosis
  - Arteriovenous (AV) fistula

Primary varicose veins (VV)	**Secondary varicose veins**
In early adolescence	Older age
Positive family history	No family history
Saphenous distribution alone is involved	Saphenous + perforators and deep veins are involved

Klippel-Trenaunay syndrome

Prominent veins along the lateral aspect of thigh mostly from very young age with dysplastic deep veins.

Classical clinical triad:

- Hemangioma
- Hypertrophy of soft tissue and overgrowth of extremity
- Varicose veins

Tests for varicose veins

Tests	*Purpose*
• Trendelenburg 1	Saphenofemoral junction (SFJ) incompetence
• Trendelenburg 2	Perforator incompetence
• Morrissey's cough impulse	SFJ incompetence
• Modified Perthe's test	Most important test before surgery to rule out DVT
• Multiple tourniquet	Perforator incompetence
• Schwartz's test	SFJ incompetence
• Pratt's test	Perforator incompetence
• Fegan's test	Perforator incompetence

Practical Tip

Easy method to complete VV examination

- Trendelenburg 2—look for filling from below then remove tourniquet—Trendelenburg 1
- Schwartz test
- Fegan's test
- Multiple tourniquet test—remove all tourniquet except at SFJ
- Modified Perthe's test
- Do not forget to look for short saphenous system.

STRIPPING

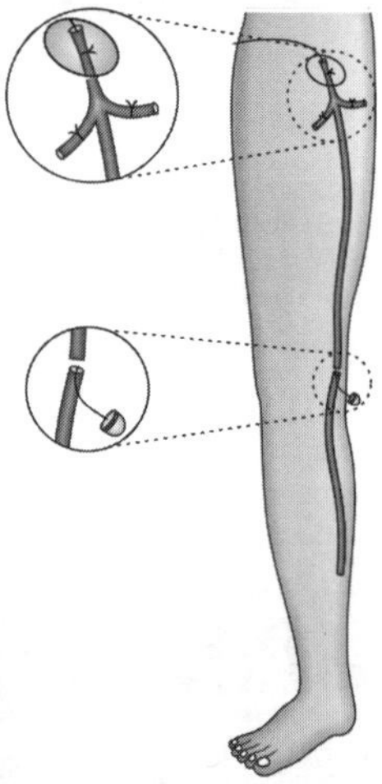

Long saphenous vein stripping

A CASE OF PERIPHERAL VASCULAR DISEASE

Pain and tingling sensation of lower limbs for 3 years.

HISTORY OF PRESENT ILLNESS

He developed cramping pain 3 years back in both calf muscles, more on right side. There is no radiation initially the pain developed after walking about 2 km and was relieved on taking rest for about 2 min. But the walking distance gradually reduced. The pain is also aggravated by cold water application. There is also associated tingling and numbness in the foot, when the pain begins. Pain is relieved on application of heat.

The ulcer appeared on dorsum of the foot and 2nd and 5th toe, following the trivial injury 8 months back. The ulcer is neither healing not progressing. There is no associated pain or discharge.

There is no history of history of swelling or redness in the affected part (seen in the Beuger's disease).

There is no history of fainting, transient blackouts, chest pain, weakness or paresthesia of upper limbs; or abdominal pain. No history of diarrhea (ulcerative colitis), athralgia (rheumatoid arthritis).

No history of trauma or impotence (Leriche's syndrome).

LOCAL EXAMINATION

Inspection

There are two triangular ulcers over 2nd and 5th toes on dorsal aspect, both measures 1.5 cm × 1 cm size. Edges are sloppy. Floor is smooth and pale. There is no discharge. There is redness over dorsum of right foot with peeling of skin. There is no edema. There is no varicosity of veins in both lower limbs. Movements of joints are present.

Beurger's test: +ve between 30° and 90° (normal –ve, i.e. no pallor or guttering of veins at 90°)
(Can be induced by active ankle dorsiflexion and plantar flexion up to the point of fatigue)
(following Beurger's test cyanotic congestion develops)

Capillary filling test—+ve
- Inference:
  - Normal limb—no change in color, remains pink.
  - Affected limb—first pallor, then pink on horizontal position or hanging down, then purple red due to filling of dilated skin capillaries (Deoxygenated blood).

Capillary filling time: Time to become pink
Venous refilling: Elevate the limb—normal limb guttering of veins at 90°: Affected limb at 0° and 10°.

Palpation

There is local rise of temperature and tenderness over the dorsum of right foot. There is mild edema.

Ulcers are tender on palpation, with well-defined margins and slopping edges, base is indurated and is formed by bone. The ulcer is fixed to bone. It does not bleed on touch.

Capillary and venous refilling are decreased.

Pulsation: Dorsalis pedis and posterior tibial are not palpable on both sides, with feeble popliteal pulsation on both side, femoral, radial, brachial, subclavian, common carotid and superficial temporal arteries palpable.
Neurological examination—there is no loss of sensation or loss of motor function.
Examination of inguinal lymph nodes—no lymph node enlargement.

Auscultation

No carotid, femoral, aortic or renal bruit.

PROVISIONAL DIAGNOSIS

- Peripheral arterial occlusion disease
- Right lower limb
- Femoropopliteal system
- Etiology atherosclerosis
- Status—critical limb ischemia
- Comorbidities — diabetes mellitus (DM), hypertension (HTN).

Peripheral vascular disease and Gangrene

- **Age and sex**
  - Atherosclerosis—old age
  - Buerger's disease—20–40 males
  - Raynaud's disease—young women.
- **Limbs affected**
  - Buerger's disease and atherosclerosis—lower limbs
  - Raynaud's disease—upper limbs.
- **Bilateral or unilateral**
  - Buerger's disease, Raynaud's disease—bilateral
  - Atherosclerosis—unilateral to start with
- **Pain**
  - Site—left thigh, buttock
  - Character—cramping
  - Radiation—along the course of artery
  - Aggravated by—walking or exercise, on application of cold
  - Relieved by—taking rest
- **Paresthesia:** Numbness, pins and needles sensation due to shunting of blood from skin to muscle.
- **History of superficial phlebitis:** Swelling, redness and minor pain in the affected part—Buerger's disease
- **Involvement of other arteries:**
  - History of fainting, transient blackouts, weakness, paresthesia—central nervous system (CNS)
  - Chest pain—cardiovascular system (CVS)
  - Abdominal pain—mesenteric ischemia
  - Impotence—Lehriche's syndrome (bilateral internal iliac artery occlusion)
- **History**
  - Past history of similar illness, history of coronary artery disease (CAD)/cerebrovascular accident (CVA)/transient ischemic attack (TIA), DM/HTN, dyslipidemia
  - Personal history of smoking
  - Family history of atherosclerosis..
- **General Examination**
  Signs of atherosclerosis
  - Arcus senilis
  - Locomotor brachialis
  - Xanthelasma
  - Palpable vessel wall
  - High volume pulse
- **Local examination**
  Inspection
  - If gangrene
    - Color and extent
    - Dry/wet (dry—mummified and shrivelled, wet—edematous)
    - Line of demarcation—zone of hyperemia and hyperesthesia on just proximal areas
    - Proximal limb
  - Edema and redness
  - Congested/pale, black patch—proximal spread.

Signs of Ischemia

- Marked pallor, purple blue cyanosed appearance
- Thinning of skin
- Loss of subcutaneous fat
- Diminished growth of hair
- Shiny nails
- Trophic changes in nail
  - Brittle
  - Transverse ridges
- Minor ulceration in the pressure areas such as heel, malleoli, ball of foot, tip of toes

Special tests:
- Beurger's postural test
- Capillary filling test
- Venous refilling test
- Crossed leg (Fuchsig's test)
- Eleveated arms test—thoracic outlet syndrome
- Allen's test—radial/ulnar artery
- Branham's sign or Nicoladoni sign—for AV fistula.
- Costoclavicular compression maneuver—1st rib
- Hyperabduction maneuver—pectoralis minor syndrome
- Adson's test—cervical rib

DISCUSSION

ABPI symptoms
> .9 none
.5 – .8 claudication
.3 – .5 rest pain
< .3 gangrene

Investigation

- Doppler
- Duplex
- Arteriography
- Digital subtraction angiography (DSA)
- Plethismography
- Lipid profile, RBS, antinuclear antibodies (ANA), venereal disease research laboratory (VDRL)
- X-ray foot, urine routine—albumin
- Swab from ulcer site.

Doppler

To find levels of occlusion.

Duplex

- Doppler + B-mode USG
- Ankle brachial pressure index (ABPI)—systolic BP at ankle to that arm
- Systolic BP at ankle is measured by applying BP cuff above ankle and using Doppler probe at dorsalis pedis

Arteriography

Retrograde percutaneous catheterization using Seldinger technique (site, extent, collaterals, distal run off)

Plethismography

Venous outflow from limb is briefly arrested while allowing arterial inflow to measure the volume change in the limb which is proportional to the arterial inflow

Treatment

- Conservative
  - Stop smoking
  - Diet
  - Control of hypertension, DM by exercise
  - Care of the foot well-fitting footwear (Cheropodry, podiatry)
  - Microcellular rubber chappal (MCR)
  - Heel rise
  - Soft sole
- Medical
  - Analgesics
  - Antiplatelet drugs—aspirin, clopidogrel
  - Pentoxiphyllin—rheo modulation
  - Cilastazol—PDE3 inhibitor
  - Naftidrofuryl oxalate

- Surgical
  - Direct arterial surgery
    - Percutaneous transarterial angioplasty (PCTA) and stenting
    - End arterectomy (short segment lesion)
    - Bypass graft (long segment lesion)
  - Lumbar sympathectomy
  - Limb amputation

Indication for direct arterial surgery
- Critical limb ischemia
- Severe intermittent claudication which is incapacitating
- To lower the level of amputation

Percutaneous Transarterial Angiography (PCTA)

During femoral arteriogram a guidewire is inserted and a balloon catheter is then inserted over the guide wire and positioned within the stenosis. Now the balloon is inflated for 1 minute and then deflated, or using metallic stent.

Endarterectomy

The occluded intima and a part of the media are removed by coring them out through an artificial plane created in the media. Done for large arteries like aorta.

Bypass graft
- A native vein (usually saphenous vein) or a prosthetic material is used for bypassing the obstruction in the vessel
- It may be
  - Anatomic—femoropopliteal bypass
  - Extra anatomic—femorofemoral crossover graft

Material used for bypass graft—polytetrafluoroethylene (PTFE), dacron.

Lumbar sympathectomy

2nd, 3rd and 4th lumbar sympathetic ganglia are removed.

Open laparoscopic method
- Open method is done by extraperitoneal approach using a loin incision
- Chemical sympathectomy—under radiographic fluoroscopic control, long spinal needle is inserted—5 mL of phenol in water (1:16) is injected.

Brown's vasomotor index

$$\frac{\text{Rise in skin temperature} - \text{Rise in mouth temperature}}{\text{Rise in mouth temperature}}$$

In case Raynaud's or Buerger's disease. Sympathectomy is advisable only when index is 3.5 or more.

Shianoya's criteria for Buerger's disease
- <40 years
- Smoking
- Distal extremity involved first (infrapopliteal)
- Absence of diabetes mellitus, hyperlipidemia.

AMPUTATION

Indication
- Dead (gangrene)
- Deadly (spreading cellulitis)
- Deadless (paralysis)

Postoperative complication of amputation
- Phantom limb
- Phantom pain
- Neuroma
- Infection
- Osteomyelitis, flap necrosis

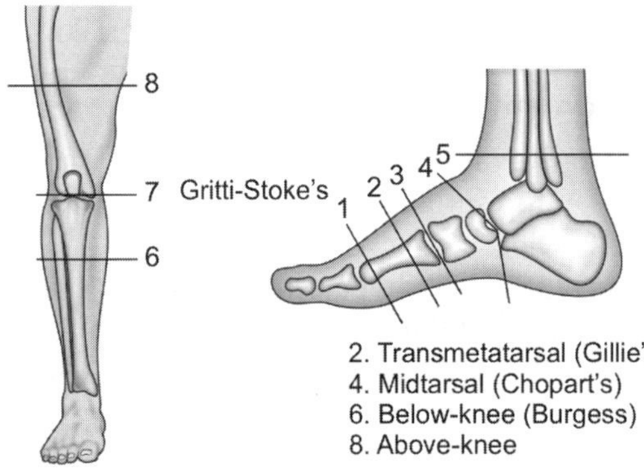

2. Transmetatarsal (Gillie's)
4. Midtarsal (Chopart's)
6. Below-knee (Burgess)
8. Above-knee

1. Ray's
3. Tarsometatarsal (Lisfrance's)
5. Syme's
7. Transcondylar

Some points

- Critical limb ischemia
  - Resting pain lasting >2 weeks
  - Ulceration/gangrene of the foot or toes with similar hemodyanamic parameters
  - Ankle brachial pressure index <0.3.
- Intermittent claudication

  Due to accumulation of the excessive P substance.

Boyd's grading

- Grade 1: Claudication pain disappears on resuming walking
- Grade 2: Can walk with effort
- Grade 3: Pain compels the patient to take rest

Raynaud's phenomenon

- **Local syncope:** Digits become cold and white with tingling and numbness—due to spasm of digital arteries
- **Local asphyxia:** White digits turns blue with burning sensation—due to slowing of circulation and accumulation of reduced Hb
- **Local recovery**
  - Bluish discoloration gradually disappears and digits gradually regain normal color due to release of spasm of digital arteries
  - Disappearing pulse
  - In arterial occlusion with well-developed collateral circulation, the distal pulses will be normal to palpation.
  - The patient is exercised to point of claudication, which may unmask the effect of arterial obstruction by disappearance of pulse
  - The exercise produce vasodilation below the obstructing lesion and arterial inflow cannot keep pace with the increasing vascular space and the pulse disappears.

Fontaine Classification for the Severity of Chronic Ischemia

Stage 1 – Asymptomatic

2 – Intermittent claudication limiting lifestyle

2a – Well-compensated

2b – Poorly compensated

3 – Rest pain due to ischemia

4 – Ulceration or gangrene due to ischemia.

Peripheral pulsations—Refer medicine general examination (vitals).

ULCER

EDGES

- Undermined edge—tuberculosis
- Punched out edge—gummatous ulcer, deep trophic ulcer
- Sloping edge—healing traumatic, venous ulcer
- Raised and pearly white beaded edge—rodent ulcer (BCC)
- Rolled out (everted edge)—squamous cell carcinoma, ulcerated adenocarcinoma.

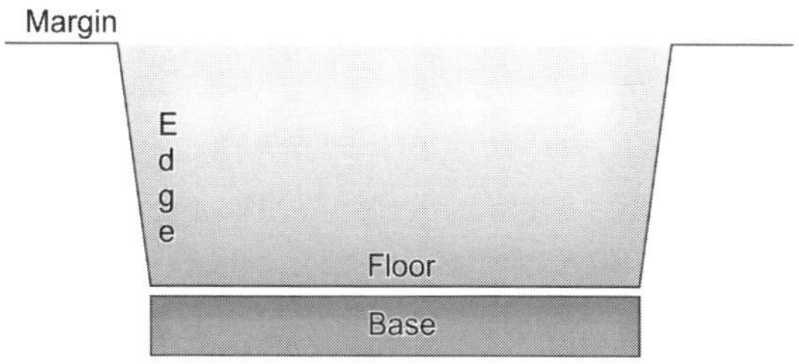

ULCER

A break in the continuity of an epithelial surface that can occur in the skin or mucosa of the alimentary or respiratory tracts.

SLOUGH

A piece of dead tissue.

ZONES OF HEALING IN A HEALTHY ULCER

- White: Fibrosed zone
- Blue: 2–3 layered epithelium
- Red: Granulation tissue.

- Margin—junction between normal epithelium and ulcer
- Edge—area between margin and the floor
- Floor—exposed surface within the ulcer
- Base—on which the ulcer rests

SURGERY

GANGRENE

Macroscopic death of a tissue with or without putrefaction.
- Dry
- Wet

Dry Gangrene

- Dry mummified shrivelled tissue
- Line of demarcation in the deeper tissue is at the same level of the line of demarcation we are seeing outside
- Separation by aseptic ulceration.

Wet Gangrene

- Edematous
- Actual line of demarcation is proximal to what we are seeing
- Separation by septic ulceration.

CLASSIFICATION OF ULCERS

Clinically
- Spreading ulcer
- Healing ulcer
- Callous or chronic ulcer

Healing Ulcer

- The surrounding skin is not inflamed
- The edge shows blue zone (bluish outline of growing epithelium) and a white zone (fibrosis of the scar)
- Floor will have reddish granulation tissue
- Minimal serous discharge.

Spreading Ulcer

- The surrounding skin of the ulcer is inflamed
- Floor is covered with slough
- No evidence of granulation tissue
- Purulent discharge.

Callous Ulcer

- Induration of the edge and surroundings
- Floor will have pale granulation tissue
- No tendency towards healing
- Copious serous discharge.

Pathologically

- Nonspecific
- Specific.

Nonspecific

- Traumatic
- Arterial—atherosclerosis, Buerger's disease, Raynaud's disease
- Venous—venous, varicose ulcers
- Neuropathic—diabetes mellitus (DM), leprosy, tabes dorsalis, spina bifida, paraplegia
- Tropical ulcers
- Metabolic—DM, gout
- 2° to disease like:
  - Rheoumatoid arthritis (RA)
  - Erythrocyanosis frigida
  - Osteitis deformans
  - Avitaminosis
- Ulcers complicating blood disease
  - Sickle cell anemia

Tropical ulcer

It is due to infection by Vincent's organisms (Bacteroides fusiformis) together with many pyogenic bacteria 2° to trauma or insect bite.

Martorell's ulcer
- Hypertensive ulcer
- Seen in old age group with atherosclerosis
- A part of skin on the outside of the calf suddenly becomes gangrenous and sloughs away producing a punched out ulcer.

Decubitus ulcer
- Bed sore
- Predisposing factors
  - Pressure
  - Injury
  - Moisture
  - Anemia
  - Malnutrition

SURGERY

- Mediterranian anemia
- Felty's syndrome.

Specific

- Tuberculosis
- Syphilitic
- Actinomycosis
- Soft sore
- Herpes simplex
- Fungal.

Diabetes

Can cause ulcer by:

- Neuropathy
- Atherosclerosis
- Hyperglycemia—infections.

Diabetic Foot Grading (Meggit Wagner)

Gr 0: Foot at risk
Gr I: Small ulcer local dressing and antibiotic
Gr II: Large ulcer/deep ulcer—up to muscle—drainage of puss
Gr III: Osteomyelitis, joint infection—wound debridement
Gr IV: Partial gangrene—partial amputation
Gr V: Whole foot gangrene—amputation.

Marjolin's Ulcer

Malignant ulcer developing in burns scar or venous ulcer or edge of any chronic ulcer or chronic discharging sinuses such as osteomyelitis (painless, radioresistant, nonmetastatic, avascular, abundant fibrous tissue).

MANAGEMENT OF ULCER

- Identify and correct comorbid factors like DM, anemia, leukemia, etc.
  - Fasting blood sugar (FBS)
  - Post-prandial blood sugar (PPBS)
  - Peripheral smear
  - Hemoglobin (Hb)
  - Total leukocyte count (TLC)
  - X-ray chest—rule out TB
- Determine the etiology of ulcer
  - Biopsy from edge of ulcer
  - If pus is present, send for culture and sensitivity and give appropriate antibiotics.
  - X-ray of the part to rule out osteomyelitis.

Treatment

- Adequate drainage and desloughing
- Care of the ulcer (foot—podiatry)
  - Daily dressing
  - Avoid antiseptic solution (impair capillary circulation)
  - Use normal saline for cleaning
  - Use nonadherent and nonadhesive dressing
  - Use microporous polyurethane film which are permeable to gases and water and impermeable to micro-organisms
- Treat the underlying cause
  - Anti-TB drugs
  - Treatment—varicose veins
  - Revascularization in case of arterial ulcer
- Excision of the ulcer and skin grafting—if ulcer is not healing

SKIN GRAFTS

THIERSCH GRAFT (PARTIAL THICKNESS GRAFT, SPLIT SKIN GRAFT)

- Removal of epidermis + part of dermis
- Donor site—thigh, arm, leg
- Graft is placed after creating window cut, to prevent seroma
- Uses—large areas of skin defects (burns).

Grafts
- Autograft
- Isograft
- Allograft
- Xenograft

WOLFE GRAFT (FULL THICKNESS GRAFT)

- Epidermis + full dermis
- Donor site—supraclavicular area, post-auricular area, groin
- Uses—repair of defect in face, eyelid, hands.

Stages of graft intake
- A stage of imbibition
- A stage of inosculation
- A stage of neovascularization

Advantages of Wolfe (Full Thickness) Graft

- Color match
- No contracture
- All sensations, sweat and sebaceous glands functions well

COMPOSITE GRAFT

Skin + fat + cartilage.

FLAPS

Transfer of donor tissue with its blood supply to the recipient area.

Types

- Cutaneous flap
- Fasciocutaneous flap
- Muscle flap
- Myocutaneous flap.

CHAPTER 8

Short Cases

INGUINAL HERNIA

INGUINAL HERNIA CASE FORMAT

Presenting Complaints

Swelling in left groin—3 weeks duration.

History of Present Illness

He noticed a swelling 3 weeks back in the left groin, extending to scrotum. He noticed it is becoming more prominent while walking and less prominent while lying down. He is able to reduce the swelling by himself. There is no associated pain, vomiting, abdominal distension or constipation. No difficulty in passing urine.

Past History

History of recurrent attacks of fever and cough for last 5 years for which he had to be hospitalized many times. No history of any surgeries (appendicectomy—damage to iliohypogastric nerve).

Local Examination

Inspection

A single oval-shaped swelling approximately of size 7 × 4 cm is present on medial part of left inguinal region with enlargement of scrotum on left side, the skin over the swelling is normal. It has smooth surface; margins are ill-defined. No visible peristalsis or pulsations. There is impulse on coughing. Penis is not displaced. External genitalia is normal. Normal rugosities of scrotal skin are present.

Palpation

There is no local rise in temperature or tenderness. A single ovoid swelling of size 7 × 4 cm is present in the medial part of inguinal region above inguinal ligament, extending down into the bottom of left side of scrotum, soft in consistency, smooth surface and ill-defined margins. It is not possible to get above the swelling. The swelling is reducible, no fluctuation, pulsation. There is expansile impulse on coughing.

- Spermatic cord and testes are separately felt
- Ring occlusion test is positive (no bulge is seen—indirect hernia) (negative in direct hernia)
- Three finger test—impulse is felt on index finger
- Invagination test—superficial ring admits little finger and impulse is felt on tip of finger
- External genitalia—normal
- Regional lymph nodes—not enlarged.

Percussion

Dull note on percussion.

Auscultation

No bowel sounds heard.

Examination of Abdomen

- No Malgaignes's bulges on straining
- No mass palpable
- No shifting dullness.

PR not Done

Respiratory System

- Normal breaths sounds
- No added sounds.

Painful inguinoscrotal swelling
- Lymphadenitis
- Strangulated hernia
- Inflamed hernia
- Torsion of undescended testis
- Inflammation of cord

CVS–CNS–WNL

Differential Diagnois

- Hydrocele
- Femoral hernia
- Inguinal LN enlargement
- Undescended testes
- Lipoma of cord.

DISCUSSION

Diagnosis

Left sided complete indirect inguinal hernia containing omentum without complications.

Preoperative Investigations

- CBC
- RBS, RFT, LFT
- Chest X-ray
- USG abdomen
- ECG
- Urodynamic study in patients with BHP.

Management
- Herniotomy
- Herniorrhaphy
- Hernioplasty

Management

Herniotomy

Indication: Hernia in infants, congenital hydrocele

It is the process of identification of sac, separation of the sac from the cord, opening the sac, reducing the content, transfixation and ligation of the neck of sac followed by excision of sac.

Herniorrhaphy

Simple repair of posterior wall alone

Bassini's herniorrhaphy

After herniotomy conjoint tendon is approximated to inguinal ligament using No.1 interrupted prolene sutures. Less foreign body—less chance of infection, but tension causes ischemic necrosis.

Shouldice's repair

6 layers by continuous suture

1. Double breasting of transversalis fascia
2. Double breasting of conjoint tendon to inguinal ligament
3. Double breasting of external oblique.

Modified Shouldice's
5 layers
Conjoint tendon and inguinal ligament – single layer.

Hernioplasty

Synthetic material is used to strengthen the posterior wall and cover the defect.

- **Lichenstein tension free hernioplasty**
  - Under LA/GA
  - An oblique inguinal skin crease incision
  - Approximately 1.5 cm above the medial 2/3rd of inguinal ligament
  - Incise the fatty layer (Camper's fascia) and membranous layers of superficial fascia (Scarpa's fascia)
  - Ligate the blood vessels
  - Divide the external oblique aponeurosis along the line of its fibers
  - In indirect inguinal hernia sac is anterosuperior to cord
  - In direct inguinal hernia sac lies behind the cord
  - Using a gauze separate the spermatic cord and hernia sac
  - Hold the cord with a cord holding forceps
  - Safeguard the ilioinguinal nerve, vas deferens and spermatic artery.

Indirect hernia

- The sac is isolated up to neck of sac until the parietal peritoneum can be seen on all sides and extraperitoneal fat is visible.
- Open the sac, reduce the contents. Neck of the sac is transfixed as high as possible and the rest of the sac is removed.

Direct hernia

No need to open the sac. Push the direct hernia sac inside. Interrupted Prolene sutures are put so that the sac will remain invaginated.

Repair

- Prolene mesh is incised laterally to fit in spermatic cord (fish tailing)
- The mesh is sutured below to the inguinal ligament, above to the internal oblique and conjoint tendon. The mesh should overlap beyond the pubic tubercle (first bite) medially
- Close the external oblique aponeurosis with catgut after placing the cord in the inguinal canal. Close superficial fascia with catgut. Close the skin with non-absorbable suture.

PHS (Prolene Hernia System)

- Inlay mesh
- Circular mesh between transversalis fascia and peritoneum
- Connector
- Onlay mesh
  - Above transversalis fascia.

Laparoscopic

- TAPP (**T**rans**a**bdominal **p**re**p**eritoneal **r**epair)
  - After entering the peritoneal cavity, the peritoneum is incised the sac reduced and mesh is secured to Cooper's ligament and to conjoint tendon.
- TEP (Total extraperitoneal repair)
  - The peritoneal cavity is not entered. Mesh is placed between under surface of abdominal wall and peritoneum fixing mesh to the Cooper's ligament
  - Ind: B/L inguinal hernia, recurrent hernia, femoral hernia
  - Disadvantages:
    Need spinal or general anesthesia
    Injury to viscera
    Mesh migration, infection.

Stoppa groin hernia repair (Giant Prosthetic Reinforcement of Visceral Sac—GPRVS)

Reinforcement of transversalis fascia in groin by large prosthesis that extends beyond myopectineal orifice
For complex hernias at risk for recurrence.

Complications of Hernia Surgery

- Hematoma
- Seroma

- Wound infection
- Infection of mesh
- Injury to testicular artery, testicular atrophy
- Injury to testicular vein
- Injury to testicular lymphatics
- Ilioinguinal/Genitofemoral neuralgia
- Obstruction of vas deferens – spermatocele
- Recurrence
- Osteitis pubis
- Mesh migration.

DOOM'S triangle
Medially – vas deferens
Laterally – testicular vessels
Inferiorly – peritoneal reflection
Content – external iliac vessels
(dangerous area in hernia repair)

Causes of Recurrence

- Preoperative
  - Chronic cough, constipation, BHP
- Operative
  - Bad surgical technique (tight suture, absorbable sutures), hematoma, infection, missed pantaloons hernia
- Postoperative
  - Infection, bleeding, poor general condition, heavy work within 3 months of surgery.

INGUINAL CANAL

It is an intermuscular slit situated between superficial and deep ring (4 cm).

Superficial Ring

- Opening in external oblique aponeurosis
- Just above and medial to pubic tubercle.

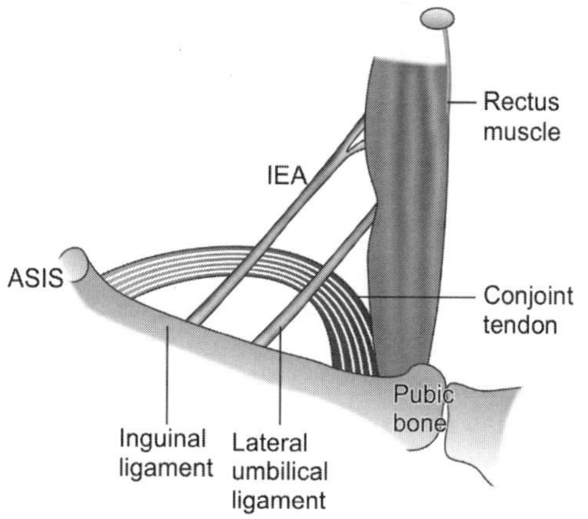

Deep Ring

It is an opening in the fascia transversalis
- ½ inch above the mid-inguinal point
- Midway between ASIS and pubic symphysis.

Femoral Artery

At mid-inguinal point—between ASIS and pubic symphysis.

Boundaries

- Anteriorly
  Whole length – Skin, superficial fascia, external oblique aponeurosis
  Laterally – Internal oblique
- Posteriorly
  Whole length – Parietal peritoneum, extraperitoneal fat, fascia transversalis
  Medially – Conjoint tendon (IO + TA), reflected part of inguinal ligament)
- Roof – IO and transverse abdominis
- Floor – Inguinal ligament
  Medially lacunar ligament.

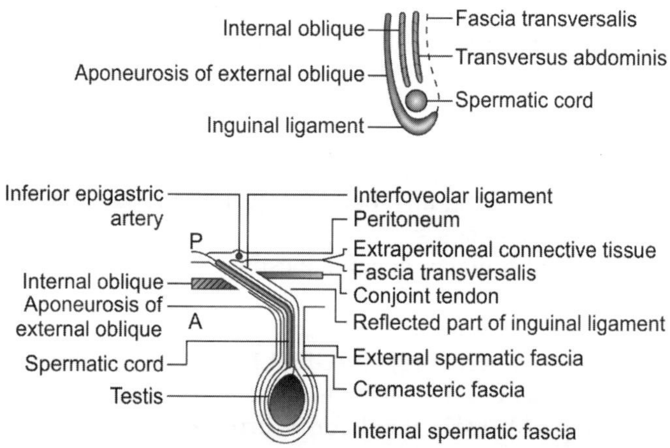

Contents

Spermatic cord/round ligament of uterus
Ilioinguinal nerve (T12–L1)
Innervates base of penis, scrotum and adjacent side.

Contents of the Spermatic Cord

- Vas deferens
- Testicular artery
- Artery to vas deferens
- Pampiniform plexus
- Lymphatics
- Genital branch of genitofemoral nerve (L1, L2, L3)
  - Motor supply to cremaster
  - Sensory supply to penis and scrotum
  - Femoral branch innervate the upper thigh
- Remnants of processus vaginalis.

Coverings of spermatic cord
- External spermatic fascia (from EO)
- Cremasteric fascia (IO+TA)
- Internal spermatic fascia (Fascia transversalis)

Mechanisms of Inguinal Canal

- Obliquity of the canal (flap valve mechanism)
- Superficial ring is supported behind by:
  a. Conjoint tendon
  b. Reflected part inguinal ligament
- Deep ring is supported anteriorly by internal oblique muscle
- Shutter mechanism by internal oblique muscle
  It forms the anterior wall, roof, posterior wall
- Ball valve mechanism
  Contraction of cremasteric muscle
- Slit valve mechanism (contraction of EO).

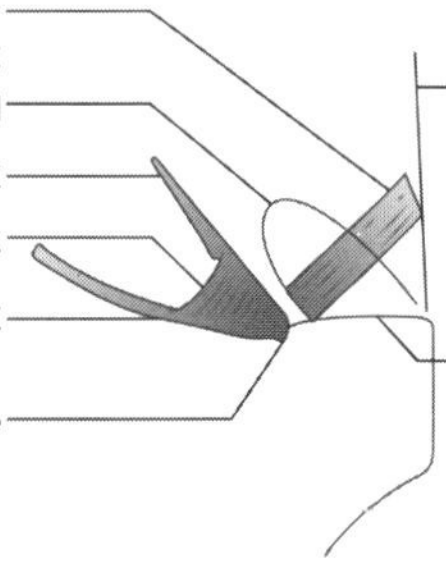

Extensions of the Inguinal Ligament

- Inguinal ligament (Poupart's ligament)
- Lacunar ligament (Gimbernart's)
- Iliopectineal ligament (Cooper's)

Myopectineal Orifice of Fruchaud

Boundaries
- Above – Conjoint tendon
- Below – Pectineal line of superior pubic ramus
- Laterally – Iliopsoas
- Medially – Lateral border of rectus abdominis
  - This space is closed off posteriorly by transversalis fascia
  - This is the site for direct, indirect and femoral hernias
  - All three can be repaired by single piece of mesh by covering this orifice (by laparoscopy).

Hernia

Definition

It is the protrusion of whole or part of viscus through the wall that contains it.

Parts
- Sac – neck, body and fundus
- Covering
- Contents

CLASSIFICATION OF HERNIA

A. Anatomical
  a. Site of exit
    i. Direct
    ii. Indirect
  b. Contents
    i. Omentocele
    ii. Enterocele
    iii. Cystocele

B. Clinical
  a. Reducible
  b. Irreducible
  c. Obstructed
  d. Strangulated
  e. Inflamed

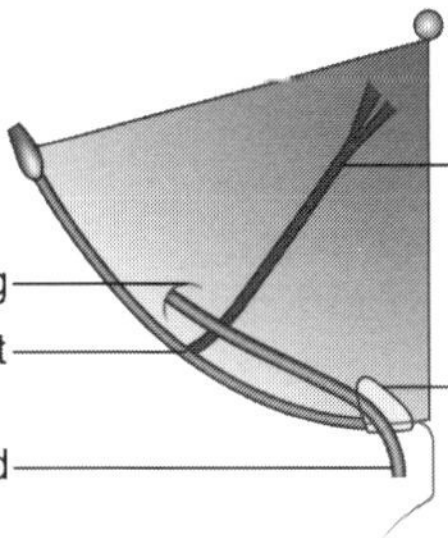

Indirect – Congenital and Acquired
- Bubonocele
  - Hernia limited to inguinal canal

Funicular hernia
- Processus vaginalis is closed just above the epididymis.

Complete hernia
- Reaches bottom of scrotum

Hernia en glissade (Sliding hernia)
Here a portion of caecum and appendix on right side, sigmoid on left side and urinary bladder on both sides will slide down behind the sac and forms the posterior wall of the sac.

If the sac is unusually thick preoperatively, one should rule out sliding hernia.

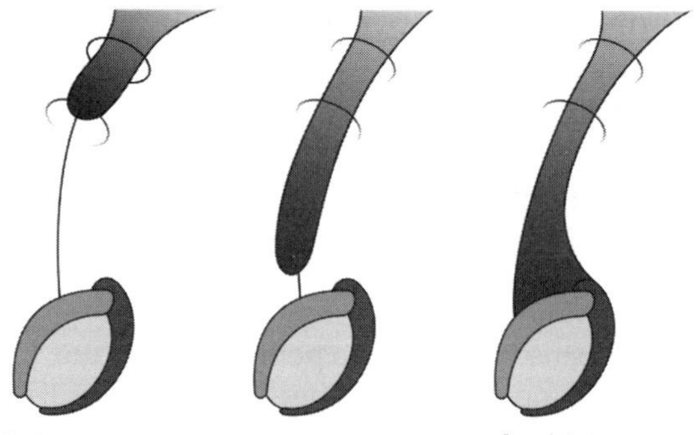

Maydl's hernia (W-loop hernia, retrograde strangulation)
- Where the small intestine forms a loop within hernia sac.
- In case of obstruction if one is not pulling out the rest of the intestine, it is likely to miss gangrene for the rest of bowel.

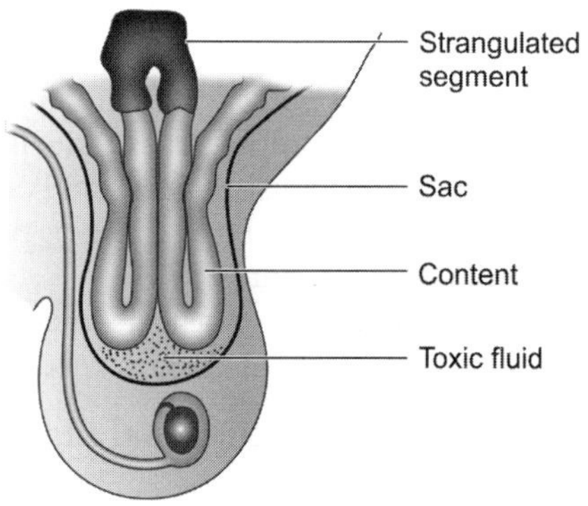

Littre's hernia
- Contents is Meckel's diverticulum

Amyand's hernia – content is appendix

Pantaloon's hernia (Dual, saddle bag hernia)
- Both direct and indirect hernia.

Richter's hernia
- Here part of circumference of the viscus is forming the content.

European Hernia Society Classification

P or R – Primary or Recurrent

M or L or F – Medial, Lateral or Femoral.

Defect size – 1.5 → 1
1.5–3 → 2
3–4.5 → 3

A primary indirect inguinal hernia with a 3 cm defect size wound be **PL2**.

Gilbert's Classification of Hernia

Type 1	Indirect inguinal hernia (IIH) – Tight deep ring
Type 2	IIH – Deep ring admits one finger
Type 3	IIH – Deep ring admits more than 2 fingers
Type 4	Direct inguinal hernia (DIH) – Entire posterior wall is defective
Type 5	DIH – Punched out defect in post wall
Type 6	Both direct and indirect hernias
Type 7	Femoral hernia.

NYHUS Classification

Type 1	Indirect hernia+ normal deep ring
Type 2	IIH + wide deep ring
Type 3	Posterior wall defect
	3A – Direct
	3B – Indirect reaching scrotum
	3C – Femoral
Type 4	Recurrent hernia
	4A – Direct
	4B – Indirect
	4C – Femoral
	4D – Combination

Hernia of Hydrocele

In long-standing cases of hydrocele, tension of fluid in tunica vaginalis causes herniation through dartos muscle.

SURGERY

Hydrocele of Hernial Sac

When neck of hernial sac is plugged with omentum, fluid accumulates in distal hernial sac.

COMPLICATIONS OF HERNIA

- **Irreducibility**
  Due to adhesions between sac and contents, sac and sac,
  - Contents to each other
  - Sliding hernia
  - Very large scrotal hernia (scrotal abdomen).
- **Obstructed hernia**
  Constriction of neck of sac leads to obstruction of loops of small bowel inside it. It will produce symptoms of intestinal obstruction.
- **Strangulated hernia**
  Irreducibility + obstruction + arrest of blood supply
  (initially venous return impaired then arterial supply—bacterial migration trans-serosally–perforation)
  Features
  - Tense tender irreducible swelling
  - No impulse on coughing
  - Abdominal distension
  - Vomiting
  - Shock, toxicity

  Treatment
  - Emergency surgery
  - Constriction ring and superficial ring is released
  - Sac opened without spillage of fluid
  - Viability of bowel is checked (by color, pulsation, peristalsis, bleeding)
  - When gangrenous, resection and anastomosis is done and drain placed.
- **Incarcerated hernia**
  Lumen of that portion of the colon occupying a hernial sac is blocked with faeces.
- **Inflammation**
  Occurs when sac contains
  - Appendix
  - Meckel's diverticulum
  - Salpinx

Coverings of indirect hernia
- Extraperitoneal fat
- Internal spermatic fascia
- Cremasteric fascia
- External spermatic fascia
- Skin

Direct hernia
- Extraperitoneal fat
- Fascia transversalis
- Conjoint tendon
- External spermatic fascia
- Skin

FEMORAL HERNIA

Why Femoral Hernia

- It is below and lateral to pubic tubercle, below groin crease
- Cannot be reduced completely
- Many do not have cough impulse
- Femoral hernia is usually irreducible.

Due to:
- Narrow neck of sac
- Contents are adhered to peritoneal sac.

Femoral hernia is common in female, elderly (30–45), after repeated pregnancies.

Most common hernia
- Inguinal hernia (both in males and females)
- Femoral hernia (most common in females)

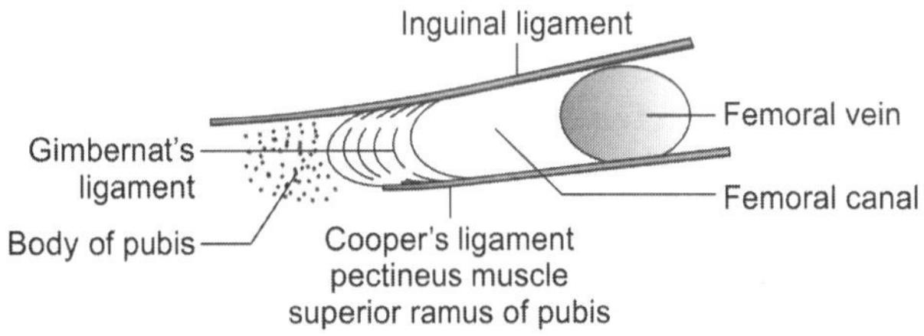

Boundaries to Femoral Canal

Medially	–	Lacunar ligament
Laterally	–	Femoral vein
Superoanteriorly	–	Inguinal ligament
Inferoposteriorly	–	Astley Cooper's ligament

Stages of Femoral Hernia

I. There is rounded reducible swelling below the medial end of the inguinal lig.
II. After passing through the femoral canal bulges into femoral triangle (Scarpa's triangle)
III. Further expansion downward is prevented by blending of fascia, the fundus mouths upward in front of inguinal ligament and overlies the inguinal canal.
By this time, it is always irreducible. Finally, femoral hernia takes the shape of a retort.

Differential Diagnosis

- Inguinal hernia
- Saphena varix (associated varicosity)
- Lymph node (focus of infection)
- Psoas abscess (cross-fluctuation)
- Lipoma.

Complications

- Obstruction
- Strangulation

Management

Principle: Suturing of inguinal to pectineal ligament after dealing with the sac.

- Low operation of Lockwood
  - Incision: 1 cm below and parallel to inguinal ligament
  - After dealing with the sac, neck of sac is pulled down and ligated as high as possible
  - Femoral canal is closed by suturing inguinal lig to iliopectineal line
- The Lotheissen's operation: Inguinal approach
- McEvedy's approach: Vertical incision: Extending from femoral canal region in the thigh upward to above the inguinal ligament.

Leugier's Femoral Hernia

Hernia through the gap in the lacunar ligament (Gimbernat's).

Narath's Femoral Hernia

In patients with CDH, the hernia lies behind the femoral vessels.

Cloquet's Hernia

Sac lies under the fascia covering pectineus muscle.

PARAUMBILICAL HERNIA (SUPRAUMBILICAL/INFRAUMBILICAL HERNIA)

Paraumbilical hernia is a protrusion through the linea alba just above or sometimes just below the umbilicus (It is not a protrusion through the umbilical scar).

Features

- Common in **females**
- Oval-shaped
- Narrow neck but large sac (increased chance of strangulation)
- Content—greater omentum, transverse colon.

Etiology
- Repeated pregnancy
- Obesity
- Flabbiness of abdominal muscles

Clinical Features

- Swelling
- Dragging pain
- GI symptoms
- Intestinal obstruction (abdominal pain, vomiting, absolute constipation).

Treatment

Always surgery
1. Mayo's operation for small defect.
2. Paraumbilical hernioplasty–For large defect (> 2 cm)

Mayo's operation – Double breasting of the defect in the rectus sheath by interrupted non-absorbable sutures.

Complications

- Strangulation
- Intertrigo
- Ulceration.

UMBILICAL HERNIA

Types

- Exomphalos
  - Major
  - Minor
- Umbilical hernia of infants and children
- Adult umbilical hernia.

Exomphalos (omphalocele): It is due to the failure of all or part of the midgut to return to the coelomic cavity during early fetal life.

Types of Exomphalos

- Exomphalos major – more than 4 cm in size
- Exomphalos minor – less than 4 cm in size (Herniation of umbilical cord)
- Contents in exomphalos major – liver, spleen, stomach, pancreas, colon, bladder
- Content of exomphalos minor–small bowel only.

Treatment

- Nonoperative therapy:
  - Indication:
    - Premature infants with gigantic intact sac
    - Associated anomalies make survival after major operations unlikely
- Operative methods
  - Skin flap closure
  - Staged closure
  - Primary closure.

Gastroschisis (not the same as omphalocele): It is the defect in the abdominal wall to the right of the normal insertion of the umbilical cord, without any investing sac).

CONGENITAL UMBILICAL HERNIA

It occurs as a result, partly from the failure of the round ligament (obliterated umbilical vein) to cross the umbilical ring and partly from the absence of rectus fascia.

Features

This hernia is common in black; symptomless, increase in size during crying.

Treatment

- Conservative and surgical
- Conservative treatment is indicated in:
  i. Less than 2 years of age (in a hope that 95% of hernia disappears spontaneously)
  ii. Size less than 2 cm.

Surgical

- Indication: failure of spontaneous closure above 4 years. Ring size more than 2 cm.
- Method: "smile" incision → skin cicatrix dissection → neck of sac is isolated → sac is ligated and transfixed → defect closed with interrupted sutures.
- Adult umbilical hernia:
- Causes:
  - Cirrhosis
  - Malignant peritoneal effusion.

INCISIONAL HERNIA (POSTOPERATIVE HERNIA)

It is the herniation through a weak acquired abdominal scar and starts as a symptomless partial disruption of the deeper layers of a laprotomy wound during the immediate or very early postoperative period.

Things to remember while history taking:

- Mention as a swelling case
- Ask history of previous surgery
- History of wound infection
- Whether postoperative drainage tube is placed through wound (increase the frequency of herniation)
- Ask for predisposing factors like postoperative coughing, vomiting, history of jaundice, COPD, steroid intake.

DISCUSSION

Points in Favor of Incisional Hernia

- History of previous lower abdominal surgery
- Swelling is seen at the site of scar
- Swelling is partially reducible in the supine position and more prominent on standing
- Expansile impulse on coughing
- Palpable defect in the lower abdomen.

Predisposing Factor for Incisional Hernia

- Method of wound closure
  - Use of absorbable suture material
  - Single layer continuous closure
- Keeping drainage tubes through wound
- Vertical incision has got higher chance
- Emergency operative procedures
- Postoperative coughing, paralytic ileus, vomiting
- General condition of the patient: obesity, jaundice, malnutrition, malignancy, anemia, COPD, on steroids.

MANAGEMENT OF INCISIONAL HERNIA

- USG abdomen – to rule out intra-abdominal pathology
- X-ray – to rule out COPD
- Blood investigations – to rule out anemia.

TREATMENT STRATEGY

Conservative management by abdominal belt.

Indications:

- Upper abdominal incisional hernia
- Patient unfit for surgery.

Surgical management by:
- Mesh repair—gold standard.
- Anatomical repair—primary fascial repair (< 4 cm)
- Autogenous repair by vascularised muscle flaps
- Complex appositions—e.g: Keel's, Catell's, Nuttall's operations.

SPIGELIAN HERNIA

Variety of interparietal hernia occurring at the level of arcuate line.

Features

- Lie beneath the internal oblique muscle and then spreads like a mushroom between internal and external oblique muscles
- Soft reducible mass lateral to the rectus muscle
- Occurs at site lateral to rectus muscle and below umbilicus
- Treatment – muscle splitting approach.

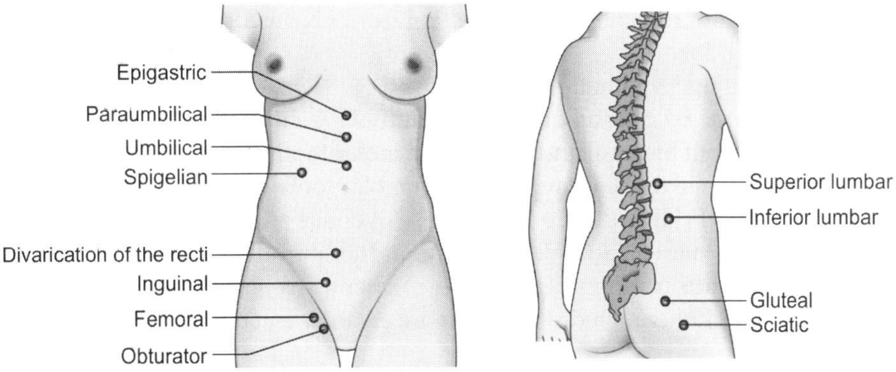

PAROTID SWELLING

A 50-year-old male presents with painless enlargement of left parotid region. On examination there is swelling of size 3 x 3 cm, irregular shape and occupying the parotid fossa, raises the left ear lobule, skin over the swelling normal on palpation size is confirmed, firm in consistency, superficial to masseter and deep to parotid facia, duct (bidigital) - normal. The facial nerve is intact and there is no palpable lymph nodes.

History:
- Swelling–site, onset, duration, U/L, B/L
- Pain–salivary colic
- Facial nerve involvement
- Deep lobe involvement–swelling in oral cavity
- Sore throat/odynophagia
- Jaw movements
- Opposite parotid and other salivary glands
- Other swellings anywhere
- Systemic symptoms (fever).

No biopsy
- Seeding
- Facial nerve involvement
- Parotid fistula

Differential diagnosis:
- Parotid swelling
- Preauricular LN (It is small swelling)
- Lipoma
- Dermoid
- Neurofibroma

Investigations

- FNAC
- CT – to know about tumor extent, LN involvement
- MRI – to know facial nerve involvement.

SURGERY

Discussion

Why you say it is a parotid swelling, because:

- Site – below, behind and slightly in front of the ear lobule and raising ear lobule (obliterates normal hollow below ear lobule)
- Deep to parotid fascia—on opening the mouth swelling become less prominent
- Superficial to masseter
- Curtain sign positive (mentioned later)—parotid gland situated in parotid fossa.

Parotid Fossa

Muscular landmark	*Bony landmark*
• Masseter	• Mastoid process
• Sternocleidomastoid	• Styloid process
• Posterior belly of digastric crossing SCM	• Angle of mandible
• Stylohyoid	

Ducts of salivary gland

- Parotid – Stensen's duct
- Submandibular – Wharton's
- Sublingual – Bartholin's

Parotid gland and SM gland are separated by stylomandibular ligament.

Two important things that will differentiate parotid swelling from LN swelling.

1. Bimanual palpation (for deep lobe)
2. Curtain sign (cannot move above zigomatic bone)
   - Bimanual palpation is done by putting one finger externally behind the ramus of mandible and one finger inside the mouth just in front of tonsil and behind 3rd molar tooth internally
   - Stensen's duct opens opposite to the crown of second molar tooth (upper)
   - Parotid is divided to superficial and deep lobe by fasciovenous plane of Patey (it is the plane, where facial nerve seen superficial to posterior facial vein in the gland) or parotid sandwich
   - Commonest cause of parotitis is mumps (it is mostly bilateral swelling)
   - Sjogren's syndrome and Mikulicz's syndrome also cause enlargement of salivary gland (bilateral enlargement).

Mikulicz's syndrome

Bilateral salivary and lacrimal gland enlargement (xerostomia, xerophthalmia)

Causes (S2L2)

S – Sarcoidosis
S – Sjogren's syndrome
L – Leukemia
L – Lymphoma

Sjogren's syndrome

Consists of keratoconjunctivitis sicca
Autoimmune disorder of exocrine gland
Xerostomia, autoimmune and CT disorder (RA)

Classification of salivary gland tumors

- Epithelial tumors
  - Adenoma: Pleomorphic adenoma
    Adenolymphoma
  - Carcinoma: Adenocarcinoma
    Squamous cell carcinoma
    Mucoepidermoid carcinoma
    Acinic cell carcinoma
- Non-epithelial tumors: Hemangioma
  Lymphangioma
- Lymphoma: NHL
- Secondary tumors: Skin and bronchus, head and neck
- Unclassified tumors
- Tumor like lesions: Salivary cyst

SURGERY

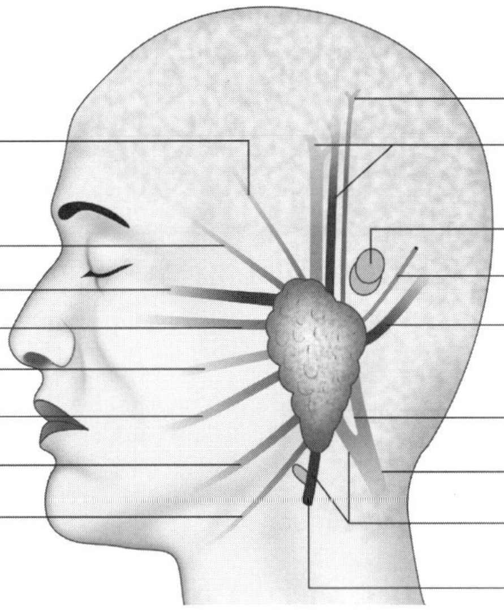

Features of Malignancy

- Swelling become painful, stony hard, starts growing rapidly, get fixed to masseter, mandible, skin.
- Facial nerve involvement (LMN type palsy)
- Temporomandibular joint involvement
- LN enlargement.

Treatment

- Superficial parotidectomy
  - Minimum operative procedure
  - Superficial lobe removed.

Radical parotidectomy
Total parotidectomy + facial nerve section
- High grade mucoepidermoid carcinoma
- Adenoid cystic carcinoma

Steps

- Lazy 'S' shaped incision (auriculomastoid cervical)–to protect marginal mandibular nerve
- Back of parotid gland, identified to expose facial nerve
- SCM is retracted and greater auricular nerve divided in avascular plane along the anterior border of muscle
- Identify posterior belly of digastric
- Identify avascular plane immediately anterior to the tragus
- Facial nerve is identified and dissected along its entire course
- Dissect the gland and required amount of gland removed
- Suction applied and wound closed

Main steps in facial nerve isolation.

- Conley's point – the facial nerve lies 1 cm deep and below the tip of inferior portion of cartilaginous canal
- Facial nerve inferomedial to tragal point
- By nerve stimulator
- Nerve lateral to styloid process
- Tracing linear distal branch to proximal (marginal mandibular, cervical branches)
- Post belly of digastric crossing SCM.
- Methylene blue injected to Stensen's duct.

COMPLICATIONS

- Infection
- Injury to facial nerve (Rx–Graft with great auricular nerve)
- Permanent numbness of ear lobule due to great auricular nerve injury
- Sialocele
- Parotid fistula (Rx–Newman-Seabrook operation)
- Frey's syndrome (gustatory sweating).

Sweating and flushing of the preauricular skin during mastication and is due to aberrant innervations of sweat gland by parasympathetic secretomotor which were destined for the parotid.

Treatment of Frey's Syndrome

- Tympanic neurectomy
- Injection of botulinum toxin
- Antiperspirants like aluminium chloride
- To prevent Frey's syndrome, place a sheet of fascia lata between skin and underlying fat to prevent secretomotor fibers reaching gland.

Some points to remember:

- Pes anserinus (goose foot)
- Fascial nerve is divided in the parotid gland into:
  - Temporofascial (temporal, zygomatic)
  - Cervicofascial (buccal, mandibular, cervical)

  These divisions in turn divide to form goose foot.

SUBMANDIBULAR SALIVARY GLAND SWELLING

INVESTIGATIONS

- FNAC
- X-ray occlusal view (to know about radiopaque stones)
- USG for demonstration of stones, lymph nodes.

Differential diagnosis
- Submandibular salivary gland swelling
- Submandibular lymph node swelling

DISCUSSIONS

Wharton's duct opens on either side of frenulum.

Stones are more common in SM gland because:

- Higher mucin content
- High Ca and P content
- Nondependent drainage of secretions. Long and tortuous course of duct

Salivary gland is differentiated from LN by bimanual palpation.

TREATMENT

- If stone is in the duct
  - If the stone lying anterior to point of which duct crosses the lingual nerve, then remove the stone, do not suture the duct (risk of stricture formation).
  - When stone is proximal to crossing the lingual nerve, then submandibular gland excision is required.
- Pleomorphic adenoma of submandibular gland–submandibular sialadenectomy
- If with malignancy–Radical submandibular sialadenectomy + modified radical neck dissection (if nodes are +ve).

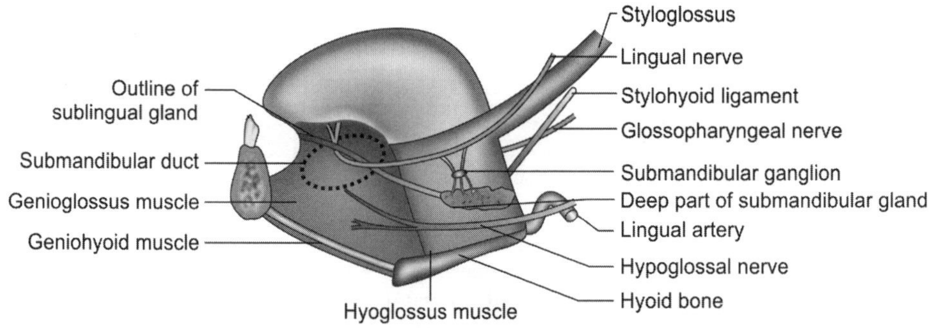

During surgery, injury to 3 nerves may occur

- Marginal mandibular nerve
- Lingual nerve
- Hypoglossal nerve.

Marginal mandibular nerve if involved

- Deviation of mouth occurs
- Dribbling of saliva.

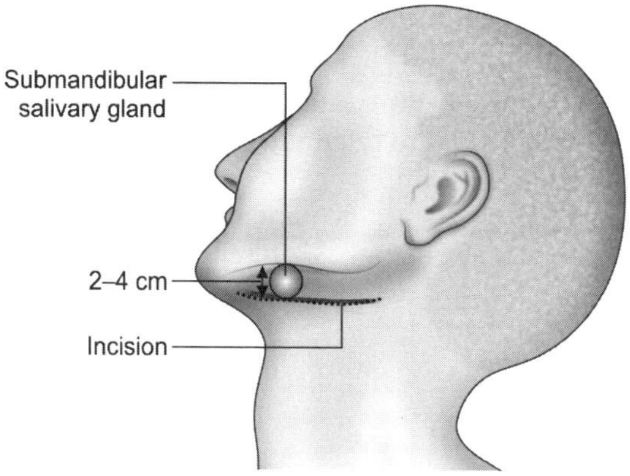

Treatment

Cut the opposite marginal mandibular nerve.
- To prevent this during surgery.
- Incision is made 2 finger breadth below the angle of mandible
- Do not flap before reaching the gland.

Complication to Surgery

- Infection
- Injury to nerves – marginal mandibular nerve, lingual nerve, hypoglossal nerve
- Hematoma
- Transection of nerve to myelohyoid muscle producing submental skin anesthesia.

> **Indication of submandibular gland excision**
> - Sialadenitis
> - Stones proximal to lingual nerve
> - Salivary tumors

MIDLINE SWELLINGS

Triangles of Neck

Anterior – Digastric
Carotid
Muscular
Posterior

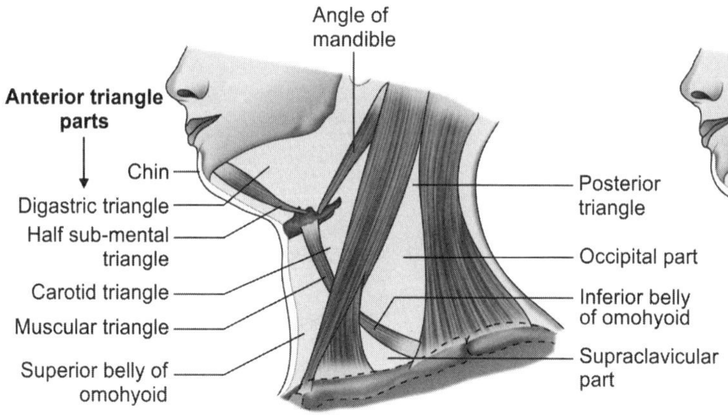

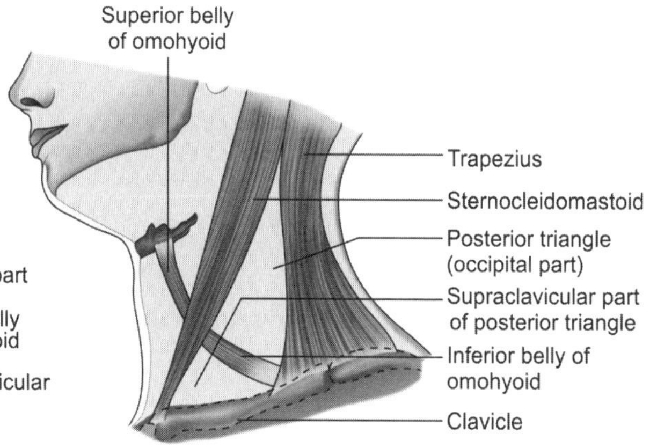

Midline Swellings of the Neck

- Sublingual dermoid
- Plunging ranula
- Thyroglossal cyst
- Pharyngocele
- Laryngocele
- Swelling from isthmus of thyroid
- Prelaryngeal LN
- Pretracheal LN
- Lymph node in the space of burns.

> **Thyroglossal fistula**
> - Skin tag (pathognomic sign)
> - Treatment: fistular tract removal

Plunging Ranula

Sometimes ranula extend into submandibular region through deeper part of mylohyoid called plunging ranula.

- Ranula—extravasation cyst arising from sublingual gland or mucous gland of Nuhn or glands of Blandin
- Initially, it is a retention cyst and later becomes extravasation cyst.
- Clinical Features
  - Bluish, soft fluctuant, brilliantly transluminant swelling in the floor of mouth
  - Cross fluctuation present in plunging ranula.

Treatment

Marsupialization or excision.

Thyroglossal Cyst

Moves with deglutition as well as with protrusion of tongue

- Smooth, soft, fluctuant, nontender
- Commonest position—subhyoid.

Treatment

Sistrunk operation—excision of cyst and full tract up to foramen cecum along with removal of center part of hyoid bone.

TB Lymph Node

Pathological stages of TB lymph node.

There are 5 stages as follows:

- Stage 1 – the lymph nodes are enlarged and solid
- Stage 2 – matting due to periadenitis
- Stage 3 – stage of caseation and cold abscess
- Stage 4 – stage of collar-stud abscess
  – abscess penetrates deep cervical fascia which leads to escape of pus beneath superficial fascia
- Stage 5 – stage of sinus formation and ulcer.

Investigation

- ESR
- CXR
- Mantoux
- FNAC of the LN
- Bx of LN for pathology and microbiology
- Aspiration of the cold abscess for abscess for AFB staining.

Bx

Take Bx for 2 nodes (1 for pathologist – send in formalin bottle) (for microbiologist – send in saline solution for AFB culture).

Treatment

ATT – triple drug therapy – rifampicin, INH, ethambutol

Treatment of cold abscess aspiration done through the nondependent part to avoid formation of sinus (zigzag aspiration, wound closure without drain).

> **Indication for Sx in cervical TB LN**
> - Bx (most important)
> - Excision of a group of nodes if it is not responding to ATT
> - Excision of offending LN in cases of collar-stud abscess
> - Excision of abscess if it is not responding to aspiration

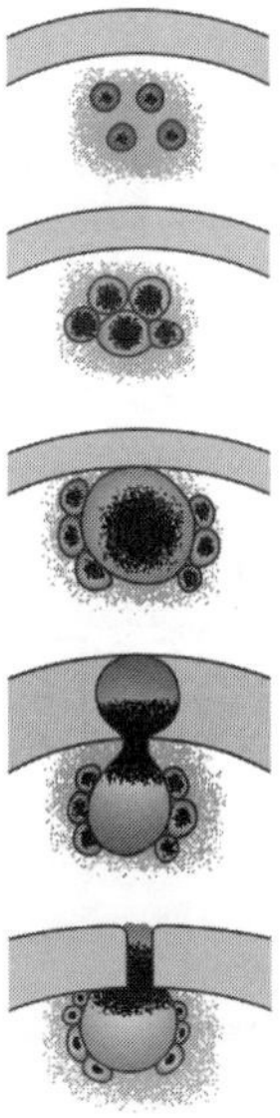

Step 1: Lymphadenitis (describe nodes, nontender fifth hard mobile)

Step 2: Melting (firm, nontender, move together en mass—due to pericarditis)

Step 3: Cord abscess deep to deep fascia

Step 4: Collar-stud abscess rupture thought deep fascia under the skin fluctuar, adherent to skin

Step 5: Shows formation

Types of neck dissection

1. Radical neck dissection
   Removal of: Fat, fascia, lymphatics, LN
   Accessory nerve
   Sternomastoid muscle
   Internal jugular vein
2. Modified radical neck dissecction
   I – preservation of acessory nerve
   II – preservation of nerve and muscle (sternomastoid)
   III – preservation of nerve, muscle and vein (internal jugular vein)
3. Selective neck dissection
   Supraomohyoid neck dissection -in tumor of oral cavity (level I, II, III)
   Central compartment neck dissecction -in carcinoma thyroid (from hyoid bone above to innominate vein below and carotids laterally)
   Posterolateral neck dissection (level II, III, IV, V)

Types of modified radical neck dissection

I	– N preservrd	N – nerve
II	– N+M preservrd	M – muscle
III	– N+M+V preservrd	V – vein

Incision used for neck dissection
- Crile's incision (Y-shaped)
- Martin incision (double Y)

LIPOMA

Universal tumor or ubiquitous tumor
Benign tumor arising from adult fat cells.
Depending on planes, lipoma may be classified as:
- Subcutaneous—commonest
- Subfacial
- Intermuscular
- Intramuscular
- Parosteal
- Intra-articular
- Subserous
- Subperitoneal
- Subpericardial
- Subperiosteal
- Subpleural
- Subsynovial
- Extradural
- Submucous.

Diagnostic Points

- Lobulations
- Slip sign
- Soft swelling with pseudofluctuation
- Transillumination positive, if it is subcutaneous.

Lobulation—due to the intervening fine strands of fibrous septa seen between the fat lobules
Slip sign: If the edge of the lump is pressed, the swelling slips beneath the finger.
Pseudofluctuation: Intracellular fat is fluid at body temperature. Therefore, the swelling will be soft and fluctuation will be elicited in one plane.

Complications

- Myxomatous degeneration
- Calcification
- Pressure effects
- Fat necrosis

SURGERY

- Ulceration
- Intussusception in submucous lipoma
- Infection
- Malignant change–liposarcoma.

Dercum's disease – multiple tender subcutaneous lipoma (adiposis dolorosa).

Investigation

1. FNAC from the swelling
2. Radiology of the part

Treatment

Excision of the swelling.

SEBACEOUS CYST

What is sebaceous cyst?

The skin is normally kept soft and oily by the sebum secreted by the sebaceous glands, mouth of which open into the hair follicle. If the mouth of a sebaceous gland is blocked, the gland will get distended by its own secretions producing sebaceous cyst (retention cyst).

Diagnostic Points

- Soft and cystic
- Sign of indentation present
- Punctum is visible at the summit of the swelling as a black spot

Plane of Sebaceous Cyst

- All sebaceous cysts are attached to the skin
- The area of attachment may be small
- There is no independent movement of the cyst of the skin
- Parts of the cyst will lie in the subcutaneous tissue.

Sign of Indentation

Cyst containing pultaceous material can be moulded. When the swelling is indented with a finger, it stays indented contradistinction to the sign of emptying.

Punctum

The cyst is arising basically from a sebaceous gland. The mouth of the sebaceous gland will open into the hair follicle or through a fine duct directly into the skin surface. This point of attachment is pulled inward as the cyst grows to form the punctum.

Classical Sites for Sebaceous Cyst

- Scalp (most common)
- Scrotum
- Back
- Shoulder
- Neck
- Face

Sebaceous cyst will not occur in palms and soles.

Complications

- Infection, ulceration, rupture, calcification, sinus formation
- Sebaceous horn
- Cock's peculiar tumor.

Sebaceous Horn

The slow discharge of sebum from a wide punctum hardens to form the horn. This will take the shape of a conical spike.

Cock's Peculiar Tumor

Suppurating and ulcerating sebaceous cyst is called Cock's peculiar tumor (Rx—excision with skin adjacent to punctum).

DERMOID CYST

- Congenital (sequestration dermoid)
- Implantation dermoid
- Tubulodermoid
- Teratomatous.

Congenital Dermoid

Sequestration of epithelial elements deep to the skin surface.
They occur along the line of embryological fusion.
For example:

- External and internal angular dermoid
- Sublingual dermoid
- Postauricular dermoid

Implantation Dermoid

They are usually traumatic. The surface ectoderm is being driven inside as a result of trauma (small cut or stab injury) and this will result in implantation dermoid.

Diagnostic Features of Dermoid Cyst

- Cystic swelling
- Nontransilluminant
- The skin can be pinched (no punctum and therefore no tethering) – they are seen deep to the skin in the subcutaneous tissue
- A bony depression of defect may be felt
- Intracranial communication may be there.

NEUROFIBROMA

Neurofibromas are benign tumor which contain a mixture of neural (ectodermal) and fibrous (mesodermal) elements.

Diagnostic Features

- They are seen in relation to a nerve (need not be in relation to named nerve)
- Patients may get tingling sensation in the distribution of the nerve
- Usually subcutaneous
- Usually fusiform in shape
- Long axis of the swelling is along the length of the limb
- Firm or rubbery in consistency
- Mobile side-to-side (not longitudinally)
- Moves at right angle to the course of the nerve.

When neurofibromas are multiple, it is called neurofibromatosis.

When they are multiple and congenital and familial and transmitted by autosomal dominant gene it is called von Recklinghausen's disease.

Investigation

- MRI: Showing gadolinium enhancing mass within a peripheral nerve
- Nerve conduction studies.

Treatment

Neurofibromas cannot be excised without resecting a segment of involved nerve.
True neurofibromas should only be biopsied to ensure that they are not malignant and should be left in place unless the parent nerve can be sacrificed without producing significant neurological deficit.

SCROTAL SWELLING (HYDROCELE)

Do not forget to look for:
- Get above the swelling
- Fluctuation
- Transluminant
- Whether testes separately palpable/not
- Lymph node (retroperitoneal, supraclavicular LN (secondary hydrocele)

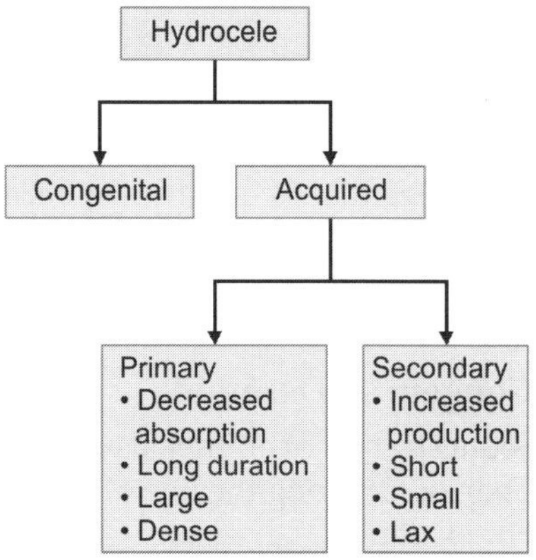

Definition

Abnormal collection of fluid in the tunica vaginalis or remnants of processus vaginalis.

TYPES

- Congenital hydrocele
  - Due to patent processus vaginalis
  - Disappears on lying down, brilliantly transilluminant
  - Direct communication between TV and peritoneal cavity
  - Associated with TB peritonitis
- Infantile hydrocele
  - Tunica and processus vaginalis are distended up to the deep inguinal ring
  - No communication with peritoneal cavity
- Funicular hydrocele – funicular process is closed just above the tunica vaginalis
- Hydrocele of the canal of Nuck—in females at the site of the round ligament
- Hydrocele of hernial sack—neck of hernial sac becomes closed by adhesions or plugged with omentum
- Encysted hydrocele of cord—cystic swelling in the inguinal or inguinoscrotal region
  - Fluctuation test, translucency test positive
  - No impulse on coughing
  - Testis felt separately
  - Traction test present
- Bilocular hydrocele en-bisac—two intercommunicating sacs, cross fluctuation is pathognomic.

Brilliantly transilluminant
- Congenital hydrocele
- Epididymal cyst
- Cystic hygroma
- Ranula
- Meningocele

Contents of Hydrocele Fluid

- Albumin
- Cholesterol
- Fibrinogen
- Inorganic salts
- Tyrosine
- Water.

Cross-fluctuation seen in: Code: CHIP
- Compound palmar ganglion
- Hydrocele en-bisac
- Iliopsoas abscess
- Plunging ranula

Differential Diagnosis of Hydrocele

- Hematocele
- Epididymal cyst
- Spermatocele, pyocele, chylocele
- Filariasis, testicular tumors.

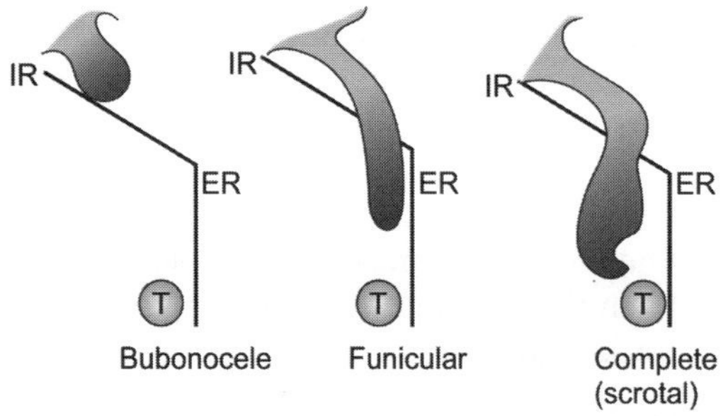

Investigations

- Blood and urine routine
- Scrotal USG
- Doppler to rule out varicocele
- Sperm count before surgery
- Aspiration—to diagnose pyocele, hematocele

Treatment

- Lords plication of TV sac—if it is small sac, and thin walled
- Jaboulay's eversion procedure—moderate sized sac

Complications of hydrocele
- Rupture
- Hematocele
- Infection
- Calcification
- Atrophy of testes
- Hernia of hydrocele
- Infertility

- Subtotal excision—large hydrocele and thick walled
- Aspiration and injecting sclerosant—if unfit for surgery
- Sharma and Javed procedure—bringing testes outside and put it in subscrotal pouch.

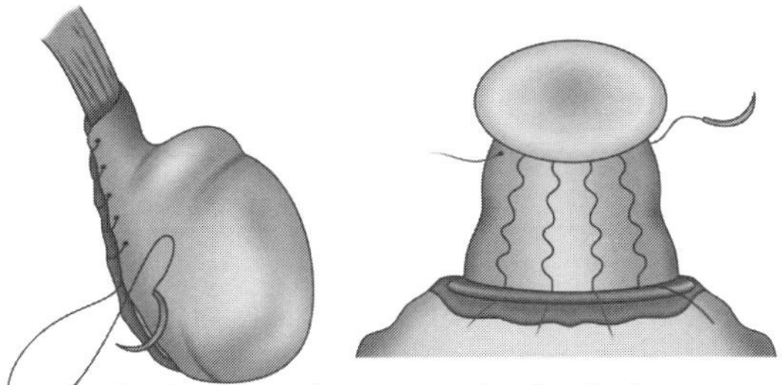

Jaboulay's eversion Lord's plication

ANATOMY

Anatomical Classification of Epididymis

- Head, body and tail
- Physiologically—Globus major and minor.

Descent of Testes

- 3rd month—iliac fossa
- Up to 7th month—deep inguinal ring
- 7th month—inguinal canal
- 8th month—superficial inguinal ring
- 9th month—bottom of scrotum.

Layers of scrotum
- Skin
- Dartos—thermoregulator
- External spermatic fascia
- Cremasteric fascia
- Internal spermatic fascia
- Tunica vaginalis
- Tunica albuginea of testis

Factors that Help in the Descent of Testes

- Differential growth of body wall
- Gubernaculum testis
- Hormones
- Processus vaginalis
- Inguinal bursa
- Testicular artery – arises at L2 level
- Lymphatic drainage – preaortic and para-aortic at L2
- Nerve supply to testis: T10
- Epididymis: T11 – L1.

VARICOCELE

Do not forget to look for:
- Side
- Bag of worm appearance
- Abdominal mass (may be secondary to renal cell carcinoma, so palpate the abdomen and renal angle)
  Definition: **Veins of pampiniform plexus becomes dilated and tortuous**
  Common side: left side.

Causes (why left side is commoner than right side)
1. Left testicular vein drains into left renal vein – high venous pressure
2. Total length of testicular vein is more on the left side (left vein drains at a higher level)
3. Left testicular artery arches over left renal vein
4. Loaded sigmoid colon presses over testicular vein
5. Left renal vein is nut-cracked between abdominal aorta and superior mesenteric artery
6. Left suprarenal vein drains into left renal vein, due to adrenalin left vein is more constricted.
   Characteristically varicocele due to renal tumors does not decompress in supine position.
   Impulse on coughing and blow test +ve—varicocele
   'Bag of worms' on palpation.

Grading of varicocele

I – on Valsalva
II – on palpation
III – on inspection

Treatment of varicocele

Conservative – scrotal support and reassurance.

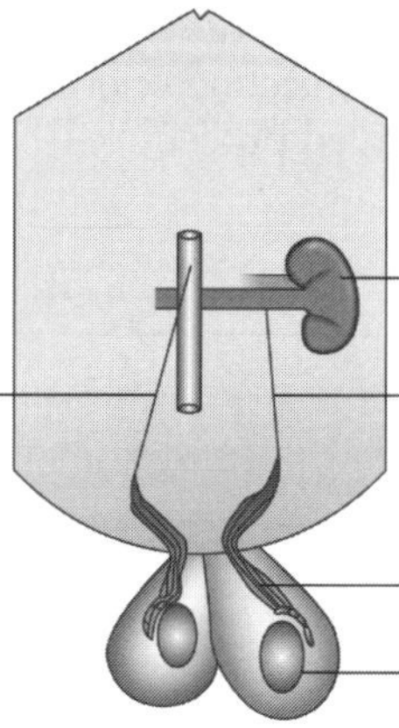

Indications for Surgery

- Painful
- Big
- Infertility
- Abnormal low levels of sperm count
- Medical unfit for job.

Treatment

- Classical varicocele operation
- Laparoscopic
- Scrotal approach
- Palomo's approach
- Embolisation of gonadal vein.

Complications of varicocele
- Dragging discomfort
- Testicular atrophy
- Infertility

EPIDIDYMAL CYST

Cystic degeneration of remnants of paramesonephric duct (epididymis) – sessile hydatid of Morgagni

Embryonic Remnants

- Pedunculated hydatid of Morgagni-Wolfian duct
- Sessile hydatid of Morgagni-Mullerian duct
- Paradidymis or organ of Giraldes-Mullerian duct
- Vas aberrans of Haller
- Multilocular cyst, brilliantly transilluminant, tensely cystic
- Chinese lantern pattern
- Excision is treatment, aspirations is useless as the cysts are multiloculated
- Marsupialization can be done in the young.

Differential diagnosis
- Encysted hydrocele
- Spermatocele
- Lipoma of cord

FOURNIER'S GANGRENE

- Idiopathic gangrene of the scrotal skin
- Uncommon vascular disaster of infective origin
- Sudden onset appearance of scrotal swelling
- Onset of gangrene leading to exposure of scrotal contents
- Testis not involved due to thick tunica albuginea
- Mostly idiopathic

Etiology: 1. Trauma, 2. Infection, 3. Instrumentation

Organism:

- *Hemolytic streptococci*
- *E. coli*
- *Staphylococcus*
- *Clostridium welchii*

Treatment:

- Ampicillin/Gentamicin/Cephalosporins
- Excision of necrotic area and exposed part closed by skin graft.

SURGERY

TORSION OF TESTES

Causes

Inversion, high investment of TV, separation of epididymis from body of testis—two and half turns are needed.
Prehn's sign: On elevation of testes, if pain decreases, it is epididymo-orchitis, while if pain increases it is torsion.

Treatment

- Early – untwist by gentle manipulation
- Late – early operative fixation within 6 hours.

Opposite testis should also be fixed, because anatomical variation may be bilateral (Angel's sign).
Deming's sign–Affected testis is positioned high.

TESTICULAR TUMORS

Clinical Features

- Sensation of heaviness in testes
- Absence of testicular sensation
- Hydrocoele (secondary)
- Back pain, jaundice, chest symptoms.

Do not forget to look for:
- Undescended testes
- LN—retroperitoneal, supraclavicular

Classification

- Seminoma
  - Spermatocytic
  - Lymphocytic
  - Anaplastic
  - Atypical
- Teratoma
  - Differentiated
  - Malignant teratoma intermediate
  - Malignant teratoma anaplastic
  - Malignant teratoma trophoblastic
- Lymphoma
- Interstitial tumors
  - Leydig cell tumor
  - Sertoli cell tumor
- Mixed tumor

Seminoma

- Arises from seminiferous tubules, compresses neighboring testicular tissue as it grows
- Macroscopy—smooth firm homogenous pinkish cream in color, areas of necrosis
- Microscopy—slightly oval cells and clear cyotoplasm and large rounded nucleus with clear nucleoli, cells
- Arranged in sheets, separated by fine fibrous stroma, lymphocytic infiltration – good host response → good prognosis
- Spread via lymphatics – para-aortic, left supraclavicular and mediastinal nodes.
  – Inguinal lymph nodes – only if scrotum involved

Teratoma

- Arise from totipotent cells in rete testis
- Small as peanut/large as coconut
- Lined by tunica albuginea hence the outline is maintained, surface slightly irregular.
- Macroscopy – yellowish, cystic, gelatinous fluid
- Microscopy
  - Teratoma differentiated – no recognizable malignancy but metastases
  - Malignant teratoma immature – most common, in type A mature tissue
  - Malignant teratoma anaplastic – embryonal Ca – yolk sac tumor – increased AFP
  - Malignant teratoma trophoblastic – most malignant, syncytial cell mass with malignant villus and papillary cytotrophoblast – increased hCG.

Interstitial Cell Tumors

Leydig
- Prepubertal
- Androgen secreting
- Masculinizing
- Opposite testis affected – so orchidectomy not much use

Sertoli
- Postpubertal
- Increased estrogen
- Feminising—gynecomastia
- Orchidectomy cures

Hurricane tumor: A ferocious malignancy which kills in a matter of weeks.

Investigations:
- FNAC and incision biopsy are contraindicated
- Blood (tumor markers) AFP, BHCG, LDH, PALP (placental alkaline phosphatase)
- CT abdomen
- X-ray chest
- If lymph node enlarged FNAC from it
- LFT
- RFT.

Why FNAC contraindicated in Ca testes?
Testes drained by para-aortic LN, while scrotum drained by superficial inguinal LN. During FNAC, tumor cells spread in to scrotal skin.

Clinical Staging

Stages 1 – Confined to testes
2 – Involvement of nodes below the diaphragm only
3 – Involvement of nodes above the diaphragm
4 – Pulmonary or hepatic metastasis.

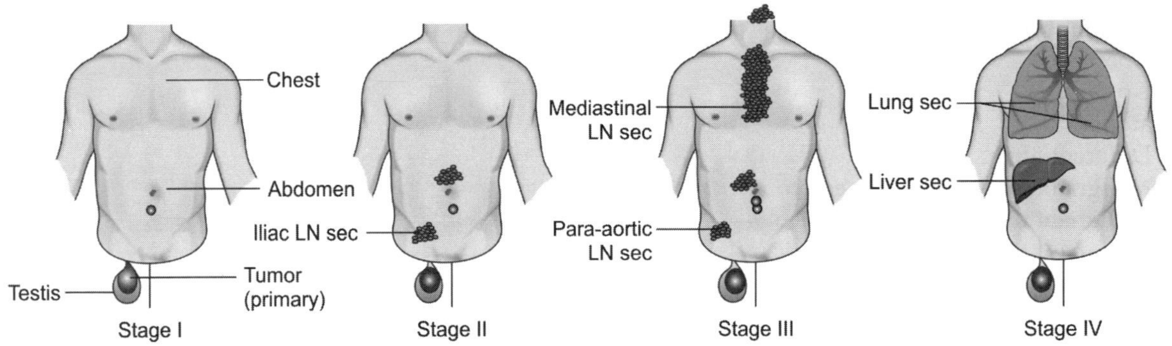

After orchidectomy, pathological staging
- T1 – testis involving tunica albuginea
- T2 – testis involving tunica vaginalis
- T3 – spermatic cord
- T4 – scrotal involvement
- N1 – <2 cm
- N2 – 2–5 cm
- N3 – >5 cm

M -
- M_{1a} – nonregional node or pulmonary metastasis
- M_{1b} – distant metastasis other than non-regional lymph node or metastasis

Treatment: High inguinal orchidectomy
- Chevasus procedure—in cases of doubt, cut open the testis and after pathology consultation, if normal, re-suture testis with tunica vaginalis.
- Radiotherapy—seminoma—3000 rads × 6 weeks stage 1 and 2 from 10th rib to pubic crest below
  Teratoma—less sensitive to radiotherapy
- Chemotherapy—seminoma—above stage 2—cisplatin highly sensitive
  - Teratoma—2–4 stage—cisplatin, MTX, bleomycin, vincristine
  - Retroperitoneal LN dissection—if retroperitoneal mass persists after chemotherapy
  - Follow-up based on tumor markers.

SEMINOMA VS TERATOMA

	Seminoma	**Teratoma**
Spread	Lymphatic	Blood
Tumor marker	-	hCG
Radiosensitivity	High	Less
Duration	Long	Short
Consistency	Firm	Variable
Surface	Smooth	Irregular
Shape	Retained	Not retained
Age	35–45	20–35

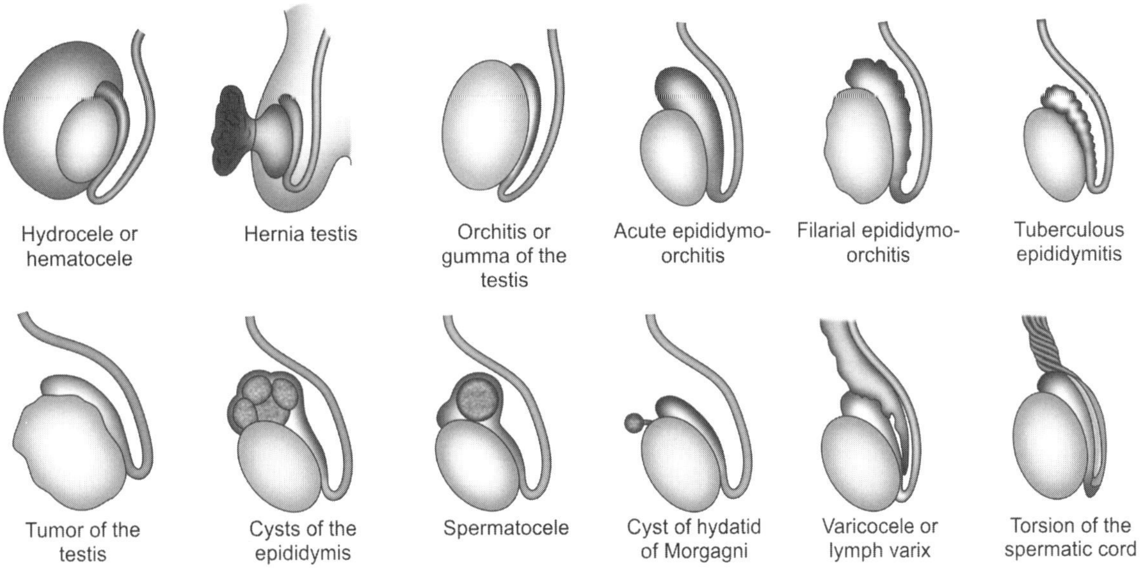

SKIN TUMORS (SQUAMOUS CELL CARCINOMA)

It arises from keratinocytes of epidermis.

ETIOLOGY

- Premalignant condition of skin.
  - Leukoplakia
  - Senile keratosis
  - Solar keratosis
  - Bowen's disease
  - Xeroderma pigmentosa
  - Junctional nevus
- Exposure to chemicals like As, vinyl chloride.
- Sunlight exposure.
  UVB is responsible for the damage by sunlight

SCC metastasis through local spread, lymphatics and blood. (SCC, but **not metastatise through lymphatics—Marjolin's ulcer)*

Common sites of SCC
- Skin
- Lip
- Mouth
- Pharynx
- Esophagous
- Glans penis

GROSS TYPES

1. Ulcerative
2. Proliferative
3. Ulceroproliferative

On microscopy epithelial pearls (***keratin pearls***) are seen.

Marjolin's ulcer
- Arise from scar
- Growth is slow
- Less malignant
- No lymphatic spread

INVESTIGATIONS

- Wedge biopsy
- If node is enlarged, then FNAC from that.
- X-ray of infected part (to rule out bone involvement)

TNM staging
T1 – tumor <2 cm in greatest dimension
T2 – tumor > 2 cm but not more than 5 cm
T3 – tumor >5 cm in greatest dimension
T4 – tumor extending to cartilage, bone tendon.
N0 – no regional lymph node enlargement
N1 – regional lymph node enlargement
M0 – no distant metastases
M1 – distant metastases

Broder's classification of SCC (Based on ratio of pleomorphic and anaplastic cell to normal cells)
- Well-differentiated
- Moderately differentiated
- Poorly differentiated
- Undifferentiated

TREATMENT

- Surgical excision—wide excision with 2 cm clear margin
- Radiotherapy
- Destructive therapy

Radiotherapy
Indications
- If tumor is small
- If patient do not wish surgery
- Affecting the face because of cosmetic problem due to surgery

Types of destructive therapy

- Electrodessication and curettage (EDC)
- Electrocautery
- CO_2 laser
- Cryotherapy
  It is done for small cancers. If used for large one it cause scarring.
  The advantage of it is to destroy and to vaporize all tissue but its disadvantage is no specimen for histopathological examination.

Prognosis

- Invasion: depth, size
- Broder's grade
- Site: Lip, ear, extremities
- Etiology: From scar, C/C ulcer–bad prognosis
- Immunosuppression
- Perineural invasion.

SURGERY

BASAL CELL CARCINOMA (RODENT ULCER)

- Most common type of skin tumor arising from pilosebaceous unit
- Etiology is same that of SCC.
- It is localy invasive and no lymphatic spread.
- Its classical area is above the line joining ear lobule and angle of mouth (Onghren's line).
- Types of BCC
  - About 26 varieties are described.
- Nodular, nodulocystic, morphic, infiltrative
- Morphic and infiltrative—worst prognosis.
- Microscopically, BCC appears as the dermis involved by basaloid cells with peripheral palisade arrangement.
- Treatment is same as that of SCC, but the excision require 1 cm clear margin and also Mohs.
- Mohs (*microscopically oriented histographic surgery*)
- Other Rx
  - Radiotherapy
  - Topical chemotherapy
  - Cryotherapy

MALIGNANT MELANOMA

- It arises from melanocytes (normally found in the stratum basale of epidermis).
- Melanin is produced in basement layer and migrated to dermis.

TYPES (Code: NASAL-D)

N – Nodular
A – Amelanotic (worst type)
S – Superficial spreading—common
A – Acro-lentigenous
L – Lentigo maligna melanoma
D – Desmoplastic

Glasgow 7 points.

1. Change in size
2. Change in shape
3. Change in color
4. Inflammation
5. Crusting and bleeding
6. Sensory changes–tingling
7. Diameter is greater than 6 mm

Satellite lesion—skin lesion within 2 cm of primary
Intransit lesion—skin lesion between primary and draining LN.

Layers of epidermis

1. Stratum corneum
2. Stratum lucidium
3. Stratum granulosum
4. Stratum spinosum
5. Stratum basale

ABCDE of melanoma

A – asymmetry
B – border irregularity
C – color variation
D – diameter >6 mm
E – elevation

Clark's Level

Level 1 – tumor confined to basement membrane
Level 2 – tumor confined to papillary dermis
Level 3 – tumor confined to interface between papillary and reticular dermis
Level 4 – tumor confined to reticular dermis
Level 5 – tumor invades subcutaneous fat

N1 – 1 node
N2 – 2–3 node
N3 – 4 or more
M1 – skin and subcutaneous tissue
M2 – lung metastasis
M3 – visceral organ other than lung.

T1 – < 1 mm
T2 – 1–2 mm
T3 – 2–4 mm
T4 – >4 mm

Breslow's thickness

Stage 1 – <0.75 mm (epidermis)
Stage 2 – 0.76 – 1.49 mm (papillary dermis)
Stage 3 – 1.5 – 3.99 mm (reticular dermis)
Stage 4 – >4 mm

Tumor marker of melanoma—LDH, melan A, 5100, HMB45
It spreads through:

- Local invasion
- Lymphatic
- Blood spread

Sentinel LN biopsy

- Carcinoma (cabana)
- Breast carcinoma
- Malignant melanoma

INVESTIGATION

- Biopsy
- FNAC from node (sentinel lymph node)
- X-ray chest/bone
- USG abdomen (secondaries in liver).

TREATMENT

- Excision biopsy—wide excision
- Subungual malignant melanoma—amputation of digit
- Malignant melanoma choroid—enucleation of eye
- Advanced and large lesion—amputation.

MANAGEMENT OF LYMPH NODE

- If LN adjacent to primary—block dissection along with primary
- If LN are away—radical block dissection
- If LN enlarged basal and fixed—radiotherapy.

MANAGEMENT OF ADVANCED MALIGNANT MELANOMA

- Radiotherapy
- Systemic chemotherapy – decarbazine, cisplatin, vinblastin
- Immunotherapy – alpha interferon, IL-2
- Hormone treatment – tamoxifen
- Isolated limb perfusion with melphalan

Clark's Level

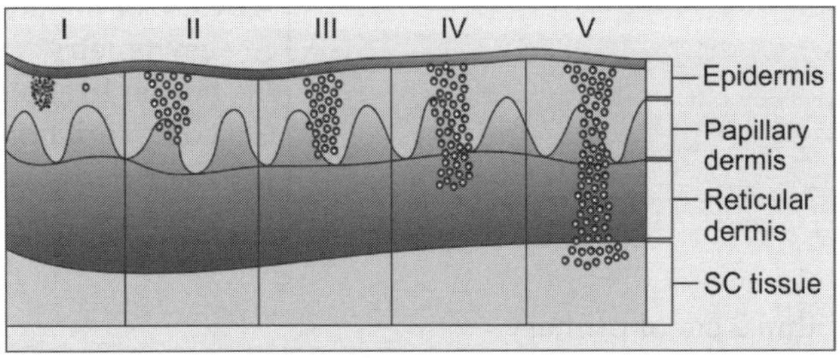

CARCINOMA TONGUE

DO NOT FORGET TO LOOK FOR

- Site
- Size
- Tobacco staining
- Dysphagia
- Excessive salivation
- Ankyloglossia
- Slurring of speech
- Induration and surrounding structures
- Lymph node
- Mandible
- Temporomandibular joint (TMJ)
- Lower cranial nerves
- Deviation of tongue.

Premalignant condition for oral cancer
- Erythroplakia, leukoplakia
- Chronic hyperplastic candidiasis
- Submucous fibrosis
- Plummer-Vinson syndrome
- Papilloma
- Syphilitic glossitis

Clinical Features of Ca Tongue

- Bleeding ulcer
- Pain in the tongue due to involvement of nerve
- Ankyloglossia—restricted mobility of tongue
- Dysphagia is common presentation from Ca of posterior 1/3rd
- Offensive smell

SCC is the most common carcinoma of tongue.

INVESTIGATIONS

- Wedge biopsy
- FNAC from LN, if it enlarged
- Chest X-ray
- X-ray spine
- Orthopantomogram
- Laryngoscopy
- CECT for staging

Etiology of oral carcinoma
- Premalignant conditions
- 6Ss (predisposing factor)
  1. Spirit
  2. Smoking
  3. Spices
  4. Sharp jagged tooth
  5. Syphilis
  6. Sepsis

TNM Staging of Oral Cavity Tumors

T1 – Tumor <2 cm
T2 – Tumor >2 cm but <4 cm
T3 – Tumor >4 cm
T4 – Tumor invades adjustment structure

N1 – single ipsilateral node < 3 cm
N2-
- N2a – single ipsilateral node > 3–6 cm
- N2b – multiple ipsilateral node <6 cm
- N2c – bilateral or contralateral node < 6 cm

N3 – Node > 6 cm
M1 – distant metastasis.

Different type of mandibulectomy
- Marginal mandibulectomy
- Sectional mandibulectomy
- Hemimandibulectomy
- Commando operation: Wide excision/ Hemiglossectomy + Mandibulectomy + Neck dissection

TREATMENT

- Surgery
  Wide excision+/–mandibulectomy+/–neck dissection
  Neck dissection – supraomohyoid neck dissection
  – Extended omohyoid neck dissection
  The mandible is reconstructed using ulna, fibula, ribs
- Brachytherapy (tentalum) or external beam radiotherapy (Co-60)
- The disadvantage of radiation is osteoradionecrosis.

Types of Glossectomy

- Wide excision–2 cm clearance
- Partial glossectomy–T3/T4
- Hemiglossectomy–T3/T4
- Total glossectomy–T4

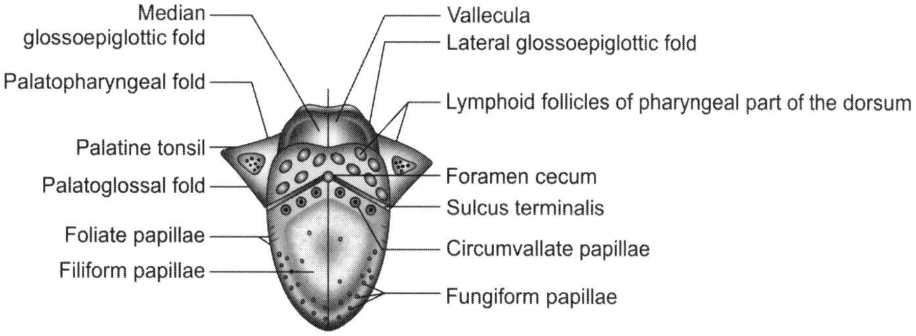

Anatomy of tongue

CARCINOMA PENIS

DO NOT FORGET TO LOOK

- Site
- Size
- Involvement of surrounding structure (scrotum, perineum)
- Lymph node
- Prerectal examination
- Any congenital anomaly (hypospadia)

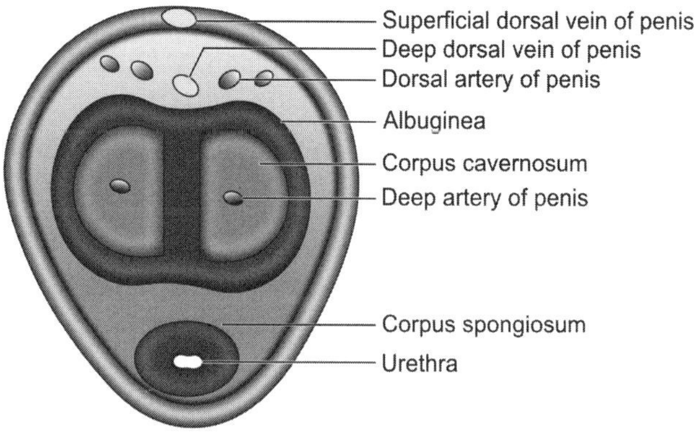

DISCUSSION

Premalignant lesion
- Genital warts—Buschke-Lowenstein tumor
- Erythroplasia of Qeuyret (Paget's disease of penis)
- Leukoplakia
- Bowen's disease.

ETIOLOGY

1. Phimosis 2. Human papilloma virus (HPV) warts 3. Balanitis xerotica (BXO) 4. Smoking, 5. Balanoposthitis, 6. Carcinoma is common in population who do not practise circumcision due to chronic irritation caused by smegma.
- *Phimosis – inability to retract prepucial skin*
- *Paraphimosis – inability to reduce previous retracted foreskin.*

CLINICAL FEATURES

- Nonhealing ulcer, indurated, everted edge
- Foul smelling discharge
- Recent phimosis
- Painless initially–2° infection–painful

Spread – direct spread and lymphatic spread

Radiotherapy indication
- Young patient who want sexual life
- Fixed/ulcerated inguinal metastasis
- Patient refuses surgery

Complicaton – radionecrosis of penis

INVESTIGATION

- Wedge biopsy
- Sentinel LN biopsy (Cabanas node)
- FNAC of enlarged lymph node
- USG abdomen–iliac nodes

TREATMENT (JACKSON STAGING)

Stage 1

Growth confined to prepuce – Circumcision
Growth involving glans – Partial amputation with 2 cm margin

Stage 2

Tumor involving penile shaft:
- Partial amputation—minimum stump size 2 cm
- Total penectomy with perineal urethrostomy.

Stage 3

Mobile regional nodal metastasis with stage 1 or 2
- Sentine lymph node biopsy,
- Illioinguinal block dissection.

Stage 4

Tumor beyond penile shaft – Radiotherapy and brachytherapy (radium wires/tantalum wires) + chemotherapy (cisplatin, MTX, bleomycin)

SOFT TISSUE SARCOMA

These are malignant tumors arising from soft tissue.

ETIOLOGY

- Genetic factors p53 mutation, NF type 1
- Exposure to radiation, chemicals
- Immunosuppression

INVESTIGATIONS

- Core biopsy—for histologic conformation and grading
- FNAC for conformation of recurrence
- Incision biopsy
  - Vertical incision is put
  - Flap should not rise
  - Prevent hematoma
- Chest X-ray (metastatic workup)
- MRI
- CT

Do not forget to look for:
- Site
- Size
- Induration
- Temperature
- Dilated veins over swelling
- Plane of swelling
- Distal neurovascular deficit
- Regional lymph node

GTNM staging of STS

Grade
Grade 1 – well differentiated
Grade 2 – moderately differentiated
Grade 3 – poorly differentiated
Grade 4 – undifferentiated

T
T1 ≤ 5 cm
T1a – superficial
T1b – deep
T2 > 5 cm
T2a – superficial
T2b – deep

N
Nx
N0
N1
M
M0
Mx

STS mainly metastasize through blood.
But some metastasize through lymphatics, which are: (code: SCREAM)
R – rhabdomyosarcoma
A – angiosarcoma
C – clear cell sarcoma
E – epithelioid sarcoma
M – malignant fibrous histiocytoma
S – synovial sarcoma

Pseudocapsule
When sarcoma grows flattening of normal tissue around them forming compression zone. Outside this zone there is edematous neovascularized area called reactive zone.
This compression and reactive zone is also called pseudocapsule.

TREATMENT

- Surgery—wide excision with 2 cm clear margin (3D excision required)
- Excision
- Intralesional excision — leave behind pseudocapsule
- Marginal excision — pseudocapsule taken
- Wide excision
- Radical excision
- Sometimes amputation is required.
- Chemotherapy — dacarbazine, doxorubicin, ifosfamide.

SUGGESTED READING

1. Bailey and Love's Short Practice of Surgery
2. A Manual on Clinical Surgery—S Das.

SURGERY

CHAPTER 9

Viva

OPERATIVE PROCEDURES—SURGERY

- **Thyroidectomy:**
  Refer chapter—Thyroid
- **Mastectomy:**
  Refer chapter—Breast
- **Parotidectomy:**
  Refer chapter—Salivary Gland Swelling
- **Hernia:**
  Refer chapter—Hernia
- **Varicose vein operation:**
  Refer chapter—Varicose Vein
- **Hydrocele operation:**
  - *Lord's plication*:
    Indication: Done for small hydrocele.
    The sac is opened and the cut edge of the sac is plicated to tunica albuginea (reflected portion of processus vaginalis). As a result, the sac gets crumpled up near the testes (so testicular secretion gets absorbed by the subcutaneous lymphatics and venous system).
  - *Jaboulay's eversion procedure:*
    Indication: Done for slightly larger hydrocele.
    Here, instead of placating the tunica vaginalis, it is everted and sutured onto itself behind the testis.
  - *Excision and eversion:*
    Indication: Done for very large hydrocele.
    Here, part of the sac is removed.

  Complications:
  - Hematoma
  - Infection
  - Injury to testes
  - Recurrence
  - Torsion of testes.
- **Tracheostomy:**
  Making an opening in the anterior wall of the trachea and converting it into a stoma on the skin surface.
  Indication:
  - Respiratory obstruction
  - Retained secretion
  - Respiratory insufficiency.

Types
• Emergency tracheostomy
• Elective tracheostomy
• Permanent tracheostomy
• Percutaneous dilatation
• Mini-tracheostomy

Steps

Position: Patient lies in supine position with a pillow under shoulder

Anesthesia: Local anesthesia (LA)/ general anesthesia (GA)/without anesthesia

- A vertical incision is made in the midline, extending from the cricoid to just above the sternal notch
  OR
  A transverse incision, 5 cm long, 2 finger breadth above the sternal notch (cosmetically better scar).
- Tissue dissected in the midline.
- Strap muscles are separated in the midline and retracted laterally.
- Thyroid isthmus is displaced upward.
- A few drops of 4% lignocaine are injected into the trachea to suppress cough when the trachea is incised.
- The trachea is fixed with a hook and opened with a vertical incision in the region of the 3rd and 4th OR 3rd and 2nd rings. This is then converted into a circular opening (Never divide the 1st tracheal ring because it can cause perichondritis of the cricoid cartilage).
- Tracheostomy tube of appropriate size is inserted.
- The skin incision should not be sutured or packed tightly as it may lead to the development of subcutaneous emphysema.

Complications:

Immediate:
- Hemorrhage
- Apnea
- Injury to recurrent laryngeal nerve
- Aspiration of blood.

Intermediate:
- Secondary bleeding
- Displacement of tube
- Subcutaneous emphysema
- Tracheitis, tracheobronchitis.

Late:
- Laryngeal stenosis
- Tracheal stenosis
- Tracheoesophageal fistula
- Keloid scar.

• **Circumcision**

Indications
- Religious
- Phimosis and paraphimosis
- Carcinoma penis stage I
- Balanitis
- Unable to retract prepuce for sexual intercourse
- Splitting of an abnormally tight frenulum.

Position: Supine

Anesthesia: LA/SA/GA (LA is preferred; Xylocaine 1 or 2% without adrenaline to the root of penis).

Procedure:
- With 2 hemostats, the prepuce is held at 3 o'clock and 9 o'clock positions and pulled forward.
- A longitudinal incision is made at the 12 o'clock position at the distal end on the prepuce up to the corona.
- At the corona, the incision is extended to either side, parallel to the coronal sulcus.
- The skin and subcutaneous tissues are removed.
- Bleeding from the frenular artery is possible and therefore should be ligated with a "Figure of 8" ligature.
- The skin is then sutured to the mucous membrane.

Complications
- Bleeding
- Infection
- Injury to the urethra and stricture.

• **Vasectomy:**

Permanent sterilization of males by removing a part of both the ductus deferens.

Anesthesia: Local anesthesia (LA).

Procedure:
- Scrotum is cleaned before the operation.
- Anesthesia is administered.
- A transverse incision of 1 cm is made at the junction of the upper and middle third of the median raphe.
- Vas is isolated and drawn out through the incision.
- The vasa are clamped at 2 sites and cut. The ends are turned backward and ligated.
- Repeat on the other side.

Postoperative counseling:
- No bath for one day
- Scrotal support for 2 weeks
- No heavy work for 3 weeks
- Psychological support
- Analgesics and antibiotics
- Report if any complication
- Advise alternate contraceptives (because it takes 30–40 ejaculations to be effective).

Complications:
- Pain
- Infection
- Hematoma
- Spontaneous recanalization
- Autoimmune response to sperms
- Sperm granuloma.

No scalpel vasectomy

Here, the advantages include: Less time; quick recovery; less pain; less postoperative discomfort, no sutures.

- **Cholecystectomy**

Indications:
- Cholelithiasis
- Cholecystitis
- Empyema gallbladder (GB)
- Carcinoma of GB
- Mucocele
- As a part of Whipple's surgery.

Complications:
- Postcholecystectomy syndrome
- Hemorrhage
- Stricture to CBD
- Injury to the liver
- Waltman Walters syndrome

Incision:

A short right upper transverse incision is made centered over the lateral border of the rectus muscle.

Steps:
- Incision
- The diagnosis is confirmed
- GB is appropriately exposed and packs are placed on the hepatic flexure of the colon, duodenum and lesser omentum (to ensure a clear view of the anatomy)
- Peritoneum is divided near the GB. Expose the cystic artery and duct and ligate (Calot's triangle).
- GB is dissected away from the GB bed.

- **Appendectomy:**

Indication: Acute appendicitis

Contraindication: Appendicular abscess

Position: Supine

Anesthesia: General anesthesia

Incision:
- Lanz incision: Transverse skin crease incision (nowadays done)
- Gridiron incision: At right angle to McBurney's point
- Rutherford Morison's: In para and retrocecal appendix.

Procedure:
- Lanz incision is made 2 cm below the umbilicus, centered along the midclavicular-midinguinal line
- The external oblique aponeurosis, IO and transversis abdominis are split in the direction of the fibers
- Peritoneum is opened

- Cecum is identified by the presence of taenia coli
- The appendix is identified and the inflammatory adhesion is broken with fingers
- The appendix is conveniently controlled using Babcock's forceps
- The base of the mesoappendix is clamped, divided and ligated
- The appendix is amputated
- A Z-suture may then be inserted into the cecum about 1.25 cm from the base
- Closure of the incision

Complications:
- Wound infection
- Intra-abdominal abscess
- Paralytic ileus
- Fecal fistula
- Intestinal obstruction.

DRUGS AND SURGERY INSTRUMENTS

DRUG

Lignocaine

Uses
- Local anesthetic
- Antiarrhythmic

Dose:
- 3 mg/kg and effect last for 90 minutes
- Lignocaine + adrenaline (1:2 lakh)—7 mg/kg
- 1% means each mL contains 10 mg of drugs
- It can be used with/without adrenaline
- Subcutaneous giddiness, headache, postural hypotension.

Contraindication

It should not be used in places, where end arteries are present (ear lobule, tip of nose, lip, fingers, toes, glans penis).

INSTRUMENTS

1. **Artery forceps**
   - To catch bleeding points
   - To pass ligature
   - To open fascial planes.
2. **Allis' tissue holding forceps**
   Used to hold skin flaps, fascia, aponeurosis.
3. **Deaver's retractor**
   - Used to retract liver, spleen, other abdominal viscera
   - It is less traumatic, gives adequate exposure of surgical fields.
5. **Morris' retractor:** To retract abdominal wall.
6. **Babcock's forceps**
   - Tip is nontraumatic
   - To hold any part of bowel, fallopian tube, etc. (tubular structures).
7. **Needle holder**
   - Needle holder held between thumb and ring finger
   - Needle is placed at the junction of proximal 2/3rd and distal 1/3rd.
8. **Toothed dissecting forceps:** To hold skin and tough structures.
9. **Nontoothed dissecting forceps:** To hold delicate structures (vessels, peritoneum, etc.).
10. **Joll's thyroid retractor:** Self-retaining retractor user in thyroid surgeries.
11. **Lister's sinus forceps:** Used in Hilton's method of draining pus from abscess cavity.

12. **Tracheostomy tube**
    - Fuller's bivalve tracheostomy tube – outer tube and inner tube
    - Jackson's tracheostomy tube – outer tube, inner tube and obturator.
13. **Foley's catheter**
    - Self-retaining urinary catheter made of latex
    - It has got balloon near tip into which distilled water is infused to make it self-retainable.

    Size
    - Adult—16 F (French unit)
    - Children—8/10 F

    Uses
    - In retention of urine (BPH, stricture, etc.)
    - Percutaneous cystotomy
    - To measure urine output
    - Epistaxis
    - Labor induction
    - Arrest bleeding after hemorrhoidectomy.

    Complication
    - Infection
    - Bleeding
    - Stricture
    - Stone formation.
14. **Ryle's tube**
    - One meter long
    - It has got 3 lead shot at its tip (radiopaque)
    - It has got 3 markings:
      1. Mark at 40 cm—at the level of gastroesophageal junction
      2. Mark at 50 cm—at the level of body of stomach
      3. Mark at 60 cm—at the level of pylorus.

    Uses

    Therapeutic
    - In acute abdominal condition
    - After abdominal surgeries
    - In upper GI bleeding
    - In pyloric stenosis
    - Decompression of stomach
    - Stomach wash.

    Diagnostic
    - For gastric function test
    - To diagnose tracheoesophageal fistula
    - Baid test for pseudocyst of pancreas.
15. **Kehr' T-tube**
    - It is used after opening CBD. CBD closed with T-tube placed in the CBD.
    - Before removal of T tube, patency of CBD should be confirmed (10 day).
16. **Humby's knife**
    - It is used to take skin graft
    - There is a screw at the end, using which exact thickness of skin removed.
17. **Myer's stripper:** Used for stripping varicose vein
18. **Proctoscope**
    - It is used to visualize rectum and anal canal.
    - In painful condition (like fissure in ano), it is contraindicated.
19. **Kocher's forceps**
    - These forceps are used to tough structures like aponeurosis, fascia.
    - During thyroidectomy, it is used to hold strap muscles for dividing them.

20. **Burr:** It is used to create opening in the cranium.
21. **Suture materials**

Classification

A. ***Absorbable***
   1. Plain catgut
      Natural
      Derived from jejunum of sheep
      Absorption time—7 days (by inflammatory Reaction and phagocytosis)
   2. Chromic catgut
      Absorption time—21 days
   3. Vicryl (polyglactin)
      Violet in color
      Multifilament and braided
      Absorption time—90 days (by hydrolysis)
   4. PDS (polydioxonone suture)

   Uses
   Bowel anastomosis
   Suturing muscle, fascia, peritoneum
   Ligating pedicle

Nonabsorbable
   1. Silk
      Natural, multifilament and braided
      Black in color
      Derived from cocoon of silkworm larva
   2. Prolene (polypropylene)
      Blue in color
      Synthetic, monofilament
   3. Ethylene
      Synthetic, monofilament
      Black in color

   Closure of abdomen
   Herniorrhaphy
   Suture the skin

B. ***Natural***
   Catgut
   Silk

Synthetic
   Vicryl
   PDS
   Prolene
   Ethylene

C. ***Monofilament***
   Prolene
   Ethylene
   PDS
   Catgut

Multifilament
   Vicryl
   Silk

22. **Needle holder**

SPECIMENS

- **Mastectomy specimen**
  - Specimen of breast showing skin and breast tissue
  - Most probably carcinoma breast
  - Investigation: Trucut biopsy or fine needle aspiration cytology (FNAC)
  - Also read about different type of mastectomy
  - Common bones affected by metastasis—lumbar vertebrae, femur, thoracic vertebrae.
- **Meckel's diverticulum**
  - Resected specimen of intestine showing diverticulum
  - Most probably Meckel's diverticulum
  - Rule of 2—it presents in 2% of cases, 2 inches long, 2 feet away from ileocecal region
  - Hernia of Littre—hernial sac consists of Meckel's diverticulum
  - Treatment – diverticulectomy.
- **Mesenteric cyst**
  - Bowel specimen showing cyst
  - Most probably mesenteric cyst
  - Types:
    - Chylolymphatic (common)
    - Enterogenous
    - Urogenital remnant
    - Dermoid
  - The sign of mesenteric cyst—lump moves in a plane right hypochondrium to left iliac fossa, but not in a plane right angles to it.

- Treatment—enucleation (chylolymphatic), resection of cyst (enterogenous)
- Enucleation contraindicated in enterogenous.

- **Intussusception**
  - Specimen showing one portion of bowel invaginated within another
  - Most probably intussusception
  - Parts: Intussusception, intussuscipiens, neck, apex
  - Common type: Ileocolic
  - Treatment: Hydrostatic reduction or operative reduction.
- **Trichobezoar**
  - Specimen showing black hairy like materials in stomach
  - Most probably trichobezoar
  - Clinical feature: Features of gastric outlet obstruction
  - Treatment: Papain, cellulose, surgical removal.
- **Splenectomy**
  - Specimen showing spleen
    - Indication of splenectomy
    - Trauma: Accidental, operative
    - Oncological: Diagnostic, therapeutic
    - Hematological: Spherocytosis, purpura, hypersplenism
    - Portal hypertension: Variceal surgery
  - Complication
  - Hemorrhage
  - Damage to adjust organs
  - OPSI (opportunistic postsplenectomy infection): *Pneumococci*, *Neisseria*, *Haemophilus*, *E. coli*
  - Splenunculi—accessory spleen, it also removed along with spleen
  - Splenosis—multiple small implant of splenic tissue on the peritoneal surface following rupture of spleen (it gives rise to adhesion).
- **Testicular tumor**
  - Cut surface of testes showing tumor in the specimen
  - Most probably seminoma
  - Seminoma spread through lymphatics
  - Treatment: High inguinal orchidectomy
  - FNAC and incision biopsy are contraindicated (read chapter on Testes)
  - Tumor marker: Beta human chorionic gonadotropin (β hCG), lactate dehydrogenase (LDH), placental alkaline phosphatase.
- **Cholecystectomy for gallstone**
  - Specimen showing gallbladder (pear-shaped) and multiple stones in the lumen
  - Most probably cholecystectomy for gallstone
  - Symptoms: Pain, dyspepsia, vomiting
  - Complication: Postcholecystectomy syndrome, bleeding, stricture of common bile duct (CBD), injury to liver
  - Gallstones: Cholesterol, pigment, mixed stones.

X-RAYS

1. **Intestinal obstruction**
   Erect abdominal film with multiple air fluid levels

Up to three fluid levels are normal
1. At fundus of stomach
2. At the duodenal cap
3. In terminal ileum

Abdomen
- Take erect and supine views
- Anteroposterior (AP) film
- Examine the entire abdomen from top of diaphragm to hernial orifices in the groin
- Look for bones
- Look for soft tissue shadows

Cause of fluid inside the intestine in obstruction
- Various digestive enzymes
- Absorption from gut is retarded
- Fluid secreted from bowel wall

Quartet of symptoms
- Vomiting
- Abdominal pain
- Abdominal distension
- Absolute constipation

- Gas – black
- Fluid – Light gray
- Metal – Intense white
- Fat – Dark gray
- Bone/calcification – White

More severe the obstruction, more distal the obstruction, more the number of fluid level.
- **Jejunum—valvulae conniventes:** Coiled spring shape folds completely pass across the width of the bowel, they are regularly spaced and give a concertina or ladder effect.
- **Ileum—characterless**
- **Colon—haustrations:** The colonic mucosal folds do not completely cross the lumen and they are placed irregularly (colon is placed peripheral and contains feces and the small bowel is central and contains fluid and gas).
- **Management:** *"The sun should not both rise and set on a case of unrelieved intestinal obstruction."*
- **Principles of Mx:**
  - Drip (IV fluids), suction (nasogastric decompression)
  - Relief of obstruction.

Etiology:
- Repeated pregnancy
- Obesity
- Flabbiness of abdominal muscles

- **Sigmoid volvulus**
  - **Pneumatic tyre appearance**—grossly distended loop of sigmoid colon—extending from the pelvis to the under surface of the diaphragm. The loop, running diagonally from right to left with two fluid levels compression, together of the two medial walls produce the **Coffee Bean sign.**
  - **Lack of haustration**
  - **Liver overlap sign**; indicative of the degree of distension of colon, the colonic loop will reach the height of the liver or above it on the right side.
  - **Left flank overlap sign**; the left limb of the coffee bean overlies the descending colon.
  - Barium enema picture produces **bird beak appearance** (point of convergence of the distended loops appearing as birds beak or bird of prey).
- **Gas under the diaphragm**
  - Plain X-ray abdomen erect posture showing dark crescent area of gas under the diaphragm other signs
  - *Double wall sign:* Both sides of the wall of a loop of bowel will become visible because air on outside and inside are demonstrated
  - *Silver sign:* Visualization of falciform ligament
  - *Football or dome sign:* Under surface of diaphragm shows dark dome like appearance.

  Causes
  - Perforated peptic ulcer
  - Appendix perforation
  - Intestinal obstruction with perforation
  - Inflammatory bowel disease (IBD)
  - Post-laparotomy
  - Drug induced.

  Differential diagnosis
  - Subphrenic abscess
  - Chilaiditi's syndrome (colonic interposition)
  - Meteorism (due to excessive air swallowing)

- **Intravenous urogram/pyelogram**
  It is carried out by intravenous injection into a vein in antecubital fossa of iodine containing dye like urografin. It is filtered from blood by the glomeruli and rapidly passes through urine.
  a. Scout film (plane X-ray abdomen taken before injection of dye)

- Nephrogram at 2 minutes, when the dye is being filtered by the glomerulus—shows the renal parenchyma opacified by the contrast medium
- Serial films thereafter at 5, 10, 15, 20 and 30 minutes
  The contrast is excreted into the collecting system opacifying the renal pelvis and calyces.
- Another film at 1 hour and 2 hours
- Post-micturition film is taken to show the details of the bladder area.

Types of urogram
- Intravenous urogram (IVU)
- Retrograde pyelography (the contrast is injected through ureteric catheter after cystoscopy)
- Antegrade pyelography (the contrast is injected to the pelvis).

Indication of IVU/IVP: Demonstration of stone, tumor, abnormal anatomy, hydronephrosis

Hydronephrosis: *Aseptic dilatation of pelvicalyceal system due to partial or intermittent obstruction.*

Features:
- Loss of cupping
- Flattening
- Clubbing of the calyces.

Causes
- Inside lumen
  - Stones
  - Sloughed papillae
- In the wall
  - Strictures
  - Tumor of ureter
  - Idiopathic pelviureteric junction
- Obstruction
  - Outside the wall
    - Ca colon
    - Retroperitoneal fibrosis

Surgical Mx: ***Anderson-Hynes pyeloplasty***

Types of renal stones
- Oxalate
- Phosphate
- Urate
- Cysteine
- Xanthine calculus.

(90% of renal stones are radiopaque and 10% are radiolucent; 90% if gallstones are radiolucent 10% are radiopaque to differentiate between two take lateral view, renal stones are near vertebral column).

- **Achalasia cardia**
  - Barium swallow showing smooth pencil-shaped narrowing at the lower end of esophagus (**bird's beak appearance**).
  - **Mx:** Heller's myotomy
  - The narrowing in carcinoma is irregular and described as '**rat tail appearance' demonstrate** stones, tumors, abnormal anatomy, hydronephrosis.
- **Barium meal, Ca stomach**
  - Persistent mucosal irregularity
  - Persistent irregular defect
  - Persistent loss of peristalsis in a particular segment
  - (In barium swallow a thick solution of barium sulfate is given to patient for swallowing mainly done for study of esophagus and pharynx, for barium meal a dilute solution of barium sulfate is used mainly for stomach, when sequential films of the small intestine after barium meal, it is called barium meal follow through).
- **Barium enema:** Showing apple core deformity with shouldering on either side in the ascending colon suggestive of carcinoma colon.
- **Ileocecal tuberculosis—barium enema**
  - Pulled up cecum
  - Obtuse ileocecal angle
  - **Fleischner sign**: Narrow terminal ileum with wide open ileocecal valve
  - **Sterlin sign:** Fibrotic terminal ileum opening into contracted cecum.
- **Barium enema, intussusception**
  - **Claw sign**: Barium seen as a claw around a negative shadow of intussusception
  - It is also called **coil spring appearance.**
- **T-tube cholangiogram**
  - With horizontal limb of the T-tube inside the CBD and the vertical limb outside the body the dye comes down the CBD and fills the duodenum. There is no evidence of any obstruction or residual stone in the CBD. The T-tube is put inside the bile duct after the exploration of the bile duct **(choledochotomy)** for removal of stone

(choledochotomy). After clearing the stones, there will be papillary edema and spasm and therefore the dye may not come to the duodenum after the preoperative cholangiogram. Therefore, a T-tube is put for drainage of the infected bile. This tube is later utilized for T-tube cholangiogram after 7 to 10 days.

- The T-tube is then connected to a drainage bottle and the 24-hour measurements are taken daily. As the edema and spasm of the papilla disappear, the quantity of bile coming to the bottle will decrease gradually over a period one week. It allows time for relief of papillary spasm.
- This tube can also be used for T-tube cholangiogram postoperatively for demonstration of residual stones.
- If residual stones are found, the tube is left in place for 6 weeks, so that a mature tract is formed. There is a chance that stone may pass to the duodenum meanwhile.
- The stone can be later removed percutaneously by an interventional radiologist (Burhenne technique).

SOME FAVORITE QUESTIONS

THYROID (THYRO-SHIELD LIKE, ID-GUTTER)

Named by Wharton.

EMIL THEODOR KOCHER

Father of Thyroid Surgery (Nobel Prize)

1. Kocher's test
2. Kocher's maneuver—for reduction of shoulder dislocation
3. Kocher's vein
4. Kocher's incision:
   - Kocher's subcostal incision for cholecystectomy
   - Kocher's collar crease incision for thyroidectomy was discovered by Bassini (father of modern hernia repair)
5. Kocher's forceps to hold tough fascia
6. Kocherization (duodenal mobilization).

BERRY

- Berry's sign
- Berry's ligament
- Berry's picking—sampling of lymph node
- Berry aneurysm.

X-RAY CHEST IN THYROID—FINDINGS

- Calcification: Fine in papillary, coarse in medullary
- Trachea: Position
- Retrosternal extension
- Cervical spondylitis.

Tremors—fine in hypothyroidism, coarse in parkinsonism, cirrhosis, drug induced, ...etc.
Cricothyroid—tuning fork of larynx (piano)—supplied by external laryngeal nerve
Strap muscles (strap = ribbon like) supplied by ansa cervicalis

PAPILLARY

Orphan Annie—cartoon caricature

MEDULLARY

- Amyloid stroma
- Calcitonin is the tumor marker
- **MNG**—follicular carcinoma
- **Thyroglossal cyst**—papillary carcinoma
- **Hashimoto's thyroiditis**—Lymphoma is an example for APUDOMA (amine precursor uptake and decarboxylation)
- **Causes of diarrhea—**hypothyroidism, medullary carcinoma
- **Cyst (=Bladder)**
  - Retention cyst, e.g. sebaceous cyst, ranula

- Inclusion cyst, e.g. dermoid cyst
- Degeneration cyst, e.g. ganglion
- Extravasation cyst
- Pseudocyst—no epithelial covering
- Demodex folliculorum is seen in sebaceous cyst
- Cysts in mandible—dentigerous (congenital), dental (acquired).

LIPOMA

- Universal tumor
- Brown fat (adult fat) is seen in lipoma.
  - Classification subcutaneous, intermuscular, intramuscular, intra-articular, intraglandular, intraosteal, subserosal, submucosal, extradural, subdural, retroperitoneal.
  - Dercum's disease—multiple painful lipomas
  - Complications: Liposarcoma, disfigurement, pressure effect, degeneration.

SPIGELIAN

- Spigelian hernia
- Spigelian lobe: Caudate lobe of liver
- Spigelian line: From 9th costal cartilage to pubic tubercle
- Spigelian fascia.

CAUSES OF GANGRENE—BREASTED

- Buerger's disease
- Raynaud's disease
- Emboli
- Arterial injection of drugs like thiopentone sodium
- Senile, syphilis
- Thrombotic
- Ergot
- Diabetes.

Paget

- Paget cell – Paget disease of nipple
- Pagetoid cell – melanoma
- Paget test – very small swelling
- Paget disease in penis
- Paget disease of recurrent desmoids.

Melanoma—ABCDE

Sailors node—epitrochlear node in syphilis

What does it mean

- Claud-I limb
- Hernia—off shoot
- Clavicle—key

Leriche sign—bilateral iliac occlusion

Renal angle—normally resonant due to colonic band

Hydrocele of breast—lymph cyst of breast

Hydatid cyst—tender coconut

Aristotle—father of embryology

Rudolf virchow—father of pathology
Virchow's node, Virchow's triad

Meleny's ulcer—necrotizing fasciitis of abdominal wall

Buruli's ulcer—*Mycobacterium ulcerans*

Bazin's ulcer?

Gas under diaphragm—Chiladiti's sign

6S in carcinoma oral cavity

SURGERY

Liver function test (LFT)—nonspecific and enzyme specific
- Enzyme (5′nucleotidase)
- Most sensitive – serum albumin (synthesized only by liver)
- Dye test (rose Bengal test, BSD test)
- Ultrasonography (USG)
- Computed tomography (CT)
- Biopsy.

In Case HIV, HBsAg Cases
- Post as a last case
- Use double glow
- Use maximum disposable instruments.

Criles
- Criles grading
- Criles method of palpation.

Breast
- CREST syndrome
- Lobular carcinoma—familial, multicentric.

House of Bassini—inguinal canal

Hunter's:
- Hunter's canal
- Hunter's operation
- Hunter's chancre
- Hunter's aneurysm
- Hunter's ligament.

Superior thyroid artery is a branch of?

Where does common carotid artery bifurcate?

Branches of external carotid art are superior thyroid, lingual, facial anteriorly, occipital and post auricular, medially ascending pharyngeal ART and terminal branches are maxillary and superficial temporal.

What is sit on VIT?

Vertebral artery enters through C6

Which are the typical vertebras? C3 to C6... Why?

Structures medial to thyroid are recurrent laryngeal nerv, external laryngeal nerve, esophagus, trachea?

Post to thyroid is carotid.

C6 level is **anatomical bonanza** because it marks the end of larynx, pharynx, recurrent laryngeal nerve and beginning of superior thyroid artery.

Patey
- MRM
- Fasciovenous plane of Patey

Mandatory Investigation in the Thyroid
- TFT (Thyroid function text)
- FNAC (Fine-needle aspiration cytology)
- Serum calcium ⎤
- Serum antibody ⎦ auxillary tests

Intern's Tumor
Renal cell carcinoma (RCC), hypernephroma, Grawitz tumor

Mayo
- Mayo's needle
- Mayo's scissors

- Mayo's vein (prepyloric vein)
- Mayo's operation.

Fibrocystic disease of breast—blue dome cyst of blood good.

Complication of Bassini's hernia repair—osteitis pubis.

$CuSO_4$
- Is a fungicide
- In phenol burn—never use water.

Halsted
- First radical mastectomy
- First used rubber glove

Dodd—mid thigh perforator—da Vinci perforator

Pan arteritis—Buerger's disease

Mantrel's appendicitis.

ORTHOPEDICS

CHAPTER 10

Short Cases

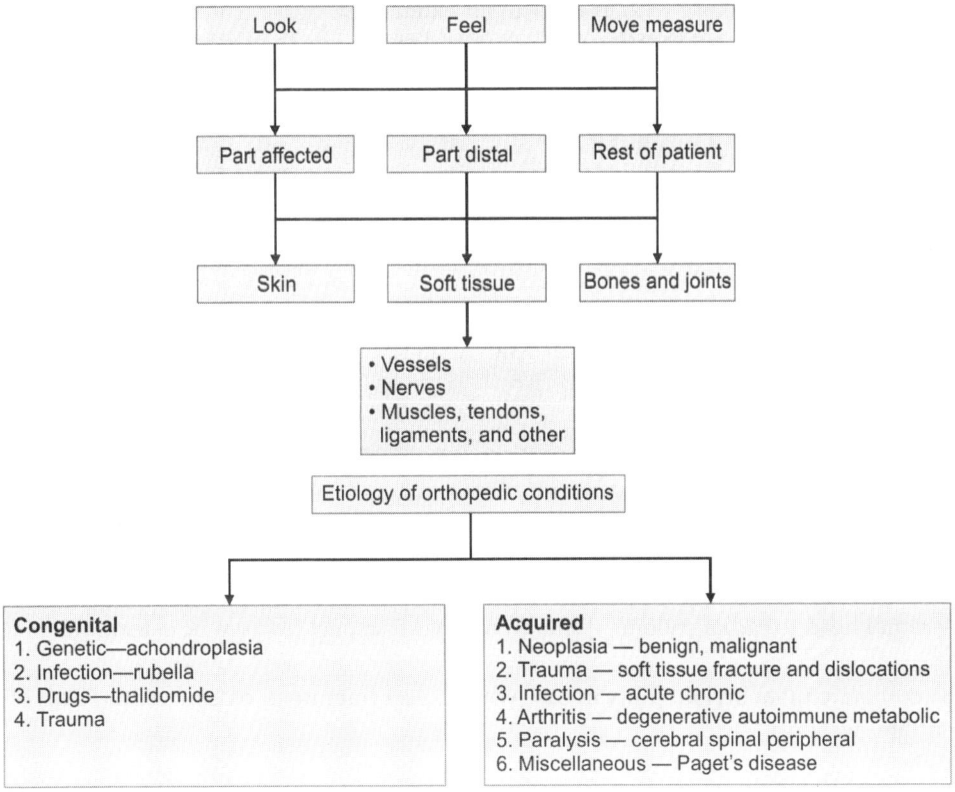

EXAMINATION OF ELBOW JOINT

INSPECTION (FROM FRONT, SIDE, BACK)

- Attitude
- Deformity—cubitus valgus, varus, etc.
- Swelling—cubital fossa, para olecranon fossa and anconeus triangle, anteroposterior thickening
- Wasting, shortening, irregularity

Cases kept

1. Cubitus varus secondary to malunited supracondylar fracture
2. Cubitus valgus secondary to malunited fracture lateral condyle

- Undue prominence of bone (olecranon—posterior dislocation)
- Effusion
- Skin over elbow and surroundings—scar, sinus, etc.
- Trophic changes of fingers.

PALPATION

- Local rise of temperature, tenderness
- Palpation of bone—look for tenderness (site), **Thickening, irregularity (suggestive of old fracture**, chronic osteomyelitis, etc.) displacements, crepitus, **myositis ossificans—bony swelling (brachialis muscle)**, referred tenderness.

  Humerus – supracondylar ridge (medial and lateral), lateral and medial condyles, epicondyle (Lateral condyle = lateral epicondyle + capitulum + lateral 1/3rd trochlea; medial condyle = medial epicondyle + medial 2/3rd trochlea)

  Radius, ulna
- **Three bony point relationship:** Maintained in supracondylar fracture. Altered in dislocation of elbow or # of condyles or supracondylar fracture with intercondylar extension.
- Ulnar nerve in cubital tunnel—subluxating on flexion and extension; thickening; tender or nodularity.

MOVEMENT

- **Range of motion**
- **Associated with pain, spasm or crepitus**
- **Deformity**
- **Abnormal mobility, e.g. varus or valgus**
  - **Active and passive**

    Flexion 0–140 Extension 0–10

    Supination 0–90 Pronation 0–80
  - **Abnormal mobility**

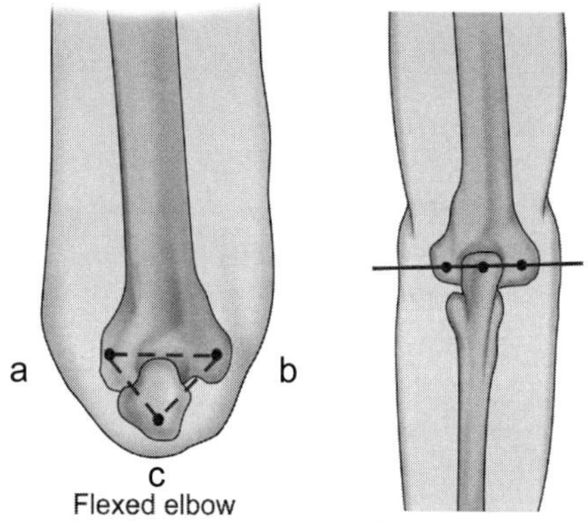

Flexed elbow (looking from behind) Extended elbow

MEASUREMENT

- **Longitudinal**
  - Arm—angle of acromion to lateral epicondyle of humerus
  - Forearm lateral column—lateral epicondyle to radial styloid
  - Medial column—medial epicondyle to ulnar styloid
  - Radius—radial head to radial styloid – [only in case you suspect fracture or osteomyelitis (OM) of forearm bones]
  - Ulna—olecranon to ulnar styloid [only in case you suspect fracture or osteomyelitis (OM) of forearm bones]
- **Circumferential**—wasting
- **Carrying angle**
  - Angle subtended by extended and supinated forearm axis with the long axis of the arm
    - Male = 5–10
    - Female = 10–15
    - <5 –varus, >15 valgus
  - Lines joining
    1. Midpoint of most prominent part of deltoid
    2. Midpoint of line joining epicondyles
    3. Midpoint of styloid processes.

SPECIAL TESTS

Valgus and varus stress test—ulnar and radial collateral ligament

One joint above and below

Distal neurovascular deficit

Proximal lymph node

EXAMINATION OF KNEE JOINT

- **Inspection** (From front, side, back)
  - Attitude (position of ease which can be brought back to anatomical position)
  - Deformity—genu valgum/varum/recurvatum
  - Position of patella—any dislocation, tilt, high riding
  - Gait
  - Swelling—fullness—parapatellar fossa, popliteal fossa
  - Wasting
  - Shortening
  - Popliteal fossa
  - Skin over knee and surroundings—scar, sinus, etc.
- **Palpation**
  - Local rise of temperature, ***joint line tenderness, site***
  - Palpation of bone—look for tenderness, thickening, irregularity, displacements, crepitus, referred tenderness Femur (condyles S/C ridges), Patella (under surface, subluxating, high riding, tracking), tibia (condyles), fibula
  - Tests for effusion
    - Minimal effusion—patellar tap (standing position)
    Stroke test (standing position)
    - Moderate effusion—patellar tap (supine position)
  - Palpate synovial thickening—medial lower femur
  - Palpate for swelling—bony (tumor)/soft tissue (ganglion/bursae)

False –ve patellar tap

- Tense effusion
- Minimal effusion
- Flexion deformity

- **Movement**
  Active and passive
  - Flexion: 0–140 (till calf touches the back of thigh)
  - Extension (till leg and thigh forms a straight line)
  - In a flexed knee only: Internal rotation—30°, external rotation—45°

  Abnormal mobility
  Locking, extension lag
- **Measurement**
  - **Longitudinal**
    - Lower limb: Anterior superior iliac spine (ASIS) to medial malleolus
    - Femur: ASIS to medial joint line
    - Tibia: Medial joint line to medial malleolus, intercondylar and intermalleolar distance
  - **Circumferential—**wasting
  - **Q angle (Quadriceps angle)**
    valgus knee angle increase: varus knee angle decrease
    - Angle between lines joining ASIS to mid patella and tibial tuberosity to mid patella (Using goniometer)
    - Normal male: 13–15
    - Female: 15–18
    - >20: chance of dislocation
  - **Special tests**
    - **Collaterals**
      - » Medial—valgus stress test
      - » Lateral—varus stress test (20°—flexion)
    - **Cruciate**
    ACL **Anterior drawer (90° flexion) – door stopper effect**
    Lachman (20° flexion)
    PCL **Posterior drawer**
    Posterior sag sign
    (pain over tibial tuberosity usually does not touch patella)
    - **Meniscus**
      - » **Mc Murray**:
        - › Medial meniscus—flex, abduct, external rotate knee then extend slowly
        - › Lateral meniscus—flex, adduct, internal rotate knee then extend slowly

ORTHOPEDICS

- » **Appley's grinding test:** (usually not done)
  - › Medial meniscus—compression and lateral rotation
  - › Lateral meniscus—compression and medial rotation

  Appley's distraction test: (usually not done)
  - – Medial collateral—pull and lateral rotate
  - – Lateral collateral—pull and medial rotate
- » **Patellar dislocation**
  - › Apprehension test—20° flex, dislocate – apprehension
  - › Patellar glide—3/4 quadrants of patella displaced
  - › Patellar grind—push patella down, flex and extend knee which causes pain
  - › Patellar tilt—tilt patella laterally
  - › Patellar tracking—on flexing knee patella takes inverted J shaped track in dislocation

- **Distal neurovascular deficit**
- **Proximal lymph node.**

OSTEOMYELITIS

HISTORY

- Age—children
- Trauma—open fracture, penetrating injury
- Acute:
  - Fever
  - Pain
  - Redness
  - Swelling
  - Limitation of movement.
- Chronic:
  - Pain only during acute exacerbation
  - Cyclical pain
  - Discharging sinus
  - Extrusion of bone fragments.

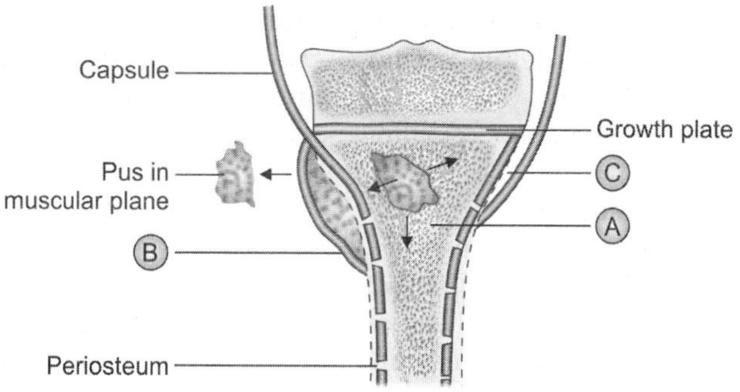

Diagnosis of Chronic Osteomyelitis

- History of tuberculosis (TB)
- History of fracture – treatment immobilization
- Diabetes mellitus (immunosuppression).

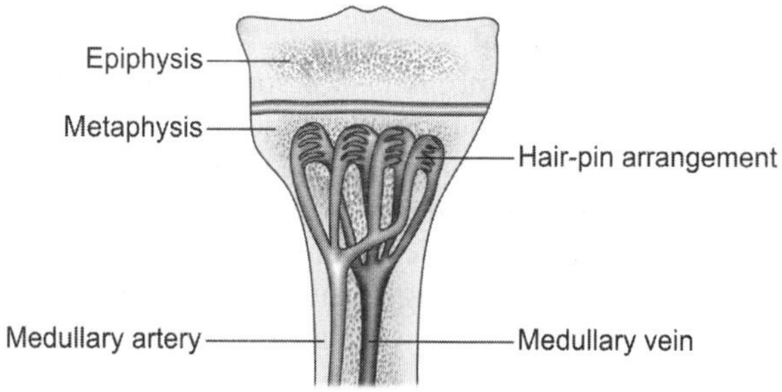

GENERAL EXAMINATION

Local Examination

Inspection

- Attitude, deformity
- Swelling, redness
- Sinus
- Discharge, granulation
- Scars
- Wasting of muscle
- In knee—any fullness of patellar fossa

Palpation

- Local rise in temperature/tenderness
- Thickening of bone, irregularity of bone
- Transmitted mobility, abnormal mobility—pathological fracture
- Scar whether adherent to bone

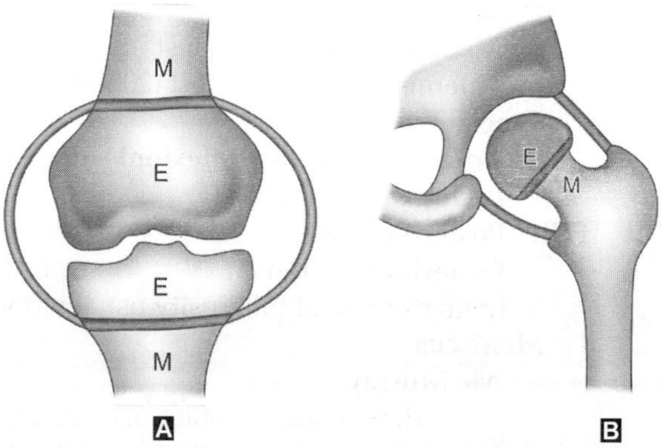

- Sinus whether adherent to bone
- **Movement**
- **Measurement**
  - Limb length
  - Wasting
- **Palpation of LN, distal neurovascular status**
- **Nearby joint—stiffness, deformity.**

INVESTIGATIONS

- X-ray—obliteration of soft tissue, sequestrum, involucrum, irregular thickening of bone, cloacae
- USG (children)
- CT and MRI
- Pus culture and sensitivity
- Biopsy (Gold standard).

> Diagnosis; chronic osteomyelitis; site (bone), topography epi-meta-or diaphysis; with complications – shortening; deformity; stiffness of nearby joint; pathology, etc.

TREATMENT

- Acute osteomyelitis:
  - Within 48 hours: Antibiotics–broad spectrums
    Ceftriaxone + vareomycin
    Ceftriaxone + cloxacillin
  - After 48 hours: Surgical explorations and drainage of pus
    Antibiotic and hydration
  - Chronic osteomyelitis: Sequestrectomy
    Sancerisations
    Curettage, debridement
    Amputations

COMPLICATIONS

- Acute osteomyelitis
  - General complications: Septicemia pyemia
  - Local complications:
    - Chronic osteomyelitis
    - Pathological fracture
    - Growth plate disturbances
- Chronic osteomyelitis:
  - Acute exacerbations or flare up
  - Growth abnormalities; deposit, shortening, lengthening
  - Pathological fracture
  - Joint stiffness.

NONUNION AND DELAYED UNION

It is a state of fracture healing in which biological process of fracture healing has come to a standstill, clinically manifested by abnormal painless mobility, radiographically by obliteration of marrow cavity, sclerosis narrowing of fracture ends even after adequate time of healing.

When a facture takes more than usual time to unite it is said to have gone in delayed union.

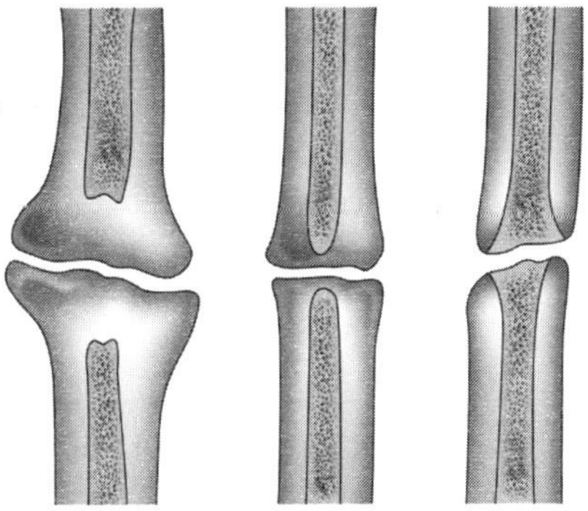

Elephant foot   Horse hoof   Oligotrophic reasons

WEBER-MULLER CLASSIFICATION OF NONUNION

- **Atrophic** (avascular, minimal/no attempt to heal)
  - Pure atrophic
  - Comminuted
  - Gap
  - Torsion wedge

ORTHOPEDICS

- **Hypertrophic** (though callus is present it does not bridge fracture site)
  - Elephant foot—exuberant callus
  - Horse hoof–poor callus due to unstable fixation with screws and plates
  - Oligotrophic—very poor callus poor internal fixation.
    - Insecure fixation of fracture (#) sites
    - Premature weight-bearing.

CAUSES OF DELAYED AND NONUNION

- Related to patient
  - Age
  - Systemic illnesses
- Related to fracture
  - Distraction at site
    - Muscle pulling fragments
    - Gravity
  - Soft tissue interposition
  - Bone loss at time of fracture
  - Infection from an open fracture
  - Damage to blood supply
  - Pathologic fracture
- Related to treatment
  - Inadequate reduction
  - Inadequate immobilization
  - Distraction during treatment.

X-ray
- Gap between the fracture fragments
- Amount of callus formed
- Decreased density of bone due to osteoporosis

Dx -It is clinicoradiological diagnosis so:
- It is better to say ununited fracture probably nonunion/delayed union
- Abnormal painless mobility—nonunion
- Abnormal painful mobility—delayed union
- **X-ray.**

MANAGEMENT

- **Infected nonunion**
  - Antibiotics—IV/Beads—as per pus, culture and sensitivity
  - External fixation
  - Sequestrectomy—only if involucrum is >2/3rd circumference
  - After infection subsides
  - Internal fixation with bone graft or Ilizarov's method.
- **Noninfected nonunion**
  - Rigid internal fixation with plate or Ilizarov's method.

Ilizarov: If there is nonunion with shortening or deformity

BONE GRAFTS

- Cancellous—for osteogenic purpose (e.g. iliac crest)
- Cortical—for stability, filling defects—fibula
- Corticocancellous, e.g. rib
- Vascular.

MALUNION

- When a fracture does not unite in proper position it is said to be malunited.
- Causes: Improper treatment
- Sites: Supracondylar fracture—gun stock deformity.
- Colle's fracture—dinner fork deformity.

Treatment

- Treatment is individualized
- Osteotomy in young active patients.

***Crossed union** Special type of malunion in fracture forearm bones, wherein the 2 bones unite with each other.

Treatment options
- Osteoclasis (refracturing the bone) under general anesthesis (GA)
- Redoing the fracture surgically
- Corrective osteotomy
- Excision of protruding bone

Stages of fracture healing

- Stage of hematoma formation
  - <7 days
  - Fracture end necrosis
  - Sensitization of precursor cells
- Stage of granulation tissue
  - Up to 2–3 weeks
  - Proliferation and differentiation of daughter cells into vessels, fibroblasts, osteoblasts, etc.
  - Fracture is still mobile
- Stage of callus formation–4–12 weeks, callus radiologically visible, no more mobile
- Stage of remodeling: 1–2 years, callus become dense.
- Stage of modeling: Many years–fracture site indistinguishable from parent bone.

SUPRACONDYLAR FRACTURE

HISTORY

- Fall—fall on outstretched hand (FOOSH) injury
- Pain
- Swelling
- Deformity
- Mobility.

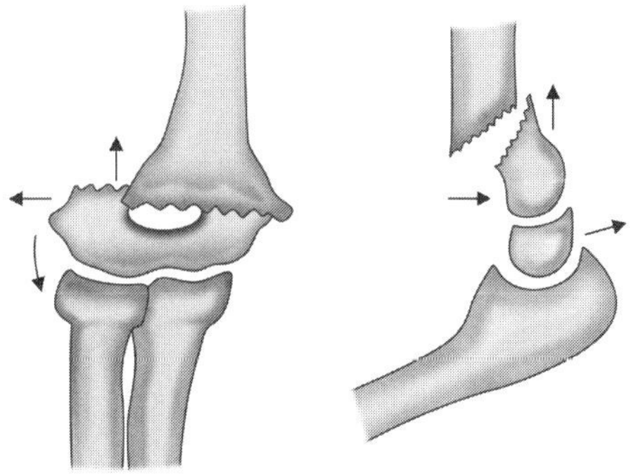

EXAMINATION

- Undue prominence of olecranon
- 3-point relationship
- Look for distal pulse
- Distal neurovascular deficit.

INVESTIGATIONS

X-ray

- Posterior shift
- Posterior tilt
- Proximal shift
- Medial shift
- Coronal medial tilt—***most important causing cubitus varus.***
- Horizontal internal rotation.

DISCUSSION

Supracondylar fracture more common in children because:

1. Periosteum loosely attached
2. Upper part of humerus round and below is flat, thin ridge.
3. Maximum remodeling occurs at this site
4. Presence of olecranon and coronoid fossae.
5. It is metaphyseal bone.

TYPES

1. Flexion type
2. Extension type

Garland's classification of extension type
- Type 1: X-ray shows fat pad sign. No break of bone, undisplaced
- Type 2: Breaks in the anterior cortex
- Type 3: Breaks in the anterior and posterior cortex—posterior medial (common) and posterior lateral.
- Type 4: Type 3 + periosteal stripping and unstable reduction.

TREATMENT

- Type 1: Sling or slab
  Type 2: CMR, correct angulation
  Type 3: Closed cross pinning using K wire or IF – K wire
- French osteotomy—supracondylar lateral closing wedge osteotomy.
- Modified French—osteoperiosteal hinge is kept.

COMPLICATIONS

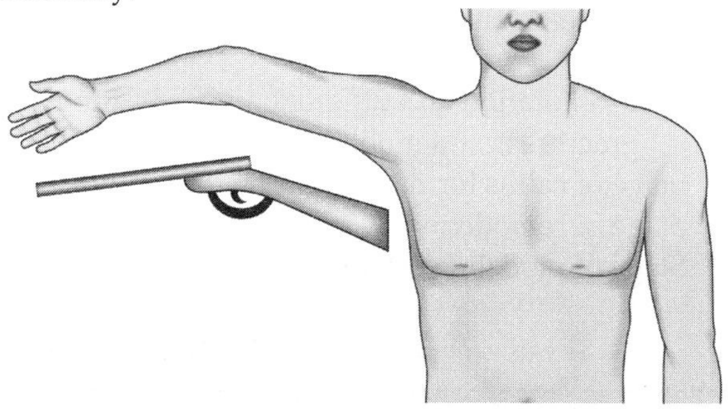

- Immediate – injury to vessels and nerves. Brachial artery, radial and median nerve
- Early—Volkmann's ischemia
- Late
  - Malunion
  - VIC (Volkmann's ischemic contracture)
  - Myositis ossificans
  - Gun-stock deformity.

COLLES' FRACTURE

Fracture occurring in adults at corticocancellous junction of distal end of radius. It is common in women due to postmenopausal osteoporosis. It results from fall on an outstretched hand.

DISPLACEMENTS

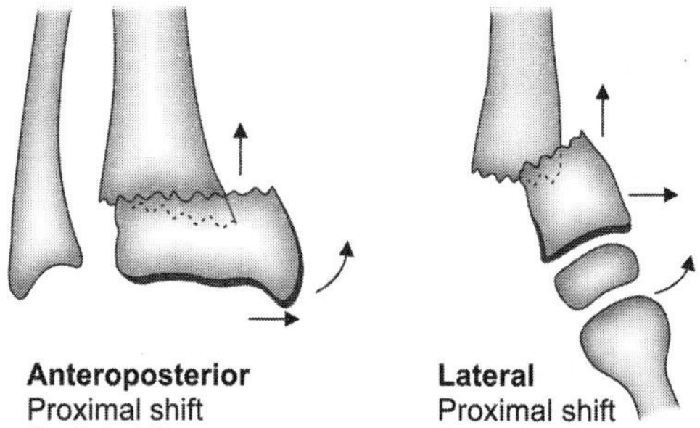

- Dorsal displacement
- Dorsal tilt
- Lateral displacement
- Lateral tilt
- Supination
- Impaction.

CLINICAL FEATURES

- History of fall
- Pain, deformity (dinner fork deformity).

INVESTIGATIONS

X-ray.

TREATMENT

Conservative treatment
- Undisplaced fracture—immobilization in a below elbow plaster cast (6 weeks)
- Displaced fracture—manipulative reduction and immobilization in Colles' cast (in palmar flexion and ulnar deviation).

COMPLICATIONS

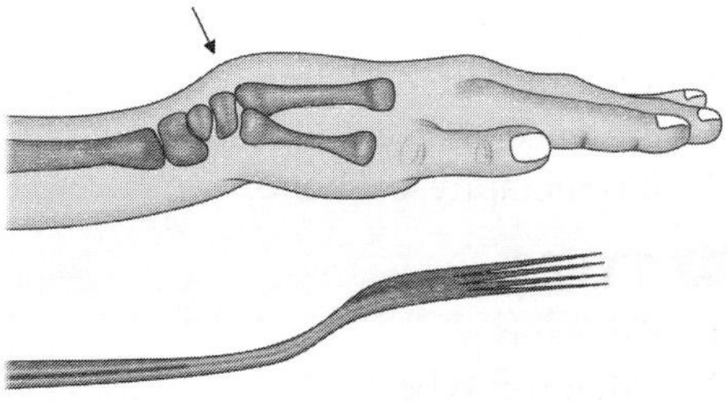

- Stiffness of joints
- Malunion
- Subluxation of inferior radioulnar joint
- Carpal tunnel syndrome
- Sudeck's osteodystrophy
- Rupture of extensor pollicis longus tendon (drummer boy palsy).

BONE SWELLING

HISTORY

- Age
  - Ewing sarcoma—young (5–15)
  - Giant cell tumor—20–30 (after epiphyseal closure)
  - Osteosarcoma—2nd decade (15–30 years)
  - Osteochondroma—growing bone (< 20 years). If swelling increases in size after 20 years suspect chondrosarcoma.
- Trauma
  - Any history of preceding trauma
  - Sudden increase after trauma may bring to notice.
- Pain
  - Acute severe pain—osteomyelitis, osteosarcoma (Ewing's sarcoma clinically simulate acute osteomyelitis)
  - Night crisis—TB or malignancy
  - Young male acute pain, more at night, relieved by aspirin—osteoid osteoma
  - Pain first—severe inflammation (infection, malignancy)
  - Constitutional symptoms—fever, discharging sinus
- Duration
  - Acute—osteomyelitis, osteosarcoma
- Pressure symptoms—distal pain, numbness, claudication
- Limitation of mobility
- Rapid increase in size
- History of chest, liver, CNS metastases
- Constitutional symptoms—weight loss, loss of appetite.

Past History

History of radiation.

Family History

Any bone diseases (osteogenesis imperfecta, achondroplasia, diaphyseal aclasis).

GENERAL EXAMINATION

- Anemia
- Cachexia
- Hepatosplenomegaly (HSM)
- LNE = rhabdomyosarcoma, angiosarcoma, synovial sarcoma.

X-ray findings
- Onion peel appearance: Ewing's sarcoma
- Sunray appearance: Osteosarcoma
- Soap bubble appearance: Osteosarcoma
- Codman's triangle: Osteosarcoma

LOCAL EXAMINATION

Inspection

- Site (EPI/META/DIA), shape, size, surface, surrounding area, pain
- Deformity
- Muscle wasting
- Pressure effects—edema
- Dilated veins, shiny stretched skin—malignancy, any scars.

Palpation

- No local rise in temperature/tenderness
- Size, shape, surface, **margin**, consistency, site, plane of swelling (translucency, fluctuation— only for soft swelling).
- Bony irregularity, abnormality, fractures, Ledge sign
- Percussion
- Auscultation—bruit in aneurysmal cyst
- Distal neurovascular defect
- Neighboring joints
- Measurements, movements

- Regional draining LN
- Similar swelling in other sites.

Epiphysis	Diaphysis	Metaphysis
• Giant cell tumor (GCT) • Chondroblastoma	• Ewing's • Multiple myeloma	• Osteosarcoma • Osteoma • Osteomyelitis • Simple/aneurysmal bone cyst

Summary: ______ year-old F/M with bone swelling of size ______ arising from ______ with loss of weight, appetite, progressively increasing in size over last _____ years.

DIAGNOSIS

- Benign/malignant
- Soft tissue/bony
- Mature/immature bone or age of patient
- Topography = Epi, meta or dia
- Complications — Pathological.

Investigations
- X-ray
- Computed tomography (CT)
- Magnetic resonance imaging (MRI)

DISCUSSION

Bony swelling with pain (e.g. osteochondroma)
- Fracture
- Bursitis
- Nerve compression
- Malignant change
- Infection

Features of malignancy
- Rapid increase in size
- Dilated veins
- Local rise in temperature
- Variable consistency

Indications for surgery in osteochondroma
- Pain (see above)
- Joint mobility impaired
- Cosmesis
- Deformity

Surgery—extraperiosteal excision (remove tumor along with periosteum)

GENU VALGUM/VARUM

PRESENTING COMPLAINTS

Bending of legs.

HISTORY

- Onset, relation with walking, weight bearing
- Progression
- Any treatment received
- Progressive/not
- Osteoarthritis/pressure effects
- Drug history—phenytoin (rickets)
- History of loose stools (malabsorption—rickets)
- Renal symptoms—renal rickets
- Current status.

Causes of genu valgum
- Idiopathic
- Post-traumatic
- Inflammatory
- Neoplastic

Genu valgum	
Unilateral	Bilateral
• Trauma • Osteomyelitis • Tumor	• Physiological (< 44) • Congenital • Rickets • Idiopathic • Paralytic • Epiphyseal dysplasia • Rheumatoid arthritis

ORTHOPEDICS

EXAMINATION

General Examination

- Craniotabes (newborn)
- AF closure delayed/not
- Frontal bossing
- Delayed eruption of tooth
- Rachitic rosary
- Pectus excavatum/carinatum
- Harrison's sulcus
- Lumbar lordosis
- Wide wrist- < 1 year
  >1 year – Ankle
- Double malleoli
- Height—***short stature***
- Weight.

} Vitamin D deficiency features

Genu varum	
Unilateral	Bilateral
• Trauma • Osteomyelitis • Tumor	• Physiological • Idiopathic • Pagets disease • Blount's disease • Osteoarthritis

Local Examination

- Attitude
- Deformity
- Any wasting of muscle
- Position of patella—subluxation if genu valgum
- Popliteal fossa
- **Movement—***during flexion of knee, if deformity disappears, deformity arising from femur. If it persists—arising from tibia*
- **Measurements**
  - Genu valgum: Intermalleolar distance >10 cm
  - Genu varum: Intercondylar distance >8 cm
  - **Q-angle**
  - Lateral thigh leg angle
  - **Special test: Ober's test if genu valgum**
  - Plumb line.

MANAGEMENT

- 6 lakh IU injection vitamin D_3
- Oral vitamin D_3, Ca^{+2}
- Take X-ray after 4 weeks treatment
  - If there is **provisional line of calcification** (PLC) between epiphysis and metaphysic vitamin D—400 IU
    Ca^{+2}—60–75 mg/kg/day
  - If X-ray has not changed then inject
    6 lakh IU and take X-ray after 4 weeks.

  If there is response give maintenance dose.
  If no response: It is resistant rickets like renal rickets, renal tubular acidosis (RTA), vitamin D resistant rickets.

Investigations
- X-ray—knee, wrist
- Serum calcium
- Serum phosphate
- Alkaline phosphatase

Conservative

Genu valgum – Osteotomy done at femur usually
Medial closing wedge osteotomy
Lateral opening wedge osteotomy

Genu varum – Osteotomy done at tibia usually
Medial opening wedge osteotomy
Lateral closing wedge osteotomy

ORTHOPEDICS

X-ray

Features of Rickets

- Loss of provision zone of calcification (earliest sign)
- Widening of epiphysis
- Metaphysis
  - Cupping
  - Splaying
  - Fraying
- Osteopenia
- Bone deformities

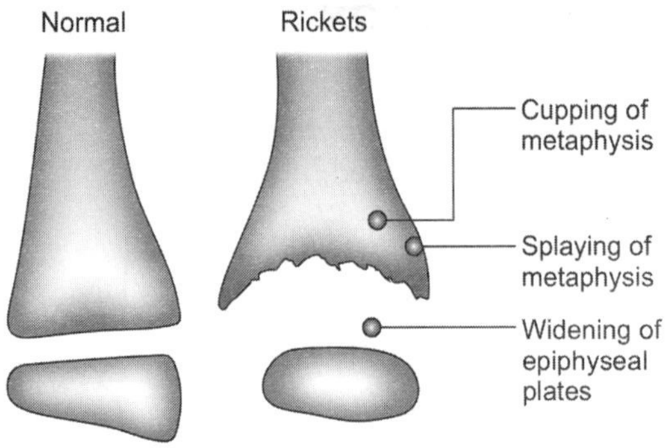

CONGENITAL TALIPES EQUINOVARUS (CTEV)

PRESENTING COMPLAINT

Deformity of the foot.

History of Presenting Complaint

- Briefly describe the history from birth onwards
- When first detected?
- Different modalities of treatment.
- Improving or not?

- Spine—tuft of hairs on the back/dimple/swelling (very very important)
- Neurological examination

GENERAL EXAMINATION

(gives clues to the etiology— syndromic or idiopathic)

- Congenital anomalies anywhere in the body (spinal anomalies)
- Café-au-lait spots
- Tuft of hairs on the back/dimple
- Congenital multiple contractures.

Diagnosis:

- Idiopathic or syndromic
- Treated or neglected
- Relapsed or recurrent
- Stiff or resistant

EXAMINATION OF FOOT

- Equinus deformity at ankle
- Varus deformity at subtalar joint
- Adduction deformity at tarsometatarsal joint
- Small foot with poorly developed heel
- Prominent lateral malleolus, convex lateral and concave medial borders
- Wasting of calf muscles
- Callosities, deep creases posterior/medial
- Deformity correctable or not
- On attempted correction, one can feel the tight structures posteriorly (tendo-Achilles) and plantar wards (plantar fascia).

INVESTIGATIONS

- **X-ray foot**—AP and lateral view with the foot in whatever corrected position possible.
  - Talocalcaneal angle (Kite's angle)
    Normal—>35°
    Reduced in CTEV
  - Tibiotalar angle
  - Talonavicular angle—25–35° (average)

  X-rays are having medicolegal importance and postoperative changes can be assessed.

TREATMENT

Principle: **Correction** of the deformity and its **maintenance.**

Methods of Correction of Deformity

- Nonoperative
- Operative.

Nonoperative Methods

- Manipulation alone
  Mother is taught to manipulate the foot after every feed
- Manipulation and plaster of Paris (PoP)
  Surgeons manipulate the foot after sedating the child
  Two philosophies:
  - Kite's philosophy
  - Ponseti's philosophy.

Kite's Philosophy

- Adduction deformity is corrected first followed by inversion deformity and then equines deformity
- Calcaneocuboid joint acting as fulcrum.

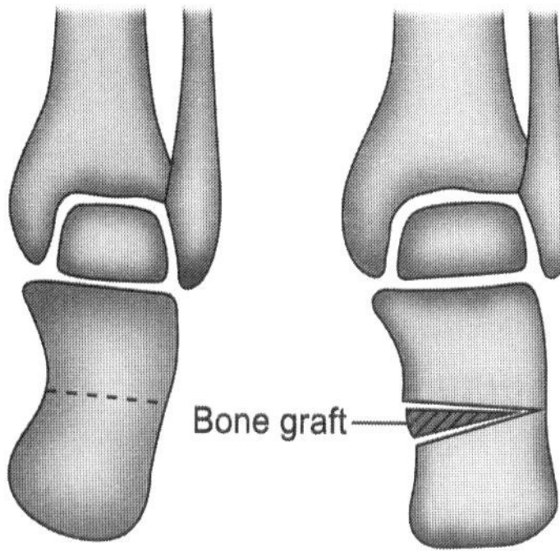

Ponseti's Philosophy

- Done by putting pressure ***over the talus head (Fulcrum)***
- Calcaneocuboid navicular complex is internally rotated (adducted) under the plantar flexed talus
- ***Ponseti's technique preferred***
  CAVE—cavus-adduction-varus-equinus—order of correction and percutaneous tenotomy if needed (if no order—Rocker bottom foot).

Operative Methods

Posteromedial soft tissue release (PMSTR)

- **Posterior side**
  - Lengthening of tendo-Achilles by ***Z plasty***
  - Release of posterior capsules
  - Release of posterior talofibular and calcaneofibular ligament.
- **Medial side**
  - Lengthening of three tendons
    - Tibialis posterior
    - Flexor digitorum longus (FDL)
    - Flexor hallucis longus (FHL)
  - Release of three ligaments
    - Talonavicular ligament
    - Deltoid ligament
    - Spring ligament
  - In severe cases three more structures
    - Interosseous talocalcaneal ligament
    - Capsule of naviculocuneiform
    - Cuneiform—first metatarsal joints
- **On the plantar side**
  - Plantar fascia release
  - Release of short flexors of the toes and abductor hallucis.
- **Limited soft tissue release**
- **Tendon transfers**
- **Dwyer osteotomy**

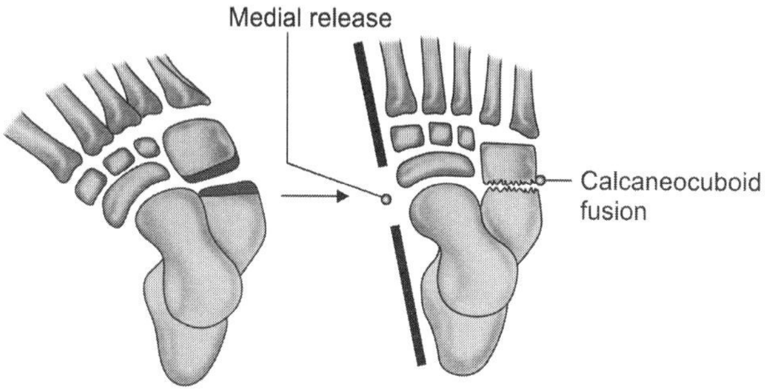

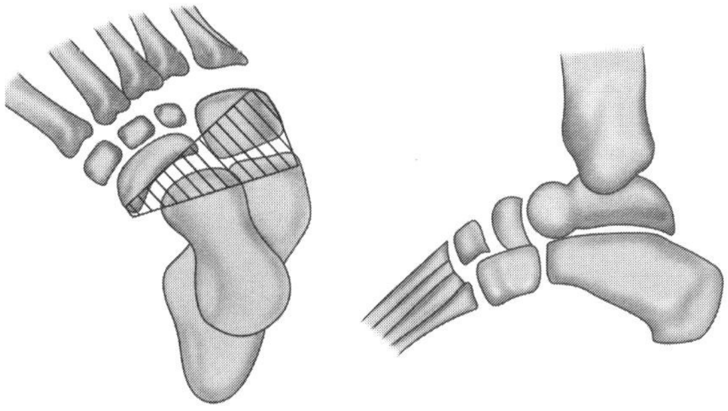

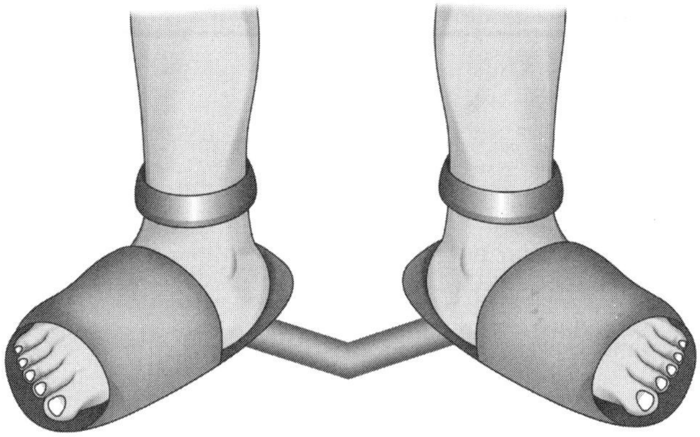

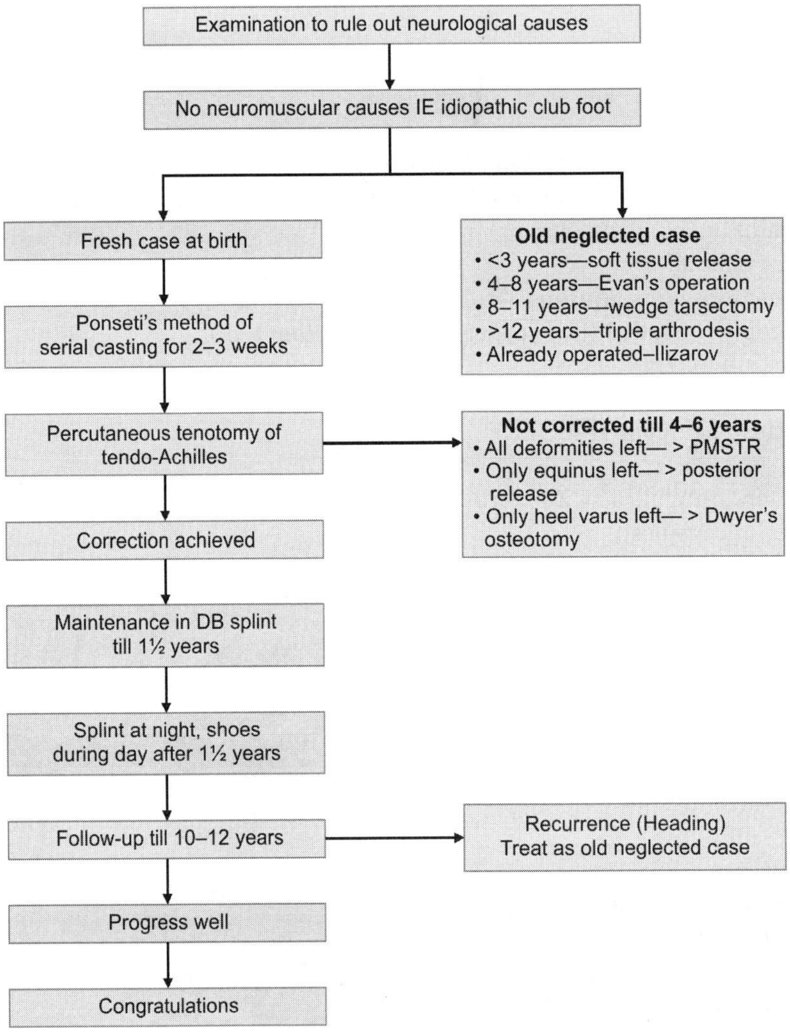

PMSTR: posteromedial soft tissue release

> **Etiology**
> - Idiopathic club foot
>   - Mechanical theory
>   - Ischemic theory
>   - Genetic theory
> - Secondary club foot
>   - Paralytic disorders, e.g. polio, spina bifida
>   - Arthrogryposis multiplex congenital

- Dillwyn Evans procedure
- Wedge tarsectomy, Jess
- Triple arthrodesis
- Ilizarov technique

METHODS OF MAINTENANCE OF CORRECTION

- CTEV splints
- Dennis Browne splint
- CTEV shows:
  - Straight inner border to prevent forefoot adduction
  - Outer show raise to prevent foot inversion
  - No heel to prevent equinus.

PATHOANATOMY

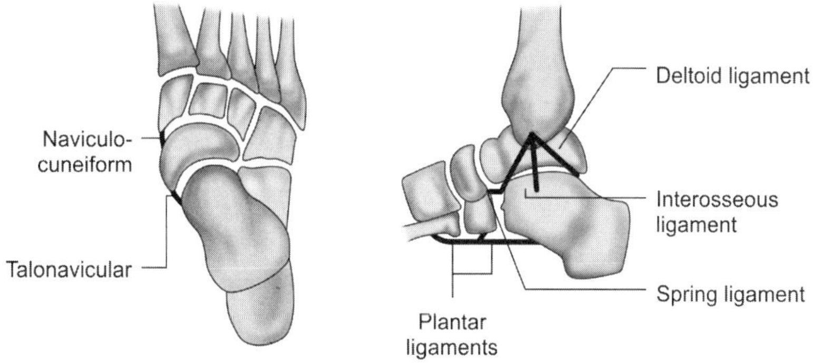

Bones

- Bones of foot small
- Neck of talus angulated
- Small calcaneum.

Joints

- **Equinus** deformity at ankle joint
- **Inversion** at subtalar joint
- **Adduction** at forefoot
- **Cavus** deformity at forefoot.

Muscles and Tendons

These are under developed, so the following groups of muscles are contracted:
- Posteriorly: Tendo-Achilles
- Medially: Tibialis posterior, FDL, FHL.

Capsules and Ligaments

These are shortened
- Posteriorly (3 structures):
  - Posterior capsule of ankle joint
  - Posterior capsule of subtalar joint
  - Posterior talofibular and calcaneofibular ligament
- Medially (3 structures):
  - Talonavicular ligament
  - Spring ligament
  - Deltoid ligament
- Plantar wards:
  - Plantar fascia and ligaments
- Interrosseous ligaments between talus and calcaneum

Skin
- Adaptive shortening on medial side of sole
- Deep creases on medial side
- Dimples on lateral aspect

Secondary changes: Callosities and bursae.

NERVE INJURY

ANATOMY

Brachial Plexus

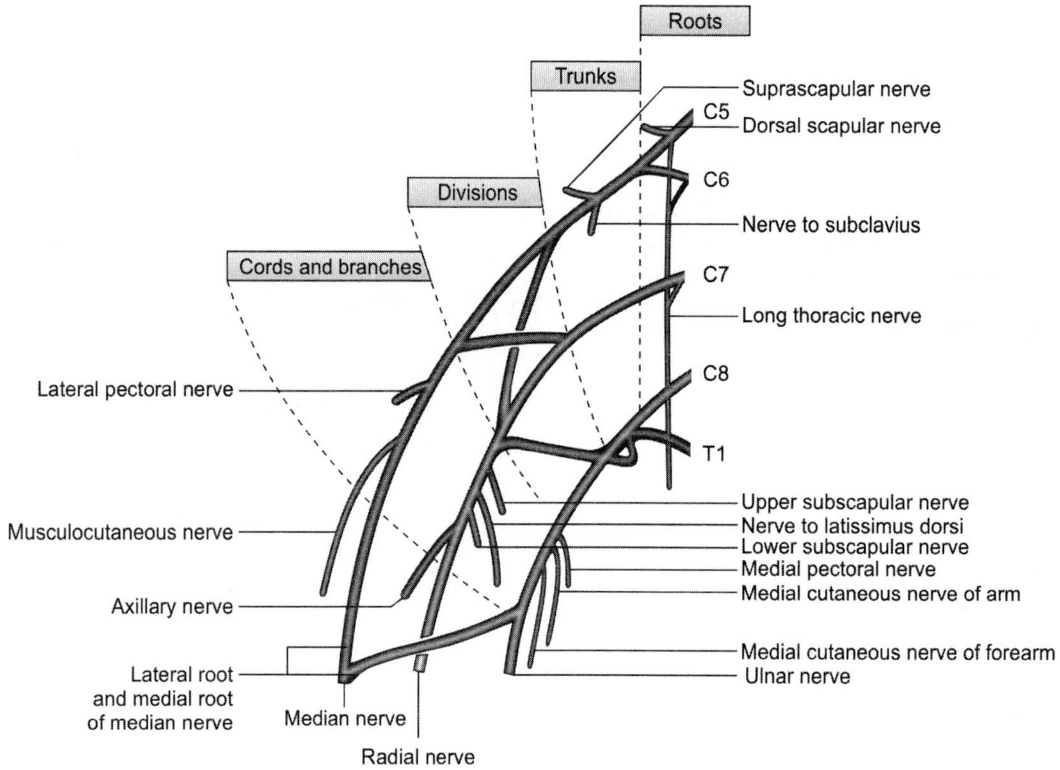

- C5–T1 – **Roots**
- C5, C6 – Upper trunk; C7– Middle trunk; C8, T1 – Lower trunk } **Trunks**
- Trunk – Dorsal, Ventral } **Divisions**
- **Cords**:
  - Lateral cord—ventral division of upper and middle trunk
  - Medial cord—ventral division of lower trunk
  - Posterior cord—union of dorsal division of all three trunks
- **Branches**
  - From roots
    - Long thoracic nerve (nerve of Bell) to ***Serratus anterior*** (C5, C6, C7)
    - Dorsal scapular nerve (C5)—Nerve to ***Rhomboideus***
  - Branches of trunk

    From upper trunk: ***Suprascapular*** nerve (C5, C6), Nerve to ***subclavius*** (C5, C6)

- **Branches from cords:**

Lateral cord (LML)	Medial cord (M4U)
• Lateral pectoral nerve • Musculocutaneous nerve • Lateral root of median nerve	• Medial pectoral nerve • Medial cutaneous nerve of arm • Medial cutaneous nerve of forearm • Medial root of median nerve • Ulnar nerve

Posterior cord (ULTRA)
- Upper subscapular nerve
- Lower subscapular nerve
- Thoracodorsal nerve
- Radial nerve
- Axillary nerve

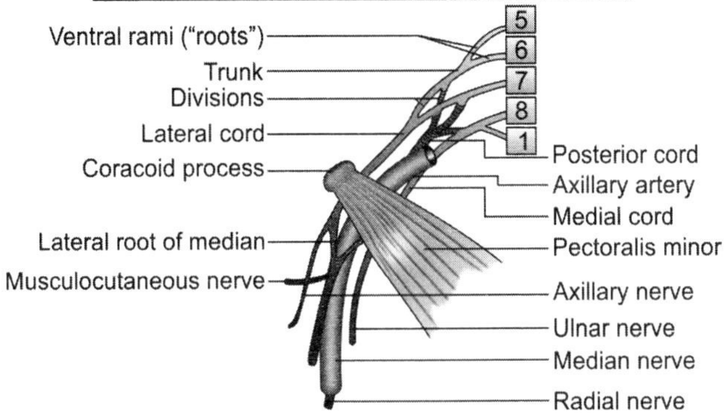

Autonomous sensory areas
Ulnar nerve–little finger tip
Median nerve–index finger tip
Radial nerve–1st web space

MEDIAN NERVE (C5–T1)

COURSE AND BRANCHES

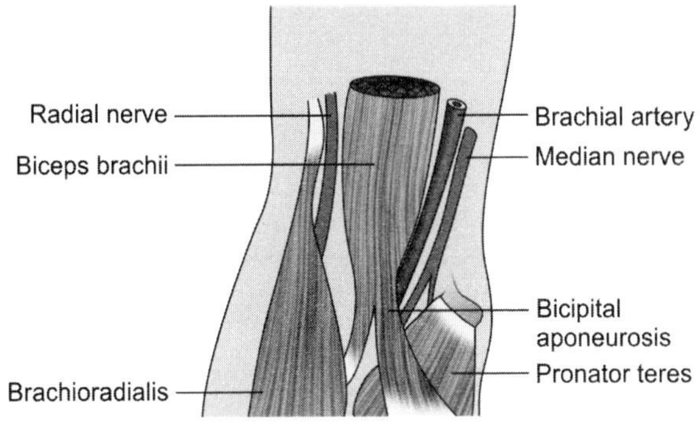

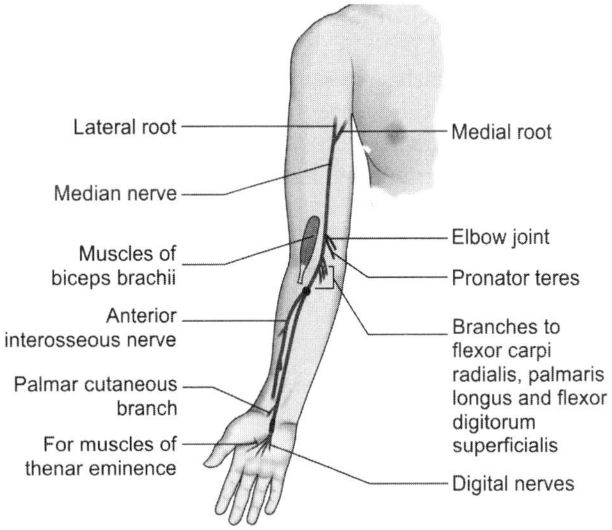

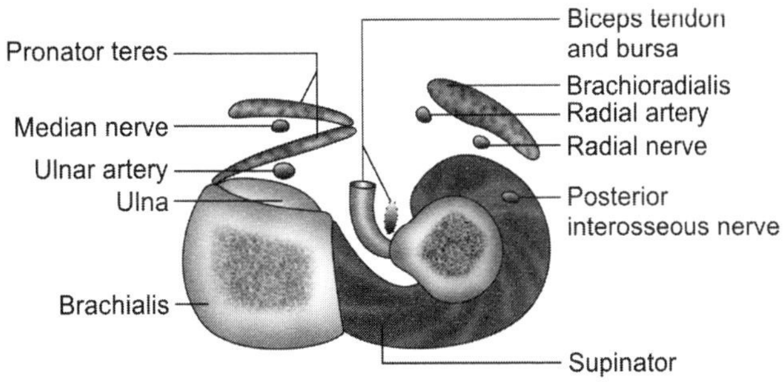

The median nerve first runs on lateral sided of axillary artery in the middle of arm and it crosses in front of artery. It gives branches to *pronator teres* and brachial artery.

In **cubital fossa**:

MBBR (medial to lateral)—***Medial nerve, brachial artery, biceps tendon, radial nerve***

It passes between two heads of *pronator teres*, then deep to *flexor digitorum superficialis*. Then it is placed deep to *palmaris longus* and enter palm under flexor retinaculum.

Branches in cubital fossa:

To Flexor carpi radialis
Flexor digitorum superficialis
Palmaris longus.

In **forearm**

Anterior interosseous nerve—supplies lateral half of flexor digitorum profundus, pronator quadratus and flexor pollicis longus

Palmar cutaneous branch—originate 5 cm above flexor retinaculum and supplies to skin over thenar eminence and also lateral 2/3rd of palm.

In **hand**

Supplies thenar muscles: via recurrent motor branch
flexor pollicis brevis
abductor pollicis brevis
opponens pollicis

Also supplies 1st and 2nd lumbricals.

Mnemonic – LOAF
L – Lumbricals
O – Opponens pollicis
A – Abductor pollicis brevis (PB)
F – Flexor pollicis brevis (FPB)

INJURY

High median nerve injury—above elbow

- Paralysis of:
  - **FDS and FDP (Lateral half)** – **Ochsner's clasping test**
    When the patient is asked to clasp the hands, the index finger of the affected side fails to flex **(pointing index)**
    Other fingers are flexed by the medial half of the profundus muscle, which is supplied by the ulnar nerve.
  - **Flexor pollicis longus** (inability to flex the terminal phalanx of the thumb
  - **Flexor carpi radialis** (hand deviates to the ulnar side when it is flexed against resistance)
  - **Thenar muscles**—wasting; Simian/ape-like hand
  - **Abductor pollicis brevis—Pen test**
    The patient is asked to lay his hand flat on the table, a pen is held above the palm and the patient is unable to touch the pen with his thumb.
  - **Opponens pollicis**
- At wrist—cut injury, carpal tunnel syndrome
- Pen test for abductor pollicis brevis
- Ape thumb deformity = Adducted and external rotated thumb.

ULNAR NERVE

Root value: C8–T1

COURSE AND BRANCHES

Lies in the axilla between axillary vein and axillary artery. At the middle of humerus, it pierces the medial intermuscular septum to lie on its back and descends on the back of medial epicondyle, where it can be palpated. Ulnar nerve enters the forearm by passing between two heads of flexor carpi ulnaris. It runs along with ulnar artery in lower 2/3rd of forearm. Finally, it lies superficial to medial part of flexor retinaculum in gyons canal then divides into its superficial and deep branch. Superficial branch supplies hypothenar muscles and deep branch ends by supplying adductor pollicis.

Branches in Forearm

Muscular

- Medial half of flexor digitorum profundus.
- Flexor carpi ulnaris

Cutaneous

- Dorsal cutaneous branch for medial half or dorsum of hand
- Palmar cutaneous branch for medial 1/3rd of palm
- Digital branches to medial 1½ and fingers, nail beds and dorsal digital phalanges.

HAND

- Superficial branch: Palmaris brevis
- Deep branch:
  - Hypothenar eminence muscles
  - Medial 2 lumbricals
  - Palmar and dorsal interossei
  - Adductor pollicis.

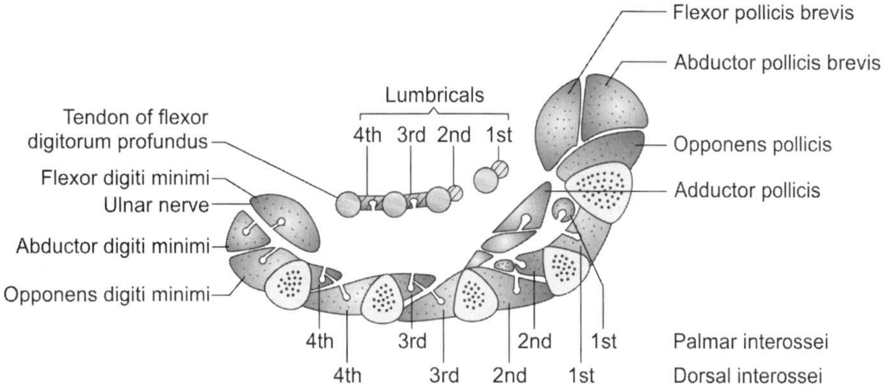

Injury to Elbow

1. Supracondylar fracture recent or late (Tardy ulnar nerve palsy)
2. Fracture of medial epicondyle of humerus

1. ***Flexor carpi ulnaris***: When the wrist joint is flexed against resistance, hand tends to deviate towards the radial side. Loss of sensation of medial side of hand, the whole of the little finger and a small part on the medial side of finger
2. ***Interossei***:
   Palmar interossei adduct (PAD) – Palmar interossei → Adduction
   Dorsal interossei abduct (DAB) – Dorsal interossei → Abduction

The patient is asked to adduct his fingers keeping straight. A card may be inserted between two fingers for grasping. The card is now pulled out against the adducted fingers to see the power of adduction of palmar interossei card test.

Egawa test: Hand kept flat on table with palmar surface down. Move the middle finger side to side–Test for dorsal interossei

Franet's sign (Book test)–Hold the book between thumb and index finger

Normally, the person will grasp the book with adductor pollicis and 1st dorsal interossei

In ulnar nerve palsy–flexor pollicis longus acts–flexion at interphalangeal joint of thumb.

RADIAL NERVE

Root value: C5–T1

COURSE AND BRANCHES

Radial nerve lies against the muscle forming posterior wall of axilla. It lies in the lower triangular space. It then reaches the radial sulcus and lies between lateral and medial heads of triceps. It leaves the sulcus piercing the lateral intermuscular septum and enters the anterior compartment of arm. It then descends between the brachialis on one side and the *brachioradialis* above and *extensor carpi radialis longus* below. In front of lateral epicondyle, it divides into 2 terminal branches—**superficial and deep**.

- Branches in **axilla**: It gives off muscular branches to medial and long head of *tricep*s and *posterior cutaneous nerve of arm.*

- **Radial sulcus**: Lateral and medial head of triceps, nerve to anconeous
- Posterior cutaneous nerve of forearm
- Lower lateral cutaneous nerve of arm.

In the arm: Brachioradialis, extensor carpi radialis longus and lateral 1/4th of brachialis.

Superficial and Deep Branch

Superficial: It runs in front of pronator teres. About 7 cm above the wrist, the nerve turns back round the lateral side of radius, pierces the deep fascia and supplies skin over dorsal aspect of hand.

Deep branch: Before it enters the supinator muscle gives a branch to *extensor carpi radialis brevis* and another to supinator. After piercing supinator, it is known as **posterior interosseous nerve.**

Then it gives branches to ***extensor digitorum, extensor digiti minimi and extensor carpi ulnaris*** and 2 long branches one to ***extensor pollicis longus and extensor indicis*** and another to ***abductor pollicis longus and extensor pollicis brevis.***

INJURY TO RADIAL NERVE

In axilla: By use of a crutch (**Crutch palsy**)
Fracture dislocation of upper end of humerus

In radial groove: Fracture of shaft of humerus
Intramuscular injection
Pressure on the arm at edge of a chair or a pavement after a deep sleep being drunk (***Saturday night palsy***)

Posterior interosseous nerve (PIN) injury: Fracture or dislocation of upper end of radius.

LOCALIZATION

In axilla: All muscles supplied by radial nerve and all cutaneous sensation by branches of radial nerve lost (elbow drop, wrist drop, finger drop, thumb drop)

In radial groove: Triceps and posterior cutaneous nerve of arm spared

PIN injury: All muscles supplied by radial nerve and cutaneous branches escape and also the supinator and extensor carpi radialis brevis

- Extension of metacarpophalangeal joint→extensors of fingers
- Extension of interphalangeal joint→interossei and lumbricals
- Flexion of metacarpophalangeal joint→interossei, lumbricals
- Flexor of interphalangeal joint
  - Flexor digitorum superficialis at proximal interphalangeal joint
  - Flexor digitorum profundus at distal interphalangeal joint
- Brachioradialis is supplied before it divides to superficial and deep branches (so can assess the level of radial nerve injury).

EXAMINATION OF PERIPHERAL NERVES

HISTORY

- Age, sex
- Occupation (painter; industrial worker; fire explosive worker, etc.)
- Numbness, paresthesia
- Diabetes mellitus, leprosy, syphilis
- Seizure disorder
- Loosening of slippers
- Areas of skin that is dry always
- Neurocutaneous markers café-au-lait spots
- Family history of neurological illness.

Disabilities
1. Walking (aided or unaided)
2. Climbing stairs, coming down
3. Taking food, washing face, brushing teeth
4. Holding and carrying objects in hand

INSPECTION

- Attitude and deformity (wrist drop, winging of scapula, claw hand, ape thumb, pointing index, foot drop)
- **Wasting of muscles**
- **Skin**
  - Dry, glossy, smooth
  - Disappearance of cutaneous folds and subcutaneous fat
  - Causalgia

- Vasomotor changes—pallor, cyanosis
- Tropic changes of nails
- Trophic ulcers
- **Scars or wounds**
- Look for Horners syndrome in all brachial plexus injuries.

PALPATION

- **Temperature**
- **Tenderness**
- **Muscles**—wasted soft flabby
- **Bone**—supracondylar ridge for old malunited supracondylar # or any myositic mass.
- **Nerves**: Thickening, tenderness or nodularity, abscess
  - Ulnar nerve at elbow

6. **Scar**
   - Common peroneal nerve (CPN) at fibula neck
7. **Tinel sign**
   - Supratrochlear nerves
   - Gentle percussion distal to proximal along course of the nerve—transient tingling sensation in distribution of the injured nerve, persists for several seconds
   - Positive Tinel sign—evidence of regenerating axonal sprouts that have not obtained complete myelinization are progressing along the endoneural tube
   - With progressive regeneration, the positive response fades proximally, progressive myelinization along more proximal part of regenerated segment (rate of regeneration 1 mm/day)
8. **Distal vascularity**
   - Movements measurements—linear and circumferential
   - Neurological examination
     - Higher function
   - Cranial nerves
     - Motor—test all muscles of individual nerve
     - Autonomic—skin, hair, nails changes
     - Spine—cervical spine/lumbar spine

   To rule out thoracic outlet syndrome – ***Adsons*** and ***Allens*** test (for radial or ulnar artery obstruction)

Diagnosis
- Nerve injured
- Level of injury
- Etiology – post-traumatic
- Type of injury
- Deformity or any complication

CARPAL TUNNEL SYNDROME

Compression neuropathy of median nerve in carpus, deep to flexor retinaculum

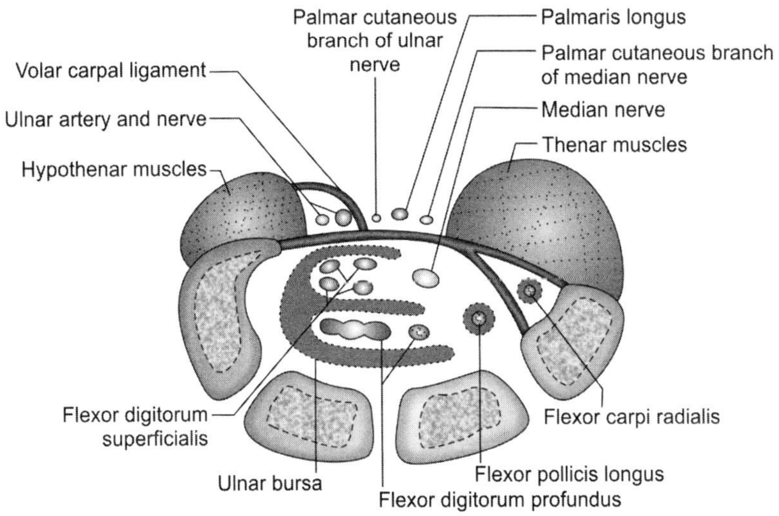

Structures passing above (U2P3)
- **U**lnar nerve
- **U**lnar artery
- **P**almar cutaneous branch of median nerve
- **P**almar cutaneous branch of ulnar nerve
- **P**almaris longus

ORTHOPEDICS

Structures passing below:
- Flexor digitorum **S**uperficialis
- Flexor digitorum **P**rofundus
- **M**edial nerve
- **F**lexor pollicis longus
- **B**ursa (radial and ulnar)

Mnemonic—SPM fully boring

Causes: (MEDIAN TRAP)
- **M**yxedema
- **E**dema
- **D**iabetes mellitus
- **I**diopathic
- **A**cromegaly
- **N**eoplasm
- **T**rauma–colles, lunate dislocation
- **R**heumatoid arthritis
- **A**myloidosis
- **P**regnancy

CLINICAL FEATURES

Women 40–60 years. Often bilateral disease

Progressive uselessness and impairment of fine movements. Pain, tingling, numbness along sensory distribution of median nerve. Symptoms worst after working at night.

ETIOLOGY

1. ***Wasting*** of thenar eminence
2. ***WEAK APB (Abductor pollicis brevis)***
3. Wrist flexion test (***Phalen's sign***): When patient is asked to flex the wrist, there will be exacerbation of symptoms and it will disappear as soon as the wrist is straightened (gravity dependent).
4. Durkan's test (Carpal compression test).

INVESTIGATION

Electrical nerve conduction study will elicit a delay motor conduction of median nerve at the wrist, RBS, TFT, EMG.

TREATMENT

Treat Medical Causes Like Hypothyroidism, Splinting

Surgical decompression of median nerve by cutting both superficial and deep part of flexor retinaculum.

CLAW HAND

Flexion of metacarpophalangeal and extension of interphalangeal joints are by extensor hood of interossei and lumbricals. It is mainly supplied by ulnar and median nerve. It there is palsy of these nerves, there is claw hand, hyperextension of metacarpophalangeal joint with flexion of interphalangeal joint.

CAUSES

- Leprosy
- Trauma
- Entrapment neuropathies
- Tardy ulnar nerve palsy
- Klumpke's palsy.

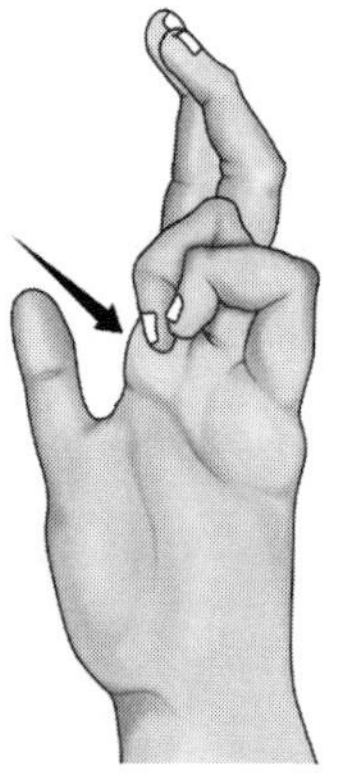

CLINICAL FEATURES

- Typical claw hand
- Loss of sensation along the distribution of the nerve
- **Card test:** Inability to grasp
- **Froment's sign** (Book test—For adductor pollicis
- **Egawa test**: For *dorsal interossei.*

TYPES

- **Ulnar claw hand:** Only medial two fingers are involved:
  - Low ulnar palsy: Here lesion is in the wrist (at ***Guyon's canal***). Here the deformity is more because of overaction of FDP.

- High ulnar palsy (at the level of elbow): Here FDP is also paralyzed and overaction is not there. So lesser deformity occurs.
- Ulnar paradox: Higher the lesion, lesser the deformity, lower the lesion more the deformity.

2. **Median claw hand:** Only lateral two fingers are involved, it is less common
3. **Combined median and ulnar claw hand:** Here all four fingers of hand are involved.

INVESTIGATIONS

• Electromyogram	Electromyogram—to know—whether injury present or not
• Nerve conduction studies	Complete/incomplete
	Any regeneration occurring or not
	Level of nerve injury

TREATMENT

Conservative (in all cases of nerve injury) and surgery

AIM: *To preserve the mobility of the affected limb while the nerve recovers*

a. **Splint—knuckle bender splint**
b. **Range of motion exercises**
c. **Care of skin and nails (to prevent trophic changes)**
d. **Physiotherapy.**

WRIST DROP

Extensors of wrist joint act at metacarpophalangeal joint which is supplied by PIN. Any lesion above the elbow will lead to wrist drop (since the radial nerve gives branches to the extensor carpi radialis longus above the elbow, which is an extensor of the wrist).

(Note: Extension of interphalangeal joint is done by interossei which are supplied by ulnar nerve). Posterior interosseous nerve lesion causes only finger drop (it supplies all the extensors of finger).

TREATMENT

- Same as above
- Splint- cock up splint—To maintain wrist in extension
- Tendon transfer—Jone's transfer
  - Pronator teres to extensor carpi radialis brevis—Correct wrist drop
  - Flexor carpi radialis to extensor digitorum—Correct finger drop
  - Palmaris longus to extensor pollicis longus—Correct thumb drop

FOOT DROP

Inability to dorsiflex and evert the foot due to paralysis of peroneal and extensor group of muscles, as a result of common peroneal nerve injury.

Sciatic nerve: Ventral rami L4 to S3

- On the back of thigh it supplies long head of ***biceps femoris, semitendinosus, semimembranosus, ischial part of adductor magnus*** Short head of ***biceps femoris***

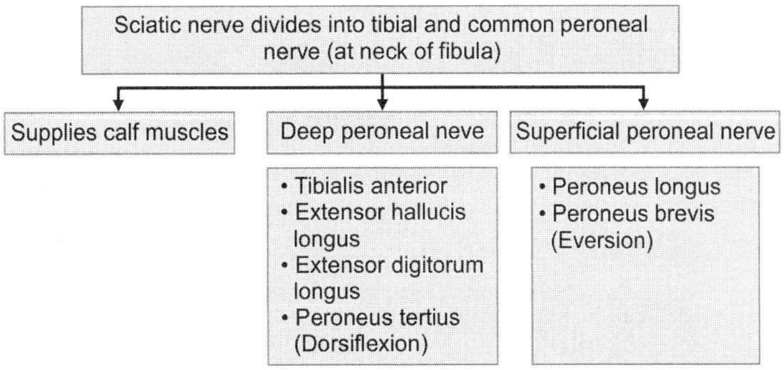

CLINICAL FEATURES

- High stepping gait
- Loss of sensation over lateral and dorsum of the foot.

Causes of foot drop
- Fracture neck of fibula
- Leprosy
- Lead poisoning
- Iatrogenic
- Direct incised wound

TREATMENT

- **Same as claw hand**
- **Splint—foot drop splint**

  Tendon transfer using tibialis posterior muscle.

  It is transferred to cuboid and cuneiform bones to get dorsiflexion and eversion.

  1. Ober's procedure

  2. Barr's procedure

MANAGEMENT OF NERVE INJURY

1. **Nerve repair: In all cut injuries and in case of failure of recovery after 3–4 weeks with investigation showing no signs of regeneration** 3 **types:**
   - **Primary**—done within 6–8 hours, and if wound is clean cut. Two ends approximated by 1 or 2 silk sutures. To prevent retraction of cut ends.
   - **Delayed primary**—between 7–8 days after injury and if wound is contaminated.
   - **Secondary**—18 days after injury, present later, signs of nerve irritation, failure of conservative management.
   - **Nerve suture**
     - **Epineural**
     - **Epiperineural**
     - **Perineural**

       (group fascicular repair)
   - **Nerve grafting**—Can be done if there is gap after injury (Graft—sural N.)
2. **Neurolysis:** Here the nerve is freed from fibrosis (in case of failure of recovery after 4–6 weeks with investigation showing no signs of regeneration).

   Two types:
   1. **External neurolysis**
   2. **Internal neurolysis**

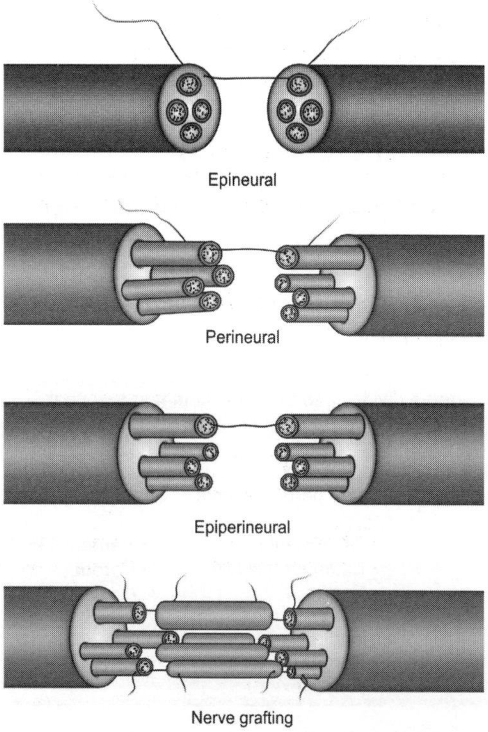

3. **Reconstruction surgery (performed when there is no hope of recovery of a nerve—usually after 18 months when the motor end plate degenerate)**
   a. **Tendon transfer—Bunnell's transfer (FDS is attached to extensor expansion)**
   b. **Muscle transfer**
   c. **Arthrodesis**

Anterior transpositioning *of ulnar nerve in case of tardy ulnar nerve palsy.*

INJURY TO LIGAMENTS AROUND KNEE

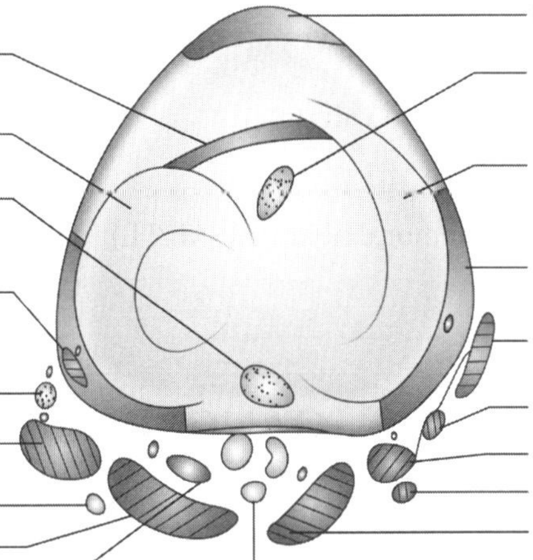

MECHANISM

- Medial collateral ligament—valgus force (abducting leg or femur)
- Lateral collateral ligament—varus force
- Anterior cruciate ligament—twisting force on a semiflexed weight bearing knee
- O'Donoghue triad—injury to ACL, medial collateral ligament and medial meniscus
- Posterior cruciate ligament—tibia is forced backward onto femur.

CLINICAL FEATURES

- Pain and early swelling (due to hemarthrosis)
- O/E – test for ligaments

Investigation – Plane X-ray
– MRI

TREATMENT

Conservative

Grade 1 and 2 injuries—cylindrical cast/Robert Jones bandage

Operative in Grade 3, athletes

1. Repair of ligament
2. Reconstruction.

MENISCAL INJURIES

- When a person standing on semiflexed knee, and twists his body to one side
- Medial meniscus is involved often since it is fixed to medial collateral ligament.

Clinical Features

- Pain
- Locking of knee
- Swelling in case of meniscal tear is due to synovial reaction, hence appears after few hours.

Treatment

Arthroscopic meniscal balancing.

RECURRENT DISLOCATION OF PATELLA

- >1 dislocation
- It dislocates laterally.

CAUSES

- Bone
  - Patella alta (high lying patella in shallower part of inter condylar groove)
  - Small patella
  - Hypoplasia of lateral condyle—genu valgum
- Soft tissue
  - Weakening of medial structures
    - Weakness of medial patellofemoral ligament (MPFL)
    - Vastus medialis wasting
    - Generalized ligament laxity
  - Contraction of lateral structures.

Treatment
- Medial plication
- Lateral release.

GANGLION

Most common cystic swelling on dorsum of wrist. It results from mucoid degeneration of the tendon sheath or joint capsule. It is usually asymptomatic, but sometimes mild discomfort or pain is there. When ganglion is arising from tendon sheath it can be moved sideways slightly, but not at all along the length of tendon particularly when tendon is made taut.

TREATMENT

Aspiration of cyst and injection of hyalase. If cyst recurs, excision of cyst is required.

MORRANT BAKER'S CYST

Herniation of synovial membrane posteriorly through the fibers of oblique popliteal ligament and forms swelling in the posterior aspect of knee slightly below joint line. This is often associated with rheumatoid arthritis or osteoarthritis of joint. Swelling become prominent on extension and disappears on flexion of joint.

TREATMENT

- Surgical excision
- Marsupialization.

- Midline
- Fluctuant
- Nontender

DIFFERENTIAL DIAGNOSIS

- Abscess (Pott's)
- Aneurysm of popliteal artery
- Bursae
- Other soft tissue swellings.

DUPUYTREN'S CONTRACTURE

CAUSES

1. Hereditary
2. Cirrhosis
3. Drugs like phenytoin

Flexion deformity of one or more fingers due to thickening and shortening of palmar aponeurosis (flexion at metacarpophalangeal joint and interphalangeal joint).

Ring finger affected mostly, less often little finger.

It may sometimes be associated with thickening of plantar fascia or Peyronie's diseases.

It can be differentiated from a similar deformity due to contracture of flexor tendon. In the former only MP and PIP are flexed, unlike the latter where DIP joint are also flexed.

TREATMENT

- **Physiotherapy**
- No need of treatment in mild cases
- Excision of palmar aponeurosis in case deformity is severe.

TRIGGER FINGER

Condition resulting from constriction of fibrous digital sheath (A1 pulley across the MCP joint). Common in middle aged women and most commonly affected finger is middle or ring finger. In children thumb is most commonly affected and often called snapping thumb.

TREATMENT

- Local ultrasonic therapy
- Local injection of hydrocortisone
- Surgical release of tight tendon sheath.

DE QUERVAIN'S TENOVAGINITIS

- It results from inflammation of common sheath of abductor pollicis longus and extensor pollicis brevis tendons (first dorsal compartment)
- It is a stenosing tenovaginitis like trigger finger.
- There is pain and swelling over radial **styloid process.**

FINKELSTEIN'S TEST

With the thumb in palm the patient is asked to make a fist by super imposing the fingers over thumb. The hand is pushed passively to medial side, pain is experienced at the radial styloid process which shoot down to thumb or upward toward elbow.

Treatment

Plain X-ray wrist to rule out tumors

- In early stages—Rest to wrist, analgesics, ultrasonic radiation
- Local infiltration of hydrocortisone
- Excision of a part of tendon sheath (de roofing)

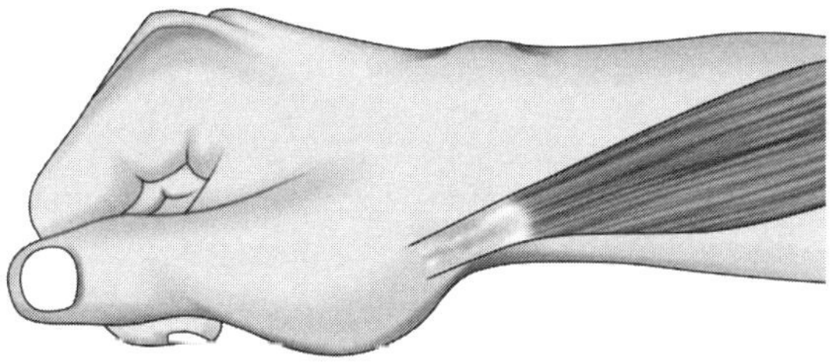

NOTES

ORTHOPEDICS

ORTHOPEDICS X-RAY AND INSTRUMENTS

1. **Fracture shaft of femur**
   Clinical features: Pain, swelling, patient bed ridden, deformity: external/internal rotation, shortening
   Treatment: A B C, closed reduction and internal fixation with interlocking nail (only proximal site is opened). If open fracture, then open reduction and internal fixation (ORIF)
   Interlocking nail—have a bend for tibia, no bend for femur
   - Holes for screws
   - Significance—provide more rotational stability

   Others – K nail (Kuntscher's nail)
   - Intramedullary nail
   - Ideal for isthmus (upper 1/3rd)
   - Clover leaf shape in cross-section
   - Principle – 3 point fixation
   - Size of K nail required:
     - Length—measure length from tip of greater trochanter to lateral joint line of knee and subtracting 2 cm from it
     - Diameter—determined on X-ray, from width of medullary cavity at isthmus
   - Technique of insertion:
     - Retrograde nailing—insert from fracture site
     - Nail introduced from greater trochanter over a guidewire passed from fracture site
   - Complications of nailing:
     - Splintering of cortex while hammering the nail
     - Proximal migration—leads to bursitis
     - Distal migration—leads to stiffening of knee
     - Infection.
2. **Nails and plates**
   Nails—load sharing device
   Plates—load bearing device
   In upper limb—plates are selected, because not weight bearing, so no compression at fracture site
   In lower limbs—nails are used, as it is a weight bearing area, compression at fracture site obtained
   Dynamic compression plate
   Used in fracture of both bone forearm, humerus, femur, tibia
   Square nail
   - Square cross-section
   - Advantage – no need to elevate the periosteum
   - For ulna – pointed tip – proximal to distal insertion, entry point—olecranon
   - For radius – arc at end – distal to proximal insertion, entry point—distal end of radius.
3. **Pins**
   - Steinmann pin – No threads
   - Denham pin – Middle thread
   - Schantz pin – Thread on ends

   Indications:
   - Skeletal traction: For example, in intertrochanteric fracture, acetabular fracture, fracture shaft of femur
   - Schantz pin, as a part of external fixator.
4. **Bohler's stirrup**
   Used for skeletal traction
5. **Bohler-Braun splint**
   Has a number of pulleys (1–3) over which the traction cord passes while giving traction for different fractures. It has no in-built system of counter traction, hence it is not suitable for transportation.
6. **Crutchfield tongs**
   For skull traction
   Indication—for cervical spine injury

7. **Skin traction/Buck's traction**
   Indication—Nack of femur (NOF) fracture, traumatic synovitis, Perthes disease
   Advantage—noninvasive
   Disadvantage—less traction, if not properly applied—skin laceration
8. **Pelvic traction**—in IVDP
9. **Halters traction**—in cervical IVDP, cervicobrachial neuralgia
10. **External fixator**
    1. *Components*
       - Schantz pin
       - Universal clamp
       - Hollow rod
    2. *Types*
       - Linear external fixator
       - Circular external fixator
    3. *Indications*
       - Open fracture type 3b (If not possible due to risk of infection and plaster application makes dressing of wound difficult)
         Classification of open fractures (Gustilo and Anderson classification)
         - Type I: Open fracture with wound >1 cm long
         - Type II: Open fracture with laceration 1–10 cm long
         - Type III: >10 cm long with soft tissue are devitalized and contaminated
           - A: With adequate soft tissue coverage
           - B: No adequate soft tissue coverage, fracture site exposed to atmosphere
           - C: Vascular damage
       - Pelvic fracture: Use EF because if abdomen is opened tamponade effect will go and it will increase bleeding
       - Temporary fixation for plastic surgery/vascular surgery.

    Tile's classification of pelvic injuries
    a. Type A: Stable
    b. Type B: Rotationally unstable, vertically stable
    c. Type C: Rotationally and vertically unstable.
11. **Ilizarov's ring**

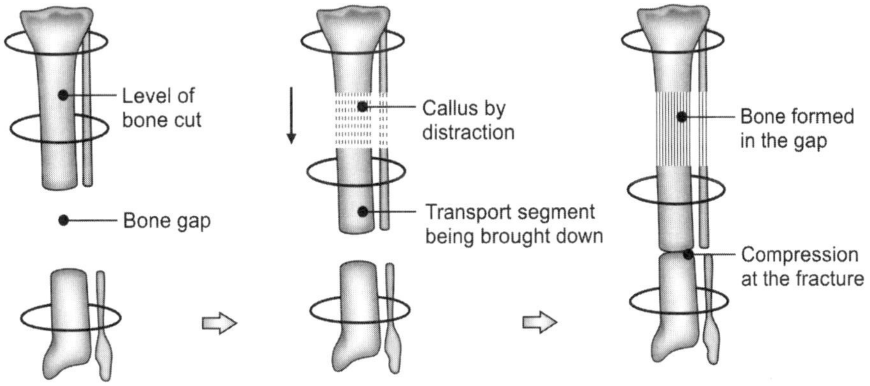

Principle: Distraction osteogenesis (slow controlled distraction at corticotomy sites)
- Uses:
  - Infected gap nonunion
    Limb lengthening or shortening
  - In deformity correction—congenital/acquired
  - In arthrodesis, osteomyelitis.
- Advantages:
  - Immediate load bearing
  - A healthy viable bone in place of devascularized bone
  - Correction of more than one problem by one stage operation

- Disadvantages:
  - Inconvenience
  - Long duration of treatment
  - Pin tract infection
  - Nerve palsy
  - Joint stiffness.

12. **JESS (Joshi's External Stabilization System)**

    Uses:
    - In CTEV principle is controlled fractional differential sequential distraction
    - In CIADER (comminuted intra-articular fracture of distal end of radius)
      - Principle is ligamentotaxis (stretching of ligaments).

13. **Plates**

    Dynamic compression plate (DCP)
    - Holes exactly mirror images of each other
    - Used for any long bone.

    One-third tubular plate
    - Indications—lateral malleolus, fracture of lower end of ulna
    - Disadvantage—no compression.

    Recon plate
    - Can reconstruct according to site by increasing or decreasing number of metal rings
    - Used in fracture of calcaneum, clavicle, iliac crest

    Locking compression plate
    - Provide compression + locking
    - Combi holes – one for locking, one for compression

    Buttress plates
    - For ends of long bones
    - L plate for upper end of tibia
    - Ellis plate for lower end of tibia
    - Cobra plate for lower end of femur or tibia.

14. **Screws**

    Parts–head, neck, shaft, tip, threads lead of screw is the distance traveled by one full turn. Pitch of screw is the distance between 2 threads.

    Types:
    1. Cortical screw—more threads. Pitch and lead is less
    2. Cancellous screw—less number of threads, threads project outwards (more bine between threads so more fixation). Pitch and lead is more
    3. Partially threaded screw/lag screw:
       - Used in fracture medial malleolus, NOF, greater trochanter
       - Lag effect of lag screw provide compression at fracture site
    4. Locking screw—thread at head.

15. **Fracture neck of femur**

		Intertrochanteric fracture
Intracapsular fracture of NOF		Extracapsular fracture of NOF
– Age	After 50 years	After 60 years
– Sex	F > M	M > F
– Injury	trivial	Significant
– Pain.	Swelling, ecchymosis—mild	Severe
Tenderness	In femoral triangle (Scarpa's triangle)	On the greater trochanter
External rotation deformity	< 45°	> 45°
Shortening	< 1 inch	More than 1 inch
Complication	Nonunion	Malunion

ORTHOPEDICS

Classifications of Fracture of NOF

A. Anatomical

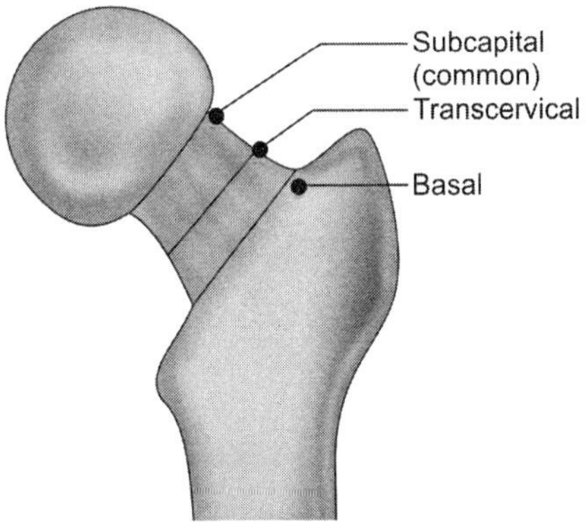

B. Pauwel' Classification

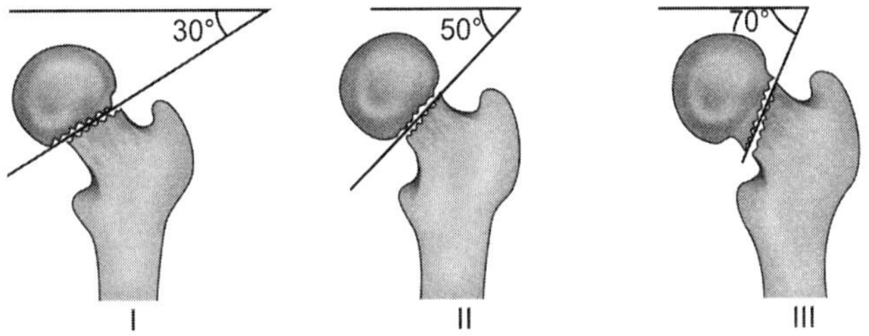

C. Garden's Classification

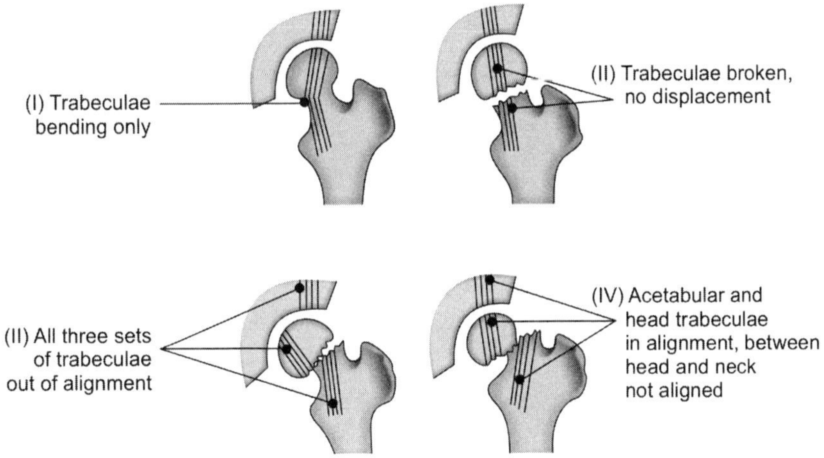

X-ray Features in Fracture NOF

- Break in medial cortex of neck
- Lesser trochanter appearing more prominent (indicate external rotation of femur)
- Overriding of greater trochanter so that it lies at the level of head of femur
- Break in Shenton's line (Shenton's line is an imaginary semicircular line joining medial cortex of femoral neck to lower border of superior pubic ramus)

Complications of fracture of NOF

- Nonunion
- Avascular necrosis
- Osteoarthritis

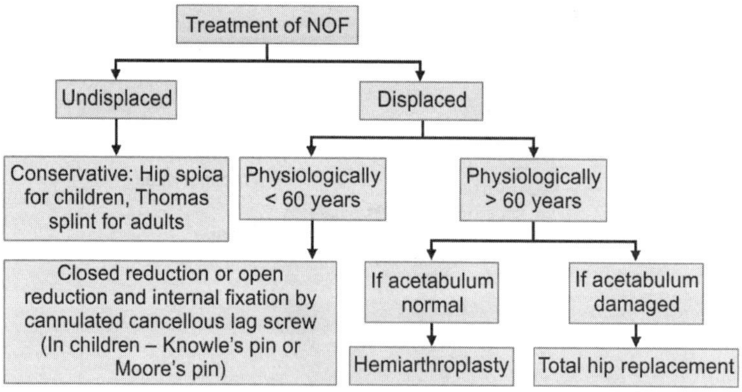

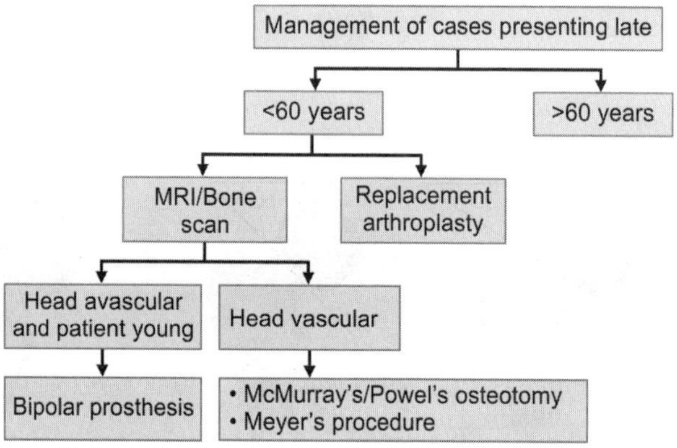

Management of Intertrochanteric Fracture
- Operative method—ORIF with dynamic condylar screw/dynamic hip screw (DCS/DHS)
- Conservative method—can be managed in traction, e.g. Russell's traction, skeletal traction in Thomas splint.

Complications
- Malunion
- Osteoarthritis.

16. **Prosthesis used in hemiarthroplasty**
   1. **Austin Moore prosthesis**
      - In fracture of NOF with calcar
      - Has a head with a small neck and a stem
      - Hole in small neck for hooking the extractor while removing
      - 2 holes on stem
        » Through which the bone supposedly grows
        » To fill with bone graft
   2. **Thompson prosthesis**
      - With large neck
      - Specially used in cases where NOF is absorbed, e.g. In old fracture of NOF without calcar
      - Can be used with or without bone cement (PMMA)
   3. **Bipolar prosthesis**
      - Two piece/bipolar (above 2 are monopolar)
      - Motion occurs between 2 parts of prosthesis itself
      - Hemiarthroplasty – only one side of joint replaced
      - Total hip replacement – both acetabulum and head of femur are replaced with artificial components.
17. **Patella fracture**
   - Types:
      - 2 part fracture
      - Stellate/comminuted

- Fracture clinical feature
  - Pain, tenderness, swelling, crepitus

  Extensor lag (cannot able to lift leg with knee in full extension).
- **Management:**
  - Undisplaced—cylinder cast for 3 weeks (from groin to just above malleoli, with knee in full extension)
  - Two part fracture—reduction and fix with tension band wiring (TBW)
  - If full reduction not achieved, patellectomy/partial patellectomy
  - Comminuted fracture—patellectomy

18. **TBW (tension band wiring)**
    - Principle—distraction force converted into compression force
    - Use stainless steel wire
    - Indicated in fracture patella, olecranon
19. **K-wire/Kirschner wire**

    Uses:
    - Internal fixation of small bones
    - For giving traction, e.g. for applying traction through olecranon
    - For fixing fractures in children
    - For Ilizarov's fixation system.
20. **Total knee replacement:**
    - Indication—disabling arthritis
    - Complications—infection, deep vein thrombosis (DVT), nerve palsy
    - Parts—femoral component, plastic spacer, patellar button, tibial base plate.
21. **Dynamic hip screw (DHS)**
    - Angle 135°
    - For internal fixation of trochanteric fractures
    - 2 components—lag screw and barrel
    - Here dynamic compression at fracture site.
22. **Dynamic condylar screw**

    Angle 90°

    Indications—subtrochanteric fracture, femoral condylar fracture.
23. **Pott's/bimalleolar fracture**

    'SASER PAPER PD'
    - **S**upination **A**dduction
    - **S**upination **E**xternal **R**otation
    - **P**ronation **A**bduction
    - **P**ronation **E**xternal **R**otation
    - **P**ronation **D**orsiflexion

    (Refer Lauge-Hanson classification of ankle injuries)

    Cotton's fracture - trimalleolar fracture
24. **Colle's and Barton's fracture**—-study **Salter and Harris classification of epiphyseal injuries:**
    - Type I – complete separation epiphysis from metaphysis (epiphyseal slip only)
    - Type II – fracture involves growth plate and triangle of metaphyseal bone attached (Thurston-Holland sign)
    - Type III – fracture through epiphysis extending to growth plate
    - Type IV – fracture extending through epiphysis, growth plate and metaphysis
    - Type V – crushing of epiphysis

      Treatment: I and II – cardiac magnetic resonance (CMR), good prognosis

      III and IV – ORIF with K-wire
25. **Monteggia fracture dislocation**
    - Fracture of proximal 1/3rd of ulna with dislocation of head of radius
      - (Monteggia – Medial side, 'MUKALIL')
    - By fall on outstretched hand
    - *Types*: flexion and extension type
    - *Treatment*: ORIF using plate (DCP)
    - *Complications*: Malunion and deformity

ORTHOPEDICS

26. **Galeazzi fracture dislocation**
   - Fracture of distal 1/3rd of radius with dislocation of distal radioulnar joint
   - By fall on outstretched hand
   - *Treatment*: ORIF with DCP
   - *Complications*: Malunion and deformity.
27. **Shoulder dislocation:**
   - The most common dislocation
   - Anteroinferior most common direction
   - *Classification.*
     - Anterior
     - Posterior
     - Luxatio erecta–head lie in subglenoid position

     Management—Reduction + immobilization in chest arm bandage for 3 weeks

     Techniques of reduction

     Kocher's maneuver– Patient came with arm in abduction
     ↓
     1st give traction
     ↓
     External rotation
     ↓
     Adduction
     ↓
     Internal rotation (code: Tea-I)

     - Hippocrates method—Complications: axillary nerve injury.
28. **Congenital dislocation of hip (CDH) or dysplastic dislocation of hip (DDH)**

   Special tests:
   - Barlow's test
   - Ortolani's test

   Attitude of limb–flexion, adduction, internal rotation (FADIR)

   Asymmetrical thigh folds

   Galeazzi's sign +ve

   X-ray features:
   - Small displaced head (with respect to Perkin's lines small epiphysis lie on outer aspect of vertical line and above the horizontal line; in normal case lie on inner aspect of vertical line and below horizontal line)
   - Shallow acetabulum
   - Break in Shenton's line.

   Treatment:
   - At birth closed reduction → if successful 1st put cast for 3 months then change to brace → physiotherapy if reduction not successful → traction → try closed reduction → if successful treat as above
   - Closed reduction failed/acetabulum does not develop → acetabular reconstruction
   - In later cases → open reduction + acetabular reconstruction + derotation osteotomy.
29. **Osteoarthritis**

   X-ray features:
   - Joint space narrowing
   - Subchondral sclerosis and cysts
   - Osteophyte formation
   - Loose bodies.
30. **Perthes' disease/coxa plana/pseudocoxalgia**
   - Osteochondritis of epiphysis of femoral head
   - Age group—5–10 years
   - Clinical feature—pain radiating to knee
   - Shortening, limitation of abduction and internal rotation

- X-ray—collapse and sclerosis of epiphysis of femoral head
  - Increased hip joint space
- Treatment – containment of head at acetabulum
  - By splint, plaster or operation (containment osteotomy)

31. **TB spine** vs **Metastasis**

TB spine	vs	Metastasis
X-ray – i. Disk space lost early ii. Bird nest appearance		X-ray—disk space initially maintained in initial stage

- Spondylolisthesis—forward displacement of a vertebra over one below it
- Spondylolysis—break in pars interarticularis of vertebra
- Spondylitis—inflammation of vertebra
- Spondylosis—degenerative change of spine

32. **Bone nibbler**: For nibbling bone
33. **Bone cutter**: Cutting bone into small pieces
34. **Bone holder**: Self-retaining or not
35. **Osteotome** vs **Chisel**

Osteotome	vs	Chisel
– Both edges are beveled		– Only one of its surfaces is beveled
– *Use*: for osteotomy		– *Uses*: a. For removing a protruding bone b. Leveling a bone surface

36. **Periosteum elevator**
    - For elevating periosteum in all operations of bone
    - Because all important structures such as vessels, nerves, tendons, etc. are outside the periosteum is, and once the periosteum is elevated surgeon is in a safe plane.
37. **Screw driver, hand drill:** Tip of screw driver is hexagonal in shape.
38. **Soft cervical collar:** Use in sprain, contusion, spondylosis
39. **Hard cervical collar:**
40. **Philadelphia collar:** With tracheostomy hole
41. **Cruciform anterior spinal hyperextension (CASH) brace/Ash brace:**
    - Restrict flexion and stabilize the spine.

SUGGESTED READING

1. A Manual on Clinical Surgery—S Das.
2. Essential Orthopedics—J Maheshwari BD.
3. Chaurasia's Human Anatomy Campell Operative Orthopedics.
4. Tachdjian's Pediatric Orthopedics.

NOTES

PEDIATRICS

Practical Examinations	Marks
Short Cases	
Case 1 (Clinical)	10
Case 2 (Nutritional)	10
OSCE	
Five Stations	10
Total	30
Viva	
Four Stations	10
(Charts, Advice and History Taking, Drugs, Nutrition, X-rays)	

CHAPTER 11

Practical Examination

PEDIATRICS—CASE FORMAT

Name: sex: address:
Age (precisely in months for small children), DOB (date of birth)
Informant (reliable or not)

Presenting Complaints

Mention in chronological order (e.g. fever—5 days, cough—3 days, breathlessness—1 day).

History of Present Illness

Onset, duration, progression, associated symptoms, aggravating or relieving factors, present status.
(You should be able to say the relevant negative history in respect to case, try to make negative history into positive)

History of Past Illness

- Any history of similar illness in past.
- Any history of vaccine preventable illness in past—measles, mumps, TB, pertussis.
- History of asthma, jaundice, seizure, previous hospitalization.

Antenatal History

- 1st trimester
- 2nd trimester
- 3rd trimester

} Look obstetrics case format—tell relevant history only

(If no relevant history, we can write as 2nd child of nonconsanguineous marriage without any previous history of abortion)
At least this should be asked—regular antenatal check up, folic acid, TT, complication (any).

Natal History

- Whether term/preterm
- Home/hospital
- Normal labor/CS, if CS—indication
- Birth weight

Postnatal History

- Baby cried soon after birth
- Put to breast immediately after delivery/within how many hours
- Any resuscitation
- Jaundice, seizure
- When was urine passed—normally within 48 hours
- When was meconium passed—normally within 24 hours

Developmental History

- Day of discharge
- Read chapters of development (milestones) (do not forget to ask hearing and vision)
- Scholastic performance.

Dietetic History

- Whether prelacteal food given/not
- When put to breast
- Exclusively breastfed/not
- Complementary feeding started at ——month with——
- Started sharing family diet at——
- Any history of food allergy
- The child has getting ... calories (expected is ... calories, and there is a gap of ... calories)
- The child has getting ... g proteins (expected is ... g, and there is a gap of ... g) as per ICMR
- Diet rich in fruits and green leafy vegetables
- Any diet modification advised.

Item	Quantity	Kcal	Protein
Cooked rice	1 cup	175	4
Uncooked rice	6 tsp	100	2
Dosa	1	70	2
Idli	1	50	2
Chapati	1	70	2
Puri	1	35	1
Upma	1 cup	250	6
Bread	1 slice	70	2
Pathiri	1	50	1
Parotta	1	100	3
Biscuit	1	20	0.5
Puttu	1	50	2
Vada	1	50	1
Banana (100 g)	100 g	116	1.2
Plantain	1	50	1
Egg	1	77	6.5
Mutton	1 oz	50	6
Beef	1 oz	30	6
Fish	1	80	6
Sardine (mathi)	1	30	3
Cow's milk	100 mL	67	3.2
Human milk	100 mL	65	1.1
Volume 6 months	600–700 mL		
Volume 1 year	400–500 mL		
Papad	1 tsp	20	0.5
Cooked dal	1 tsp	8	0.5
Smash potato	50 g	40	0

Item	Quantity	Kcal	Protein
GLV	100 g	33	1
Upperi	1 cup	10	0.5
Sambar	100 g	50	2.5
Fruits	100 g	60	0.5
Coconut	1 tsp	444	4.5
Sugar/Jaggery	1 tsp	20	0
Oils/ghee	1 tsp	36	0
Lactogen	100 g (6 tsp)	100 kcal	2 g
Ragi	100 g (6 tsp)	100 kcal	3 g
Amritham	100 g (6 tsp)	130 kcal	3.5 g
Pulse	100 g	345	24

Lactogen: In 100 mL (½ glass) boiled and cooled water add 3 spoon of lactogen (for 30 mL water 1 tsp)
Working formula for calories (bedside calculation)
At 1 year 1000 calories, after that add 100 calories for every year.

1 cup of tea/coffee containing ½ glass milk and 1 tsp sugar will give 90 kcal 3.5 g protein.
1 cup tea containing ¼ glass milk and 1 tsp sugar will give 55 kcal and 1.75 g protein.

Holliday-Segar formula for calculation of calories and fluid
- RDA—> for expected weight of child, Fluid—> for present weight
- Up to 10 kg – 100 kcal or mL/each kg
- 10-20 kg – 1000 + 50 kcal or mL/kg for each kg >10 kg
- >20 kg – 1500 + 20 kcal or mL/kg for each kg >20 kg

- 1 teaspoon – 5 mL
- 1 table spoon – 15 mL
- 1 cup – 200 mL
- 1 tumbler – 250 mL

NEW ICMR—2010

0–6 months		1.16 g/kg	92 kcal/kg
6 months to 1 year		1.69 g/kg	80 kcal/kg
1, 2, 3 years		16.7 g	1060 kcal
4, 5, 6 years		20.1 g	1350 kcal
7, 8, 9 years		29.5 g	1690 kcal
10, 11, 12	Male	39.9 g	2190 kcal
	Female	40.4 g	2010 kcal

Immunization History

- Fully immunized to date according to National Immunization Schedule
- Look for BCG scar
- Last vaccine taken
- Any optional vaccine
- If not taking vaccine, why?, pulse polio?

Family History

- Draw pedigree chart
- Age of parents, consanguinity
- Similar illness in family
- Chronic illness in family.

SES

- Occupation of parents
- Income
- Housing
- Education of parents
- Sanitation, environment, APL or BPL
- Financial supports (RSBY, thalolam).

GENERAL EXAMINATION [CODE—GVHAD]

I. General survey

Conscious, cooperative, bedridden, playful and active.

II. Vitals

a. Pulse: Rate, rhythm, volume, character, other peripheral pulses, femoral pulse palpable/not, radiofemoral delay

Age	Pulse rate
Newborn	120–160
Up to 1 year	120/min
Up to 5 years	100/min
Up to 10 years	90/min
>10 years	80/min

For practical purpose tachycardia is
1. Newborn >200/min
2. Infants >150/min
3. Older child >120/min

b. Blood pressure: Refer AGN

c. Temperature:

d. Respiratory rate:

Age	Normal RR
Newborn	40/min
Up to 1 year	30/min
Up to 5 years	20/min
Up to 10 years	18/min
>10 years	18/min

Tachypnea

Age group	RR
<2 months	60 or more
2–12 months	50 or more
12 months to 5 years	40 or more
>5 years	>30

Up to 6 years in female and all males—abdominothoracic, >6 year in females → thoracoabdominal

III. Head to foot examination

Head: Size
Shape
Anterior fontanelle—size, closed/not, bulging/depressed
(measured by the lines joining the midpoints of the opposite sides)
Try to include PICCLE in head to foot examination

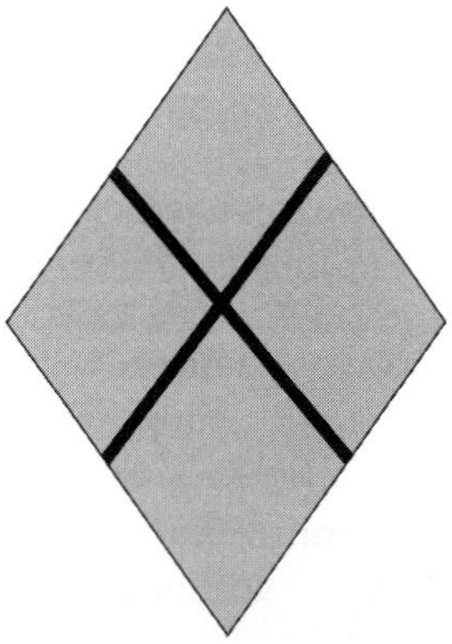

Hair: Hyperpigmentation, sparseness, alopecia (PEM features—refer in heading **Nutrition**), low hair line, pyoderma.

Face: Any dysmorphism

Eyes: Pallor, jaundice, signs of vitamin A deficiency, cataract, hypertelorism, slant

Ears: Any anomaly, low set ears

Nose: DNS, polyp, depressed nasal bridge

Oral cavity: Hygiene, dentition, cheilitis, glossitis, stomatitis, tonsils, caries, lips, palate

Neck: Lymph nodes, JVP, short neck, webbing

Chest: Shape, widely-spaced nipples

Limbs: U/L—pallor, clubbing, flat nail, L/L—edema, (look for BCG scar)

Abdomen: Distended, dilated vein

Genitalia: Undescended testes

Skin: PEM, neurocutaneous markers, pyoderma, rash

Spine: Any deformities.

Notes:

- **Macrocephaly**: Causes (>2 SD)
  Hydrocephalus, rickets, achondroplasia, hemolytic anemia, familial, hydranencephaly
- **Microcephaly:** (>3 SD)
  - *Primary*: Present since birth and causes are inherited—for example, Down's syndrome, craniosynostosis
  - *Secondary*: Due to an insult to growing brain—for example, TORCH infections, malnutrition, IU toxin
  - *Drugs*: Phenytoin, steroid.
- **Anterior fontanelle:** Time of closure of anterior fontanelle is 9–18 months
  - *Early closure:* Craniostenosis or craniosynostosis, primary microcephaly
  - *Delayed closure of AF:* Rickets, hypothyroidism, hydrocephalus, mucopolysaccharidosis
  - *Bulging AF:* Newborn on crying, hydrocephalus, increased intracranial pressure, pseudotumor cerebri
- **Posterior fontanelle:**
  - Closes completely by 2 months
  - It may be open in Down syndrome, congenital hypothyroidism.
- **MacEwen's sign**: Make sure that fontanelle is closed
  Cracked pot sound on percussion of the skull. Present in hydrocephalus, increased intracranial pressure or suture separation.
- **Canthal index:** Ratio of the distances between the inner and outer canthi of both eyes multiplied by 100. Normal is 33–38.
  - **Interpupillary distance**: Distance between centers of the pupils of both eyes measured with child looking upward.
  - **Hypotelorism:** Spacing between eyes is less than normal, canthal index <33.
  - **Hypertelorism:** Abnormally wide spacing of the eyes with broadened bridge of nose, usually due to maldevelopment of the sphenoid bone. Canthal index >38.
  - **Slanting of eyes:** Difference in levels between inner and outer canthi of the eyes.
  - **Mongoloid slant**: Slanting downward from lateral to medial canthus/upward slanting of eyes, for example, Down syndrome.

Antimongoloid slant: Noonan syndrome, Apert syndrome.

- **Low set ears:** With patient standing straight, an imaginary line is drawn from the inner canthus, parallel to floor. Normally, this line crosses the ear in such a way that superior attachment of pinna should be at or above that line, e.g. Down, Turners, Cri-du-cat syndromes.
- **High arched palate:** Ask the child to stand straight, look forward and open the mouth. Normally, the posterior part of the palate is easily visualized. In high-arched palate one cannot visualize the posterior part of the palate. For example, Marfan's syndrome, Down syndrome.
- **Hess test:** To assess the capillary fragility. The sphygmomanometer cuff is tied on the arm and the pressure is elevated to a point in between the systolic and diastolic BP for 5 min. The appearance of purpura on the forearm should be noted. The test is said to be positive if >20 petechiae appear in a 2.5 cm^2 area. Test is positive in—poor platelet function, thrombocytopenia, scurvy.
- **Lymphadenopathy:**
  - Significant LNE—if any of the following factors are present
    - Size—inguinal nodes >1.5 cm diameter, cervical and axillary nodes >1 cm diameter, epitrochlear nodes—any size
    - Site – multiple sites
    - Matted nodes
    - Nodes which are red/tender/ulcerated
    - Associated with focus of infection
    - Associated with systemic signs and symptoms
  - Generalized LNE—involvement of >2 non-contiguous lymph node areas due to systemic disease.

IV. Anthropometry

- **Weight:** (most reliable criterion of assessment of the health and nutritional status of children)
  - Beam type weighing scale, electronic weighing scale for infants, bathroom type.
  - In field conditions, Salter spring scales are used.

PEDIATRICS

Birth weight—3 kg
- Newborns loses 10% of weight during 1st 7 days
- By 7–10th day regains birth weight
- Weight doubles—5/6 months
- Triples—1 year

Quadruples—2 years
- 5 times – 3 years
- 6 times – 5 years
- 7 times – 7 years
- 10 times – 10 years

Weight gain
- 0–3 months—25–30 g/day
- 3 months—1 year – 400 g/month
- 3 years—7 years – 2 kg/year
- 7 years—puberty – 3 kg/year.

Formulas
- 3 months to 1 year: (x in month + 9)/2
- 1–6 years: 2 x in year +8
- 7–12 years: (7 x in year–5)/2

(**Weech's formula**)

1 SD = 12.5% of value

IAP classification:

	Weight for age
Normal	>80%
Grade I (mild malnutrition)	71–80%
Grade II (moderate)	61–70%
Grade III (severe)	51–60%
Grade IV (very severe)	< 50%

+ k = edema

Wellcome trust classification:

Weight for age	Nutritional status
60–80 % + no edema	Undernutrition
60–80% + edema	Kwashiorkor
<60% + no edema	Marasmus
<60%+ edema	Marasmic Kwashiorkor

- **Height:**

  (Length—below 2 years—infantometer)

  (Height—above 2 years—stadiometer)

  – Make the child stand bare feet on a level floor, feet slightly separated.
  – Heels, buttocks and back are brought in contact with the wall.
  – Head is so positioned so that the child looks directly forward with the **Frankfurt plane** (line joining floor of external auditory meatus to the floor of the orbit) and the biauricular plane horizontal.
  – A firm card/long scale is kept firmly over vertex to compress the hair and the point using pencil.
  – Remove the child
  – The 0 of the tape is fixed at the floor and is measured upward to the fixed drawn point.

Birth—50 cm
3 months—60 cm
6 months—65 cm
9 months—70 cm
1 years—75 cm
2 years—90 cm
3 years—95 cm
4 years—100 cm
12 years—150 cm

Rate of height	Velocity
1, 2, 3 months	3.5 cm/month
4, 5, 6 months	2 cm/month
7, 8, 9 months	1.5 cm/month
10, 11, 12 months	1.2 cm/month
1 – 2 years	1.2 cm/month
2–3 years	1 cm/month
4–12 years	6 cm/year

1 SD = 4% of value

Short stature—reduction in height by >2 SD from normal

Weech's formula

Ht (2–12)

= Age × 6 + 77

Waterlow grading of wasting based on weight for height

>90% No wasting
80–90% Mild wasting
70–80% Moderate wasting

Waterlow grading of stunting based on height for age

>95%	Normal
90–95%	Grade I stunt
85–90%	Grade II stunt
< 85%	Grade III stunt

PEDIATRICS

WHO classification	Moderate malnutrition	Severe malnutrition
Symmetrical edema	NO	YES (edematous malnutrition)
Weight for height	SD score between –2 to –3 (70–79%)	SD score < –3 (<70%) (severe wasting)
Height for age	SD score between –2 to –3 (85–89%)	SD score < –3 (<85%) (severe stunting)

$$\text{SD score(Z)} = \frac{\text{Observed value – median reference value}}{\text{SD of reference population}}$$

	Weight	Height
Double	5/6 months	4 years
Triple	12 m	12 years

- **Head circumference:**
  - Ideally use a fiber glass tape
  - Tape should encircle the most prominent part of the occiput and the supraorbital frontal area
  - The occipitofrontal HC is measured by the overlapping technique

Birth	34 cm	0–3 months	2 cm/month
3 months	40 cm		
6 months	43 cm	4–6 months	1 cm/month
1 year	46 cm		
3 years	49 cm	6–12 months	0.5 cm/month
4 years	50 cm	1–2 years	2 cm/year
5 years	51 cm		
12 years	52 cm	2 years	0.5 cm/year

Dines formula—for estimating HC in first year of life

$$\left[\frac{\text{length in cm}}{2} + 9.5\right] +/- 2.5$$

> adult size reached between 5–6 years

Microcephaly: Reduction in HC by >3 SD from normal

1 SD = 2.5% of value (approx 1 SD = 1.25 cm)

Macrocephaly: Increase in HC by >2 SD from normal

- **Chest circumference:**
  - Keep the child in recumbent position
  - Measure at the level of the nipple, midway between expiration and inspiration

At birth	31 cm [Hc > cc by 3 cm]
HC = CC	1 year
After 1 year	CC >HC

In malnourished case CC is < HC even beyond 1 year.

- **Mid-arm circumference:**

Measure using fiber glass or steel tape, use the overlapping tape. While the child sitting, semiflex his **left** upper limb at the elbow and mark the midpoint between acromion and olecranon process.

Then take measurement in extended position

Age independent criteria between 1–5 years

At birth 11–12 cm
At 1 year 15–16 cm

Arnold's classification:

>13.5 cm	– Normal
12.5–13.5 cm	– Moderate PEM
< 11.5	– Severe PEM

Shakir tape: Plastic tape with colored zones—green, yellow and red

Green – >13.5 cm
Yellow – 12.5–13.5 cm
Red – <12.5 cm

PEDIATRICS

Other age independent indices:

1. ***Bangle test***: Done by slipping a bangle with an inner diameter 4 cm up the forearm if crosses elbow—malnourished
2. ***Skinfold thickness:*** Triceps skin fold is the most representative of the total subcutaneous fat up to sixteen years of age. Usually, above 10 mm in normal children whereas in severely malnourished, it may fall below 6 mm.

3. **Ratios:**	
a. Kanawati and McLaren's index	Mid-arm circumference/head circumference
b. Rao and Singh's index	[weight (in kg)/height^2 (in cm)]×100
c. Dugdale's index	weight (in kg)/height$^{1.6}$ (in cm)
d. Jeiliffe's ratio	HC/CC

4. ***Quack stick:*** Quacker arm circumference stick. It is a rod with 2 sets of markings, one indicating height and other MAC for the corresponding height. The arm circumference is measured and the stick placed behind the standing child. If height is more than expected height for measured AC, child is malnourished.

- **Upper segment: Lower segment ratio**
  - Should be taken if the patient is too short or too tall
  - LS – from pubic symphyasis to sole of foot
  - US = Height–LS
  - Proportionate short stature—US:LS ratio is normal for age

At birth	1.7:1
6 months	1.6:1
1 year	I.5:1
2 years	1.4:1
3 years	I.3:1
4 years	1.2:1
6 years	1.1:1
10 years	1:1
Adult	.9:1

Causes—familial, constitutional
— Intrauterine growth restriction (IUGR), nutritional deficiency
— Endocrine disorders – GH deficiency,
Cushing's syndrome: Misc—McCune Albright syndrome

Disproportionate dwarfism—S:LS ratio is not normal for age

Types:
1. Short limbs – Achondroplasia, rickets, osteogenesis imperfecta, cretinism, hypochondroplasia, chondrodysplasia
2. Short trunk – Mucopolysaccharidosis, mucolipidoses, spondyloepiphyseal dysplasia, caries spine

- **Arm span:** It is the distance between tips of middle fingers of both arms when the arms are outstretched at right angles to the body facing away from wall.

Below 5 years	2 cm < height
5–10 years	1 cm < height
At 10 years	arm span = height
Above 10 years	arm span > height by 2 cm

Arm span > height—Marfan's syndrome, Klinefelter's syndrome, Homocystinuria
Arm span < height—achondroplasia, cretinism

V. Developmental assessment

Systemic examination: Refer medicine case format...

NUTRITION

It is the process by which organism utilizes food.
1. Macronutrients
2. Micronutrients

Macronutrients (Proximate principle or major nutrients)

Main components are: 1. Carbohydrate
2. Protein
3. Fat

CHO and protein will provide 4 kcal/g
Fat will provide 9 kcal/g

Food
1. Energy yielding—CHO
2. Body building—protein
3. Protective—vitamins and minerals

PEDIATRICS

Protein

Nitrogen intake → Nitrogen absorbed → Nitrogen retained

$$\text{Digestibility coefficient} = \frac{N_2 \text{ absorbed}}{N_2 \text{ intake}} \times 100$$

$$\text{BV (Biological value)} = \frac{N_2 \text{ retained}}{N_2 \text{ absorbed}} \times 100$$

$$\text{NPU (Net protein utilization)} = \frac{TD \times BV}{100} \text{ or } \frac{\text{Retained N} \times 100}{N_2 \text{ intake}}$$

$$\text{Amino acid score} = \frac{\text{No. of mg of particular amino acid per gram of protein}}{\text{No. of mg of that AA per gram of egg protein}}$$

$$\text{Protein energy ratio} = \frac{\text{Energy from protein}}{\text{Energy (total) derived from food}} \times 100$$

Kilocalorie—amount of heat necessary to rise temperature of 1 kg of water by 1°C from 14.5 to 15.5°C

Egg has highest Br and NPU
∴ Reference protein

Essential Amino Acids

TT HALLIM VP
- T – Threonine
- T – Tryptophan
- H – Histidine — only in infancy
- A – Arginine — only in infancy
- L – Lysine
- L – Leucine
- I – Isoleucine
- M – Methionine
- V – Valine
- P – Phenylalanine

Fats
- *Essential fatty acids*:
  1. Linoleic acid (ω_6)
  2. Linolenic acid (ω_3)
  3. Arachidonic acid
- *Functions:*
  1. Antithrombotic
  2. Antivasorestrictive
  3. Antihypertensive
  4. Antiarrhythmic
  5. Anti-inflammatory

Fiber

- Fiber includes polysaccharides such as cellulose, hemicellulose, pectin and lignin.
- *Functions*:
  - Maintains growth of normal intestinal flora
  - Elimination of waste
  - Essential for normal functioning of gut
  - Bile acid binding capacity.
- [RDA: Range of acceptable or safe intake levels has been formulated based on the current knowledge of nutritional requirement of different age and sex].

[**Balanced diet:** One which contains a variety of food in such quantities and proportion that the need for energy, amino acid, vitamins, minerals, carbohydrate, fat and other nutrients adequately met for maintaining health vitality and general well-being and also makes a small provision for extra nutrients to withstand short duration of leanness].

COMPLEMENTARY FEEDING (WEANING)

Giving the child other food in addition to breast milk (exclusive breastfeeding up to 6 months). Ideal weaning food—Ragi.

Criteria for complementary food:
- Culturally acceptable
- Physiologically suitable
- Easily prepared at home with the existing facilities
- Adequate to provide all nutritional requirements of the infant with respect to energy, proteins, vitamins and minerals.

Benefits of breastfeeding:

- *Benefit to baby*:
  - Nutritional superiority
  - Immune superiority
  - Higher IQ
  - Protection from allergy
- Benefit to mother:
  - Protection from pregnancy (lactational amenorrhea)
  - Reduced severity of PPH
  - Helps in uterine involution
  - Prevents cancer (ovarian and breast cancers)
  - Helps in shedding of extra weight of mother
- Contraindication for breastfeeding is when mother is on anticancer drugs, galactosemia, phenylketonuria, active varicella, herpes zoster, radioactive I_2 intake.

Ragi per 100 g		
Calorie	–	328 kcal
Protein	–	7.3 g
Fat	–	1.3 g
Fe	–	3.9 mg
Ca	–	34 mg

Protein Energy Malnutrition (PEM)

Definition: Range of pathological condition arising from coincidental lack in varying proportions of proteins and calories occurring most frequently in infants and young children and commonly associated with infection

Clinical Findings of Marasmus and Kwashiorkor

Occurrence	More common	Less common
Edema	-	+
Activity	Active	Apathetic
Appetite	Good	Poor
Liver enlargement	-	+
Mortality	Less than kwashiorkor	High in early stage
Recovery	Recover early	Long to recover
Infection	Less prone	More prone

Marasmus—Monkey facies, Baggy pants appearance, wasting of muscles and fat

Grading of marasmus
- Grade I – wasting axilla and groin
- Grade II – I+ thighs and buttocks
- Grade III – II+ chest and abdomen
- Grade IV – III+ buccal pad of fat

Grading of Kwashiorkor or
1. Pedal edema
2. 1+ facial edema
3. 2 + paraspinal and chest edema
4. 3 + ascites

Kwasiorkor—Hair changes:
- Hypopigmentation (light colored hair)
- Sparse hair (alopecia)
- Easily pluckable hair
- Flag sign
- Straight/Brittle/Coarse/Lusterless/Dry

Nail changes: Brittle nails, paronychia/platonychia/koilonychias

Skin changes:
- Pigmentation, desquamation, dyspigmentation
- Marbling/Mosaic pattern
- Crazy pavement sign
- Flaky paint dermatoses
- Enamel paint dermatoses (buttock, perineum, upper thigh)
- Edema
- Shiny skin
- Infection (like scabies, pyoderma)
- Ulceration

General appearance: Sugar baby appearance, pitting edema, weak, hypotonic.

MANAGEMENT

Mild and Moderate

Treatment—giving adequate amount of:

Protein and energy

150 kcal/kg/day—frequent high density food

Protein—3 g/kg/day

Severe

10 step management

Usage of oil and fat rich foods
Give milk (if the child drinks tea without milk, add milk to it)

SAM (severe acute malnutrition)

WHO and UNICEF criteria [Any 1 of the following]

- Weight <3 SD of the median WHO reference
- Visible severe wasting
- Bipedal edema
- MAC <11.5 cm [Not required in child < 6 month]

10 step management

Steps	**Stabilization**	**Rehabilitation**
	Days 1–2 to days 3–7	Weeks 2–6
1. Hypoglycemia (<54 mg/dL)		
2. Hypothermia (<35°C axillary)		
3. Dehydration		
4. Electrolytes		
5. Infection		
6. Micronutrients	No iron	With iron
7. Initiate feeding		
8. Catch up growth		
9. Sensory stimulation		
10. Prepare for follow-up		

1st 6 steps can be easily studied by the mnemonic: "SHIELDED"

S – Sugar deficiency, i.e. hypoglycemia
H – Hypothermia
I – Infection
EL – Electrolyte imbalance
DE – Dehydration
D – Deficiency of micronutrients

CEREALS

- Deficient in lysine, threonine and tryptophan
- Rice—100 g gives 350 kcal, 7 g proteins. It is deficient in **lysine**. Polished rice causes **beriberi**
- Wheat—100 g gives 350 kcal, 11 g proteins. It is deficient in **lysine and threonine**
- Ragi—100 g gives 325 kcal, 7 g proteins, 3.44 mg Ca, 3.9 mg Fe and Iodine. It is a **weaning** food.
- Maize—it has high **leucine** content. It interferes with the absorption of niacin, vitamin B_2: causes **pellagra.**

PULSES

- Deficient in **methionine, vitamin C** (but germinated pulses contain vitamin C)
- Combined in the ratio of 1:4 with cereals (complementary action of food)
- Green gram (cherupayar) 348 kcal, 24 g protein
- Red gram (unakka payar) 350 kcal, 22 g protein
- Black gram (uzhunnu) 347 kcal, 24 g protein
- Bengal gram (kadala) 360 kcal, 17 g protein
- Soybean 440 kcal, 44 g protein

Egg deficient in:
- CHO
- Vitamin C

EGG

- Reference protein (BV = 100)
- 50 g egg contains 77 kcal energy, 6 g protein, 5.3 g fat, 1.5 mg iron, 30 mg calcium, 250 mg cholesterol
- (Duck egg has increased amount of avidin which decreases the availability of biotin)

MILK

- Deficient in vitamin C and Fe
- Rich in Ca

PEDIATRICS

VITAMINS

Fat soluble vitamins: (A, D, E, K)

VITAMIN A

RDA Infant 350 μg (300–400)
Children 550 μg (400–600)
Adolescent 750 μg

Deficiency
- Defective dark adaptation
- Night blindness
- Conjunctival xerosis
- Bitot spot
- Corneal xerosis
- Keratomalacia.

Extraocular manifestations: Follicular keratosis, anorexia, growth retardation, infection (respiratory, intestinal), infertility.

Functions of Vitamin A
- Vision
- Maintenance of epithelial tissue
- Tissue differentiation

Source
- Animal—liver, egg, fish, liver oil
- Plants—spinach, amarnath carrot
- Fortified vanaspati

Treatment

Oral vitamin A: 0, 1 day, 1 month (3 doses)
<6 months – 50,000 IU
6 months to 1 year – 1 lakh IU
>1 year – 2 lakh IU

Prevention

Vitamin A prophylaxis program

1–5 year old children (give vitamin A, total = 9 doses 6 months apart)
[Nowadays 1 lakh given along with measles (at 9 months), 2 lakh given with DPT booster (at 15 months)]

WHO classification

Primary signs		*Secondary signs*	
X1A	Conjunctival xerosis	XN	Night blindness
X1B	Bitot spots	XF	Fundal changes
X2	Corneal xerosis	XS	Corneal scarring
X3A	Corneal ulceration (<1/3 of cornea)		
X3B	Corneal ulceration (>1/3 of cornea)		

Hypervitaminosis A
- A/c—Pseudotumor cerebri
- C/C—Dermatitis, Alopecia, HSM
- In pregnancy—fetal anomaly.

VITAMIN D

Source a. Sunlight
b. Food—animal origin (liver, egg yolk, butter, cheese)

RDA Infant—5 μg (200 IU)
Children—10 μg (400 IU)

Deficiency: Rickets in children
Osteomalacia in adults.

Metabolism
7 dehydrocholesterol
↓ Sunlight
Cholecalciferol
↓ Liver
25-hydroxycholecalciferol
↓ Kidney
1, 25-dihydroxycholecalciferol

Clinical Features

- Soft skull—craniotabes
- Delayed closure of AF
- Rachitic rosary
- Harrison's groove
- Widened wrist
- Genu valgum/genu varum

PEDIATRICS

- Double malleoli due to metaphyseal hyperplasia
- Spinal and pelvic abnormality
- Growth disturbance
- Green stick fracture
- Bone pain/tenderness
- Muscle weakness
- Dental problems.

Radiological features (findings mainly seen in the lower end of ulna and radius)
- Loss of normal zone of provisional calcification—earliest sign
- Widened epiphysis
- Cupping
- Fraying metaphyseal end
- Splaying.

Treatment—Oral vitamin D 6 lakh IU given followed by 400 IU/day and oral Ca supplements.

VITAMIN E (Tocopherol)

Deficiency leads to:
- Hemolytic anemia
- Spinocerebellar ataxia

VITAMIN K

- Vitamin K_1 is called phylloquinone.
- Function—cofactor in the post-translational carboxylation of glutamic acid to form glutamate (takes place in liver).
- Vitamin K dependant factors in coagulation system—II, VII, IX, X
- RDA: 5 µg (newborns)
  10 µg (children)
- Deficiency causes hemorrhagic disease of newborn.

WATER-SOLUBLE VITAMINS (VITAMIN B AND C)

VITAMIN B

Vitamin B_1 – Thiamine
Vitamin B_2 – Riboflavin
Vitamin B_3 – Niacin
Vitamin B_5 – Pantothenic acid
Vitamin B_6 – Pyridoxine
Vitamin B_9 – Folic acid
Vitamin B_{12} – Cobalamin.

> Biotin—vitamin H

VITAMIN B_1

- Polished rice deficient in B_1 and leads to beriberi
- *Biological action*: Active form is TPP (Thiamine pyrophosphate) and is involved in:
  - Oxidative decarboxylation of pyruvate to form acetyl CoA (pyruvic acid → acetyl CoA)
  - Pentose pathway (transketolase)
  - Decarboxylation of a-ketoglutaric acid to succinic acid—Korebs cycle.

Deficiency: Beriberi
- Dry beriberi—nerve involvement like peripheral neuritis (no edema, muscle wasting)
- Wet beriberi—involvement of heart—peripheral edema, cardiomegaly,
- Infantile beriberi and Wernicke's encephalopathy

Diagnosis is made by 24 hours thiamine urinary excretion [decreased in beriberi <15 mg/day)].

> **Treatment**
> - Mild disease—5 mg vitamin B_1/day
> - Severe disease—10 mg IV BD

PEDIATRICS

VITAMIN B_2

- **Function:** It is the constituent of two coenzymes (FAD and FMN)
- **RDA:**
  - *Infants*: 0.4 mg/1000 kcal
  - *Children*: 0.8 mg/1000 kcal

Deficiency (Ariboflavinosis)

Photophobia, glossitis, angular stomatitis, seborrheic dermatitis, cataract.

Treatment

1 mg vitamin B_2 tid for few weeks.

VITAMIN B_3

- **Function:** Constituent of two coenzymes, i.e. NAD and NADP
- **RDA:** 6.4–8 NE/1000 kcal [NE= Niacin equivalent]

Deficiency: Seen in children who take maize
- Pellagra
- Diarrhea, dermatitis, dementia (3 Ds)

Treatment: 10 times the RDA.

VITAMIN B_{12} and B_9.

- Deficiency causes megaloblastic anemia
- Refer Pediatrics
- **RDA** of vit B_{12}
  - *Infants*: 0.3 µg/day
  - *Children*: 0.5–1.5 µg/day
  - *Adolescent:* 2 µg/1 day.

VITAMIN C (ASCORBIC ACID)

- Rich in citrus fruits, cauliflower, cabbage
- **Functions:**
  - Strong reducing agent
  - Required for normal functioning of leukocytes, fibroblasts, microsomes, osteoblast
  - Affects immune response, wound healing, collagen synthesis, detoxification.
- **RDA**
  - *Infants*: 30–40 mg/day
  - *Children*: 40–70 mg/day.

Deficiency: Scurvy

In infancy clinical features of scurvy (***Barlow's disease***) are:

1. Pallor	P
2. Anorexia	A
3. Diarrhea	D
4. Irritability	I
5. Pseudoparalysis	P
6. Infections	I
7. Subperiosteal hemorrhage	S
8. Tenderness of bone	T

In older children, hemorrhagic signs usually predominate with bleeding gums, conjunctivae and intestinal tract. It is diagnosed by X-ray of long bones. [Ground glass appearance, thinning of cortex].

Rx—100-200 mg vitamin C oral or 100 mL orange juice daily.

PEDIA

SOME IMPORTANT MINERALS

Zinc

'Zn' dependant enzymes:
- Thymidine kinase
- DNA polymerase
- RNA polymerase
- Carbonic anhydrase

Macrominerals—conc >0.01% body weight Ca, K, Na, Mg Microminerals (trace elements) Fe, I, Cu, Cr, Zn, Se, Mn, Ni, Si

RDA

3.5–5 mg/day

Deficiency

Typical syndrome of Zn deficiency includes
1. Hypogonadism
2. Anemia
3. Growth retardation

Other manifestations include diarrhea, dermatitis, hair loss and anorexia.

Acrodermatitis enteropathica
- AR condition of Zn deficiency
- Due to defective Zn absorption—transporter defect
- Anorexia is a prominent feature

Treatment: 0.5–1 mg/kg/day for several months.

Selenium (Se)

Function: Component of glutathione peroxidase (an antioxidant which scavenges free radicals)

Deficiency: Severe deficiency—***Keshan disease*** (presents as cardiomyopathy)
Mild deficiency of Se presents as macrocytosis and loss of hair pigment.

Iodine (I)

RDA 90 mg (0–5 years)
120 mg (6–12 years)
150 mg (>12 years)
200–250 mg (pregnant and lactating women)

The term **iodine deficiency disorders (IDD)** refers to all the ill-effects of iodine deficiency in a population that can be prevented by ensuring an adequate intake of iodine.

Fetus	Abortions, stillbirths, congenital anomalies, increased perinatal mortality, endemic cretinism
Neonate	Neonatal goiter, neonatal hypothyroidism, endemic mental retardation
Child and adolescent	Goiter, subclinical hypothyroidism, impaired mental function, retarded physical development

Rx—Legol's iodine, iodized salt. [1:25000–50000]

ADDITIONAL POINTS

Baby-Friendly Hospital Initiative (BFHI)

Ten steps to successful breastfeeding:

1. Have a written breastfeeding policy that is routinely communicated to all health staff.
2. Train all healthcare staff in skills necessary to implement this policy.
3. Inform all pregnant women about the benefits and management of breastfeeding.
4. Help mothers to initiate breastfeeding within half an hour of birth.
5. Show mothers how to breastfeed, how to maintain lactation even if they should be separated from their infants.
6. Give newborn infants no food or drink other than breast milk, unless medically indicated.
7. Practice rooming in—allow mothers and infants to remain together 24 hours a day.
8. Encourage breastfeeding on demand.
9. Give no artificial teats or pacifiers (also called dummies or soothers) to breastfeeding infants.
10. Foster the establishment of breastfeeding support groups and refer mothers to them on discharge from the hospital or clinic.

SAT MIX

It is a combination of roasted and powdered rice, wheat, black gram and powdered sugar in the ratio 1:1:1:2. 100 g mix give 380 kcal energy and 8 g protein.

Etiology of Kwashiorkor and Marasmus

- Classical theory of deficiency
- Gopalan's theory of dysadaptation
- Golden theory of free radicals.

ICDS Program—Refer New ICDS Guidelines

Norms for supplementary nutrition in ICDS

Beneficiaries	Calories (kcal)	Protein (g)
Children <6 years	500	12–15
Severely malnourished children <6 years	800	20–25
Pregnant and lactating women	500	18-20

Mid-day Meal Program

For LP-450 kcal/12 g proteins, UP-700 kcal/20 g protein

a. The meal should be a supplement and not a substitute to the home diet.
b. The meal should supply at least one-third of the total energy requirement, and half of the protein needed.
c. The cost of the meal should be necessarily low.
d. The meal should be such that it can be prepared in schools; no complicated cooking process should be involved.
e. As far as possible, locally available foods should be used; this will reduce the cost of meal, and
f. The menu should be frequently changed to avoid monotony.

National Nutrition Anemia Prophylaxis Program

For expecting/nursing mothers, give 100 mg elemental 'Fe' and 0.5 mg folic acid for a period of 100 days. Children (1–5 years) are given one tablet containing 20 mg elemental 'Fe' and 0.1 mg folic acid daily for a period of 100 days.

Amrutham powder

- Protein
- CHO
- Sodium, potassium, calcium
- Iron, vitamin C
- Cholesterol
- Moisture
- Ash
- Calorie: 395.06

Breast milk vs Cow's milk

	Breast milk Vs (per 100 g)	Cow's milk
Calorie	65 kcal	67 kcal
Protein	1.1 g	3.2 g
Fat	3.4 g	4.1 g
Calcium	28 mg	120 mg
Iron	Zero	0.2

GROWTH AND DEVELOPMENT

Growth: Increase in size or mass of tissue.

Development: Maturation of function and related to maturation and myelination of nervous system and indicate acquisition of various skill for the functioning of individual.

LAWS OF GROWTH

- Its continuous and orderly process
- Growth pattern of every individual is unique (cephalocaudal and distal to proximal)
- Different tissue of body grow at different rates.

PERIODS OF GROWTH

Prenatal Period

Ovum	0–14 days
Embryo	14 days to 9 weeks
Fetus	9 weeks to birth
Perinatal period	22 weeks of gestation to 7 days after birth

Postnatal Period

Newborn	1st 4 weeks after birth
Infancy	First year
Toddler	1–3 years
Preschool child	3–6 years
School age child	6–12 years
adolesence	*Early*: 10–13 years *Middle*: 14–16 years *Late*: 17–20 years

Principles of Development

- Development is a continuous process from conception to maturity.
- Sequence of development is same in all children but rate of development varies from child to child.
- Development is intimately related to maturation of nervous system.
- Generalized mass activity is replaced by individual response.
- Development is in cephalocaudal direction.
- Certain primitive reflexes have to be lossed before the corresponding voluntary movement is acquired.

Functional developmental estimation

Main domains	*Extended neurological examination*
• Gross motor	• Vision
• Fine motor	• Hearing
• Social, adaptive	• Muscle tone
• Language	• Primitive reflexes

DEVELOPMENTAL MILESTONES

Gross Motor

Main domains	*Extended neurological examination*
3 months	Neck holding
5 months	Rolls over
6 months	Sit in tripod fusion prone to supine
7 months	Supine to prone
8 months	Sitting without support
9 months	Standing with support crawling
10 months	Walk with support with creeping
12 months	Standing without support, creeps well
15 months	Walks alone, creeps upstairs
18 months	Runs, explores drawers
2 years	Walks up and downstairs [feet/step] jumps
3 years	Rides tricycle, 1 feet per step upstairs
4 years	1 feet per step down Hops on one foot

Fine Motor	
Up to 3 months	Grasp reflex
4 months	Bidextrous approach
6 months	Unidextrous, transfer objects
9 months	Immature pincer grasp
12 months	Mature pincer grasp
15 months	Imitates scribbling tower of 2 blacks
18 months	Scribbles tower of 3 blocks
2 years	Tower of 6 blocks vertical and circular stroke
3 years	Tower of 9 blocks draws circle
4 years	Bridge with blocks draws cross
5 years	Gate with blocks draws triangle

Social and adaptive	
2 months	Social smile
3 months	Recognition smile, anticipate feed
6 months	Mirror smile, stranger reaction
9 months	Bye bye
10 months	Peek a boo
12 months	Comes when called, play simple ball games
15 months	Jargon
18 months	Domestic mimicry and follow orders
2 years	Ask for toilet, food and drink
3 years	Know sex and age and handedness, share toys
4 years	Imaginative play and go to toilet himself
5 years	Helps in household tasks, dresses and undresses

Language milestone	
1 months	Alert to sound
3 months	Cooing
4 months	Lough loud
6 months	Monosyllables – ma, ba
9 months	Bisyllables – mama, baba
12 months	1–2 words with meaning
15 months	Jargon speech
18 months	10 words with meaning
2 years	100 words with meaning (2–3 word sentence)
3 years	Ask questions, knows full name and gender
4 years	Tell story and poems
5 years	Ask meanings of words

Vision	
At birth	Fixation follow 45°
1 month	Fixation follow 90°
3 months	Fixation follow 180°
4 months	Binocular vision
6 months	Fix only on interest
1 year	Fix rapid moving objects

Hearing	
At birth	Respond to sound by cry, blink
5–6 months	Child turn head to one side then downward if the sound is made below the level of ears
7 months	Is able to localize sound by turning head to one side then upward if sound made above the level of ears
10 months	Child directly looks at source of sound directly

Global development delay—delay in 2 or more spheres of milestone, e.g. Downs, CP, galactosemia
Dissociated development delay—difference between rate of development of 2 spheres
Development regression—loss of previously attained milestone. It is seen in degenerative disorder (In CP, there is no development regression).

*Development quotient DQ = A/O*100*
A–Average age of attainment
O–observed age of attainment
If <70% evaluation should be needed.

DISORDERS OF GROWTH

SHORT STATURE

Height below 3rd percentile or more than 2 SD below the median height for the age and sex according to standard population.

CAUSES

Physiological or normal variant short stature

- Familial
- Constitutional.

Pathological Short Stature

- Undernutrition
- Chronic systemic illness:
  - *Renal*: Renal tubular acidosis, chronic renal failure, steroid dependent nephrotic syndrome
  - *Cardiopulmonary*: Congenital heart disease, cystic fibrosis, asthma
  - *Gastrointestinal and hepatic*: Malabsorption
  - *Chronic severe infections*
- Endocrine causes
  - *Growth hormone deficiency*
  - *Hypothyroidism*
  - *Cushing syndrome*
  - *Pseudohypoparathyroidism*
  - *Precious or delayed puberty*
- Psychosocial dwarfism
- Children born small for gestiaional age
- Skeletal dysplasias, e.g. achondroplasia, rickets
- Genetic syndromes, e.g. Turner syndrome, Down's syndrome.

Failure to Thrive

- Term used in children below 5 years of age.
- It refers to weight below 3rd or 5th percentile, or failure to gain weight over a period of time, or change in rate of growth that has crossed two major centiles.

PEDIATRICS

Causes

Organic causes:
- *Gastrointestinal*—gastroesophageal reflex, malabsorption, inflammatory bowel disease, pyloric stenosis
- *Neurological*—mental retardation, cerebral palsy
- *Renal*—renal tubular acidosis, chronic renal failure
- *Cardiopulmonary*—congenital heart disease, cystic fibrosis, asthma
- *Endocrine*—hypothyroidism, DM, adrenal insufficiency
- *Infections*—chronic parasitic or bacterial infections of gastrointestinal (GI) tract, tuberculosis, infection with HIV virus
- *Genetic*—inborn errors of metabolism, chromosomal anomaly
- *Miscellaneous*—lead poisoning, malignancy, collagen vascular disease.

Nonorganic causes
- Poverty
- Misperception or lack of knowledge about diet and feeding practices.
- Lack of breastfeeding, feeding diluted formulae.
- Dysfunctional parent child relationship with child abuse and neglect.

Treatment

Treat the cause and nutritional rehabilitation.

ABNORMAL DEVELOPMENT

Red Flag Sign in Child Development

Milestone	Age
No visual fixation or following by	2 months
No vocalization by	6 months
Not sitting without support by	10 months
Not standing alone by	17 months
Not walking alone by	18 months
No single words by	18 months
Loss of imaginative play	3 years
Loss of comprehension, single words or phrases	At any age

Ponderal index

$$\frac{\text{Weight in grams}}{\text{Length in cm}} \times 100$$

>2.5 – normal

if <2 – asymmetric (malnourished)

if 2-2.5 – symmetric (hypoplasia)

IMMUNIZATION

- Vaccination—process of administration of a vaccine
- Immunization—induction of immune response
- Vaccine failure—if disease occurs despite immunization.

Vaccine Failure

- Primary—when administration of recommended dose of vaccine does not result in adequate protection against disease.
- Secondary—disease occurs despite of immunization.

Adjuvant

Substance given along with antigens in order to enhance immunological efficiency of vaccine. For example, aluminum salt used in DPT vaccine.

PEDIATRICS

TYPES OF VACCINE (live, killed, toxoid, subunit)

Live vaccine

Advantages

- Single dose enough (exception-OPV)
- Produce local immunity
- Induce cell mediated immunity
- Given as combined vaccine of virus
- More convenient for mass immunization

Disadvantages

- Reversion to virulence
- Difficulty in storage
- Toxoid—modified toxin, and are nontoxic to recipient
- Subunit vaccine—capsular polysaccharide and viral or bacterial subunit

Killed vaccine

Advantages

- No danger of spread
- Stability and safety

Disadvantages

- Multiple injection may be required
- May be contaminated with dangerous infectious agent

Description	Example
Live attenuated vaccine	
Bacterial	BCG, oral typhoid
Viral	OPV, measles, MMR varicella, JE
Killed or inactivated organism	
Bacteria	DTPw, whole killed vaccine, typhoid,
Viral	inactivated polio vaccine, rabies, Hep A
Modified bacterial toxins or toxoids	dT
Subunit	
Bacterial capsular polysaccharide	*S. typhi*, *Haemophilus influenzae* type b meningococcal, pneumococcal
Viral (surface antigen)	Hepatitis B

National Immunization Program

Age	*Vaccines*
0 (at birth)	BCG, OPVO, Hep BO
6 weeks	DTwP1, OPV1, Hep B1, Hib 1
10 weeks	DTwP2, OPV2, Hep B2, Hib 2
14 weeks	DTwP3, OPV3, Hep B3, Hib 3
9 months	Measles, Vitamin A1
15 months	MMR
16–24 months	$DTWPB_1$, OPVB1, Vitamin A_2, JE
5 years	$DTWPB_2$
10 years	TT
16 years	TT

*Pregnant woman 2 doses of TT 1 month apart

COLD CHAIN

It is the system of transporting, storage and distributing vaccine at recommended temperature from manufacture site to which it administered:

- OPV stored in freezed compartment (0–4°C)
- In the main compartment (4–10°C)
- Top rack (below freezer)—BCG, measles, MMR
- Middle rack—DPT, Hep A, typhoid, DT, TT
- Lower rack—Hep B, varicella.

BCG VACCINE

It should contain at least type of vaccine, dose, schedule, route, contraindication

- Live attenuated vaccine administered intradermally in the left arm on insertion of deltoid (site is selected for universal equality).
- *Dose*: 0.05 mL in neonate and 0.1 mL in all others
- Protect against miliary TB and TB meningitis (efficacy 50–80%)
- Contraindicated in immunocompromised
- Complication—ulceration, lymphadenitis, osteomyelitis, local abscess, keloid, vaccine failure
- *Strain used*: Copenhagen and Pasteur (Danish 1331)
- Vaccine reconstituted with normal saline.

POLIO VACCINE

Two type of vaccine:

1. Live—sabin
2. Killed—salk.

Oral Polio Vaccine

- Contain 10^5–10^6 median cell culture infectious dose of type I, II, III viruses
- *Dose*: 2 drops in India (look NIP)
- Contraindication—in immunocompromised, diarrhea, infectious fever
- $MgCl_2$ is the stabilizing agent
- Mopping up
- Pulse polio immunization—giving 2 doses 1 month apart
- Vaccine vial monitors—to know potency of vaccine
- Reverse cold chain
- Complications:
  - Vaccine associated paralytic polio (VAPP) (due to type 2)
  - Vaccine derived paralytic polio—due to mutation of virus in the vaccine.

Injectable Vaccine

- Formaldehyde killed and purified polio virus
- Contain 40D, 8D, 32D units of types 1, 2, 3 polio viruses, respectively (40 – 8 = 32)
- 6, 10, 14 weeks according to IAP 0.5 mL IM, or SC, booster at 18 months.

DTPw *Vaccine*

- D,T-toxoid, pertussis –killed, whole cell
- Give IM in the anterolateral aspect of thigh (0.5 mL)
- *Complications*
  - Prolonged screaming episodes
  - Progressive neurological diseases/encephalopathy
  - Complication is due to pertussis component in these situation give DT or TT.
  - Absolute contraindication—immediate anaphylaxis, encephalitis lasting >24 hours within 7 days of vaccination.

DTPa Vaccine

- Here pertussis vaccine is acellular pertussis vaccine
- It contains inactivated pertussis toxin and one or more additional pertussis antigen like filamentous hemagglutinin (FHA), fimbrial protein, nonfimbrial protein
- *Advantage*: Fever systemic and local side effect less
- *Disadvantage*: High cost.

MEASLES

- Live attenuated vaccine (Edmonston-Zagreb strain)
- Given 0.5 mL right upper arm or thigh SC

- Given at 9 months (because at that time maternal antibody wean off)
- *Contraindications:*
  - Malignancy
  - Therapy with alkylating agent/corticosteroid
  - Immune deficiency
- *Side effect:* TSS (toxic shock syndrome) due to bacterial contamination, fever, rash, measles like syndrome.

MMR

- Measles—Edmonston-Zagreb strain
- Mumps—Jeryl-Lynn strain
- Rubella—RA 27/3 strain
- Dose is 0.5 mL (2 dose one at 15 months and another 8 weeks later) (S/C).
- Each dose contain 1000, 5000, 1000 TCID 50 of measles, mumps, rubella, respectively.
- Contraindication—pregnancy, immunosuppression
- *Side effects*: Fever, arthralgia, aseptic meningitis.

HEPATITIS B VACCINE

- Recombinant DNA vaccine (in yeast)
- 0.5 mL IM in <1 year and 1 mL >1 year, anterolateral/thigh.
- 3 doses at 0, 1, 6 months
- HBIG gives passive immunity} dose—0.5 mL in newborns and 0.6 mL/kg for all other ages
- HBIG should be given preferably within 48 hours of exposure.

TYPHOID VACCINE

- 2 doses
- 0.5 mL SC 1 month interval (killed vaccine)
- Typhoral—oral live vaccine (stable mutant *S. typhi* strain type 2 Ia)
- Typhim—give SC or IM single dose.

Hib VACCINE

- Capsular polysaccharide used as antigen
- Given particularly prior to splenectomy
- 3 dose below 6 months
- 2 dose between 6–12 months
- 1 dose between 12–15 months, and a booster dose should be administered in this children at 18 months.
- >15 months—only one dose.

Pentavalent vaccine
Contains D, P, T, Hib, Hep B
Schedule—6, 10, 14 weeks

HPV Vaccine

- **0.5 mL** IM deltoid
- Recommended age for initiation of vaccine is 10–12 years—3 doses at 0, 2,6 months.

Pneumococcal Vaccine

- High-risk group (children <2 years, congenital immunodeficiency, HIV, immunosuppressive therapy, asplenia, hyposplenia, nephrotic syndrome), sickle cell, DM, c/c cardiac, renal, liver disease.
- *Currently **two types:***
  1. Polysaccharide vaccine
  2. Conjugate vaccine
- Unconjugated polysaccharide vaccine (**PPV 23**)—0.5 mL IM: S/E—poorly immunogenic in <2 years, immunological memory is low.
- Pneumococcal conjugate vaccine—**PCV 10, PCV 13**
- Dose—0.5 mL IM 3 doses 6, 10, 14, with a booster at 15–18 months.

Japanese Encephalitis Vaccine

- Dose 0.5 mL S/C

- S/C—anaphylaxis
- Can be given up to 15 years.

Chickenpox

Dose—0.5 mL S/C 2 doses at more than 3 months apart.

IMMUNIZATION OF AN UNIMMUNIZED CHILD

Visit	At evaluation	After 1 month	After 2 months	After 6 months
Age ≤7 years	BCG, OPV DTwP/DTaP Hep B	OPV DTwP/ DTaP Hep B	MMR or measles, typhoid	DTwP/DTaP Hep B
Age ≥7 years	Tdap Hep B	dT Hep B	MMR Typhoid	Hep B

CHAPTER 12

Congenital Heart Diseases

DIAGNOSIS

- Congenital heart disease
- Cyanotic/acyanotic
  L → right shunt
- ± Features of cardiac failure
- ± Features of infective endocarditis
- ± Features of pulmonary hypertension
- In sinus rhythm
- Protein-energy malnutrition (PEM), developmental delay.

NADA's criteria (1 major or 2 minor indicates heart disease)	
Major	*Minor*
• Systolic murmur grade 3 or more • Diastolic murmur • Cyanosis • CCF	• Systolic murmur more than grades • Abnormal S2 • Abnormal electrocardiogram (ECG) • Abnormal X-ray • Abnormal blood pressure (BP)

PRESENTING COMPLAINTS

- **Cough and breathlessness:**
  Differentiate congestive cardiac failure (CCF) and respiratory infection
  – *Congestive Cardiac Failure (CCF):*
    - Poor feeding (suck-rest-suck cycle), interrupted feeding
    - Breathes better when held against shoulder (equivalent to orthopnea)
    - Excessive head sweating. Due to increased sympathetic activity and large surface area of head to maintain tissue perfusion
  – Respiratory infection:
    - Fever, cough, sputum production.
- **History of increased precordial activity**
- **History of failure to thrive**
- **Cyanosis:**
  Bluish discoloration of skin, mucous membrane due to increased amount of reduced hemoglobin >5 g%, methemoglobin >1.5 g/dL or sulfur Hb > 0.5 g/dL.
  – Look at tongue, nail bed, ear lobule, tip of nose, cyanosis/pigmentation.
    Diascopy: Blanch with a slide, cyanosis will blanch, pigmentation will not
  –

Central	**Peripheral cyanosis**
Due to hypoxic hypoxia	Stagnant hypoxia
Tongue and periphery cyanosed	Not on tongue
Limb warm	Limb cold
On warming cyanosis remains	Cyanosis disappears
On breathing 100% O_2 cyanosis disappears	Cyanosis persists

  – Cardiac vs. respiratory
    - Associated symptoms
    - During crying cyanosis will improve in respiratory causes and worsens in cardiac causes.

- If due to cardiac disease:
  Cyanotic or acyanotic
  ↓
  Cyanotic (Eisenmenger)

I. Cyanotic heart disease:

A. With increased pulmonary blood flow:
- Transposition of great arteries (TGA)
- Total anomalous pulmonary venous circulation (TAPVC)
- Truncus arteriosus
- Tricuspid atresia without pulmonary stenosis
- Double outlet right ventricle without pulmonary stenosis (PS).

5Ts of cyanotic heart disease
1. Truncus arteriosus
2. Two vessel parallel—TGA
3. Tricuspid atresia
4. Tetralogy of Fallot
5. TAPVC

Clinical Features: Mild cyanosis.
- Recurrent respiratory tract infection (RTI)
- CCF—develop early
- Do not survive long (80% die in 3 months due to CCF/pulmonary infection).

B. With decreased pulmonary blood flow:
- Tetralogy of Fallot (commonest cyanotic heart disease above 2 years)
- TGA with ventricular septal defect (VSD) and PS
- Corrected TGA, VSD and PS
- Double outlet right ventricle (RV) with PS.
- Tricuspid atresia with decreased pulmonary blood flow

Clinical Features: Fallot's physiology
- More cyanosis, cyanotic spells, squatting episode, less dyspnea
- CCF late
- Survive more
- *In decreased PBF*
  - Time of cyanosis:
  - At birth – severe tetralogy of Fallot (unlikely to survive without associated patent ductus arteriosus (PDA)
- Tricuspid atresia with decreased pulmonary blood flow (PBF)
  - 1 year—Double outlet right ventricle
  - Teenage—Ebstein's anomaly (Lithium cause it)

II. Acyanotic heart disease:

(ASD/VSD/PDA) Recurrent RTI, CCF
↓
Pulmonary hypertension
↓
Period of quiescence
↓
Cyanosis

- **Infective endocarditis (Not seen if <2 years)**
  - History of high-grade fever with chills
  - Petechial hemorrhage
  - Dental procedures/surgery.
- **History of complications:**
  - Fever, vomiting, seizure, focal neurological deficit (cerebral abscess in congenital cyanotic heart disease, thromboembolism)
  - Protein-energy malnutrition
  - Recurrent respiratory tract infections—>6/year.

Causes of Loss of Weight in CHD

- Increased respiratory rate
- Respiratory infection
- Increased metabolism

Normal feeding:
- Continue up to 15–20 min
- In first 5–7 min—90% feeding completed
- Rest—for satiety

Suck-rest-suck cycle—after 1–2 min → breathlessness → stop feeding

- Poor feeding
- Gastric congestion—poor absorption
- Tissue anoxia
- Brain (pituitary) blood flow decreases.

Past History

- History of lower respiratory tract infection (LRTI)
- Any treatment (Digoxin, Lasix)
- Prophylaxis (rheumatic fever)
- Cyanosis.

Antenatal History

- Intrauterine infection
  - Fever with rash
  - Rubella—PDA, PS
- Diabetes mellitus—asymmetrical septal hypertrophy, VSD, TGA, caudal regression syndrome
- Drug:
  - Phenytoin or valproate (septal defect) (Safe drug—phenobarbitone)
  - Lithium: Ebstein anomaly
  - Thalidomide: Phocomelia
  - Alcohol (Fetal alcoholic syndrome)

Natal history

Prematurity—PDA
(Delivery at high altitude—PDA, ASD)
Low birth weight (LBW)—TGA

Postnatal history

Cyanosis in newborn period
Birth asphyxia—PDA

Developmental History

- Gross motor delay: Congenital heart disease
- Global delay: In systemic anomalies

GENERAL EXAMINATION

- Pallor
- Cyanosis
- Clubbing
- Polycythemia

(Pallor, Cyanosis, Clubbing, Polycythemia — Congenital cyanotic heart disease)

Pedal edema, presacral edema

Infective endocarditis features like:

- Splinter hemorrhage, pallor, clubbing, splenomegaly
- Osler's nodes
- Janeway lesion
- Roth's spot

Down syndrome:

- Endocardial cushion defects
- Atrial septal defect (ASD), ventricular septal defect (VSD).

Turner syndrome:

- Bicuspid aortic valve, coarctation of aorta, aortic stenosis, pulmonary stenosis
- Syndactyly, polydactyly, VSD
- **Holt-Oram syndrome:** Familial atrial septal defect + Limb anomaly
- **Marfan syndrome**: Aortic regurgitation (AR), pulmonic regurgitation (PR), mean platelet volume (MVP).

Triad of infective endocarditis
- Splenomegaly
- Tender clubbing
- Pollar

Head to Foot

- Microcephaly, cataract—congenital rubella
- Signs of infective endocarditis
- Signs of vitamin deficiency

PEDIATRICS

Pulse

- PDA, AR: Water hammer pulse
- Pulsus bigeminus: Digitalis toxicity
- All peripheral pulses: To rule out emboli in infective endocarditis (IE)
- Left ventricular failure (LVF): Pulsus alternans.

Blood Pressure

Apex beat:

Outer most and lower most part of precordium (part of anterior chest wall overlying the heart) where definite cardiac impulse is felt.

Position of apex:

<4 years	4th intercostal space 1 cm lateral to midclavicular line (MCL)
4–6 years	5th intercostal space on MCL
>6 years	5th intercostal space 1 cm medial to MCL

Types:

- Tapping: MS
- Forceful: VSD, PDA, MR, AR
- Heaving: AS

Investigations:

- Complete blood count (CBC)
- Erythrocyte sedimentation rate (ESR)
- Chest X-ray
- ECG
- Echocardiogram

Gastrointestinal System

- Hepatomegaly: CCF
- Splenomegaly: IE

X-ray

- TGA: Egg on side appearance
- TOF: Boot shaped heart
- TAPVC: Figure of 8

Respiratory System

Features of infecton

Extracardiac anomalies	Likely congenital cardiac lesion
Down syndrome	ASD (endocardial cushion type), VSD
Turner syndrome	Coarctation of the aorta
Rubella syndrome	PDA, PS
Marfan's syndrome	Aortic or pulmonary artery dilatation
Holt-Oram syndrome	Familial ASD
Hurler syndrome	MR or AR

VENTRICULAR SEPTAL DEFECT

Differential Diagnosis of Pansystolic Murmur

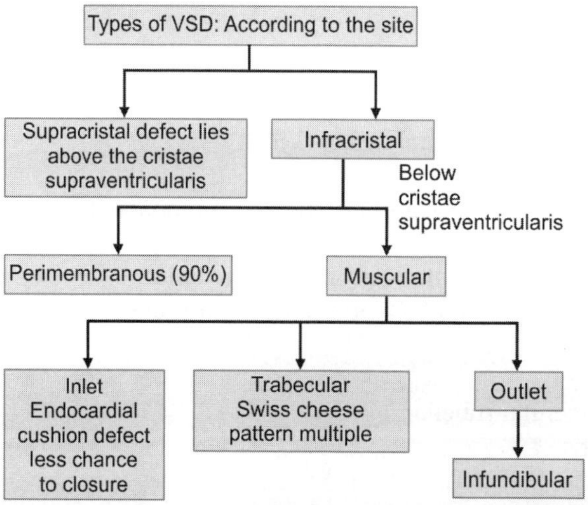

- According to size—small (<.5 cm^2/m^2 of body SA)
  - Moderate (0.5-1 cm^2/m^2 of body SA)
  - Large (>1 cm^2/m^2 of body SA)
- According to flow—restrictive VSD and nonrestrictive VSD
  - Spontaneous closure:
    - 80% chance in muscular VSD
    - 35% chance in perimembranous VSD
- Vast majority of defect that close do so below the age of 3 years.
  - Commonest cardiac lesion complicated by IE–VSD
  - **VSD reversal:** Eisenmenger complex
  - **Roger's VSD:** small VSD
  - **Gazul VSD:** Right ventricular infundibular hypertrophy leading to reversal.
  - **Benjamin VSD:** Right ventricular outflow obstruction = due to development of ventricular aneurysm.
  - **Gerbodes VSD:** Left ventricle to right atrial shunt.
  - Why L to R shunt manifest at 8 weeks?
    - Before birth pulmonary vasculature is closed. RV pressure > LV pressure.
    - After crying pulmonary vasculature opens and pulmonary vascular resistance decreases.

    Gradually RV pressure < LV pressure by 6 weeks.
    - Then L to R shunt become apparent.

    Gradually pulmonary blood flow increases → pulmonary vascular resistance → pulmonary HTN → right ventricular pressure increases → reversal of shunt → Eisenmenger.

Complications of VSD
- Pulmonary stenosis (PS)
- Pulmonary arterial hypertension (PAH)
- Aortic regurgitation (AR)
- Infective endocarditis (IE)

Indications of Surgery in VSD

- Congestive cardiac failure in infancy
- Left to right shunt is large
- Pulmonary stenosis, pulmonary arterial hypertension, aortic regurgitation.

PATENT DUCTUS ARTERIOSUS

Functional closure: Soon after birth

Anatomical closure: 3 weeks to 3 months.

Ductus arteriosus:
- In fetal life, most blood from right ventricle flows into descending aorta via ductus – as lungs are non-functioning (less blood flows to pulmonary circulation)
- At birth: After clamping cord there is sudden increase in the systemic vascular resistance due to the loss of low resistance placental circulation. When the baby breathes lung expand → pulmonary artery pressure decreases → flow reverse from aorta to pulmonary trunk.

Differential Diagnosis of Continuous Murmur

- Arteriovenous (AV) fistula—coronary, pulmonary, systemic
- Ruptured sinus of Valsalva (RSOV)
- Aorticopulmonary septal defect
- Venous hum (TAPVC)
- MR/TR + AR
- VSD + AR

Differential Cyanosis

Differential cyanosis – PDA reversal + coarctation of aorta.

TETRALOGY OF FALLOT

Components

- Valvular/infundibular pulmonary stenosis—most important
- Large VSD
- Overriding of aortic root over the ventricular septum
- Right ventricular hypertrophy—concentric

Cyanotic spells: During crying (in infundibular PS) there is muscle spasm leading to more right to left shunt usually seen from 2nd month to 2nd year. Uncommon after 2 years due to fibrosis of muscle undergoing spasm.

Why spells in early morning?

During sleep respiratory center is suppressed. After waking and crying the center becomes active, tissue hypoxia to brain so respiratory center becomes unstable leading to hyperventilation.

Squatting Episodes

During squatting:

- Femoral artery kinks – systemic pressure increases – pressure of LV increases LR shunt increases and pulmonary flow increases—cyanosis decreases.
- Decreased venous return of high unsaturated blood to right side of heart by trapping blood in lower extremities → decreased R to L shunt at ventricular level.
- Increased intrathoracic pressure, thereby helping in decreased venous return.

Why cyanosis around first year:

- Infundibular stenosis is progressive
- CCHD with decreased pulmonary blood flow ductus arteriosus close late.
- Amount of fetal Hb is more in early life. So more oxygen carrying capacity and cyanosis at later age (Pink Fallot)

Management of Cyanotic Spells (Tet Spells or Hypercyanotic Spells)

Immediate

- Check airway, O_2 by mask
- Knee chest position
- Sedate with morphine (0.2 mg/kg SC)
- Sodium bicarbonate if cyanosis persists
- Correct hypovolemia
- Keep child warm
- β blocker metoprolol (0.1 mg/kg IV slowly)
- Maintain saturation, BP, heart rate

Persistent/No significant improvement

- Vasopressor—methoxamine
- If spell persist—paralyze the patient – intubate – ventilate – plan for surgery
- Seizure are managed with diazepam

Following spell

- CNS examination, imaging
- Initiate therapy with β-blocker
- Palliative or corrective surgery

Prevention

Counsel parents to avoid precipitating factors like fever, dehydration.

Investigation:

- Hb—increased
- PCV—increased
- TC—decreased
- Platelet decreased
- CXR
- ECG
- Echo

- Fallot's monology—VSD
- Triology—single ventricle + PS
- Pentology—+ASD

PINK FALLOT

In TOF, if PS is less severe, it acts like VSD. So there is little cyanosis and hence name.

CONGESTIVE CARDIAC FAILURE

Inability of heart to maintain an output at rest or during stress, necessary for the metabolic needs of body (systolic failure) and inability to receive blood into ventricular cavities at low pressure during diastole (diastolic failure).

Cases of CCF

- **Infants**
  - CHD
  - Myocarditis
  - Anemia
  - Kawasaki
  - Arrhythmia
- **Children**
  - RF, RHD
  - CHD + anemia/injection/endocarditis
  - Systemic HTN
  - Myocarditis

(CCF: Congestive cardiac failure; CHD: Congestive heart disease; RHD: rheumatic heart disease; RF: rheumatic fever; HTN: hypertension)

Symptoms

- Poor weight gain
- Difficulty in feeding
- Baby is more comfortable on shoulder (orthopnea)

- Persistent cough
- Suck-rest-suck cycle
- Edema.

Signs of CCF

Right heart failure	*Left heart failure*	*Failure of either side*
Elevated JVP	Tachypnea	Cardiomegaly
Tender hepatomegaly	Tachycardia	S3
Edema	Basal crepts	Small pulse volume
		Gallop rhythm

Treatment

- Reduce cardiac work
- Augmenting myocardial contractility
- Improving cardiac performance
- Correcting underlying cause

7 Steps of Management of CCF

1. Frusemide + digoxin + ACE inhibitor.
2. Add isosorbide nitrate (if there is pulmonary congestion) or carvedilol (if HR is fast).
3. Involves addition of nitrate or carvedilol which not used in previous step.
4. Intermittent use of dobutamine or dopamine with dobutamine if BP is low.
5. Make sure that patient get all medications mentioned above.
   - If the patient is not adequately controlled either have medical/surgical correction of cause of CCF
   - If the patient is not controlled and do not have a correctable cause would be patient with myocarditis. For them,
6. Take myocardial biopsy and treat with corticosterol if there is myocarditis
   - In the absence active myocarditis therapy with β-blocker should be increased maximum.
7. Ventricular assist device or cardiac transplantation

Why wide fixed split in ASD?

- Since the right ventricle is fully loaded, further increase in right ventricular volume during aspiration cannot occur.
- Most common congenital cyanotic heart disease in newborn period is TGA.
- If one sibling affected or if 1 parent affected, then 2–6% chance of CHD. If 2 primary relative affected—20–30% chance.
- Hyperoxia test.

RHEUMATIC FEVER

- Immunologic disorder caused by group A beta-hemolytic streptococci
- Antibodies produced against streptococcal antigen cross react with connective tissue of body and heart
- Most common age group is 5–15 years
- Poor socioeconomic status is a predisposing factor.

Criteria to Diagnose RF

Duckett-Jones criteria.

Major criteria

- Carditis
- Arthritis—migratory fleeting polyarthritis
- Erythema marginatum—serpiginous form
- Subcutaneous nodule—on bony prominence
- Chorea

(Carditis, arthritis, erythema marginatum, subcutaneous nodule: Early)

Minor criteria

Clinical

- Fever
- Arthralgia

Laboratory

- Increased ESR
- CRP, leukocytosis
- Prolonged PR interval

Essential Criteria (Evidence of Recent Streptococcal Infection)

- Increased ASO titer
- +ve throat culture
- Recent scarlet fever
  [(2 major) or (1 major + 2 minor)] along with one essential criteria

Management

Symptomatic + Suppressive therapy.

Symptomatic

- Bed rest—for 2–3 weeks. Patient with carditis can be rested for 1–3 months
- Diet—if there is carditis then salt should be restricted, otherwise no need of salt restriction
- Penicillin—oral penicillin or single IM benzathine penicillin (12 lakh) or erythromycin 250 mg QID for 10 days.

Suppressive Therapy

- If the patient has carditis with CCF, corticosteroid is mandatory (prednisolone)
- Carditis without CCF, either steroid or aspirin is used. Steroids are preferred
- Without carditis, use aspirin (100 mg/kg/day in 4 divided doses for 10 weeks).

Prevention

- Primary prevention (antibiotic for sore throat)
- Secondary prevention
  Give benzathine pencillin 1.2 million units every 21 days or 0.6 million units every 15 days or daily oral penicillin
  - RF without carditis—5 years or until 18 years whichever is longer
  - RF with carditits without residual features—10 years or 25 years whichever is longer
  - RF with carditis with residual features—at least 10 years since last episode or at least 40 years, sometime life-long.

Management of chorea

- Phenobarbitone 30 mg thrice daily

Arthritis: Usually large joints (knee joint), lasts for 3–7 days and migratory. Younger the patient, lesser is arthritis.
Carditis: Commonest manifestation—50–60%, pancarditis
Pericarditis: Pericardial pain and rub
Myocarditis: Cardiomegally, soft S1, S3 gallop, Carry-Coomb's murmer, CCF
Endocarditis: Regurgitation murmers
Erythema marginatum: Rare in Indians, red rash with pale center (serpiginous outline)
Subcutaneous nodule: 6 weeks after the onset of acute renal failure, occupies bony prominences like elbow, shin, occiput. Almost always have carditis.
Chorea:

- Sydenham's chorea—late feature (3 months after onset of acute renal failure)
- Teacher scolds due to handwriting
- Mother scolds dropping object
- Grandmother scolds grimace

Why streptococcal skin infection do not produce RF?
More lipase content in skin.

Features	*VSD (30–35%)*	*PDA (6–8%)*	*TOF (5–7%)*	*Eisenmenger's syndrome*
GE and Pulse	Usually normal	High volume collapsing pulse	Cyanosis, clubbing, polycythemia	Cyanosis, clubbing, polycythemia
BP		Wide pulse pressure and features of high volume		
JVP			Large a wave	
Apex	LV apex, hyperkinetic (down and outward)	LV apex, hyperkinetic	RV apex (outward)	
LPH, palpable P2				Yes
S1	Loud (masked by murmur)	Loud	Normal	
S2	Wide variable split, loud P2	Single/paradoxical split, normal	Single S2 is only audible soft, delayed P2 inaudible	PDA: Normal (loud P2) VSD: Single
Other sound	S3 (with small shunt)	S3, ejection click in aortic area	Pulmonary ejection click (if associated valvular PS)	
Murmur flow shunt	Pulmonary: ESM Mitral: DDM Pansystolic murmur on left 3, 4, 5th intercostal space	Mitral: DDM Aortic: ESM Continuous machinery murmur	Pulmonary ESM	Intensity of murmer decrease ESM—pulmonary
ECG	LVH: Biventricular hypertrophy (later)	LVH	RVH	RVH, right axis deviation
X-ray	Pulmonary plethora: Left atrial enlargement (LA), LVH Cardiomegaly–LV type	LVH, prominent aortic knuckle, pulmonary plethora	Upturned apex (RVH) Boot-shaped heart (Coeur-en-sabot), absence of main pulmonary trunk, aortic arch enlargement, oligemic of lung field	Feature of pulmonary artery, HTN, oligemia of lung field
Severity	Early symptoms, marked symptoms, CCF, cardiomegaly, S3, DDM	Wide pulse pressure, cardiomegaly	Severe stenosis, more cyanosis, less murmur	
	Very small: ESM (functional) Small: PSM + normal S2 (no DDM)	S3 - moderate, DDM—S3 large		

Contd...

PEDIATRICS

Contd…

Features	***VSD (30–35%)***	***PDA (6–8%)***	***TOF (5–7%)***	***Eisenmenger's syndrome***
	Large: ESM loud P2, Pulmonary stenosis ESM + Soft P2			
Complications	Recurrent RTI, CCF Growth failure Pulmonary artery hypertension Infective endocarditis Aortic regurgitation Aneurysmal dilation of aorta	CCF, IE, pulmonary hypertension Diastolic component is lost	Anoxia, infarction hemiplegia Paradoxical embolism Infective endocarditis Brain abscess [Rasy CCF if associated with (AIIMS) anemia, IE, AR, myocarditis, systemic hypertension]	
Management	*Medical treatment:* CCF, IE, anemia, respiratory infection *Surgical treatment:* Patch closure (via RA/RV) Device closure *Indication for surgery:* CCF not responding to medical *Treatment:* If pulmonary blood flow twice that is systemic flow: Before, development of PA HTN Complications of surgery: RBBB, residual block	*In preterm:* Indomethacin 0.1 kg/kg/dose orally 12th hourly 3 doses *Indication for surgery:* Small infants with large duct—preterm infants Ducts which are larger than available device *Surgery:* Triple ligation Coil/umbrella closure under cardiac catheterization Ligation and division	*Management of anoxic spell:* • Knee chest position • Humified oxygen • Morphine 0.1 mg/kg SC • Propranolol 0.1 mg/kg IV methoxamine $NaHCO_3$ (If acidosis) correct anemia, surgery *Palliative surgery:* Blalock-Taussig shunt (BT shunt) (Subclavian—pulmonary) Pott's shunt: Descending aorta and right pulmonary artery Definitive surgery: *Indications:* • Severely symptomatic • Hypoxemia with PaO_2 <75% • Hypercyanotic spell	

NOTES

CHAPTER 13

Respiratory System

APPROACH TO A CASE OF RESPIRATORY SYSTEM (PNEUMONIA)

PRESENTING COMPLAINTS

- Fever
- Cough
- Breathlessness in the form of fast breathing
- Chest pain
- Feeding difficulty, fits, cyanosis, head nodding – features of severe pneumonia

HISTORY OF PRESENT ILLNESS

1. **Cough**
   - Productive/nonproductive
   - Color, amount, smell
   - Nature of cough (brassy, barking, etc.)
   - Diurnal variation, foreign body aspiration
   - Complications of cough
     a. Posttussive vomiting
     b. Affects feeding
     c. Disturbs sleep
     d. Whoop
     e. Complications – subconjunctival hemorrhage, ulceration of frenulum, appearance of umbilical/femoral hernia, cough syncope, rib fracture.

Nocturnal Cough
- Asthma
- Gastroesophageal reflux disease (GERD)
- Left ventricular failure (LVF)
- Post nasal drip

2. **Fever**
   - Onset—gradual/sudden
   - Type—continued/intermittent
   - Fever with rashes, arthritis
   - Relieved by medication
   - Diurnal variation
3. **Breathlessness**
   - "Mother noticed breathlessness in the form of fast breathing"
   - Severity—unable to speak
     - Words
     - Phrases
     - Sentences
   - Not able to drink
   - Not able to eat
4. **Chest pain**: Pleuritic
5. **Respiratory sound**
   - Rattling

- Grunt
- Wheeze
6. **Running nose, nasal obstruction**
7. **Poor feeding, fits, cyanosis, head nodding**—very severe pneumonia
8. **Predisposing factors**
   - Pyoderma—staphylococcal pneumonia
   - Rash—predisposing measles
9. **Conjunctivitis, arthralgia, myalgia**—viral pneumonia

PAST HISTORY

If recurrent respiratory tract infection
- Bronchial asthma—history of nebulization which relieved symptoms
- Cardiac symptom
- Foreign body aspiration
- GERD—symptom following food intake followed by vomiting
- History of seizure (aspiration)

Antenatal
Natal
Postnatal

DIETETIC HISTORY

GLV—vitamin A

IMMUNIZATION

- Bacillus Calmette Guerin (BCG)
- Diphtheria-tetanus-pertussis (DPT)
- Measles—giant cell pneumonitis
- *Haemophilus influenzae* type b (Hib)
- Pneumococcal.

FAMILY HISTORY

- History of bronchial asthma/TB
- Overcrowding
- Passive smoking

Predisposing conditions
- History of measles
- History of skin lesions
  - Chickenpox, abscess in axilla or anywhere in the body—staphylococcal pneumonia

Respiratory sounds
- Snoring—oropharyngeal obstruction
- Grunting—ejection of air through partially closed glottis
- Rattling—secretion in trachea/bronchi
- Stridor—obstruction of larynx/trachea
- Wheeze—lower airway obstruction (Inspiratory—ISSR)

SOCIOECONOMIC STATUS

- House nearby roads
- Pets in the house
- Sleeping on the floor
- Cooking with firewood
- Floor, wall
- Paddy field
- Factory
- Pest
- Perfume

O/E general assessment—tachypneic, position of comfort, conscious, alertness

In a case of bronchial asthma:
- Presenting complaint—cough, breathlessness—for which he was underwent nebulization from home/hospital – symptoms relieved
- In past history—first episode of symptom at the age of:
  - Number of episodes per month
  - Whether he was on inhaler
  - Family history of bronchial asthma, allergy, atopy
  - Socioeconomic status in detail

Recurrent Respiratory Tract Infection

- Lower respiratory tract infection ≥ 6 years

- Causes

Surgical
- CHD: L to R shunt
- Foreign body aspiration
- Cleft palate
- Tracheoesophageal fistula
- Congenital lobar emphysema
- Congenital cystic malformation

Medical
- Bronchial asthma
- Immunodeficiency – congenital/acquired
- Ciliary dysfunction (Kartagener syndrome) (cystic fibrosis)
- Aspiration–GERD, seizure disorder

DEFINITIONS

- Recurrent pneumonia — ≥ 2 episodes in 1 year or >3 episodes at any time with radiological clearance between 2 episodes
- Persistent pneumonia — persistence of symptoms and X-ray abnormalities >4 weeks.

BRONCHIOLITIS

First episode of expiratory wheeze of acute onset in a child less than 2 years of age which has signs of viral respiratory illness like coryza, otitis media or fever with or without indication of respiratory distresses, pneumonia or atopy. RSU is implicated in most cases.

Bronchial asthma	Bronchiolitis
– Unusual below 1 year	– Age greater than 6 months
– Recurrent episodes	– First episode
– Positive family history	– Negative
– Responds to bronchodilators	– No much response

MANAGEMENT OF BRONCHIOLITIS

- OP management
- Admit in ICU in case of danger signs
  - Humidified oxygen
  - Tepid sponging – using lukewarm water
  - IV fluid
- Then do investigation:
  - Hb
  - Tc, Dc
  - CXR – overinflation
  - Homogenous opacity
- If not improving, superadded infection – start antibiotic
  - Nebulization with racemic epinephrine or bronchodilator
  - Ribavirin—indication:
    - Impending respiratory failure
    - Congenital heart disease
    - Immunodeficiency

DD's of bronchiolitis
- Bronchial asthma
- Congestive heart failure (CCF)
- Foreign body
- Bacterial pneumonia

PNEUMONIA

Investigations

1. **X-ray**
   - Consolidation—opacity with air bronchogram
   - Bilateral patchy opacity—bronchopneumonia
   - Pneumatocele—*Staph. aureus, Klebsiella*
2. **Microbiological examination**
   - Sputum
     - Gram- and Ziehl-Neelsen staining
     - Culture and sensitivity

Types of pneumonia

Anatomical
- Lobar or lobular
- Bronchopneumonia
- Interstitial pneumonia
- Multilobar pneumonia

Duration
- Persistent
- Recurrent

PEDIATRICS

- Blood culture—positive in pneumococcal pneumonia
- Gastric aspirate
- Serology—*Mycoplasma, Chlamydia, Legionella* and viral infection
- Throat and nasopharyngeal swab—influenza

3. **Blood test**
   - Neutrophil leukocytosis—bacterial pneumonia
   - WBC count marginally raised—atypical pneumonia

Etiological
- Infective—bacterial, viral, atypical
- Noninfective—chemical

Source
- CAP
- HAP

Immunity
- Primary—high virulent organism in good immunity
- Secondary—low virulent organisms in immunodeficient

	Bacterial pneumonia vs	Viral pneumonia
Onset	Abrupt	Gradual
Epidemic	Not seen	Common
Associated conditions	Infection at other sites, septicemia	Associated with URI, coryza
Fever	High grade	May be present
Toxemia	Common	Absent
Respiratory distress	Common	Common in infants
Lung signs	Crackle	Wheeze
X-ray	Confluent infiltrate	Diffuse in peripheral areas
Prognosis	Complication—empyema, pneumatocele	Self-limiting

	Typical vs	Atypical (walking pneumonia)
Causative organisms	*S. pneumoniae* *H. influenzae* *Staph. aureus*	*M. pneumoniae* *Chlamydia* *Legionella*
Onset	Sudden	Gradual
Age	Any age	>4 years
Fever	Common	May be present
Cough	Productive	Dry
X-ray	Localized	Diffuse

DEFINE ACUTE RESPIRATORY INFECTION

- Acute infection of respiratory tract including ear, nose, throat, paranasal sinus, and pleura of less than 30 days and in case of ear infection, less than 14 days.
- Acute URI—common cold, otitis media, pharyngitis
- Acute LRI—croup (epiglottitis, laryngitis, laryngotracheitis), bronchitis, bronchiolitis, pneumonia.

ACUTE RESPIRATORY INFECTION CONTROL PROGRAM (2 MONTHS – 5 YEARS)

Clinical category	*Essential features*
Very severe pneumonia	• Central cyanosis or feeding difficulty or convulsion or lethargy or unconsciousness or severe respiratory distress (e.g. head nodding)
Severe pneumonia	• Lower chest indrawing or nasal flaring and no signs of very severe pneumonia
Pneumonia	• Fast breathing – age—newborn >60/min 2–12 months—> 50/min, 12 months to 5 years >40/min • No signs of severe or very severe pneumonia
No pneumonia	• Cough or cold • No fast breathing, chest indrawing or indicators of severe illness

PEDIATRICS

Infants less than 2 months

I. Very severe pneumonia
II. Severe pneumonia
III. No pneumonia

Treatment According to ARI Control Program

No Pneumonia

- Paracetamol for fever 15 mg/kg
- Saline nasal drops
- Lemon + honey

Pneumonia

- Oral cotrimoxazole for 5 days is recommended
- Now using amoxicillin 15 mg/kg/dose 8th hourly – 5 days
- Review after 2 days.
- If improved – continue for 5 days
- If not improved – treat as severe pneumonia.

Severe Pneumonia

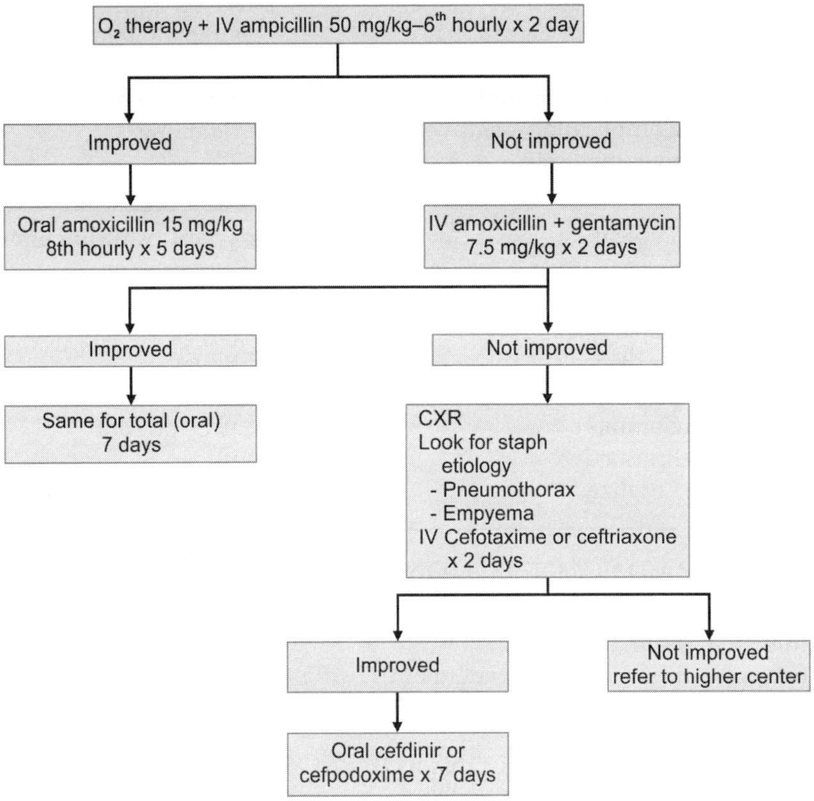

Signs indicating admission in hospital (Danger signs)
- Central cyanosis
- Inability to drink or take food
- Convulsions
- Lethargy or unconsciousness
- Severe respiratory distress (head nodding) or grunting
- *Lower chest indrawing
- Nasal flaring
- Stridor in a calm child
- Severe dehydration or shock
- Severe malnutrition or severe anemia

*Lower chest indrawing means definite inward movement of lower chest wall.

Very severe pneumonia

- Hospitalization, O_2 therapy, X-ray
- IV fluids
- IV ampicillin + Gentamicin × 2 days

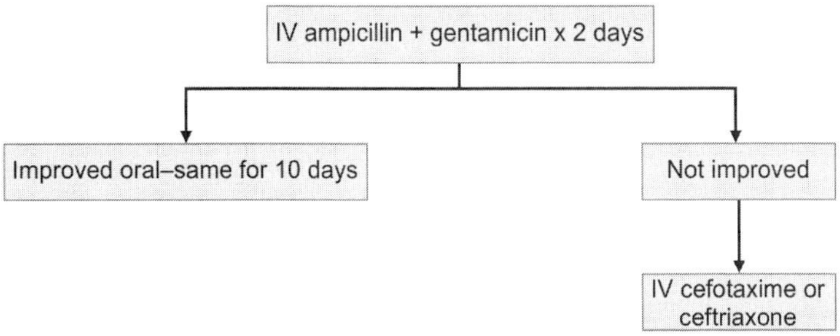

Infants less than 2 months

- Admit the child
- Ampicillin + Gentamicin + supportive care
- Add ceftriaxone if meningitis present.

Causes of recurrent pneumonia

Same lobe	*Different lobe*
• Congenital anomaly	• Aspiration
• Tumor	• Asthma
• Foriegn body	• Immune deficiency
• Tuberculosis (TB)	• Cystic fibrosis
	• LR shunt

❖ **Indicators of good response to antibiotics in severe and very severe pneumonia**
  - Subsiding fever if initially present
  - Less severe chest indrawing, it should disappear by 48 hours
  - Decreasing respiratory rate
  - Child begins to drink and eat better.

❖ **Discharge from the hospital**
  - The clinical condition has improved markedly
    - No lower chest indrawing or fast breathing
    - Afebrile
    - Alert
    - Eating and sleeping normally
  - Oral antibiotic treatment has been started
  - In case the patient is a malnourished infant or child or is a nonbreastfed infant weight gain on 2 consecutive days has been observed.

❖ **Causes for delayed resolution**
  - Underlying immunosuppression
  - Resistance to antibiotics
  - Inadequate dose and duration of treatment
  - Noncorrected predisposing LR shunt
  - Underlying TB
  - Underlying congenital anomalies, TOF
  - Underlying osteomyelitis of rib

Prevention of ARI

- Proper antenatal care, exclusive breastfeeding
- Nutrition and proper hygiene

- Vaccination
  - Measles
  - < 3 years – *H. influenzae* vaccine
  - 3 – 5 years – Pneumococcal vaccine.

Additional Discussion

- Lobar pneumonia
- Bronchopneumonia
- Intestinal pneumonia

Pneumonia – Etiology

- <2 months → gram –ve—Klebsiella, *E. coli*
  - *Staph. aureus,* pneumococci
- 3 months – 3 years
  - *H. influenzae,* pneumococci
  - *Staph. aureus*
- >3 years
  - Pneumococci
  - *Staph. aureus*

❖ Gram –ve organism cause pneumonia in early infancy, severe malnutrition and immunocompromised children.

1. **Pneumococcal pneumonia**
   - Associated herpes labialis
   - Can diagnose by blood culture
   - Treatment – IV or IM penicillin G
   - Most common
   - Rusty sputum
2. *Staph. pneumoniae*
   - Rapidly progressive
   - Associated pyoderma
   - Pneumatocele – on X-ray
   - Blood culture may be positive.

   Treatment
   - Penicillin G, cloxacillin, vancomycin, ticoplanin, cephalosporin
   - Usually longer duration (6 weeks) of therapy, bacteria persist in the necrotic area.

   Specific treatment
   - Intercostals drainage – empyema
   - Intercostals decompression – for large pneumatocele causing respiratory distress.

Complications of *Staph. pneumoniae*
- Empyema
- Pericarditis
- Arthritis
- Osteomyelitis
- Mastoiditis

3. *H. influenzae* **pneumonia**
   - Treatment – Ampicillin + Chloramphenicol

     Or
   - Cefotaxime/Ceftriaxone
4. **Streptococcal pneumonia**
   - Interstitial pneumonia, may be hemorrhagic
   - Secondary to measles, chickenpox, influenza or whooping cough
5. **Primary atypical pneumonia**
   - Mycoplasma
   - Constitutional symptoms—fever, sore throat, myalgia, cough

     O/E
   - X-ray poorly defined hazy or fluffy exudates which radiate from the hilar region.

   Rx—macrolides - azithromycin, erythromycin
6. **Viral pneumonia**
   - Constitutional symptoms—fever, myalgia, arthralgia, conjunctivitis, rash
   - Always B/L
   - Signs minimal, symptoms more, no features of consolidation
   - Complication is less

- *Precipitating factors*: Otitis media, pyoderma
- Leukopenia
- *X-ray*: Interstitial pneumonia

❖ *Pseudomonas* may colonize airways of patients with cystic fibrosis and cause recurrent pulmonary exacerbation

❖ **Pneumatocele**

1. Staphylococcal pneumonia
2. *Klebsiella*

*Why ampicillin is preferred over CP in smaller children? Ans: *H. influenzae* coverage is for ampicillin
*When can child expectorate sputum? Ans: 4 years
*Most common congenital anomaly of lung—congenital lobar emphysema
*Normal amount fluid in pleural cavity – <1 mL
*Most common cause of community acquired pneumonia – pneumococci
*Why asthma is common in children?
*MOA of co-trimoxazole?

BRONCHIAL ASTHMA

Bronchial asthma is characterized by an increased responsiveness of the airway to various stimuli; it manifests by widespread narrowing of the airways causing paroxysmal dyspnea, wheezing or cough (mucosal hypertrophy, edema, secretions, bronchospasm).

Pathophysiology

- Early reaction
- Late reaction

5 P's in Asthma

- Pest
- Pets
- Pollen
- Perfumes
- Passive smoking

Trigger of an attack of asthma

a. Allergens in the environment
b. Viral infections
c. Exercise
d. Weather change
e. Emotional factor
f. Food
g. Endocrine factor

In case of bronchial asthma your diagnosis will be, e.g. acute exacerbation of mild persistent asthma.

Classification	*Day symptoms*	*Night symptoms*	*PEFR*
Severe persistent	Continuous, limited physical activity	Frequent	< 60% predicated variability > 30%
Moderate persistent	Daily, affect activity	> 1 times a week	> 60% – < 80% predicated; variability > 30%
Mild persistent	> 1/week, but < 1 time/day	> 2 times a month	< 80% predicated; variability > 20–30%
Intermittent	< 1/week	< 2 times a month	< 80% predicated; variability > 20%

*Classification of asthma severity (Nelson)

Stepwise treatment of asthma

Step 1: Intermittent — Inhaled β_2 agonist (short acting)
If needed more than 3 times per week move to step II

Step II: Mild persistent — Inhaled short acting β_2 agonist + inhaled corticosteroid (100 – 200 mg/day)
Or
Cromolyn sodium
Or
Leukotriene modifiers
Or
Theophylline [sustained release]

Step III: Moderate persistent — Inhaled short acting β2 agonist
\+
Inhaled corticosteroid [200 – 400 mg/day]

PEDIATRICS

	If needed, add Long acting β_2 agonist and/or sustained release theophylline
Step IV: Severe persistent	Inhaled short acting β_2-agonist + Inhaled corticosteroid [400 – 800 mg/day] + Long acting β2-agonist and/or Sustained release theophylline + Oral low dose prednisolone

What is Life-threatening Asthma?

Presence of any of the following indicates a life-threatening asthma:

- Cyanosis
- Silent chest
- Poor respiratory effort
- Exhaustion
- Fatigue
- Altered sensorium
- PEFR < 30% of predicted
- Oxygen saturation of <90%.

Treatment of Mild Acute Asthma

Beta-2 agonist nebulizer (0.5 mL salbutamol respiratory solution in 3 mL saline water)

- MDI + spacer + or – Mask (every minute – 1 puff for 10 puff)
- Then discharge
- Repeat MDI or oral β_2 agonist every 8 hours
- Follow-up after 2 weeks.

Moderate and Severe Asthma

O_2 inhalation (full O_2 saturation >95%)
+
Inhalation of β_2 agonist (repeat every 20 minutes – for 1 hour)
+
Oral prednisolone (1–2 mg/kg – 7 days)

a. *If improvement after 1 hour*
Repeat inhalation of β_2 agonist every 30 minutes then every 4–8 hours
Patient discharged when,
- Patient need for bronchodilator is every 4–6 hourly
- Able to speak well and feed
- Maintains O_2 saturation of >95% in room air

Discharged patients are educated about the disease, need of regular follow-up, avoidance of triggers

b. *If no improvement after 1 hour*
Inhalation of beta 2-agonist is continued and ipratropium 250 µg is also added every 20 minutes
+
Injection hydrocortisone 10 mg/kg
If no response
Injection theophylline
+
Inj $MgSO_4$ (50 mg/kg in dextrose over 30 min)

PEDIATRICS

Treatment of Life-threatening Asthma

O_2 inhalation
+
Inhalation of salbutamol + ipratropium bromide
+
Subcutaneous injection of adrenaline/terbutaline
+
Hydrocortisone 5 mg/kg
(Shift to ICU with accompanying physician)

If improved
Repeat inhaled salbutamol + ipratropium every 30 minutes
Injection hydrocortisone 5 mg/kg every 8 hours, till patient can take orally

If no improvement
Loading dose of theophylline
OR
Injection $MgSO_4$ – 50 mg/kg over 30 minutes

If there is no improvement with this management, patient is prepared for mechanical ventilation

In case of poor response, suspect:
- Acidosis
- Pneumothorax
- Electrolyte imbalance
- Infection

Effective Long-term Management of Asthma

- Identification and elimination of exacerbating factors
- Pharmacological therapy
- Education of patient and parents about the nature of disease and the steps required to avoid acute exacerbation

Pharmacotherapy

- Bronchodilators
- Corticosteroid
- Mast cell stabilizers
  - Cromolyn sodium
  - Nedocromil
  - Ketotifen
- Leukotriene modifiers
  - Zileuton – decreasing synthesis of leukotriene
  - Montelukast and Zafirlukast – antagonizing receptors
- Theophylline
- Immunotherapy

This consists of giving gradually increasing quantities of air allergen extract to a clinically sensitive subject so as to ameliorate the symptoms associated with subsequent exposure to causative allergen.
- Pharmacological Mx
- Assessment of sensitivity
- Stepwise treatment of asthma

Goals of therapy
- Maintain (near) normal pulmonary function
- Minimal use of short-acting inhaled β2-agonist
- Minimal or no adverse effects from medications
- Prevention of exacerbations

Monitoring and Modification of Treatment

(Step up, Step down)
After starting appropriate treatment patient should be seen every 4–12 weeks
On each visit detailed history is taken regarding

Selection of appropriate initiation device
- MDI—>12 years
- MDI + spacer—4–12 years
- MDI + spacer + Mask—< 4 years
- Dry powder inhaler – Rotahaler, diskhaler, spinhaler, turbohaler, accuhaler
- Nebulizers

(How to use these..? study in detail from OP Ghai)

PEDIATRICS

- Frequency of symptoms
- Sleep disturbance
- Physical activity
- School absenteeism
- Visit to a doctor
- Need for bronchodilator

If a child examine, look for:

- Adverse effect of drugs
- Records height, weight, PEFR
- Assessment of control of asthma?
- Step up and step down of treatment? refer OP Ghai

Four components of optimal asthma management

1. *Regular assessment and monitoring*
   - Asthma checkups
   - Lung function monitoring
2. *Control of factors contributing to asthma*
   - Eliminate or reduce problematic environmental exposures
   - Treat comorbid conditions: rhinitis, sinusitis, gastroesophageal reflux
3. *Asthma pharmacotherapy*
   - Long-term control vs quick-relief medications
   - Step-up, step-down approach
4. *Patient education*

CHAPTER 14

Gastrointestinal System

Practical Approach to a Child with Jaundice

Jaundice

Definition (refer Medicine)

- Is it true jaundice?
- If jaundiced, is it conjugated/unconjugated jaundice?
- Assess severity of functional state
- Identify complication
- Establish etiology

1. **Is it true jaundice?**
   - To rule out pseudo-jaundice—drugs, carotenemia
   - Ask history of ingestion of drugs antitubercular drugs (ATT), nonsteroidal anti-inflammatory drugs (NSAIDs)
   - Sclera would not be discolored in carotenemia
2. **Conjugated**—staining of clothes **Unconjugated**—clear urine

   If unconjugated—bilirubin more, enzymes absent
   - Bilirubin normal enzymes normal
   - Increased bilirubin—hemolytic anemia—**hemolytic facies, pallor, splenomegaly**
   - If no splenomegaly
     a. Sickle cell anemia—autosplenectomy
     b. Postsplenectomy—look for scar
   - If no pallor—compensated synthesis
   - Enzyme problem
     - Gilbert syndrome
     - Crigler-Najjar syndrome
   - **In a case of conjugated hyperbilirubinemia**
     - Sructural problem—like a block
     - Bilirubin transport from cell to canaliculi affected—Dubin-Johnson syndrome.
   - In a structural problem; clinical features due to:
     a. Accumulation of bile—itching, xanthelasma
     b. Deficiency of nutrients carried via bile are:
        - Vitamin A, D, E, K deficiency, steatorrhea,
        - Rickets, bleeding—take longer time to appear
   - In **Dubin-Johnson syndrome**—only bilirubin transport from cell to canaliculi affected, no other deficiency manifestations
3. **Assess severity of functional stale**
4. **Complications**
5. **Any signs of liver failure**
   - Edema (abdominal, pedal, facial puffiness)—chronic liver failure
   - Bleeding manifestations—acute liver failure
   - Altered sensorium, sleep rhythm—fulminant hepatic failure.

JAUNDICE—CASE TAKING

Presenting Complaints

- Yellowish discoloration of urine
- Yellowish discoloration of eye
- Itching
- Pale stools.

History of Present Illness

- Jaundice—onset, progress, duration, waxing and waning
- Color of stool
- Color of urine
- Itching
- In hemolytic jaundice—urine and stool—normal
- In hepatocellular jaundice—high colored urine and normal stools
- In obstructive jaundice—high colored urine and pale stools.

If hemolytic jaundice (acholuric jaundice)
- History of exertional dyspnea, fatigue, palpitation, pallor—anemia
- History of blood transfusion—transfusion dependant anemia
- Abdominal distension, abdominal pain—splenomegaly
- Antimalarial drug intake—G6PD deficiency
- Foot ulcer, chest, bone pain—sickle cell anemia
- Oliguria, hematuria, diarrhea, dysentery—HUS

In hepatocellular jaundice
- Infection
- Drugs
- Malignancy
- Collagen vascular diseases
- Metabolic disease—Wilson's disease, galactosemia

Infection

Viral
- Hepatitis A—prodromal symptoms—anorexia, fatigue
  - Fever → subsides → jaundice
  - History of contact, clustering of cases
- Hepatitis B, C—history of blood transfusion
- Others—cytomegalovirus (CMV), infection mononucleosis, mumps, measles, rubella, human immunodeficiency virus (HIV), herpes simplex virus (HSV).

Bacterial
- Leptospirosis—high-grade fever, rigor
  - Conjunctival injection, myalgia
  - Bleeding tendencies
- Enteric fever—mild icterus
  - 1st week—constipatioin
  - 2nd week—diarrhea
  - 3rd/4th week—complication
- Disseminated TB—history of contact
- Malaria

Malignancy
- Loss of appetite
- Weight loss

PEDIATRICS

- Hematological
  - Leukemia—bleeding manifestation
  - Lymphoma
    - Joint pain
    - Petechial rash
    - Progressive pallor
- Other malignancies
  - Hepatoblastoma
  - Neuroblastoma
  - Wilms tumor.

Collagen vascular disease [polyarteritis nodosa (PAN), Kawasaki disease]
- Rash
- Arthralgia.

Drugs
- Paracetamol
- Anti-TB drugs
- Sodium valproate

If we suspect obstructive jaundice
- Fever with rigor, colicky pain—cholangitis
- Itching.

HEPATIC FAILURE

- Edema (abdominal, pedal, facial puffiness) – chronic liver failure
- Bleeding manifestations—acute liver failure
- Altered sensorium, sleep rhythm—fulminant hepatic failure.

History of Past Illness

- History of similar complaint (Hepatitis B)
- History of transfusion
- Drugs
- Travel to endemic area—malaria
- History of treatment for TB—history of contact with open case of TB.

Antenatal History

- Fever with rashes—toxoplasmosis, CMV
- Natal low birth weight (LBW) in intrauterine infection (IU). In biliary atresia weight is normal
- Postnatal.

Developmental History of Delaying in Intrauterine Infection

Dietetic History

Immunization history
- Hep A
- Hep B
- BCG scar

Family History

- History of similar illness
- Metabolic diseases—Wilson disease

Alpha-1 antitrypsin deficiency
- Abdominal surgeries in the family (gallstones).

GENERAL EXAMINATION

- Irritable, less active — hepatic encephalopathy
- Sick child — malignancy
- Pallor — hemolytic jaundice
- Jaundice
- Significant/generalized lymphadenopathy—tuberculosis (TB), malignancy
- Pedal edema — Chronic liver failure
- Socioeconomic status (SES) — income, boiled water usage, sanitations, etc.

Head to Foot Examination

- Hemolytic facies (Chipmunk facies)
- Head
  - Microcephaly—intrauterine infection
  - Open A-F—hypothyroidism
- Eyes
  - Cataract—galactosemia
  - Kayser-Fleischer (KF) ring—Wilson disease
- Features of hepatic failure
  - Bleeding manifestation
  - Spider naevi
  - Palmar erythema, flapping tremor
  - Abdomen—ascites, dilated veins.

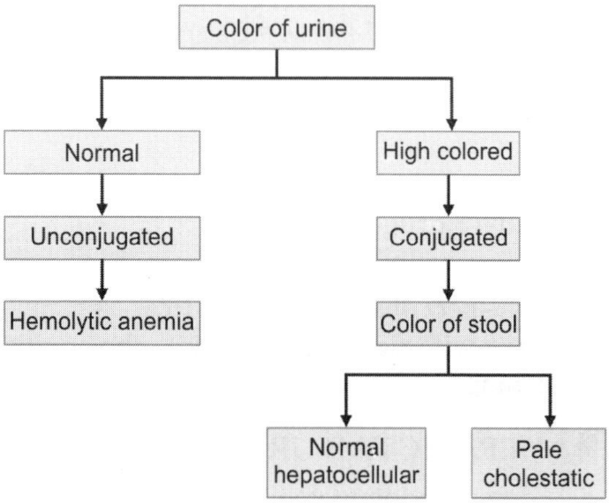

Investigations

- Hemoglobin (HB)—anemia
- Total count (TC)—increased (leukemia)
- Differential count (DC)—lymphocytosis—TB
- Blood indices
- Red cell distribution width (RDW)
- Peripheral smear
  - Type of anemia, hemolysis
  - Malaria
  - Malignancy—lymphoblast/myloblast
- **Liver function test (LFT)**
  - Conjugated bilirubin
  - Unconjugated bilirubin
  - Serum glutamic-pyruvic transaminase (SGPT), Serum glutamic oxaloacetic transaminase (SGOT)
  - Alkaline phosphate (ALP)
  - Total protein/albumin
  - Prothrombin time and international normalized ratio (PT/INR)
- **Urine**
  - Bilirubin
  - Urobilinogen
- **USG abdomen**
  - Hepatomegaly
  - Focal mass
  - Lymph node
  - Other organomegaly
  - Ascites
- Lymph node biopsy
- Bone marrow aspiration
- Gastric aspirate for acid-fast bacilli (AFB).

> SGPT = ALT
> SGOT = AST

> - Modified Fouchet's test—bile pigment
> - Ehrlich's test—urobilinogen
> - Conjugated hyperbilirubinemia—if conjugated bilirubin >15–20% of total
> - Hay's test—bile salt

PEDIATRICS

Bilirubin Metabolism

Reticuloendothelial system
↓
Hemoglobin
↓
Globin
↓
Heme
↓ Heme oxygenase
Biliverdin
↓ Biliverdin reductase
Bilirubin
↓ UDP-glucuronosyl transferase
Bilirubin diglucuronide
↓ Reaches gut
Deconjugation by gut bacteria
Bilirubin
↓
Urobilinogen → urobilin → urine
↓
Stercobilinogen
↓
Stercobilin → feces

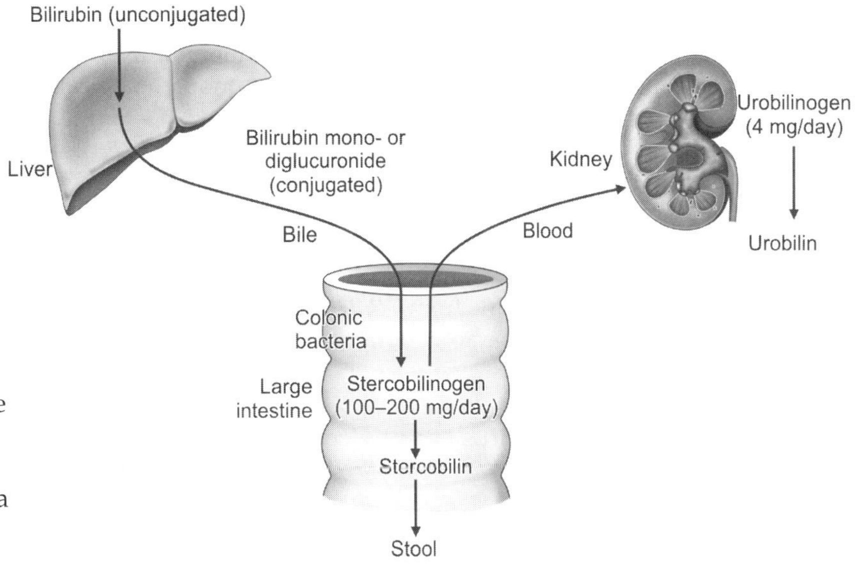

Urine

Hemolytic	**Hepatocellular**	**Obstructive**
Urobilinogen – 3+	Urobilinogen – 2+	Urobilinogen – 0
Bilirubin – 0	Bilirubin – 2+	Bilirubin – 3+

*__Pale stools__—due to absence of stercobilin

Hepatitis A

- Hepatitis A in water is sterilized by:
  - Boiling <5 min
  - Autoclaving
  - Chlorination (1.5–2.5 mg/L for 15 min)
  - Formaldehyde
- Feces are infective in 2 weeks before and 1 week after onset of jaundice.

Differential diagnosis of viral hepatitits
- Entenic fever
- Falciparum malaria
- Leptospirosis
- Viral hemorrhagic fever

Clinical Features

Four phases

1. Incubation or preclinical period
   - 30 days
   - Asymptomatic in spite of active multiplication of virus
2. Prodromal or preicteric period
   - Loss of appetite, fatigue, abdominal pain nausea and vomiting
   - Fever, diarrhea, dark urine and pale stools
3. Icteric period
   - Fever subsides and jaundice develops
4. Convalescent period.

Laboratory Investigation

- Alanine aminotransferase (ALT), aspartate aminotransferase (AST), alkaline phosphatase (ALP), Gamma-glutamyl transferase (GGT)
- Immunoglobulin M (IgM), anti-hepatitis A virus (anti-HAV)
- Polymerase chain reaction (PCR)—HAV, ribonucleic acid (RNA)

Treatment

Supportive treatment—maintain adequate nutrition (monitor liver span, signs of liver failure)
(Antivirals have no role because hepatic injury is immunopathologically mediated)

- Prevention
  - Passive immunization—pooled immunoglobulin 16%–0.02 mL/kg given within 2 weeks of contact (efficacy —6 months)
  - Active immunization:
    - Killed formalin inactivated vaccine from 9 R 326, HM 175 (efficacy – 10 years)
    - Live attenuated vaccine from CR 326
- Avoid hepatotoxic drugs (paracetamol).

Hepatitis B

- DNA virus (all hepatitis virus except Hep B virus are RNA viruses)
- Spread through serum, saliva, semen
- In case of HbsAg +ve mother only 5–10% is infected in utero and the rest is infected at the time of delivery

Extrahepatic manifestation of hepatitis B

- Serum sickness like syndrome
- Essential mixed

Cryoglobulinemia

- Polyarteritis nodosa
- Aplastic anemia
- Pleural effusion, myocarditis, pericarditis

Clinical Features

- Acute hepatitis
- Chronic active hepatitis
- Chronic persistent hepatitis
- Fulminant hepatitis

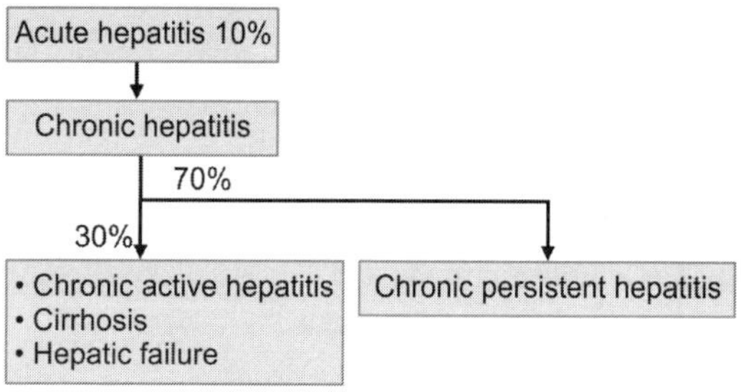

Laboratory Investigation

- HbsAg
- Anti-Hbs
- Anti-Hbc
- HbeAg
- Anti-Hbe
- Anti-Hbs—after immunization, previous infection
- Anti-Hbs + anti-Hbc—previous infection.

Treatment

- **Acute hepatitis**—bed rest
  (prolonged bed rest should be avoided and early ambulation is preferred)
- **Chronic active hepatitis**
  a. IFN-alpha—5–10 million/m^2; 3 times a week for 4–6 months
  b. Lamivudine—3 mg/kg/day for 1 year
- **Fulminant hepatitis**
  - Antibiotic—neomycin, ampicillin
  - Carbohydrate rich diet/protein elimination
  - Lactulose—10–15 mL/day × 3 doses
  - Exchange transfusion/plasmapheresis

ACUTE DIARRHEAL DISEASE

Name: Age: Sex: Address: Information:

Presenting Complaints

Loose watery stool (duration)

History of Present Illness

Loose stools:
- Onset
- Duration
- Number of episodes
- Whether blood stained/not
- Consistency—watery/solid
- Whether frothy/not, smell.

Associated symptoms
- Abdominal pain, tenesmus
- Vomiting
- Fever (in parenteral diarrhea), seizures or other foci of infection
- Abdominal distension.

Signs of Severe Dehydration

- Thirst
- Urine output
- Seizures
- Tears, appearance of eye (sunken)
- Altered sensorium
- Malnourishment (↓ weight).

Also ask about (to know the cause)
- History of weaning, artificial feeding
- History of similar illness in family
- Any travel to outside/food from outside
- Any history of previous infections like UTI, pneumonia, otitis externa (parenteral diarrhea)
- Any drug intake (antibiotics—cause loss of normal intestinal flora and cause diarrhea).

From the history we should get answers for 4 questions:
1. Is the child dehydrated ?
2. Is the child malnourished?
3. Is the child have other disease than loose motion?
4. Dysentery or not?

Past History

- Similar illness in the past (if present child is malnourished)
- Ask about food from outside
  - Travel outside
  - Any history of infection

  } We are already asked in presenting complaint
- History of measles and TB

Antenatal

Natal

Postnatal

Developmental history

Dietetic history
- Any history of prelacteal food, breastfeeding adequate or not
- Any history of bottle feeding, cow's milk
- Any weaning problems.

Immunization

Any special vaccine taken like typhoid vaccine, rotavirus vaccine.

Family History

Similar illness in the family or neighborhood.

Socioeconomic Status (SES)

Hygiene of food, water should be asked like source of water, whether boiled/cooled water, latrines, whether food material washed before cooking (clean hand, clean container, clean environment).

GENERAL EXAMINATION

Playful/alert/lethargic/unconscious (to know severity of dehydration).

Vitals

Head to Foot Examination

Look for sign of nutritional deficiency and sign of dehydration, also about perianal excoriation if any comment on anterior fontanelle in infants.

Anthropometry

If the child has recurrent illness, then there is malnourishment, so anthropometry is important.

Systemic Examination

- Gastrointestinal tract (GIT)
- Respiratory—to rule out any infection (pneumonia)
- Cardiovascular system (CVS)
- Central nervous system (CNS)—to rule out meningitis.

DISCUSSIONS

Diarrhea: It is the passage of watery stools at least three times a day with recent change in consistency (recent change in consistency is more important).
- Acute diarrhea—<2 weeks
- Persistent diarrhea—acute onset and last for >2 weeks
- Chronic diarrhea—incidocious onset and last for >2 weeks

Dysentery: Presence of gross blood and mucous in stool usually associated with tenesmus.

Etiology

Bacterial infections
- *Salmonella*
- *Shigella*
- *E. coli*
- *Vibrio cholerae.*

Viral
- Rotavirus
- Corona virus
- Norwalk virus
- Astrovirus, adenovirus.

Protozoa
- Cryptosporidium
- Amoebiasis
- *Giardia, Isospora belli*

Organism causing dysentery: Enterohemorrhagic *E. coli* (EHEC), *Shigella*, *Campylobacter*, amoeba.

Danger Signs

- Drowsiness
- Not able to drink

PEDIATRICS

- Not able to feed
- Urine output nil for last 6 hours
- Blood in stools
- Fever
- >3 episodes of/hours of stools.

Assessment of Dehydration Status

Clinical signs (key signs)

General conditions	Well alert	Restless, irritable	Lethargic or unconscious
Eyes	Normal	Sunken	Sunken
Thirst	Drinks normally not thirsty	Drinks eagerly thirsty	Drinks poorly or not able to drink
Skin pinch	Goes back quickly	Goes back slowly	Goes back 'very slowly'
Mouth and tongue	Moist	Dry	Very dry
Tears	Present	Absent	Absent
Decide	No signs of dehydration	Some dehydration*	Severe dehydration*
Treatment plan	Plan-A	Plan-B	Plan-C

*If child has 2 or more signs.

Star Signs in Acute Diarrheal Disease (ADD)

- General condition
- Skin pinch—not reliable in child with malnutrition and obese children.

Causes of convulsions in ADD
- Hypo- and hypernatremia
- Febrile seizures
- Hypoglycemia
- Vertebral venous/sagittal sinus thrombus
- *Shigella* encephalopathy
- Meningitis
- Reye's syndrome

- Vomiting in ADD
- Gastritis/gastroenteritis
- Oral rehydration salt (ORS)
- Drug induced

Abdominal Distension in ADD

- Hypokalemia
- Necrotizing enterocolitis
- Septicemia.

Content	Low-osmolarity ORS (new)
Na	75
K	20
Cl	65
Citrate	10
Glucose	75
Total	**245**

MANAGEMENT

Principles

- Rehydration and maintaining hydration
- Ensuring adequate feeding
- Oral supplementation of zinc
- Early recognition of danger signs and complications.

Plan A

Give Oral Rehydration Therapy (ORT)

a. ORS solution
b. Solution made from sugar (40 g) + salt (4 g)
c. Food-based solution—rice water + salt
d. In the presence of continued feeding, a variety of commonly available, structurally fluid irrespective of presence of sugar and salt (Coconut water, rice kanji).

NaCl	—	2.6 g
KCl	—	1.5 g
Glucose	—	13.5 g
Sod.citrate	—	.9 g

- It is given in sips (10 mL/kg)
- If large gulps given, it stimulates gastric colic reflex and results in quick passage of stools
- In addition to this, continue breastfeeding

- Give 1 teaspoon of ORS every 1–2 minute (<2 years)
- Give frequent sips (older child)
- If the child vomits, then stop for 10 minutes and continue feeding
- ORS solution is prepared by taking boiled, cooled water (1 L or 5 cup) then add one packet ORS into it and use within one day
- If the child is not better in 3 days or develops danger sign then take to hospital.

Plan B

Rehydration Therapy

- 75 mL/kg ORS given within 4 hours.
- If signs of dehydration presist after 4 years—repeat one more course.

Maintenance Therapy

- ORS should be given in volume equal to diarrhea (10–20 mL/kg) for each stool
- Breastfeeding continue
- Semisolid food.

ORS will be ineffective if:

- High stool purge rate >5 mL/kg/hr
- Persistent vomiting >3/hr
- Paralytic ileus
- Incorrect preparations of ORS.

Plan C

Start IV fluid (RL + 5% dextrose) 100 mL/kg

Age	Initially give	Then give
<1 year	30 mL/kg in 1 hour	70 mL/kg in 5 hours
1–5 years	30 mL/kg in 30 minutes	70 mL/kg in 2½ hours

Look for radial pulse, if it is still very weak repeat it
If there is improvement, change to Plan B and then to Plan A, respectively.

INDICATION OF ANTIBIOTICS

- Dysentery
  - Co-trimoxazole
  - Nalidixic acid
  - Ciprofloxacin
- Cholera
  - Tetracycline (adult)
  - Furazolidone (child)
- Systemic infection
- Probiotics: Lactobacillus – not preferred
- **Zn**
  - <6 months old child—10 mg/day × 14 days
  - >6 months old child—20 mg/day × 14 days
- It decreases the severity and helps in faster recovery, improves immune function.

If IV route not getting, we can infuse fluid through interosseous route (upper end of tibia).

Rehydration Solution for Malnourished Child (RESOMAL)

- It is different from ORS by increased K^+ concentration and decreased Na^+ concentration
- It is prepared by:
  - Standard ORS + 4 g potassium + 50 g sucrose in 2 L water.

RESOMAL

Contents	*Amount*
Glucose	125
Na	45
K	40
Cl	70
Citrate	7
Mg	3
Zn	0.3
Ca	0.05

PEDIATRICS

APPROACH TO HEPATOSPLENOMEGALY

LIVER EXAMINATION

Conventional Method

Place the palm of the hand over the abdomen with fingers parallel to the right subcostal region. Start from the right iliac fossa. The radial border of index finger is used to palpate liver. Ask the child to take deep breath, the enlarged liver will be felt by the fingers. If not felt, keep moving the hand upward till it becomes palpable. The lower border is defined by palpation. The upper border is defined by tidal percussion. The size is measured in midclavicular line.

Age	Liver span
Infants	5 – 6.5 cm
1 – 5 years	6 – 7 cm
5 – 10 years	7 – 9 cm
10 – 15 years	8 – 10 cm

Preferred Method

Sit on the couch beside the patient. Place both hands side by side flat on the abdomen in the right subcostal region lateral to rectus, with fingers pointing toward the ribs. If resistance is encountered, move the hands further down until the resistance disappears, exert gentle pressure and ask the patient to breath in deeply. Concentrate on whether the edge of the liver can be felt moving downward and under the examining hand. Normally in infants liver palpable is 2 cm below coastal margin (it is normal). So liver span is important.

SPLEEN

- Start from the right iliac fossa and move toward left hypochondriun, with palm of right hand with fingers pointing toward the left costal margin. The left hand is kept posterolaterally over the left lower rib cage to support it from below.
- Patient in right lateral position and fingers should be insinuated below the left subcostal margin.
- **Hooking method**: The examiner should stand on the left side facing the foot end of the child, palpate with hooked fingers of the left hand.
- **Dipping method**: In the presence of ascites, sudden pressure is exerted by their palpating fingers to displace the fluid and palpate any enlarged organ.
- Percuss the Traube's space.

Features	Spleen	Kidney
Site	Located anteriorly behind 9th, 10th, 11th rib	Located posteriorly in the L1 vertebral region
Plane	Intra-abdominal	Retroperitoneal
Notch	Present	Absent
Finger insinuation	Fingers cannot be insinuated between spleen costal margin	Can be insinuated
Bimanual palpation	Not possible	Possible ballotable
Movement with respiration	Moves freely	Restricted mobility
Direction of enlargement	Toward right iliac fossa	Toward lumbar fossa
Band of colonic resonance	Absent	Present
Loin	Free and resonant	Full and dull

Grading of splenomegaly (cm)	Palpable spleen below left costal margin
• Mild	< 3
• Moderate	3–7
• Massive	>7

Hepatosplenomegaly (HSM) with Pallor

- Infections
  - Bacterial
    - Infective endocarditis
    - Disseminated TB
  - Protozoal
    - Chronic malaria
    - Kala-azar
- Hematological
  - Hemolytic anemia
- Malignancy
  - Leukemia
  - Lymphoma
- Collagen vascular diseases
  - Systemic lupus erythematosus (SLE)
  - Juvenile rheumatoid arthritis (JRA)
- Metabolic
  - Wilson's disease
  - Gaucher's disease
- Other causes
  - Extreme protein–energy malnutrition (PEM)

Massive splenomegaly >8 cm/crosses umbilicus

- Portal hypertension (HTN)
- Hematological malignancies, chronic myeloid leukemia (CML), lymphoma
- Osteopetrosis
- Hemolytic anemia—thalassemia major
- Storage disorder
- Injection: Kala-azar, chronic malaria

HSM with jaundice

- Infections
  - Viral
    - Hepatitis
    - IMN
    - Neonatal hepatitis
  - Bacterial
    - Leptospirosis
    - Septicemia
  - Protozoal
    - Malaria
    - Kala-azar
- Hemolytic anemia
- Congestive cardiac failure (CCF) leading to cardiac cirrhosis
- Metabolic
  - Galactosemia
  - Cystic fibrosis
- Malignancy
  - Metastasis liver
- Storage disorders leading to cirrhosis

HSM with fever

- Infection
  - TB, kala-azar, chronic malaria, IMN
- Malignancy
  - Leukemia
  - Lymphoma
- Collagen disorder
  - SLE, JRA

NEONATAL JAUNDICE

Neonatal jaundice is the visible manifestation in skin and sclera of elevated serum concentration of bilirubin in neonate.

PHYSIOLOGICAL JAUNDICE

Causes

- Increased bilirubin synthesis
- Loss of effective binding and transportation
- Inefficient conjugation
- Decreased efficiency of excretion
- Enhanced enterohepatic circulation.

Criteria to Rule Out Physiological Jaundice

- Jaundice in first 24 hours of life
- Jaundice extending beyond 1 week in term baby and 2 weeks in preterm
- Total serum bilirubin increasing more than 5 mg/dL/day
- Total serum bilirubin is more than 12.9 mg/dL in term and more than 15 mg/dL in preterm.

PATHOLOGICAL JAUNDICE

Causes of Unconjugated Hyperbilirubinemia

- Excess bilirubin production
  - ABO and Rh incompatibility
  - RBC enzyme abnormality (G6PD, pyruvate kinase deficiency)
  - RBC membrane defect (hereditary spherocytosis)
  - Extravasated blood (cephalohematoma)
  - Polycythemia
- Impaired conjugation or excretion
  - Hormone deficiency—hypothyroidism, hypopituitarism
- Disorders of bilirubin metabolism
  - Crigler-Najjar syndrome
  - Gilbert's syndrome
- Enhanced enterohepatic circulation
  - Intestinal obstruction
  - Meconium plugs
  - Cystic fibrosis

Causes of Conjugated Hyperbilirubinemia

- Obstruction to bile flow
  - Biliary atresia—extrahepatic and intrahepatic
  - Choledochal cyst
  - Inspissated bile syndrome
- Hepatocellular injury
  - Infection
    - Bacterial—TB
    - Viral—rubella, CMV
    - Parasitic—toxoplasmosis
  - Idiopathic—neonatal hepatitis
  - Toxic—bacterial sepsis
- Metabolic—galactosemia, Rotor syndrome, Dubin-Johnson syndrome.

APPROACH TO NEONATAL JAUNDICE

- Mother and baby's blood group—incompatibility
- Antenatal
  - Fever with rash—TORCH (toxoplasmosis, other agents, rubella, cytomegalovirus, and herpes simplex)
  - Gestational diabetes mellitus (GDM)—hyperbilirubinemia
- Natal
  - Instrumental delivery (cephal hematoma—extravasated blood)
  - Delayed cord clamping—polycythemia
- Postnatal
  - Preterm
  - Birth trauma
  - Asphyxia
- Family history
  - Anemia
  - Gallstone
  - Splenectomy.

ASSESSMENT OF NEONATAL JAUNDICE

- Physiological or pathological
  - Age of onset—< 24 hours or not
  - Duration of jaundice

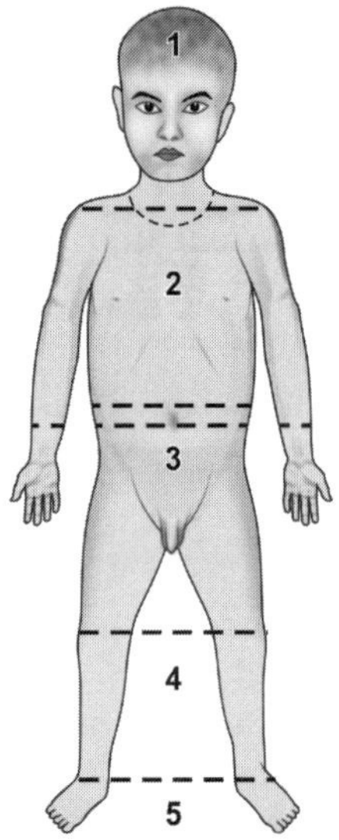

1. 4–6 mg/dL
2. 6–8 mg/dL
3. 8–12 mg/dL
4. 12–14 mg/dL
5. > 15 mg/dL

Dermal zones for estimation of serum total bilirubin levels

- Severity
  - Krammer's rule

Danger signs present	**Etiology of jaundice**
• Vomiting • Lethargy • Poor feeding • Fever • High pitched cry • Dark urine • Light stool • Hepatosplenomegaly (HSM)	• Premature/small for gestational age (SGA) • Evidence of infection—microcephaly, microphthalmia, chorioretinitis • Evidence of birth trauma—cephalohematoma, bruising • Pallor, polycythemia—evidence of hypothyroidism • Evidence of neonatal infection/sepsis

INVESTIGATION

- **Cord blood**
  - Blood group and Coombs test in Rh negative mother
  - Serum bilirubin, Hb
- **Serum bilirubin** (total and direct)
- **Other hemolytic conditions** other than Rh, ABO incompatibility
  - PS
  - Glucose-6-phosphate dehydrogenase (G6PD) assay
- Evaluation for sepsis
- In cholestatic jaundice
  - Bacterial culture
  - Ultrasonography (USG)
  - Radionuclide scan— hepatobiliary iminodiacetic acid (HIDA) scan
  - Liver biopsy
    - Biliary atresia—ductular perforation and fibrosis
    - Neonatal hepatitis—alteration in lobular architecture, focal hepatocellular necrosis and
    - Giant cell with ballooning of their cytoplasm.

TREATMENT

- **Hydration**
  - Correct dehydration

PEDIATRICS

- Increase intestinal motility
- Enhanced removal of photoproducts in urine and stool
- **Phototherapy**

  Procedure:
  - Undress the baby completely
  - Cover the eyes and genitalia to prevent damage by bright light
  - Keep baby at a distance of 30–45 cm from light source [blue-green light (460–490 nm)]
  - Turn the baby after each feed to express maximum surface area of baby to light
  - Ensure adequate breastfeeding
  - Record body weight daily and ensure that baby passes adequate amount of urine (6–8 times per day)

  Phototherapy acts by several way:
  - Configurational isomerization: Zisomer → Eisomer
  - Structural isomerization: Bilirubin → Lumirubin
  - Photo-oxidation: Photo products are excreted in urine.

  Side effects:
  - Rash, overheating
  - Dehydration, diarrhea
- **Exchange transfusion**

  Procedure:
  - Push—ball technique via umbilical vein
  - Blood drawn <72 hours preferred.

Complications of exchange transfusion
- Bacterial sepsis, thrombocytopenia
- Portal vein thrombosis
- Arrhythmias, cardiac arrest
- Hypocalcemia, hypoglycemia, hypomagnesemia
- Hep B and Hep C infection

Features	Neonatal hepatitis	Extrahepatic biliary atresia (EHBA)
Onset	Any time in neonatal period	Usually end of first week
Sex	More in males	More in females
Gestation	Preterm, IUGR	Term
Family history	+ve in 15%	Absent
Cataract	May be present	Absent
Stools	Pale/normal	Clay colored
General condition at birth	Looks sick	Healthy initially
Hepatosplenomegaly (HSM)	Early	Late
Urine urobilinogen	Increased	Absent
Transaminases	Very high	High
Alkaline phosphatase (ALP)	High	Very high
TORCH screen	May be +ve	Negative
Serum lipoprotein X	High	High
AFP	High	Normal
USG	GB imaged	GB usually not imaged
Liver biopsy	Giant cells predominate; no bile ductular proliferation; no bile lakes	Very few giant cells; Marked proliferation; Bile lakes +++
Biliary scintigraphy	Radioactivity in gut +	No radioactivity in gut
Operative cholangiogram	Normal	Block may be visualized
Prognosis	Better	Poor

PEDIATRICS

Nervous System

CEREBRAL PALSY

CASE FORMAT

Presenting Complaints

Causes of – Delayed milestones
– Fever and cough
– Seizures
– Say as not attaining age appropriate milestones

History of Present Illness

1st child of a nonconsanginous marriage with normal/abnormal antenatal history, detected to have difficulty in attaining age appropriate milestones from 4th month onward, now presented with fever and cough for 6 days.

Explain history of fever and cough (briefly).

History of Past Illness

Since the child as having problem from early infancy, I am starting from antenatal history.

Antenatal History

- Conceived 2 years after marriage
- No history of abortions or treatment for infertility (more chance for genetic abnormality)
- No history of any drug intake other than Iron (Fe) and folic acid
- No history of urinary tract infection (UTI) or radiation exposure
- No history suggestive of rubella like fever with rash and associated swelling behind neck
- She has taken regular antenatal check-ups
- Ultrasonography (USG) taken at 4th, 6th and 8th months and no abnormalities detected
- Quickening felt at 4th month (absent in congenital anomalies), decreased fetal movements (hypotonia)
- No history of gestational diabetes mellitus (GDM), Pregnancy-induced hypertension (PIH), intrauterine grwoth restriction (IUGR) detected or antepartum hemorrhage (APH)
- No history of polyhydramnios (open neurol take defect NTD)
- No history of trauma during pregnancy, prolonged 2nd stage.

Natal History

- Hospital/home delivery
- Term/preterm
- Cesarean section (CS) (indication)/Full time normal delivery (FTND), birth weight
- Induction (indication)
- History of passage of foul smelling liquor

- Maternal pyrexia
- History of chorioamnionitis/premature rupture of membrane (PROM)
- History of instrumentalization/intrapartum convulsions.

Postnatal History

- Cried soon after birth (CSAB)
- Birth weight was ... [low birth weight—most important single risk factor for cerebral palsy (CP)]
- If asphyxia ask
  - When child handed over, when does child discharged
- When breastfeeding (BF) started
- Mechanical ventilation
- Whether taken to neonatal intensive care unit (NICU)
- If neonatal jaundice ask:
  - Detected at
  - Color of urine/stool
  - Sites of jaundice
  - Phototherapy/exchange transfusion done

  (to know whether it is unconjugated and severity of jaundice)
- No history suggestive of bilirubin encephalopathy like shrill cry, hypotonia, poor suck, seizures and opisthotonic posture during these days.
- Neonatal meningitis [21 day intravenous (IV) drugs]
- Neonatal seizures
- No history of detection of any congenital malformations (hydrocephalus)
- Started hand preference at:
- History of drooling of saliva or pooling of secretion (pseudobulbar palsy)
- Abnormal arching of body detected at
- Mother detected stiffening of upper limb (UL)/lower limb (LL)
- Detected hand preference at
- History of cortical thumb/constant fisting > 2 months
- Had history of difficulty in changing diapers
- History of commando crawl detected
- History of chewing movements/lip masking
- History of inconsolable cry
- Increased sensitivity to light and noise
- Bowel and bladder control attained at.

Developmental History

- Say the development of child as a story touching all spheres
- Ask whether on regular physiotherapy
- Gross motor
- Fine motor
- Language
- Social
- Vision
- Hearing

> - Developmental age in each sphere
> - Global or dissociative developmental delay
> - Whether child is attaining milestone (suggestive of CP)
> - Any regression in milestones (suggestive of neurodegenerative disorder)

- There is no history of regression of any attained milestones.

Immunization History

- Whichever vaccines given?
- Diphtheria, pertussis and tetanus (DPT) how many?
- DPT can be given/if not advice
- Optional vaccines/[Hepatitus B and haemophilus influenzae type b (Hib) are must due to rehospitalization)]

Dietetic History

- Prelacteal feeds not given
- Put to breast within ___hours of birth

- Exclusive breastfeeding (EBF) up to ___months
- Weaned at ___months by ____
- Breastfeeding up to ___years
- History of feeding difficulties (recurrent aspiration, nasal regurgitation) pseudobulbar palsy
- Started giving solid foods/family diet at ___years
- Calorie intake is ____and protein______ per day
- There is a gap of ____kcal protein adequate.

Family History

- 1st child of nonconsanguinous marriage (NCM)
- Maternal age at gestation was 30 years
- No history of abortions
- No history of any mental retardation (MR) in family
- No history of any congenital anomalies
- No history of any developmental delay
- No history of any neonatal death in family
- Younger brothers development is normal and he is fully immunized to age and healthy.

Socioeconomic status (SES)

- Economic status
- Who is looking after child
- Impact of illness in the family.

Head to Foot Examination

- Head size appears to be decreased
- Facial dysmorphisms +
- Anterior Fontanelle
- Hairline
- Brownish hair, bushy
- Occipital flattening
- Ridging of sutures
- No receding of forehead
- Single circular parietal whorl/microcephaly
- Vitamin deficiency
- Eyebrows
- Eyes
  - No cataract (crs)
  - No microphthalmia (crs)
  - Squint, type
  - Nystagmus
  - Hypertelorism
  - Eye lashes
  - Eye slants
  - Epicanthal folds

Mouth
- Open mouth with drooling of saliva
- Angular stomatitis
- Cheilitis
- Teeth
- Dysplastic teeth/kernicterus
- Poor oral hygiene
- Glossitis
- High-arched palate

- Ear
  - No low set ears
  - Pinna
- Webbing or short neck
- Flexion contracture of elbow
- Cortical thumb or constant fisting
- Simian crease
- Scissoring (Delagae sign)
- Plantar flexion
- Achilles tendon contractures
- Nail not trimmed (muddy)

- Contractures
- *Chest*
  - No pectus excavatum or carinatum
  - Kyphosis or scoliosis
- Spinal deformities
- Tuft of hair at low back (spina bifida)
- Evidence of dehydration
- Evidence of malnutrition on skin
- Callus/bed sores
- Perineal excoriation
- IV cannulated
- Nasogastic tube (NGT) put
- External genitalia
- 180° deviation assessment (only after consent)—180° flip method in small infant
- *Supine*
  - Asymmetrical Tonic Neck Reflex (ATNR)
  - Hand open
  - Reaching out
  - Mouthing.
- Pull to sit
  - Grasp
  - Head lag +/Back
  - Round or not.
- Vertical suspension
  - Scissoring
  - Slipping through
  - Bearing weight.
- Ventral suspension
  - Head lag
  - Head same plane/head
  - Raise above body/parachute+
  - Landau.
- Prone
  - Head off the couch
  - Crawling
  - Sitting up
  - Forearm support
- Motor system
- Bulk
  - Wasting+
  - Measurements
- Tone
  - Explain posture
  - Palpate muscle—flabby or firm
  - Hypertonia of UL/LL all joints
- Power
  - Bed movements
- Reflexes

Reflex	**Appearance**	**Disappearance**
Moro	Birth	3–6 months
ATNR	1 month	3–5 months
STNR	2 months	6 months
Sucking and rooting	Birth	4 months—awake 7 months—sleep
Parachute	9 months	Persists for life
Palmar grasp	Birth	2 months
Landau	10 months	2 years

Superficial
- Conjunctival
- Corneal
- Gag/palatal
- Abdominal + in CP
- Cremasteric
- Plantar – extensor bilateral

Deep
- Jaw jerk
- Biceps jerk
- Triceps jerk
- Supinator
- Knee jerk
- Ankle jerk

- Clonus

NEONATAL REFLEXES

- Glabellar tap
- Rooting/sucking
- Palmar grasp
- Plantar grasp
- Asymmetrical tonic neck reflex
- Moro reflex

Coordination

Abnormal movements

Gait

Sensory

Spine and skull

Diagnosis (should include physiologic, topographic, etiology, +mental retardation, seizures, hearing, vision, squint, etc. + complication)

It is a case of spastic quadriparesis CP with pseudobulbar palsy due to perinatal asphyxia and having MR, seizures, speech, visual and hearing impairment, microcephaly, grade III protein-energy malnutrition (PEM) and fully immunized + bronchopneumonia.

It is a case of spastic diplegia due to prematurity and having microcephaly, grade II PEM, no MR, seizures, speech, visual or hearing impairment and is fully immunized.

CEREBRAL PALSY—DISCUSSION

It is a dynamic disorder of posture and mobility being motor manifestation of a nonprogressive brain damage occurring during the period of brain growth.

Incidence: 1-2/100 live births

In LBW: 15/100 live births.

Classification

Topographical
- Paraplegia
- Diplegia (quadriplegia with more involvement of LL)
- Hemiplegia

Neurologic classification
- Spastic
- Hypotonic
- Choreoathetoid
- Cerebellar
- Mixed type

Funtional classification (grade)
- Mild
- Moderate
- Severe

Pathological
- Infective—intrauterine infection, meningitis
- Genetic
- Vascular problem—thrombophilia
- Periventricular leukomalacia (PVL)
- Metabolic

Causes of Cerebral Palsy

- Antenatal cause (80%)
- Birth asphyxia
- Cerebral malformation
- Acid-base imbalance
- Thrombophilia
- Infection (IU, acquired)
- Indirect hyperbilirubinemia.

Treatment

Participation of parents—they should be explained about the prognosis of disease

Multidisciplinary team approach [pediatrician, pediatric neurologist, occupational therapist, physiotherapist, child psychologist, counselor, orthopedic surgeon, ophthalmologist, ear, nose and throat (ENT) surgeon].

Methods to decrease spasticity

- **Nonpharmacological**: Physiotherapy, occupational therapy, electrical stimulation, use of orthoses, manipulative methods
- **Pharmacological:**
  Oral – Diazepam or nitrazepam
  – Dandrolene sodium
  – Tizanidine, baclofen, levodopa
  Parenteral – Alcohol or Phenol injections
  – Botulinum toxin injection
  – Intrathecal baclofen
- **Surgical**
  - Tenotomy
  - Osteotomy, tendon lengthening, arthrodesis, etc.
  - Selective posterior rhizotomy—selective sectioning of 20–40% of dorsal nerve roots

Treatment of associated features—epilepsy, visual disturbances, hearing, speech, behavioral problems special education

Nursing care and nutritional management

Rehabilitation

Spastic Type

For example, Periventricular leukomalacia (PVL)

- Ventricle is very vascular and controls motion of lower limb (mainly) in addition to upper limb, so it produce **diplegic** type of cerebral palsy
- PVL clinicaly seen in preterm babies with asphyxia.

Clinical Features

- Here LL involvement is more (PVL)
- Increased stiffness of LL
- Limb position—scissoring position due to adductor
- Spasm (difficulty in changing diapers)
- Paucity of movement
- Commando crawling
- Abnormal posturing

(Sometimes, we think developmental milestones are early attained, it is due to false impression).

Hemiplegia

- Paucity of movement on one side of body
- Early hand preference, persistent fisting
- Cortical thumb
- Limb length deformity (sometime, affected limb is small).

Choreoathetoid

- Cause
  - Birth asphyxia
  - Kernicterus
- There is abnormal deposition of myelin in place of gray matter of basal ganglia (status marmoratus).

Complications

- Neurological
  - Mental retardation
  - Visual loss
  - Hearing problem
  - Communication disorder
- Gastrointestinal tract-gastroesophageal reflux disease (GIT- GERD)
  - Constipation

- Orthopedic
  - Contractures (Achilles contracture)
  - Scoliosis, kyphosis
  - Equinus deformity
- Miscellaneous
  - Respiratory problem
  - Learning problem

Early Marker of Cerebral Palsy

- Episodes of inconsolable cry. Chewing movement, excessive sensitivity to light and voice
- Persistent neck tonic posture >4 weeks
- Clenched fist and thumb adducted and flexed cross plan >8 weeks
- Paucity/absence of limb movement 6–12 weeks
- Persistence of primary reflux beyond 4–5 months
- Absence of parachute reflex
- Slow head growth
- Early hand preference <1 year.

Investigations

- Visual and hearing evaluation
- IQ
- Rule out other causes
  - Hypothyroidism
  - Chromosomal abnormality
  - Inborn errors of metabolism
- Imaging—Computed tomography (CT), magnetic resonance imaging (MRI)
- Electroencephalogram (EEG) – if there is seizures
- Fundus examination

Differential diagnosis

- Neurodegenerative disorders
- Ataxic telangiectasia
- Subdural effusion
- Hydrocephalus
- Muscular disorders

FEBRILE SEIZURES

APPROACH

Presenting Complaints

- Fever
- Seizures.

History of Present Illness

- Detailed history of fever
- Seizures – onset: Within 24 hours of fever
- Duration
  - <10 minutes (typical febrile seizures)
  - >15 minutes (atypical febrile seizures)
- Type
  - Focal/generalized
  - Associated history of:
    - Fever
    - Head trauma [Subarachnoid hemorrhage (SAH)]
    - Aura
    - Frothing
- Number of episodes: Single/repeated episode (atypical FB)
- Similar history of among siblings
- To rule out other causes of febrile seizures (FS):
  - Frontal headache
  - Projectile vomiting
  - Photophobia

  } meningitis
- Motor system—history of any weakness (Todd's paralysis)
- Sensory system—history of any pins and needle sensations, numbness
- Autonomic system—bladder and bowel disturbance
- Cranial nerves—mention as negative history.

Past History

- Previous episode in the past
- History of any seizure drug intake

Developmental History

Any delay in attaining milestones (atypical seizures)

Examination of a Central nervous system (CNS) case

1.	Attitude—active in FS Irritable/apathetic in meningitis
2.	Posture
3.	Head to foot examination
4.	Cranial nerves system examination 2-blinks to light Menace reflex
3, 4, 6	No ptosis, squint, nystagmus Reflex—direct/indirect
5	No deviation on opening mouth for food Jaw jerk Corneal/conjunctival reflex
7	No facial dysmorphism No history of drooling No facial deviation
8	Startle response +/–
9 and 10	Whether baby feeds normal History of any regurgitation Position of uvula Palatal reflex, gag reflex
11	Shrugging of shoulders +/–
12	Position of tongue Strength of movements Any fasciculation/tremor

MOTOR SYSTEM PROPER

- Bulk—wasting +/–
- Tone
- Power
  - For babies mention power as 'Child move his limb actively and appears to be normal'
- Reflexes
  - Superficial
  - Deep
  - Primitive
- Any involuntary movements
- Any signs of meningeal irritation
  - Kernig's sign
  - Brudzinski's sign
  - Neck stiffness
- Mention other systems within normal limits [cardiovascular system (CVS), gastrointestinal tract (GIT), respiratory (RESP)]

DIAGNOSIS

First/recurrent episode of seizure probably FS probably typical/atypical FS.

DISCUSSION

Management: Investigation to rule out other causes of seizures:

- Hemoglobin (HB), total count (TC), differential count (DC), erythrocyte sedimentation rate (ESR)
- Blood glucose
- Blood calcium

Indications of LP in FS

- <1 year
- Suspecting meningitis
- Atypical FS
- 1st episode of FS
- Immunization status not known
- Not immunized to Hib and pneumococci

- Serum electrolytes
- Cerebrospinal fluid (CSF) study—lumbar puncture—meningitis
- Blood culture
- EEG and neuroimaging have no role in FS

Q1. Why you said it is a cause of FS?
- Seizure started within 24 hours of onset of fever
- Duration < 15 minutes
- Single episode, generalized
- Positive family history
- No developmental delay in milestones
- On examination: Child is active
  : No signs of meningeal irritation

Q2. What is FS?
Febrile seizures: Seizures during fever occurring between 6 months and 5 years age in the absence of injection of the central nervous system in a neurologically normal child.

Q3. Differential beween typical FS and atypical FS.

	Typical FS	Atypical FS
• No of febrile episode	Single	Recurrent
• Onset	Within 24 hours	Any time
• Duration	<15 minutes	>15 minutes
• Type	Generalized	Focal
• Postictal phase	No postictal confusion	Focal neurological deficit in postictal period
• Chance of epilepsy in future	No	Yes

Q4. Treatment of FS.
1. Supportive measures— nurse in semiprone position
   ABC—Airways, breathing, circulation
2. Fever—paracetamol—15 mg/kg tid
   Tepid sponge
   Hydrotherapy
3. Seizure—Intramuscular (IM) diazepam—0.3 mg/kg/dose.

Febrile seizure prophylaxis
- **Intermittent prophylaxis**
  - Indicated 3 or more FS in 6 months, FS lasting >15 minutes, or requiring pharmacological therapy to control seizures.
  - Drugs Clobazam (0.75–1 mg/kg/day) gives for 3 days during fever episodes.
- **Continuous prophylaxis**
  - Indicated
    - Recurrent atypical seizures
    - Failure of intermittent prophylaxis
    - Not able to recognize the onset of fever
  - Drugs
    - Sodium valproate: 10–20 mg/kg/day or
    - Phenobarbitone: 3–5 mg/kg/day
    - Until 5 years of age or 1–2 years, whichever comes earlier.

ACUTE FLACCID PARALYSIS

- Acute onset of (<4 weeks) flaccid paralysis
- A case of acute fluid paralysis (AFP), in any child <15-year-old who has acute onset of flaccid paralysis for which no obvious cause is found or paralytic illness of any age in which polio is suspected.

Causes
- Poliomyelitis
- Guillain-Barre' syndrome (GBS)

- Transverse myelitis
- Traumatic neuritis
- Post-diphtheritic neuropathy
- Non-polio enterovirus illnesses.

Polio

- Fever present alongwith the paralysis
- Asymmetrical paralysis, proximal muscle weakness more
- Bladder dysfunction absent.

Spectrum of polio
- Inapparent (90–95%)
- Abortive
- Nonparalytic
- Paralytic

Guillain-Barré Syndrome

- History of fever, diarrhea prior to the onset of weakness (*Campylobacter jejuni*)
- Symmetric, ascending paralysis with involvement of distal muscle is more
- Complication is respiratory failure.
- Affecting cranial nerves 7, 9, 10, 11, 12
- Bladder dysfunction transient
- CSF show cytoalbumino dissociation
- Asbury criteria used
- Treatment—Intravenous immunoglobulin (IVIG), plasmapheresis, supportive care

Cytoalbummino dissociation
1. GBS
2. Froin's syndrome

AFP Surveillance

All cases of AFP should be reported regardless of final diagnosis.

Step 1 – case identification

Step 2 – inform nodal officer

Step 3 – line listing – detailed history including immunization along with particulars (age, name, sex, address) is taken.

Step 4 – stool samples are collected (2 specimen) at least 24 hour apart, collected within 14 days of paralysis onset, each having adequate volume (8–10 g or thumb size) and it is sent to WHO accredited laboratory in reverse cold chain.

Step 5 – active search of similar illness.

Step 6 – Outbreak response immunization (ORI)
Single dose of OPV is given to 500 children below 5 years residing around the cases (5 km radius)

Step 7 – manage the cases

Step 8 – the case should be followed up for 60 days, look for residual paralysis.

Laboratories
- Pasteur Institute of India, Coonoor
- National Institute of Communicable Disease, New Delhi
- King Institute of Preventive Medicine, Chennai.

HYDROCEPHALUS

- The accumulation of CSF within ventricle either due to increased production, obstruction of flow or decreased absorption.

DIFFERENTIAL DIAGNOSIS

- Megalencephaly
- Chronic subdural hematoma
- Hydranencephaly
- Achondroplasia
- Rickets
- Hemolytic anemia
- Pseudotumor cerebri.

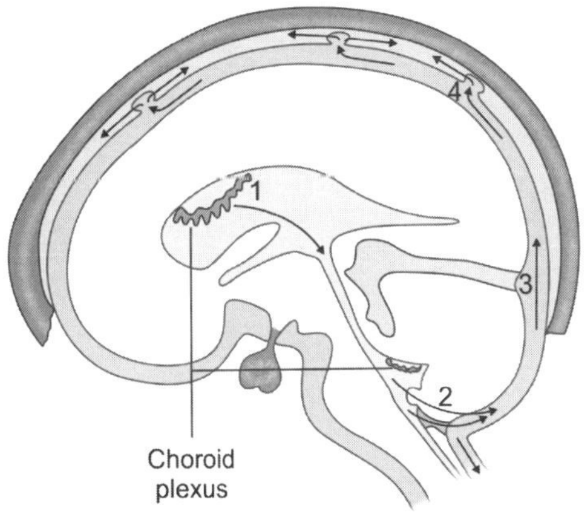

CLASSIFICATION AND CAUSES

- Communicating hydrocephalus (nonobstructive/external)
- Noncommunicating hydrocephalus (obstructive/internal)

PEDIATRICS

Congenital hydrocephalus

- Intrauterine infections: Rubella, CMV, toxoplasma
- Congenital malformations: Aqueductal stenosis, Arnold-Chiari malformation
- Midline tumor obstructing: CSF flow

Acquired hydrocephalus

- Pyogenic meningitis
- Posterior fossa tumor
- Intraventricular hemorrhage
- Intracranial hemorrhage

CLINICAL FEATURES

- Enlarging head size, suture separation
- Delayed closure of fontanelle
- Headache, nausea, vomiting, irritability, head banging, diplopia
- Forehead prominent
- Scalp vein become prominent
- Cracked pot sound on skull percussion (only if fontanelle closed), transillumination (+ve)
- Sclera above the cornea visible (sunset sign)
- Difficult in delivery of head during labor
- Spasticity of lower limb
- Upward gaze impaired.

INVESTIGATIONS

- Serial recording of head circumference
- USG
- CT/MRI (periventricular ooze)

Look for

- Neurofibroma
- Cataract, CHD, deafness – *Klebsiella*
- Spina bifida, meningocele, mylomeningocele (Arnold-Chiari malformation)

TREATMENT

- *Medical*
  - Acetozolamide
  - Glycerol
- *Surgical*
  - Ventriculoatrial/ventriculoperitoneal shunt—Upadhyaya shunt, Chopra shunt
  - Third ventriculotomy.

CHAPTER 16

Hematology

APPROACH TO BLEEDING DISORDERS

CLOTTING FACTORS

I—Fibrinogen
II—Prothrombin
III—Tissue thromboplastin
IV—Calcium
V—Proaccelerin
VI—No factor
VII—Stable factor
VIII—Hemophilia A
IX—X-mas factor, Hemophilia B
X—Stuart-Prower
XI—Plasma thromboplastin, Hemophilia C
XII—Hageman factor
XIII—Fibrin stabilizing factor

Petechiae: <2 mm Purpura: 2–5 mm Ecchymosis: >5 mm

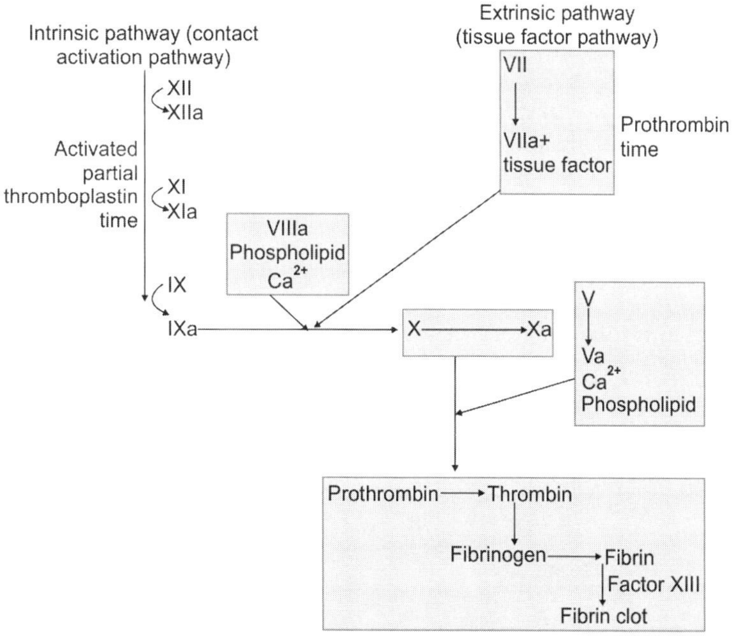

	Bleeding disorder	*Coagulation disorder*
Site	Skin, mucous membrane (epistaxis, oral, GIT)	Deep (soft tissue, joint, muscle)
Petechiae	Yes	No
Ecchymoses	Small, superficial	Large, deep
Hemarthrosis	Extremely rare	Common
Bleeding after minor trauma	Yes	No
Bleeding after surgery	Immediate	Delayed (1–2 days)
Example	vWD, ITP	Hemophilia

Bleeding Disorders: Causes

I. Vessel wall abnormality
- *Infection*: Meningococcemia
  Infective endocarditis (IE), Rickettsiae
- Drug—sodium valproate, warfarin
- Scurvy
- Henoch-Schönlein purpura
- Hereditary hemorrhagic telangeictasia
- Vasculitis: Systemic lupus erythematous (SLE)
- Ehlers Danlos syndrome

II. Platelet abnormality
- Decreased number
  1. Decreased production
     i. Diseases of bone marrow
        – Aplastic anemia
        – Leukemia, disseminated cancer
     ii. Selective destruction of platelets
        – *Drug*: Alcohol, thiazide
        – *Infection*: HIV, measles
     iii. Ineffective megakaryopoiesis
        – Megaloblastic anemia
        – Myelodysplastic syndrome
  2. Increased destruction
     – Idiopathic thrombocytopenic purpura (ITP), SLE
     – Quinidine, sulpha drug
     – Disseminated intravascular coagulation (DIC), Thrombotic thrombocytopenic purpura (TTP), Microangiopathic hemolytic anemia (MAHA)
- Qualitative defects
  1. Inherited
     – Glanzmann thrombasthenia (GpIb)
     – Bernard-Soulier syndrome (GpIIb-IIIa)
  2. Acquired
     – Nonsteriodal anti-inflammatory drug (NSAID), Uremia

III. Coagulation disorders

Inherited
- Hemophilia A
- Hemophilia B
- Von Willebrand disease (vWD)

Acquired
- Liver disease
- Vitamin K deficiency
- Warfarin overdose
- DIC

HISTORY

- Sex (hereditary)
- Onset, mucosal bleed
  – Like epistaxis, gum bleed

PEDIATRICS

- Joint swelling, muscle hematoma
  - History of transfusion
- History of trauma
- Drug intake
- Henoch-Schönlein purpura (HSP) – Arthralgia, abdominal pain, palpable, purpura, oliguria, edema, hematuria
- Hemolytic-uremic syndrome (HUS) – Oliguria, diarrhea
- Anemia
- Recurrent infection
- Bone pain, loss of weight, loss of appetite—malignancy
- *Complications*: Intracranial (IC) bleed
  - Increased intracranial tension (ICT) – vomiting, seizures, focal neurological deficit, melena, hematuria.

Steps of coagulation

i. Vasoconstriction
ii. I° hemostasis
Platelet adhesion, activation (release of ADP, TXA_2), aggregation
iii. II° hemostasis
Thrombin formation, fibrinogen clot

Past History

- First episode and each episode
- History of blood transfusion
- History of prior viral infection (usually 1 month in ITP)
- History of bleeding
  - From umbilicus at birth
  - During vaccination, circumcision, tooth extraction
- History of drugs
  - NSAID
  - Anticoagulants
  - Cephalosporin
  - Anticonvulsive—Sodium valproate
- Jaundice—in liver disease
- SLE—rash, arthralgia

Antenatal

- Maternal drug
- History of infection: CMV, rubella, neonatal thrombocytopenia

Natal

Bleeding from cord—factor XIII deficiency

Postnatal

Blood in stool—hemorrhagic disease of newborn
Cephalhematoma

Developmental Delay

If IC bleeds

Immunization

- Bleeding during vaccination
- Hep B
- MMR—ITP like illness

Decrease number of injections

- IM injections into S/C
- Use smallest diameter needle
- Use ice packs after vaccination

Family History

Three generation
1. X-linked recessive—hemophilia
2. AD–vWD
3. Family history of menorrhagia.

Socioeconomic Status

- Literacy
- Income

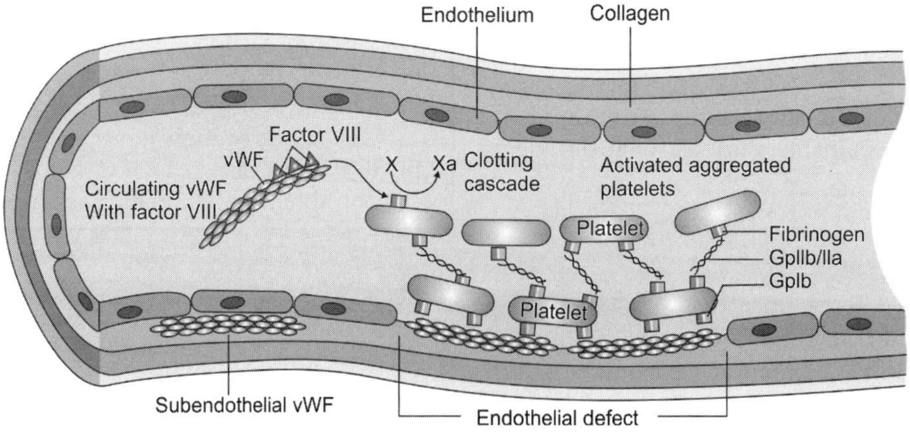

GENERAL EXAMINATION

- Pallor (proportionate or disproportionate)
- Jaundice – liver disease, HUS, hepatitis B
- Lymph node enlargement – malignancy
  - Edema – HUS, HSP

Respiratory Rate

- Tachypnea – Congestive cardiac failure (CCF)
- Fever – malignancy (due to infection)

Head to Foot Examination

- Any bleeding manifestation
- Facies – due to hemolytic anemia
- Mouth
  - Blebs in lips and oral cavity, ITP
  - Palate-ITP
  - Gum hypertrophy (Leukemia)
  - Oral thrush
- Malar rash – SLE
- *Purpura*: Nontender, nonblanching (Diascopy) purpura
- Bone tenderness, eczema
- Abdominal distension
- Limbs – absent radii, thumb (TAR), thumb hypoplasia with anemia (Fanconi's), hyperextensibility of joints (Ehlers–Danlos Syndrome)
- External genitalia (testis).

Examination of Joint (refer Orthopedics)

- **Inspection**
  - Attitude
  - Deformity
  - Any wasting, shortening of limbs
  - Any swelling (site, size, shape, surface, skin over swelling)
  - Redness
- **Palpation**
  - Local rise of temperature, tenderness
  - Swelling
- **Movement: Flexion, extension, etc.**
- **Measurements:**
  - Linear
  - Circumferential

PEDIATRICS

Gastrointestinal System

- HSM

CNS: Rule out intracranial bleed.

CVS: CCF

Respiratory: Respiratory infections
Fundoscopy: Not done – retinal bleed, papilledema.

Investigations

Hb: Decreased in aplastic anemia, leukemia
TC, DC: To rule out infections, leukemia

Platelet count

>50,000	– Easy bruisability
20,000–50,000	– Petechiae
<20,000	– Spontaneous bleeding
<10,000	– Intracranial bleed

Bleeding time: Normal: 2–3 minutes
Increased in any platelet function defect, decrease in number, vWD
Clotting time: Normal: 8 minutes
Elevated in coagulation disorders
Then,

i. aPTT (Normal: 35–45 sec)
   – Elevated in intrinsic pathway
ii. PT (Prothrombin time: 12–14 sec)
   – Elevated in extrinsic pathway

Peripheral Smear

- Anemia
- Leukemia – blast cells
- Low platelet count

Bone marrow:
Indications

- Before starting steroid therapy
- If suspecting malignancy, aplastic anemia
- In ITP bone marrow shows increased megakaryocytes

X-ray joint – in hemophilia

- Factor assay VIII, IX – in hemophilia
- Ristosectin co-factor assay – vWD disease

Hess test: Positive in:

- HSP, ITP, dengue
- Elevate BP between systolic-diastolic pressure
- If >20 petechiae/inch in forearm after 5 min.

IDIOPATHIC THROMBOCYTOPENIC PURPURA

Acute Idiopathic thrombocytopenic purpura (ITP)

- Sudden onset
- Duration: 2–4 months
- Age: 1–7 years old
- Spontaneous remission in 80% cases

Newly diagnosed ITP – <3 months duration
Persistent ITP – 3–12 months duration
Chronic ITP – >12 months duration

Relapsing ITP: Relapses and remission during disease course

Course of ITP
- 60–80% – spontaneous remission
- 20% – becomes chronic ITP
- <1% – produce complications

The presence of lymphadenopathy or splenomegaly suggests other causes of thrombocytopenia.

LABORATORY DIAGNOSIS

- ITP is a diagnosis of exclusion
- Platelet count <1 lakh
- BT – prolonged
- CT, PT, aPTT normal
- ESR normal
- Eosinophilia may be present

Peripheral smear

Varying number of large platelets

Bone marrow aspirate

Increased number of megakaryocytes with budding

Indications for bone marrow examination in ITP
- Chronic ITP
- Abnormal TC/DC
- Moderate, severe anemia (disproportionate)
- Atypical history
- Before steroid treatment
- Failure to respond to steroids

Differential diagnosis of ITP
- VWD
- Platelet function disorder
- Aplastic anemia
- Drug induced thrombocytopenia

MANAGEMENT

Supportive care
- Bed rest
- Avoid IM injections
- Avoid trauma

Treatment
- Steroids
  - Mechanism of action
    - Reduced antibody production
    - Antigen-antibody reaction delayed
    - Delayed platelet destruction
    - Capillary stability increased
  - CI – malignancy
  - Prednisolone 1-4 mg/kg/day × 2-4 weeks, then tapered
- IVIG
  - Mechanism of action
    - Block Fc receptor
    - Protect platelet from Abs induced phagocytosis
      1 g/kg/day × 1–2 days
- Anti-Rh D therapy—only in Rh +ve patients
  - Block fc receptors by antibody coated RBC in place for platelets
  - 50–75 mg/kg
- Platelet transfusion
  - If significant IC bleed
  - For surgical procedures

Management of Chronic ITP
- Alternate day low dose steroids
- Cyclophosphamide, vincristine, azathioprine, danazol

PEDIATRICS

- Splenectomy
  - Reduced antibody production
  - Increased platelet destruction
- Anti-CD20 – Rituximab
- Thrombopoietin receptor-binding agents.

HEMOPHILIA

- Most common clotting disorder
- X-linked recessive
  - Hemophilia A – Factor VIII deficiency
  - Hemophilia B – Factor IX deficiency
  - Hemophilia C – Factor XI deficiency—AR
  - Parahemophilia—Factor V deficiency

Mild hemophilia	5–40% factor
Moderate hemophilia	1–5% factor
Severe hemophilia	<1% factor

Treatment

- Factor replacement
  - Cryoprecipitate – contains all factors except IX (not useful in hemophilia-B)
  - Fresh frozen plasma – contains all factors including IX
    1 unit of factor VIII/kg rises factor level by 2%
    - To prevent hemarthrosis target level = 30–50%
    - Needs = 15 U/kg factor VIII
    - To prevent IC bleed 80–100%
    1 unit of factor IX rise factor level by 0.7%
  - Adjuvant therapy
    - Epsilon aminocaproic acid
    - Tranexamic acid
- Physiotherapy for joint diseases
- Advise for injury prevention
- Supportive care.

Prevention

- Genetic counseling and prenatal diagnosis
- Most common cause of death are:
  - AIDS
  - IC bleed

Most common muscle involved in bleeding
- Flexors of arm
- Gastrocnemius
- Iliopsoas

HEMORRHAGIC DISEASE OF NEWBORN

Hemorrhagic disease of newborn (HDN) results from transient deficiencies of vitamin K and hence vitamin K dependent coagulation factors II, VII, IX, X leading to bleeding from various sites.

Types

a. **Early onset**
  - *Age*: 0–24 hours
  - *Etiology*: Malarial drugs, phenobarbitone, phenytoin, warfarin

  Sites of hemorrhage
  - Cephalohematoma
  - Subgaleal
  - Intracranial
  - Gastrointestinal
  - Intra-abdominal

b. **Classic diseases**
  - *Age*: 2–7 days
  - *Etiology*: Vitamin K deficiency, breastfeeding

c. **Late onset**
   - *Age*: 1–6 months
   - *Etiology*: Cholestasis – malabsorption of vitamin K.

Investigations

- Prothrombin time, aPTT
- Protein induced vitamin K absence (PIVKA) – tends to be positive for longer period and even after blood transfusion.

Treatment

Injection vitamin K 2–5 mg IV.

Prevention

- Inj vitamin K
- 1 mg IM (if >1 kg)
  0.5 mg IM (if <1 kg).

LEUKEMIAS

ACUTE LYMPHOCYTIC LEUKEMIA (ALL)

T-cell: Adolescence (boys)
B-cell: 2–5 years (Common ALL)

French-American British (FAB) Classification

	L1 (85%)	*L2 (15%)*	*L3 (2%)*
Cell size	Small, homogeneous	Large, heterogeneous	Large, homogeneous
Cytoplasm	Scanty	Variable	Moderately abundant
Nucleoli	Small, inconspicuous	One or more, after large	One or more, prominent

Clinical Features

- Short duration pyraxia of unknown origin (PUO), pallor, lymphadenopathy, hepatosplenomegaly (HSM), bleeding manifestations
- Joint pain

Myeloblast vs	**Lymphoblast**
• Abundant cytoplasm	• Scanty cytoplasm
• Auer rods present	• No Auer rods
• Fine chromatin	• More condensed chromatin
• 3–5 nucleoli, distint	• Nucleoli 1–3, indistinct

Investigations

- CBC—increased total count
- Decreased lymphoblast
- Bone marrow
  - >20% blasts
- Stained by periodic-acid Schiff and terminal deoxy peroxidase
- *Flow cytometry*: Look for specific CD (in blood)
- Immunochemistry: To see CD in solid tissue like liver and spleen
  Precursor B-cell - CD18, CD19, CD20, CD79a
  Mature B-cell - CD19, CD20, CD 21
  T cell – CD2, CD3, CD5, CD7
- Cytogenetics

Management

- **Induction phase:** For remission

– **VAPA**	**Adverse effects**
– Vincristine	– Neuropathy
– Adriamycin	– Cardiotoxicity
– Prednisolone	– Pancreatitis
– Asparaginase	

- **Consolidation phase**: Intensification
  MECA
  - Methotrexate

Good Prognostic Factors
- Age at diagnosis (2–10 years)
- Initial leukocyte <50,000/mm^3
- Female sex
- B cell type (4)
- Hyperdiploidy
- Trisomy 4, 10 (Translocations 8:14, 4:11, 9:22 – bad prognosis features)
- Response to treatment with prednisolone
- No LNE, HSM, CNS involvement

- Etopside
- Cytarabine
- Adriamycin
- *Maintenance phase:*
  - 6 mercaptopurine
  - Methotrexate
  - Prednisolone
  - Vincristine

CNS preventive therapy
- Intrathecal methotrexate and cranial irradiation.

AML (ACUTE MYELOID LEUKEMIA)

Clinical Features

- Short duration, fever, pallor, bleeding tendency, sternal tenderness
- Gum hypertrophy (AML – M4 M5)
- Chluroma (AML – M2)
- Oral petechiae
- Fundal hemorrhage
- Diffuse bone pain
- HSM, lymph node enlargement not common.

FAB Classification

1.	AML M0	– Undifferentiated	
2.	AML M1	– Acute myeloblastic leukemia with minimal maturation	
3.	AML M2	– AML with maturation – Most common, t(8:21)	
4.	AML M3	– Acute promyelocytic leukemia – t(15:17) – Increased risk of DIC – PML – RARα translocation	
5.	AML M4	– Acute myelocytic leukemia	Gum hypertrophy, organomegaly
6.	AML M5	– Acute monocytic leukemia – t(9:11)	Gum hypertrophy, organomegaly
7.	AML M6	– Acute erythrocytic leukemia (Di Guglielmo's syndrome)	
8.	AML M7	– Acute megakaryocytic leukemia – Associated with Down's syndrome	

Investigations

- CBC – TC
- PS – Myeloblast
- BM – Blast >20%
- Stained by – Sudan black, myeloperoxidase and nonspecific cytometry

Treatment

- Cytosine arabinoside + Daunorubicin
- AML M3 – All transretinoic acid (ATRA) and As_2O_3

TRANSFUSION DEPENDENT ANEMIAS

CLASSIFICATION OF ANEMIA

Due to Blood Loss

Increased destruction (hemolytic anemia)

- Intrinsic (intra-corpuscular)
  - Acquired
  - Hereditary

- RBC membrane defect, e.g. hereditary spherocytosis, hereditary elliptocytosis
- RBC enzyme defect, e.g. G6PD deficiency
- Disorder in Hb synthesis
  - Decreased globin
  - Abnormal globin
- Extrinsic (extra-corpuscular)
- Autoimmune hemolytic anemia, micro-AHA, DIC

Impaired Production

- Proliferation and differentiation of stem cell
  - Aplastic anemia, aplasia, pure red cell
- Proliferation and maturation of RBC
  - Decreased DNA synthesis, e.g. B_{12} deficiency, folate deficiency
  - Decreased Hb
    - *Heme*, e.g. Fe deficient anemia
    - *Globin*, e.g. thalassemia
  - Bone marrow (BM) infiltration

> - Pallor
> - Jaundice
> - Rule out SCA, Fe deficient anemia, G6PD
> - Rule out leukemia, aplastic anemia

HISTORY

- Pallor and its severity
  - Easy fatigability, tiredness, decreased concentration, breathlessness, progressive/not
  - Paroxysmal nocturnal dyspnea (PND), pedal edema, PICA, hookworm
- Jaundice
  - Time of appearance
- Abdominal distension

– AD – HS	<4 months
– AR – Thalassemia	6 months–2 years
SCA	1–5 years
– XR – G6PD	drug

- Leg ulcer (Sickle cell anemia)
  - Chest pain (Acute chest syndrome)
  - Extremity pain (Dactylitis)
  - Repeated left sided abdominal pain (Acute splenectomy)
  - Sudden increase in depth of pallor and jaundice (Hemolytic crisis)
  - Features of shock (sequestration crisis)
- History of drug intake, e.g. G6PD deficiency
- History of bleeding tendencies
  - (Aplastic anemia, leukemia, aplastic crisis, sequestration crisis)
  - Bleeding from orifices
  - Nasal bleed
  - Gum bleed

> **Triad to hemolytic anemia**
> - Pallor
> - Jaundice
> - Splenomegaly

APPROACH TO HEMOLYTIC ANEMIA

	Urine	**Stool**
Hemolytic	Normal	Normal
Obstructive	Cola colored	Pale
Hepatocellular	High colored	Normal

Associated Symptoms

- History of recurrent infection—leukemia
- History of bone pain

PAST HISTORY

- Blood transfusion and its complications.
- Age of onset

PEDIATRICS

- Frequency of blood transfusion
- Pretransfusion and post-transfusion changes
- Transfusion reactions
- Drug intake – folic acid
- Chelation therapy (History of chemotherapy/RT (aplastic anemia)
- Surgery – splenectomy, cholecystectomy

(*Gallstone risk*: HS > SCA > Thalassemia)

Complications of Transfusion

- Hep B – Fever + Jaundice
- Malaria
- Cardiomyopathy – CCF (arrhythmias is the most common cause of death around 10–20 years)
- Hypothyroidism – constipation, somnolence
- Hypoparathyroidism – tetany
- Diabetes mellitus/diabetes insipidus – polyuria, polydipsia
- Hypogonadism – delayed 2° sexual character , 1° amenorrhea
- Growth retardation
- Recurrent bacterial infection

Complication of Disease

- Sequestration crisis
- Hemolytic crisis
- Vasoocclusive crisis
- Aplastic crisis

Antenatal History

Anemia in pregnancy.

Natal

- Neonatal jaundice
- Sepsis
- Exchange transfusions

Developmental Delay

Diet

- Intake of Fe rich food
- Cooking in steel container
- Tea, chocolate decreased, Fe intake
- Milk cause Fe deficiency and poor in folate

Immunization

- HBV
- Pneumococcal (4 weeks prior to splenectomy)
- Meningococcal

Family History

- Consanguinity
- Similar illness
- History of splenectomy.

Socioeconomic Status

GENERAL EXAMINATION

- Hemolytic facies (Chipmunk facies)
  - Prominent frontal and parietal eminences
  - Flattened vault

- Straight forehead
- Hypertrophied muscles
- Prominent maxillae
- Prominent malar eminence
- Depressed nasal bridge

- Pallor, jaundice (Hepatitis B, hemolysis, Fe overload)
- Clubbing (CLD)
- Edema (CCF)
- LNE (Malignancy)
- Oral cavity (gum hypertrophy in leukemia)
- Eye (subconjunctival hemorrhage, proptosis in leukemia)
- Skin (Hyperpigmentation in Fe overload)
- Mucocutaneous bleed
- Thyroid swelling
- Skeletal deformity
  - Absent thumb – Fanconi's anemia
  - Thrombocytopenia absent radius (TAR) syndrome, (Diamond-Blackfan syndrome)
  - Abdominal distension
  - External genitalia (size of penis, scrotum, pubic hair)
  - External genitalia
  - Signs of liver failure

Pulse

- Tachycardia – CCF, anemia
- High volume – anemia
- Low volume CCF
- Peripheral pulsations embolism (sickle)

ANTHROPOMETRY

- Head circumference increases (frontal bossing)
- Height decreased (short stature)

Gastrointestinal System

- HSM
- **Cardiovascular system (CVS)**—CCF
- **Central nervous system (CNS)**—Compression myopathy

Examine parents for HSM (any hereditary disease)

Respiratory System

Chest syndrome

Diagnosis

- Transfusion dependent anemia
- Probably thalassemia
- With/without features of Fe overload
- With/without complications
- Protein-energy malnutrition

• Elevated reticulocyte count – Hemolysis – Recovery from vitamin/Fe • Deficiency – Hemorrhage – Sepsis, splenic sequestration – RHS • Low reticulocyte count – Fe deficiency anemia – Pure red cell aplasia – BM infiltration	• Feature of a post-splenectomy – Howel-Jolly bodies – Basophilic stippling – Anisopoikilocytosis – Heinz bodies – Normoblast • Immediate • Thrombocytosis and leukocytosis

PEDIATRICS

INVESTIGATIONS

- Hemoglobin and red cell indices
  - Low MCV and MCH
  - RDW – elevated
  - Fe deficiency anemia
  - Normal—thalassemia
- Total count
  - Leukocytosis – shift to left
  - Low platelet and WBC – hypersplenism
- ESR – elevated in all anemias except sickle cell anemia
- Reticulocyte count—elevated
  - Using supravital staining—crystal blue
  - Corrected reticulocyte count = patient's reticulocyte count × (patient hematocrit/Normal hematocrit)
- Peripheral smear
  - Microcytic hypochromic anemia (thalassemia, Fe deficiency anemia, sideroblastic anemia)
  - Anisopoikilocytes (different size and shape of RBC)
  - Polychromasia
  - Normoblast
  - Sickle cell (drepanocytes) in SCA
  - Spherocytes (HS, autoimmune hemolytic anemia)
  - Bite cell—G6PD deficiency
- Definitive diagnosis
  - In thalassemia, SCA – high performance liquid chromatography (HPLC)
  - Thalassemia major – HbA absent, HbF elevated
  - Thalassemia trait – HbA2 elevated, HbF normal/increased
- Sickling test: Using 2% Na metabisulphite
- Osmotic fragility
  - Using Kahn tube
  - Normally starts at 0.45% and ends at 0.35.
  - Increased in hereditary spherocytosis
  - Decreased in thalassemia
  - NESTROF (Naked Eye Single Tube Rapid Osmotic Fragility Test) – used for mass screening
- G6PD estimation – in G6PD deficiency
- Coombs test – AIHA (Autoimmune hemolytic anemia)
- Paroxysmal nocturnal hemoglobinuria (PNH)
  - CD55/C59 assay
  - Ham's test
  - Sucrose hemolysis
- Serum bilirubin
  - Elevated unconjugated bilirubin
  - Elevated LDH

  (Serum bilirubin, elevated unconjugated bilirubin, elevated LDH: Hemolytic anemia)
- Urine
  - Urobilinogen—elevated
  - Bile salt and bile pigment—absent
- CT, BT: If bleeding tendencies.
- Indication for bone marrow examination
  - Bone tenderness
  - Bleeding manifestations
- X-ray
  - Hair on end appearance on skull—thalassemia
  - Earlier X-ray change—metacarpal tuberculations

MANAGEMENT

- Blood transfusion
- Fe chelators

- Splenectomy
- Diet
- Drugs
- BM transplants
- Prenatal diagnosis and genetic counseling.

Aims of Management

- Limit size of spleen by suppressing extramedullary erythropoiesis
- Limit facial change by suppressing medullary erythropoiesis
- Promote normal growth and development
- Limit Fe overload
  If the Hb low—body absorb more Fe
  If transfused—decreased Fe absorption

1. **Blood transfusion**
   OP Ghai – Pretransfusion level 9–10 g/dL
   Types:
   - Low transfusion
     Pretransfusion level is maintained (6–10 g%)
   - Hypertransfusion
     - Keep pretransfusion level >10 g%
     - Transfuse blood to raise Hb to 12–13 g% when Hb<10 g%
     - Check Hb every 2–3 week

   Advantages
   - Maintain normal growth
   - Limit size of spleen
   - Supertransfusion

   Keep pretransfusion Hb> 12 mg%
   Give blood to keep Hb 14–15 g%
   - Transfusion reaction can be minimized by the saline wash (deplete leukocyte and plasma protein) using leukocyte filters
   - Allergic reaction can be prevented by giving hydrocortisone and antihistamines
   - Fe overload occurs after 10–20 transfusions due to:
     a. Increased GI absorption
     b. Transfusional siderosis

   Diagnosis: Serum ferritin > 1000 μg/L (ng/mL)
   Monitoring of Patient
   - Hb
   - Size of spleen (for Fe overload)
   - Serum ferritin (normal—300 ng/mL)
   - TFT
   - Serum calcium
   - FBS/PPBS
   - LFT, liver biopsy, USG abdomen, MRI liver
   - Chest X-ray, ECG, Echo, Cardiac T2 MRI
   - Evaluate height, hypogonadism
   - HBV, HIV
2. **Fe chelation**
   After 1–2 years of transfusion when ferritin level 1000–1500 μg/L
   a. **Deferoxamine**
      - *Dose*: 40–60 mg/kg/day S/C /over 8–12 hours. Daily night over 5–6 days/week by mechanical pumps
      - IV if cardiac failure occurs
      - Chelate Fe from ferritin and hemosiderin (not from transferrin).

      Adverse effect
      - Red discoloration of urine due to iron-deferoxamine complex excretion
      - Hypersensitivity

PEDIATRICS

- *Contraindication*: Renal failure, sensorineural hearing loss, visual toxicity
- *Monitoring*: Slit lamp, RFT, audiometry

b. Deferiprone
- 75 mg/day oral
- Mobilize Fe from transferrin, hemosiderin and ferritin
- Adverse effect:
  - Arthritis
  - Agranulocytosis
- Monitoring:
  - Joint examination
  - Total count

c. Deferasirox
- Oral 30 mg/kg/day
- Tridentate ligand finds Fe from intracellular and extracellular Fe throughout the body including liver, heart, reticuloendothelial system and circulation
- Adverse effect:
  - Rashes
  - GI toxicity, nausea, vomiting
  - Renal and hepatic toxicity

Monitoring: RFT, LFT

Shuttle Hypothesis
- Combination of oral and parenteral drugs is more effective

ICL-670
- New synthetic oral chelator
- It chelates Fe from parenchymal organs and RES
- Remove Fe directly from myocardial cell

Role of vitamin C

Vitamin C converts hemosiderin to ferritin from which Fe can be easily chelated 100 mg/daily

3. Splenectomy

Indications:
- Hypersplenism
- >12 whole blood transfusions/year
- >24 packed cell transfusion/year, >200–250 mL/kg/yr
- Splenic sequestration crisis in sickle cell anemia
- Hereditary spherocytosis (After 5 years is curative)

Hypersplenism criteria
- Splenomegaly
- Pan/bicytopenia
- Corrected by splenectomy
- BM normal/ hypercellular

Causes of cytopenia in hypersplenism
- Sequestration
- Increased splenic function
- Splenic phagocytosis
- Increased antibodies

Before splenectomy
- Pneumococcal vaccine
- Meningococcal vaccine
- Influenza
- Anti-malarial prophylaxis in endemic areas

After splenectomy
- Penicillin prophylaxis <5 years – 125 mg bd orally
>5 years – 250 mg bd orally
- Overwhelming post-splenectomy infection (OPSI)
- Fever in splenectomized patients should be considered as sepsis.

4. Diet
- Supplements of folic acid, ascorbic acid and vitamin E
- Fe preparation should not be given
- Drinking tea with meals decrease Fe absorption
- Avoid cooking in steel vessel

5. Drugs
- Folic acid – 5 mg/day
- Hydroxyl urea (15–20 mg/kg/day)
  - Increase production and reduce need for transfusion
  - It is leukemogenic

6. **Hematopoietic stem cell transplantation**
   - It is the only known curative treatment of thalassemia.
   - Poor outcome:
     - If hepatomegaly, portal fibrosis
     - Inadequate chelation prior to treatment
   - Types of stem cell transplantation
     a. Autologous – from patient
     b. Allogeneic – HLA matched sibling
7. **Prenatal diagnosis**
   - Genetic counseling
   - To create awareness and prevent thalassemia major in offspring
8. **Others**
   - Bone problem: Chipmunk facies
     - Osteoporosis
     - Bisphosphonate
     - Calcium
     - Vitamin D
   - Compression fractures of spine
   - Psychological counseling.

THALASSEMIA

Autosomal Recessive (AR)
- α - Decreased α globin synthesis
- β - Decreased β globin synthesis

β-thalassemia Major

- β^+/β^+ or β°/β° — β^+ decreased synthesis of β chain
- TDA — β° – absence of β

β-thalassemia Intermedia

- β^+/β°
- Monitor patient
- Blood transfusion not needed.

β-thalassemia Minor (Thalassemia trait)

- β/β^+ or β/β°
- Mild anemia
- HbA_2 increases

HbA – $\alpha_2\beta_2$	95%
HbA_2 – $\alpha_2\delta_2$	2–3%
HbF – $\alpha_2\gamma_2$	traces

α-thalassemia

- Absent/decreased α chain
- Newborn — Adult
- γ_4 (Hb Bart) (Hydrops fetalis) — β_4 Hb H

α-thalassemia Trait

α/α, -/- or α/-, α/-

Silent Carriers

-/α, α/α

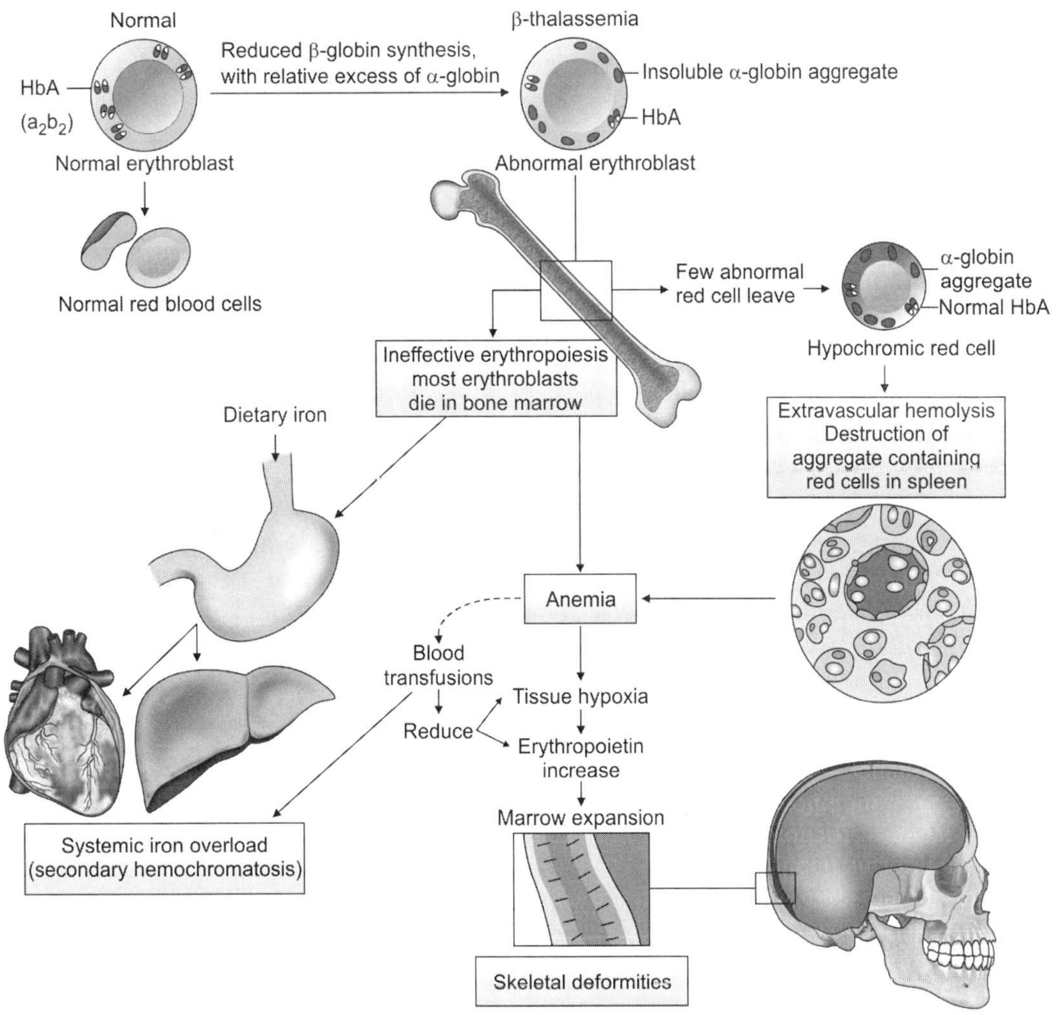

Complications of Thalassemia

- Iron overload
- Transfusion reactions
- Infections
- Hypersplenism
- Bone disease
- Extramedullary erythropoiesis
- Psychosocial complications

HEREDITARY SPHEROCYTOSIS

- Autosomal dominant (AD)
- Due to membrane protein defect in ankyrin/spectrin molecules
- Decrease membrane stability → loss of membrane fragment → spherocytes → less deformable → destruction in spleen.

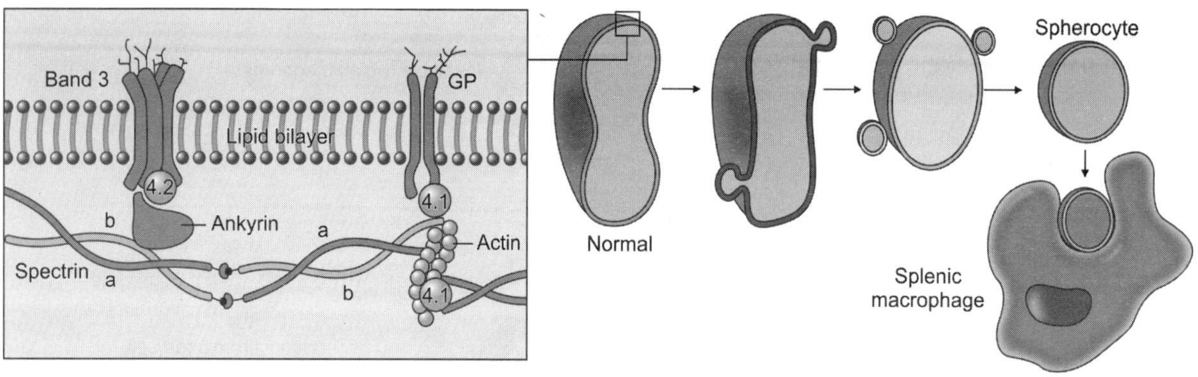

Clinical Features: Jaundice, splenomegaly, gallstones

Diagnosis

- Family history
- Increase osmotic fragility
- Decrease MCV
- Increase MCHC (very important) due to cellular dehydration

Treatment

- Folic acid 1–5 mg/day
- Splenectomy
- Cholecystectomy

THALASSEMIA VS HS

Thalassemia	HS
After first 6 month (6 months to 2 years)	Neonatal period (or at any time)
Jaundice—very minimal	Mild jaundice
Reticulocytes—2–8%	5–15%
Site of RBC destruction – bone marrow	spleen
Osmotic fragility—decreased	Increased

SICKLE CELL ANEMIA

Autosomal Recessive (AR)

6th position in beta chain, valine for glutamic acid (glutamic acid go)

Deoxygenation of heme moiety in HbS → interaction between adjacent HbS molecule → large polymer less deformable → obstruct microcirculation → increases hypoxia → increases sicking.

Life span RBC with HbS – 10–20 days.

Clinical Features

Pain, icterus, pallor, mild splenomegaly, tachypnea, infections, etc.

Crisis

V – Vaso-occlusive → pain dactylitis, hand foot syndrome, CVA, acute abdomen, priapism
A – Aplastic → in viral infection, folate deficiency
S – Sequestration → sudden fall of the hemoglobin >2 g/dL from baseline
I – Infiltration
A – Acute chest syndrome → chest pain, cough, tachypnea

Investigations

- Anemia
- Thrombocytosis

- Leukocytosis
- *Peripheral smear*: Sickle cell, target cell.

Howell-Jolly bodies (if asplenic)
- Sickling test
- Hb electrophoresis.

Management of Crisis
- Analgesics nacrotics
- Hydration
- Oxygen
- Blood transfusion—aplastic crisis/sequestration crisis
- Ventilation in CVA
- Exchange transfusion in CVA, chest syndrome

Preventive Care
- Penicillin prophylaxis at least until 5 year
- Pneumococcal, meningococcal, influenza vaccine
- Folate supplementation
- Hydroxy urea to increase HbF and to decrease crisis episodes
- Gallstone screening
- Genetic counseling.

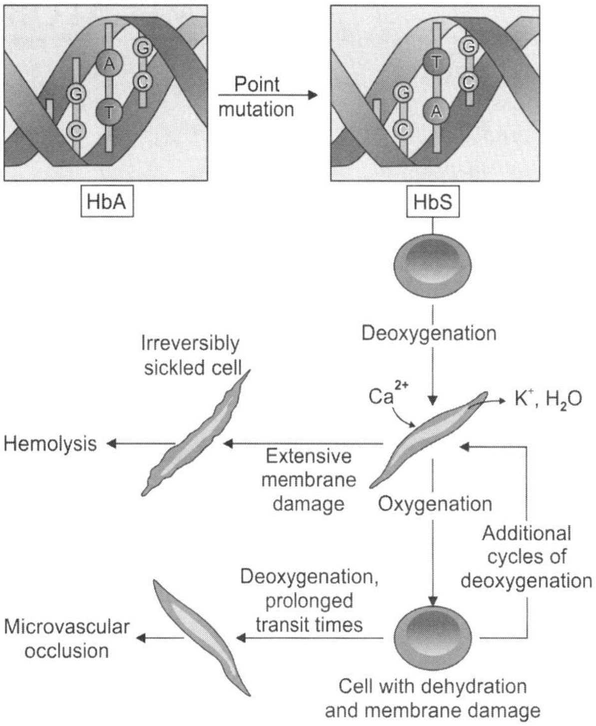

Fe DEFICIENCY ANEMIA

CLINICAL FEATURES

- Pica
- Koilonychia
- Angular stomatitis
- Glossitis

Investigations
- Low Hb
- Decreased MCV
- Decreased MCH
- Increased RDW

- Peripheral smear
  - Microcytic hypochromic anemia
  - Anisopoikilocytosis
- Serum Fe decreased,
- Serum ferritin decreased,
- Increased total iron binding capacity

Management

a. Ferrous sulfate
   - 3–6 mg/kg/day Fe
   - After correction of anemia
   - Continue oral Fe for 4–6 months to replenish Fe stores

b. Parenteral Fe
   - IV Fe sucrose preparation
   - Dose:

   Fe required = wt (in kg) × 2.3 × (15-patient's Hb) + 500 to 1000 mg
   - Given as divided doses

   Indications
   - Intolerance to oral iron
   - Malabsorption states
   - Rate of ingoing blood loss is more so that cannot be replenished by oral Fe.

c. Blood trasnfusions

   Indications:
   - Urgent surgery
   - Hemorrhage
   - Severe anemic with CCF

PEDIATRICS

MEGALOBLASTIC ANEMIA

Clinical Features

- Glossitis
- Stomatitis
- Oral ulcer
- Hyperpigmentation of skin, knuckle
- HSM (40%)
- Petechiae (25%)
- Neurological: Memory loss, confusion, loss of position and vibration sense.

Peripheral Smear

Macrocyte, cytopenia, hypersegmented neutrophil >6 lobe.

Bone Marrow

Cellular increased precursors.

Treatment

- Folate 1–5 mg/kg
- B_{12} 1 mg IM

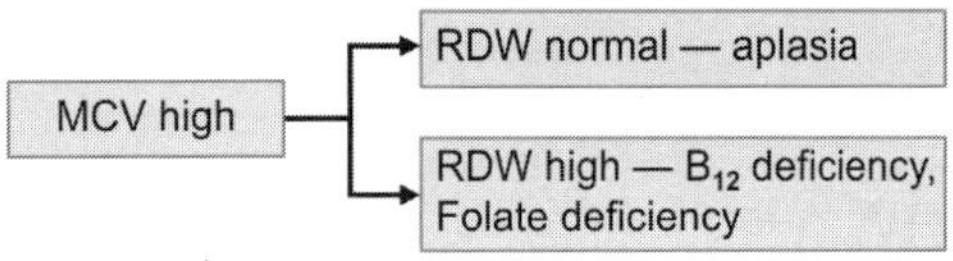

M – malaise, memory loss
E – easy fatigability
G – gray hair, a glossitis
A – anorexia
L – loss of weight
O – optic atrophy
B – bleeding manifestations, breathlessness, beefy tongue
L – liver and spleen enlargement
A – angular stomatitis
S – skin pigmentation SCD
T – thrombocytopenia
I – impotence
C – change in personality, confusion, CCF

CHAPTER 17

Renal, Arthritis and Pediatric Surgery

RENAL SYSTEM

APPROACH

- Renal edema
  - First on face, then lower limbs → ascites → hydrocele → scrotal edema
  - More in early morning
- History of acute glomerulonephritis
  - Hematuria (if present rule out drug history (rifampicin), colored food (Beetroot), bleeding manifestations, muscle injury—myoglobinuria)
  - Oliguria
  - Pyoderma, sore throat
- History of nephrotic syndrome
  - Frothy urine
  - Generalized edema
- History of Henoch-Schonlein purpura (HSP)
  - Abdominal pain, fever, rash, arthritis

  History of hemolytic-uremic syndrome (HUS)
  - Abdominal pain, diarrhea
- Rule out other causes of edema
  - Localized—insect bite reaction, lymphedema, angioedema
  - Generalized
    a. Cardiac cause
       First on dependant parts [Lower limb (LL), presacral edema]
       More in the evening
       Cardiac symptoms—orthopnea, paroxysmal nocturnal dyspnea (PND)
    b. Hepatic cause
       Early abdominal distension (ascites)
       Jaundice, bleeding manifestations
    c. Nutritional causes
       Associated growth retardation
       Recurrent infections
       History of nutritional deprivation
    d. Endocrine—hypothyroidism
- Complications
  - Nephrotic syndrome
    a. Spontaneous bacterial peritonitis—abdominal pain, fever
    b. Pleural effusion—breathlessness
    c. Pericardial effusion—pain on leaning forward
    d. Thrombosis
       » Pulmonary embolism—dyspnea, chest pain
       » Renal vein thrombosis—flank pain, hematuria

Edema causes
Cardiac
Hepatic
Endocrine
Renal
Inflammatory
Angioedema
Nutritional

  e. Steroid toxicity—peptic ulcer, Cushing syndrome, growth retardation
  f. Infection
- Acute glomerulonephritis (AGN)
  a. Acute renal failure (ARF)—oliguria, anuria
  b. Hypertensive encephalopathy—headache, vomiting, seizures, altered sensorium
- Left ventricular failure (LVF)—exertional dyspnea
  a. IgA nephropathy—recurrent hematuria, 2–5 days after respiratory illness.
  b. Alport's syndrome—family history of deafness.

Past history

- History of similar episodes in the past
  Number of episodes, treatment taken, monitoring in case of relapse, precipitating factors like urinary tract infection (UTI), respiratory tract infections. Response to drug
- Sore throat 1—2 weeks prior—strain 4, 12
  Pyoderma 2—4 weeks prior—strain 49
- Jaundice (Hep B, C), malaria—2° nephrotic syndrome
- TB → Steroid treatment→ Flaring up of TB.

Antenatal History

Oligohydramnios, fever with rash.

Developmental History

Gross motor delay, hearing—Alport's syndrome.

Diet

Any diet modification.

Immunization

Hep B, pneumococcal vaccine.

Family History

- Hearing loss—Alport's syndrome
- Systemic lupus erythematosus (SLE), renal diseases.

GENERAL EXAMINATION

- Pallor due to hemodilution (AGN)
  - Hemolytic-uremic syndrome
  - Severe hematuria
  - Chronic renal failure (CRF)
- Jaundice—Hep B, Hep C, hemolysis
- Edema.

$$\text{95th percentile BP (>1 year of age)} = \frac{100 + (\text{age in year} \times 3)}{70 + (\text{age in year} \times 1.5)}$$

Vitals

- Respiratory rate—effusion
- Blood pressure (BP)
- Jugular venous pressure (JVP)—right heart failure.

Head to Foot Examination

- Cushingoid facies—steroid toxicity
- Oral candidiasis—steroid treatment—immunosuppression
- Malar rash—SLE
- Features of liver disease(s)
- Skin—pyoderma scars
- Edema
- Vitamin D deficiency features.

PEDIATRICS

Anthropometry

Height decreased in:
- Steroid treatment
- Recurrent infections
- Hypothyroidism.

Examination of gastrointestinal system
- Abdominal wall edema—hold for 30 seconds
- Scrotal edema—very important finding
- Renal mass
- Henoch-Schonlein purpura
- Ascites.

Examination of respiratory system
- Effusion
- Basal crepitations
- Pneumonia.

Examination of cardiovascular system (CVS)
- Congestive cardiac failure
- Central nervous system (CNS)—Cortical vein thrombosis.

Diagnosis

- Generalized edema
- Due to renal disease(s)
- Probably nephrotic (relapse, which episode, treatment failure, etc.)
- Without complications.

ACUTE GLOMERULONEPHRITIS

1. Hypertension (HTN)
2. Hematuria
3. Oliguria
4. Edema
   (code H_2O_2)
   - Type 3 immune reaction following infection by Group A beta hemolytic streptococci
   - Intravascular fluid overload.

Causes of acute glomerulonephritis node (AGN)
- Post-infectious—streptococcal, staphylococcal, Hep B and C
- Systemic vasculitis—HSP, SLE, polyarteritis nodosa (PAN)
- Membranoproliferative glomerulonephritis (GN)
- IgA nephropathy
- Familial—Alport

INVESTIGATIONS

- Complete blood count (CBC)—Hb is low due to hemodilution
- Urine
  - Protein 1+/2+
  - Red blood cell (RBC)
  - White blood cell (WBC) due to glomerular inflammation [not intrauterine insemination (IUI)]
  - RBC cast, granular cast
- Renal function test (RFT)—in acute renal failure increased blood urea and serum creatinine
- Serum electrolytes—low Na, elevated K
- Low C3—singlemost important investigation (post-streptococcal)
- Antistreptolysin O (ASO) titer increased in >80% pharyngitis cases
  DNAase B >50% pyoderma cases
- Chest X-ray—hypervolemia
- Renal biopsy—indications
  - Hypertension, oliguria beyond 1 week (7–10 days)
  - Gross hematuria beyond 3–4 weeks
  - Low serum C3 beyond 12 weeks
  - Those with features of systemic illness
  - Nephrotic range proteinuria beyond 2 weeks
  - Mixed features of nephrotic and nephritic syndrome
  - Persistent proteinuria beyond 6 months.

MANAGEMENT

- Diet
  - Limit sodium, potassium, proteins
  - Avoid pickles, bakery items, pappads, salted fish, fruits rich in potassium, muringa leaves, tender coconut water
  - Carbohydrates and fats are allowed
    Calories = RDA + 10% extra
- Fluid intake—renal output + insensible water loss (400 mL/m^2/day)
- Weight (monitor daily) should lose 0.5% daily.
  Gain indicates fluid overload
  In severe oliguria, there is 0.5% loss of weight due to endogenous catabolism.
- BP—frequent monitoring (labile HTN)
  Mild—salt and water restriction, nifedipine, atenolol
  (Spironolactone, ACE inhibitors contraindicated)
  Hypertensive emergency—intravenous (IV) nitroprusside or labetalol
- Diuretics—oral frusemide
  IV frusemide in pulmonary edema
- Left ventricular failure
  - Propped up position
  - IV frusemide
  - Respiratory support with positive end expiratory pressure
- Prolonged oliguria
  Dialysis if
  - Severe renal failure
  - Fluid overload
  - Life-threatening electrolyte concentration
- Management of hyperkalemia (>5.5 mEq)
  - Stop intake of potassium and offending drugs
  - Glucose insulin infusion
  - $NaHCO_3$ infusion
  - IV calcium gluconate
  - IV salbutamol or nebulization
  - Dialysis
  - Potassium binding ion exchange resin
- Pyoderma lesions—even if healing, penicillin for 10 days (prophylaxis).

Course of AGN
- Urinary protein excretion and HTN becomes normal by 4-6 weeks
- Persistent microscopic hematuria may persist for 1–2 years after the initial presentation

MONITORING

- Intake output chart daily
- Monitoring pulse, frequent BP measurement, respiratory rate (labile HTN)
- Daily temperature chart
- Daily weight monitoring.

Hematuria—presence of more than 5 RBC/HPF

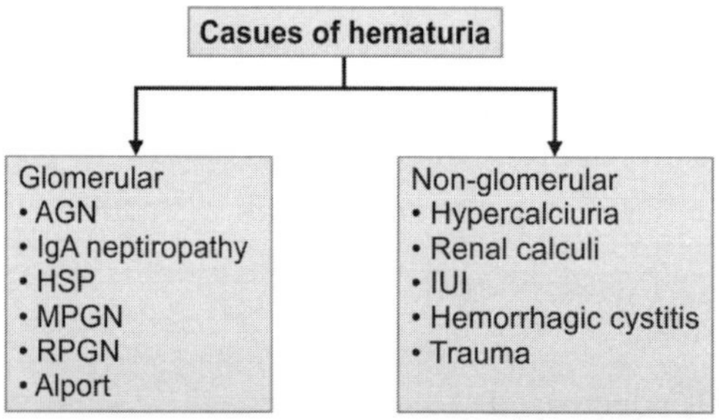

(AGN: acute glomerulonephritis; IgA: immunoglobulin A; HSP: Henoch-Schonlein purpura; MPGN: membranoproliferative glomerulonephritis; RPGN: rapidly progressive glomerulonephritis; IUI:intrauterine insemination)

LOCALIZATION OF BLEEDING SITES IN HEMATURIA

- Glomerular
  - Cola colored
  - Proteinuria
  - RBC cast
  - Deformed RBCs
- Ductal convoluted tubule (DCT) and collecting duct
  - WBC and epithelial casts
- Lower urinary tract
  - Gross hematuria
  - Terminal hematuria
  - Normal RBCs.

Complications
- Acute renal failure
- LVF, pulmonary edema
- Hypertensive encephalopathy

Blood pressure
- Length at least 80% of arm circumference
- Width 40–50% of arm circumference.

FLUSH METHOD IN INFANTS

Mean BP = diastolic + 1/3rd pulse pressure

Doppler method is accurate.

Hypertension:
- Average systolic/diastolic BP
- 95th percentile for that age and sex in at least 3 occasions, 50th percentile of spontaneous bacterial peritonitis (SBP) in children more than 2 years = 90 + 2 × age in years.

On discharge:
- BP should be normal
- Renal output should be normal
- No complications.

NEPHROTIC SYNDROME

INVESTIGATIONS

- Hb—elevated if there is contracted plasma volume due to hypoalbuminemia
  - Total count (TC), and differential count (DC) increased even in the absence of infections
  - Erythrocyte sedimentation rate (ESR) to rule out TB.
- Urine:
  - 24 hour urine protein more than 40 mg/m^2/h or 1 g/m^2/day
  - Protein-creatinine ratio more than 2
  - Pus cells >5/hpf—UTI in males
  - >10/hpf—UTI in females
  - RBC >5/hpf—hematuria.
- RFT—if abnormal indicates different histology or acute renal failure
- Liver function test (LFT)
  - Serum albumin <2.5 g/dL
  - Serum globulin normal or elevated
- Lipid profile
  - High density lipoprotein (HDL) decreased
  - Low density lipoprotein (LDL), Very low density lipoprotein (VLDL), total cholesterol increased
- Serum C3 low in atypical presentation, otherwise normal

Etiology
- Idiopathic—90%
  Minimal change—85%
  Mesangial proliferative—5%
  FSGS—10%
- Secondary (10%)—membranous
  Membranoproliferative glomerulonephritis (MPGN)

- Chest X-ray—to rule out tuberculosis (TB), effusion
- USG abdomen—kidney size, ascites
- Mantoux—TB
- Indication for renal biopsy
  - Age <1 year, >8 year
  - Hematuria
  - Low C3
  - Hypertension
  - Impaired renal function
  - Frequent relapses
  - Steroid resistance.

	Acute glomerulonephritis	**Nephrotic syndrome**
• Age group	Older (school going)	2–6 years
• Preceding illness (skin, throat infection)	Present	Not
• Pathogenesis	Immune complex	Minimal-T cell dysfunction
• Onset	Acute	Insidious
• Hematuria, HTN	Present	Absent
• Edema	+	+++
• Recurrence	Rare	Present
• Urine	RBC cast, granular cast	Fat laden cells
• Albuminuria	Moderate	Massive
• Serum cholesterol	Normal	Increased
• Hb	Hemodilution	Hemoconcentration

MANAGEMENT

- Diet
  - No added salt
  - High normal good quality protein diet
  - High cholesterol, low fat
  - No water restriction
- Treat any associated infection
- Diuretics:
  - If significant edema
  - Frusemide 1–4 mg/kg/day in 2 divided doses
  - Spironolactone 2–3 mg/kg/day
  - Should be cautious since plasma volume contraction may already be present and may lead to hypovolemic shock
- Specific management

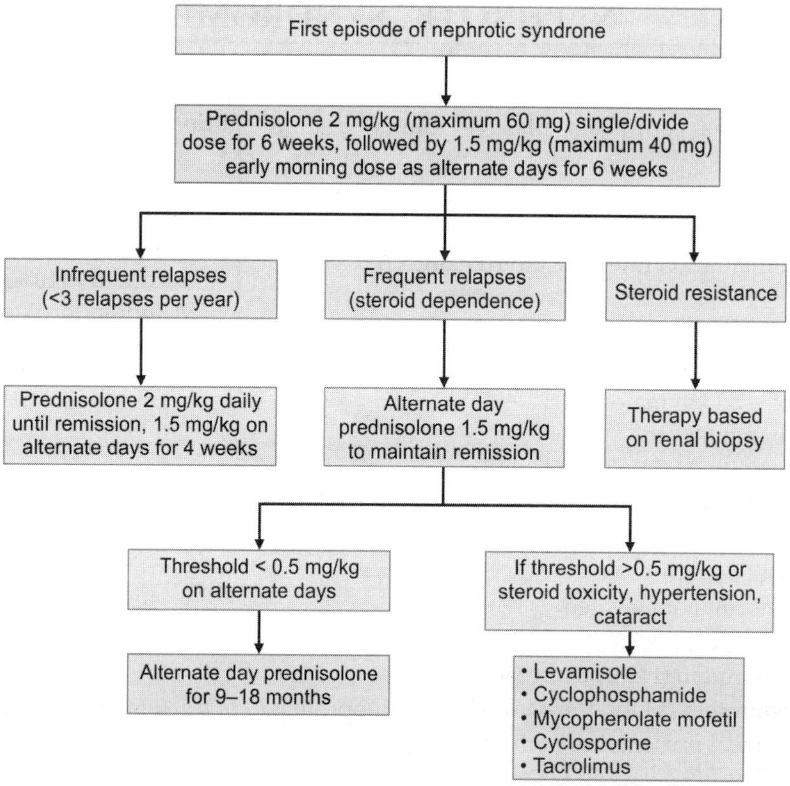

- Remission: Urine albumin nil or trace (or proteinuria <4 mg/m²/hr) for 3 consecutive days in early morning specimens.
- Relapse: Urine albumin 3+/4+ (or proteinuria <40 mg/m²/hr) for 3 consecutive days in a patient who was in remission.
- Frequent relapses: 2 or more relapses in 6 months or 4 or more in 12 months.
- Steroid dependence: Two consecutive relapses when on alternate day steroids or within 14 days of its discontinuation.
- Steroid resistance: Absence of remission despite therapy with daily prednisolone for 4 weeks and alternate day for next 4 weeks.

- Human albumin:
  - If serum albumin <1.5 g%
  - Symptomatic ascites
  - Symptomatic hypovolemia
  - Dose: 1g/kg over 30–60 minutes followed by frusemide.

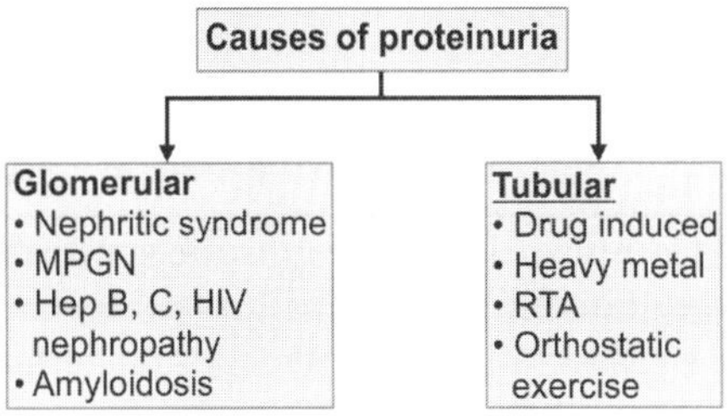

(MPGN: membranoproliferative glomerulonephritis; HIV: human immunodeficiency virus; RTA: renal tubular acidosis)

MONITORING

- Blood pressure, temperature
- Input output chart
- Daily weight
- Urine albumin

Nephrotic syndrome is defined as a clinical state characterized by:

- Edema
- Proteinuria >40 mg/m²/hr
- Hypoalbuminemia <2.5 g/dL
- Hypercholesterolemia.

1. ***Edema—causes***
   - Proteinuria → hypoalbuminemia → decreased oncotic pressure → extravasation of fluid in interstitial spaces
   - Increased secretion of renin-angiotensin system → sodium and water retention
   - Increased secretion of antidiuretic hormone (ADH) → water retention
   - Blunted responsiveness to atrial natriuretic peptide.
2. ***Proteinuria:***
   - Normal protein excreted in urine <150 mg/day, normal protein excretion <4 mg/m²/hr, abnormal 4–40 mg/m²/hr, nephrotic range >40 mg/m²/hr
   - *Transient proteinuria*—after fever, exercise, etc. does not reach 2+, no evaluation or treatment needed
   - *Orthostatic proteinuria*—if child with persistent asymptomatic proteinuria to rule out orthostatic proteinuria,
     - Supine—normal/slight proteinuria
     - Upright position—up to 10 fold
     - Diagnosis—absence of proteinuria (p:c <.2) in first morning urine sample for 3 consecutive days.

   Causes of proteinuria:
   - Loss of fixed negative charges from glomerular basement membrane
   - Abnormality of epithelial foot processes (podocytes)

   Heat and acetic acid test:

   Fill 2/3rd of test tube with urine and heat upper part of test tube. A coagulum is formed at the top. Add few drops of 3% acetic acid and compare with the lower part.

   Other method useful—sulphosalicylic acid test.

Proteinuria	While reading newspaper across test tube
Trace	Clear (0.1 g/dL)
1+	Can read bold and small letter (0.3 g/dL)
2+	Can read bold letters, not small ones (1 g/dL)
3+	Can read bold letters, not small ones can (3 g/dL)
4+	Nothing is seen (10 g/dL)

3. ***Hypoalbuminemia***
   - Due to selective proteinuria
   - <2.5 g/dL
   - Edema appears when serum albumin <2 g/dL
   - Pleural and pericardial effusion may appear when serum albumin <1.5 g/dL

4. *Hypercholesterolemia*
   - Due to hepatic synthesis of lipoproteins 2° to hepatic synthesis of albumin (due to closely related pathways)
   - Increased loss of lipoprotein lipase in urine.

   Lipid profile—VLDL and LDL increased
   HDL normal or increased in MCNS.

Causes of 2° Nephrotic Syndrome

- Collagen vascular disease—rheumatoid arthritis, SLE, polyarteritis nodosa (PAN)
- Infections—hepatitis B, *P. malariae*
- Malignancies—leukemia, lymphoma
- Endocrine—diabetes
- Drugs—captopril, nonsteroidal anti-inflammatory drugs (NSAIDs), penicillamine

Complications of nephrotic syndrome
- Edema
- Infections—spontaneous bacterial peritonitus (SBP)
  - Pneumonia
- Thrombotic complications
  - Due to hemoconcentration
  - Loss of antithrombin, protein C, S
  - Increased fibrinogen
  - Immobilization
- Steroid toxicity
- Acute renal failure
- Abnormal growth and nutrition

Henoch-Schonlein Purpura

Palpable purpura in the presence of at least one of the following four features:
1. Diffuse abdominal pain—intermittent, colicky, periumbilical
2. Any biopsy showing predominant IgA deposition
3. Arthritis or arthralgia
4. Renal involvement (any hematuria +/– proteinuria).

Treatment—supportive with maintenance of hydration and pain relief.
Oral corticosteroid + cyclophosphamide initially followed by maintenance steroid and azathioprine.

Hemolytic-Uremic Syndrome

Characterized by microangiopathic hemolytic anemia, thrombocytopenia and acute (a/c) renal insufficiency
- D+ HUS in 2–3 years old follows *Shigella dysentriae*
- D- HUS any age lacks history of diarrhea/dysentery.

IgA Nephropathy

- IgA deposits in mesangial cells and capillary wall
- Hematuria/proteinuria, recurrent episodes
- Biopsy—IgA deposition
- Treatment
  - ACE inhibitors
  - Corticosteroid + cyclophosphamide.

APPROACH TO ARTHRITIS

Arthritis is swelling/effusion in joint or,
Two out of the following four:
1. Joint pain (arthralgia)
2. Tenderness

Swelling is not a must to diagnose arthritis

PEDIATRICS

3. Warmth
4. Limitation of range of movements.

HISTORY

- **Onset**
  - Acute <2 weeks
    a. Acute rheumatic fever
    b. Transient synovitis
    c. Kawasaki disease
    d. Septic arthritis
    e. Henoch-Schonlein purpura.
  - Subacute 2—6 weeks
    a. Reactive arthritis
    b. SLE, PAN
    c. Dermatomyositis
    d. Lyme disease, brucellosis.
  - Chronic > 6 weeks
    a. Juvenile idiopathic arthritis (JIA)
    b. Ankylosing spondylitis
    c. Tuberculosis
    d. Psoriasis
    e. Legg-Calve-Perthes disease
- **Site**
  - Peripheral joints—SLE, vasculitis
  - Axial—JIA
- **Number of joints**
  - Monoarthritis
    - Post-traumatic
    - Septic arthritis
    - Hemarthrosis
    - TB arthritis
    - Oligoarticular—4 joints or less
    - Polyarticular—5 joints or more, e.g. acute renal failure (ARF), reactive arthritis, rheumatoid arthritis, SLE, PAN, e.g. viral, ARF, poncet, lyme disease, Kawasaki disease
- **Additive:** JIA, Migratory—ARF, gonococcal
  - Distal interphalangeal joints – psoriatic arthritis
  - Knee, ankle, elbow—Acute rheumatic fever
    - Pauciarticular
      » Type 1—knee, elbow, ankle
      » Type 2—large joints of lower limb
    - Polyarticular
      » RF +ve—Metacarpophalangeal (MCP) joint, proximal IP joint, cervical spine, temporomandibular joint (TMJ)
      » RF -ve—knee, hip, wrist.
- **Time**: Night pain, disturbing sleep—malignancy
  - During activity mechanical pain
  - Morning stiffness—JIA
- **Fever:** Quotidian fever with twice daily peak – Systematic onset juvenile idiopathic arthritis (SOJIA)
- **Rash**
  - Salmon colored transient, evanescent with spike of fever with central clearing, more common in trunk (SOJIA)
  - Erythema marginatum—ARF
  - Erythema chronicum migrans—lyme disease
  - Dermatomyositis—Heliotropic rash + Gottron papules.
- **Recurrent ulcer**: Behcet's disease.

PEDIATRICS

- **Disability:**
  - Daily activities limitation
  - School days lost
  - Deformities.
  - **Arthritis mimickers**:
    - Growing pain (4–8 year)—localized to calf muscle, occurs in night
    - Benign hypermobility of joint
    - Chondromalacia patella.

HEAD TO FOOT EXAMINATION

- Eye
  - Non-purulent conjunctivitis—Kawasaki disease (KD)
  - Uveitis—JRA
- Oral cavity—ulcer in Behcet's disease
  - Strawberry tongue in KD.
- Skin
  - Psoriatic patches
  - Malar rash
  - Erythema marginatum, subcutaneous nodules—ARF
  - Subcutaneous nodules—over occipital protuberance, spine of scapula, medial and inferior borders of scapula, spinous process of vertebra, extensors of forearm, dorsum of hand, iliac crest, shin, foot
- Nail pitting, onycholysis—psoriasis
- Malignancy features—petechiae, pallor, lymph node (LN) enlargement.

EXAMINATION OF JOINTS

1. Inspection
2. Palpation
3. Range of movements
4. Measurements.

- Cervical spine—whether able to touch the ear on either shoulders
- TM joint—opening of mouth (able to pass 3 fingers in mouth)
- Shoulder—whether able to touch opposite shoulder with hand
- Elbow—refer orthopedist
- Wrist
- Hip
- Knee
- Ankle—inversion and eversion
- Ankylosing spondylitis (AS)
  - Mark a vertical line (10 cm) on the skin overlying lumbar spinous process and sacral dimples, and measuring the increase in line length on flexion, normally this should be 5 cm or more (Modified Schober's test)
  - Draw a line 10 cm above and parallel to iliac crest and 5 cm below
  - Ask the patient to flex
  - Normally the distance between these two = 21 cm
  - In AS, it is <21 cm.

Other Systems

- **Gastrointestinal tract (GIT)**—hepatosplenomegaly (HSM) (to rule out malignancy, SOJIA)
- **Cardiovascular system (CVS)**—to rule out ARF
- **Respiratory system**—dyspnea
- **Renal**—HSP
- **Nervous system**—chorea, fits, psychosis.

Grades of joint tenderness
I—patient says
II—patient winces
III—patient winces and withdraws the affected part
IV—will not allow to touch

JUVENILE RHEUMATOID ARTHRITIS

Investigations

- Complete blood count (CBC)
  - Hb—anemia

- DC—increased (neurophils)in Sojia
- Thrombocytosis
- Erythrocyte sedimentation rate (ESR)—elevated
- C-reactive protein (CRP)—for follow-up (note RF is for prognosis)
- Antinuclear antibodies—to rule out collagen vascular disease
- Slit lamp examination:
  - ANA +ve—3 months follow-up
  - ANA –ve—6 months follow-up
- Joint X-ray—early soft tissue swelling, cortical erosion
- Synovial aspiration—in monoarthritis to rule out septic arthritis
- Bone marrow—to rule out leukemia, before steroid treatment
- ECHO—to rule out ARF
- Ultrasonogaphy (USG) abdomen.

Management

- NSAIDs
  - Naproxen
  - Ibuprofen
  - Indomethacin
  - Diclofenac
- Disease modifying anti-rheumatoid drugs (DMARDs)
  - Methotrexate 15–25 mg/m^2/week + folic acid
  - Gold
  - D-penicillamine
  - Hydroxychloroquine
- Steroids
  - Intra-articular—triamcinolone
  - Topical—in uveitis
  - Systemic—in unremitting arthritis, systemic manifestations (prednisolone)
- Biological
  - Etanercept—tumor necrosis factor (TNF) receptor fusion protein
  - Infliximab—monoclonal antibody (MAB) again TNF alpha

JIA definition according to American College of Rheumatology (ACR):
- Criteria of JIA
- Age <16 years
- Arthritis in more than or equal to 1 joint
- Duration $\geq$ 6 weeks
- Onset type defined by articular involvement in 1st, 6 months of age—poly, oligo, SOJIA
- Exclusion of other causes of juvenile arthritis

ACR Classification

- Pauciarticular-onset JIA (< or = 4 joints)—hip never involved
  - Type 1—young girls, uveitis
  - Type 2—boys may develop AS
- Polyarticular onset JIA (> or = 5 joints)
  - Rheumatoid factor +ve—similar to rheumatoid arthritis
  - Rheumatoid factor –ve
- Systemic onset JIA

1970—ACR - JRA 3 types
1977—EULAR - JCA 6 types
1997—ILAR - JIA 6 types

International League of Association for Rheumatology (ILAR)

Use term—juvenile idiopathic arthritis

PEDIATRICS

ILAR-JIA	SOJIA
• Onset <16 years arthritis	• Daily fever—for 2 weeks
• Duration >6 weeks	• Quotidian for at least 3 days
• Types • Systemic onset	• 1 or more of following:
• Oligoarticular-< or = 4 joint	– Evanescent erythematous rash
• Polyarticular > or = 5 joint	– Generalized lymphadenopathy
• Psoriatic	– HSM
• Enthesitic arthritis	– Serositis

DOWN SYNDROME

- Trisomy of chromosome 21
- Incidence increases with maternal age (exposure of maternal oocyte to harmful environmental influences for longer period, since Graafian follicles are present in the fetal life).

CAUSES

- Miotic non-disjunction of chromosome 21 (94%)
- Translocation—4% (14, 21)
- Mosaicism—1%

HISTORY

Presenting Complaints

- Delayed milestones
- Recurrent urinary tract infection (UTI)
- Motor clumsiness
- Complaints related to other system abnormality like CVS, GIT, etc.

Antenatal

Age of mother at conception, polyhydramnios, 1% risk in mother > 35 years old.

Natal

Flailness at birth.

Postnatal

Prolonged jaundice (hypothyroidism), poor activity.

Developmental Delay

Delay in milestone, decreased in scholastic performance.

Family History

History of Down syndrome in siblings.

HEAD TO FOOT EXAMINATION

- Skull appears small, brachycephalic with flat occiput
- Epicanthic eyefold, upward slant eye, cataract, nystagmus
- Flat facies
- Small nose with flat nasal bridge
- Furrowed and protruding tongue, small teeth, narrow short palate (mouth)
- Ears are small, conductive hearing loss and prone to serous otitis media
- Clinodactyly (hypoplasia of middle phalanx with single flexion crease of 5th finger), simian crease, sandle gap (wide gap between 1st and second toe)
- Thorax—small sternum
- Genitals—small external genitals

Other Examination

- CVS—congenital heart disease [endocardial cushion defects, ventricular septal defect (VSD), mitral valve prolapse (MVP)]
- Respiratory—RTI, obstructive sleep apnea, hypoplastic lung
- GIT malformation—duodenal atresia, Hirschsprung's disease, gastroesophageal reflux disease (GERD), tracheoesophageal fistula (TEF)
- CNS—Mental retardation (MR), hypotonia, weak reflexes, spinal cord compression (atlantoaxial dislocation), Alzheimer's like dementia
- Musculoskeletal—Congenital dislocation of hip (CDH), lax joints
- Endocrine—thyroid dysfunction—hypothyroidism, diabetes mellitus (DM), short stature, obesity, annular pancreas
- Immune—decreased T cell immunity
- Hematological—leukemia, transient myeloproliferative disorder.

MANAGEMENT

- Early stimulation
- Physiotherapy
- Speech therapy—visual and hearing
- Nutritional support, immunization
- Treat complications
- Prenatal diagnosis (karyotyping of cell done by):
  - CVS (10–12 weeks)
  - Amniocentesis (16–18 weeks)
  - Cordocentesis (after 18 weeks)
  - Triple test—AFP (decreased), BHCG (increased), estriol (decreased)
    Quadruple test—tripple + inhibin A (increases)
  - USG
    - 1st trimester—nuchal translucency
    - 2nd trimester—nuchal fold thickness
    - Short femur length
    - Short humerus length
    - Duodenal atresia.

PYREXIA OF UNKNOWN ORIGIN

Fever 101°F for which no cause is identifiable after 1 week of inpatient investigation and duration lasting 3 weeks or more.

CAUSES

- Infection
  - Tuberculosis
  - Brucellosis
  - Enteric fever
  - Infective mononucleosis (IMN)
  - Infective endocarditis (IE)
  - Malaria
  - Urinary tract infection (UTI)
- Collagen vascular diseases—SOJIA, SLE, Kawasaki disease (KD), polyarteritis nodosa (PAN)
- Malignanacy—lymphoma, leukemia
- Abscess—subdiaphragmatic abscess, hepatic abscess
- Factitious—drug intake (anticholinergic)
- Munchausen by proxy syndrome
- Familial dysautonomia (anhidrotic ectodermal dysplasia).

History

- Travel history
  - Enteric fever
  - Malaria
- Sore throat—IMN
- History of contact with TB
- Evening rise of temperature—TB
- History of heart disease—IE
- Arthritis—collagen vascular disease
- Anemia, bleeding manifestation—malignancy—lymphoma, leukemia
- Recurrent infection—HIV
- Dysuria, urgency—UTI
- Animal contact—brucellosis.

General Examination

- Pallor—malaria, malignancy, IE
- Icterus—malaria
- Clubbing—IE
- Lymph node
- Rash—KD, SOJIA, SLE
- Petechiae—leukemia
- Features of IE
- Malar rash
- Oral ulcer
- Coated tongue—enteric fever
- **CVS**—murmurs—IE
- **Abdomen**—HSM.

INVESTIGATION

- CBC, Hb, TC, DC
- ESR
- Widal
- Peripheral smear—cells, malaria
- LFT
- Blood culture
- URE, culture
- CXR, Mantaux
- Echocardiography
- Antinuclear antibody (ANA)
- Paul Bunnel/Monospot test
- Bone marrow (BM)

PEDIATRIC SURGERY

RESPIRATORY DISTRESS IN NEWBORN

Medical Causes

- Respiratory distress syndrome
- Meconium aspiration syndrome
- Pneumonia
- Transient tachypnea of newborn
- Persistent pulmonary hypertension

Surgical Causes

- Tracheoesophageal fistula
- Lobar emphysema
- Congenital diaphragmatic hernia.

Congenital Diaphragmatic Hernia

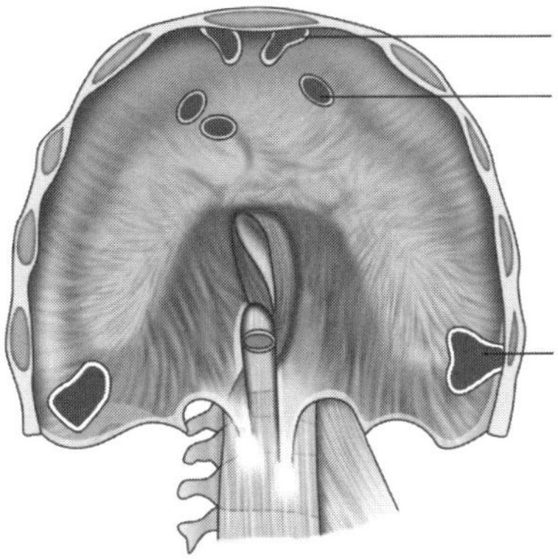

Types

- Esophageal hiatal hernia
- Through foramen of Morgagni
- Posterolateral—most common (Bochdalek hernia)
- Paraesophageal hernia.

Pathology

- Lung hypoplasia
- Surfactant deficiency
- Failure of fusion of pleuroperitoneal canal.

Clinical Features

- Respiratory distress
- Scaphoid abdomen
- Mediastinal shift
- Bowel sounds in chest
- It is a medical emergency
- Pulmonary hypoplasia → persistent pulmonary hypertension → cyanosis → hypoxia
- Prenatal diagnosis—USG at 16–24 weeks
- Investigations—chest X-ray neck to knee and abdomen with nasogastric tube.

Contraindication for bag and mask ventilation
- Diaphragmatic hernia
- Meconium stained liquor

Management

- Ventilation (no bag and mask ventilation)
- Nitric oxide—pulmonary vasodilator
- Surgery—transabdominal approach (subcostal approach)
  - Reduction of contents
  - Repair of sac
  - Increase the volume of abdominal cavity by stretching.

Tracheoesophageal Fistula

Types

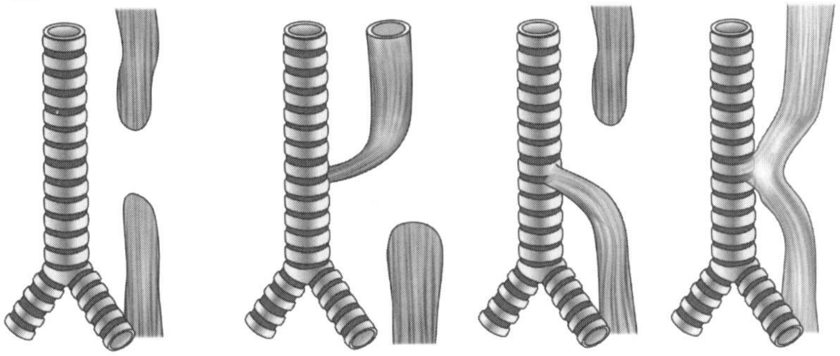

A **B** **C** (Most common) **D** (H type)

- Clinical features—respiratory distress
- **Complications**
  - Pneumonia
  - Gastroesophageal reflux disease (GERD)
  - Atelectasis
- **Prenatal diagnosis**
  - Polyhydramnios in mother
  - Single umbilical artery

- **Investigations**
  - Orogastric tube cannot be passed to stomach
  - Plain X-ray shows coiled feeding tube.

Management

- Prone head down position
- Chest physiotherapy
- Frequent suction
- IV fluid
- Surgery—Right thoracotomy
  - Via 4th space
  - Identify and disconnect
  - Anastomosis of upper and lower pouch
- Associations (VACTERL)
  V—vertebral anomalies
  A—anorectal atresia
  C—cardiac anomalies
  T—trachea
  E—esophageal fistula
  R—renal anomalies
  L—limb anomalies.

NON-BILIOUS VOMITING

- Hypothyroidism
- Septicemia
- Maternal drugs
- Congenital adrenal hyperplasia
- Infantile hypertrophic pyloric stenosis (IHPS)
- Gastric volvulus
- Gastroesophageal reflux.

Infantile Hypertrophic Pyloric Stenosis

Rule of 4

- Incidence 4 in 1000
- Male : female 4:1
- Presentation 4 days–4 months
- Symptoms
  - Non-bilious vomiting—progressive, projectile, persisting
  - Visible gastric peristalsis—left to right
  - Palpable pyloric mass in right hypochondrium
  - Voracious appetite
- Metabolic derangement
  - Hyponatremia
  - Hypokalemia
  - Hypochloremic metabolic alkalosis
- Signs
  - USG
  - Muscle thickness >4 mm (Doughnut sign)
  - Canal length >14 mm
  - Barium meal
    - String sign/double track sign
    - Shoulder sign
    - Beaking

PEDIATRICS

- Surgery—Ramstedt's pyloromyotomy
  Four approaches:
  1. Via linea alba
  2. Lateral to rectus
  3. Supraumbilical
  4. Rectus splitting
- Recurrence: 4%
- Mortality: 0.4%.

BILIOUS VOMITING

Causes

- Duodenal atresia—6 hours after food
- Jejunoileal atresia—24 hours after food
- Meconium ileus—48 hours after food
- Necrotizing enterocolitis
- Malrotation
- Volvulus
- Intussusception.

INTUSSUSCEPTION

Rule of 6

- Most common
  - Idiopathic: 94%
  - Secondary causes: 6%
- Age: 6 months
- Six symptoms
  1. Abdominal distension
  2. Lump
  3. Abdominal pain
  4. Vomiting
  5. Bleeding per rectum (red currant jelly stool)
  6. Rectal prolapse.
- Six signs
  1. Sausage shaped mass with concavity towards umbilicus
  2. Sign de dance—empty right iliac fossa
  3. Target sign in USG
  4. Pseudokidney sign in USG
  5. Claw sign in barium meal
  6. Coiled spring in barium meal
- Management
  - Conservative (6% resolves)—in vitro fertilization (IVF), nasogastric tube, antibiotics
  - Hydrostatic saline
  - Barium
  - Pneumatic reduction
  - Squeezing
  - Resection and anastomosis.

> - Single bubble sign: Pyloric stenosis
> - Double bubble sign: Duodenal atresia
> - Tripple bubble sign: Jejunoileal atresia

DELAYED PASSAGE OF MECONIUM

Causes

- Prematurity
- Sepsis
- Hypothyroidism
- Birth asphyxia
- Hirschsprung's disease

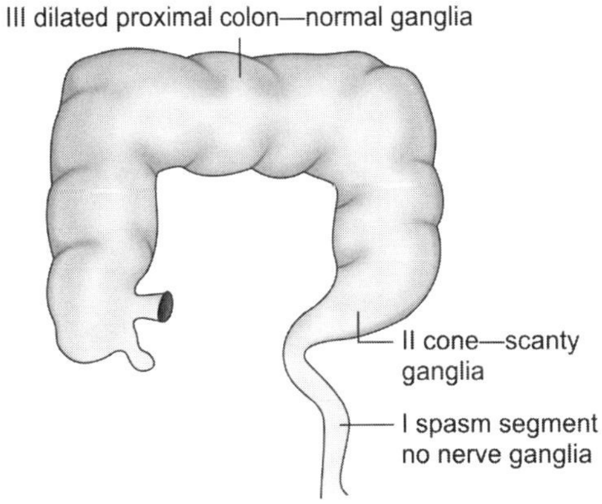

- Anorectal malformation
- Meconium ileus
- Atresia.

HIRSCHSPRUNG'S DISEASE

- Congenital megacolon
- Absence of Auerbach's and Meissner's plexus
- Arrest of descend of neural crest cell
- Mutation in the RET proto-oncogene in chromosome 10
- Male: female 4: 1
- Associated diseases—Down syndrome, ventricular septal defect (VSD).

Three Zones

I. Distal immobile spastic segment (aganglionic zone)
II. Middle transitional zone—with sparse ganglion
III. Normal hypertrophied dilated segment (normal ganglionic area).

Types

- Ultrashort segment—anal canal and terminal rectum
- Short segment—anal canal + rectum
- Long segment—anal canal + rectum + part of colon
- Total colonic—anal canal + rectum + whole colon.

Clinical Features

- Delayed passage of meconium, fail to pass within <8 hours, bilious vomiting, abdominal distension, constipation
- Introduce rectal thermometer and withdraw gradually, there will be a spurt of meconium.

Investigations

- X-ray abdomen—absence of rectal gas shadow
- Barium enema—transition zone, abnormal rectosigmoid ratio
- Rectal biopsy—gold standard—shows hypertrophy of nerve terminals with increased acetyl choline (Ach) esterase activity
- Anorectal manometry—absence of rectoanal inhibitory reflex.

Management

- After diagnosis
  - Antibiotics
  - Decompression
  - Temporary colostomy
- Definite management
  - Swenson's procedure—removal of aganglionic segment and coloanal anastomosis
  - Duhamel operation—remove distal part, bring proximal colon behind rectum, crush wall between rectum and colon
  - Soave operation—mucosectomy and endorectal pull through
- Complications
  - Enterocolitis and sepsis
  - Perforation
  - Constipation.

ANORECTAL MALFORMATIONS

Imperfect fusion of allantoic gut with proctodeum.

Types (Wing Spread Classification)

- High
  ± fistula

- Anorectal agenesis
- Rectal atresia
- Rectovaginal fistula
- Intermediate
  - Anal agenesis
  - Males—rectovesical, rectourethral fistula
  - Females—rectovaginal, rectovestibular fistula
- Low
  - Anal stenosis
  - Anocutaneous fistula.

Clinical Features

- High—flat perineum, absence of dimple, associated with fecal incontinence
- Low—meconium in perineum, anal membrane through which meconium is visible, associated with constipation.

Associations

VACTERL (or VATER syndrome)

Investigations

- Invertogram
  - 2 line in invertogram
- Prone cross-table lateral radiograph (PCTLR).

Management

- Low
  - Anoplasty
  - Incision of anal membrane
- High
  - Initial colostomy
  - Followed by posterior sagittal anorectoplasty (PSARP).

POSTERIOR URETHRAL VALVE

- Congenital symmetrical valve in posterior urethra just below verumontanum
- It allows passage of catheter
- But obstruct urine outflow
- Proximal urethra enormously dilated with obstructive pathology in bladder
- Hypertrophied
- Sacculation and diverticula
- Cricket ball bladder (palpable in suprapubic area).

Clinical Features

- Poor urinary stream
- History of infections
- Hydronephrosis.

Investigations

- Micturating cystourethrography (MCU)
- Intravenous urogram (IVU)
- USG abdomen
- Blood urea, serum creatinine—renal failure
- Antenatal USG—bilateral hydronephrosis.

Treatment

- Initial suprapubic catheterization

- After several weeks, resection of posterior valve
- Endoscopic ablation, fulguration.

VESICOURETERIC RELUX

Causes

- Congenital—associated with posterior urethral valve
- Acquired—trauma, after surgery
- Primary—isolated
- Secondary—associated with other anomalies

Grading on Micturating Cystourethrography

I. Ureters seen
II. Ureters and pelvis seen
III. Ureters, pelvis, calyces seen with no or mild blunting of calyceal fornices
IV. With grossly distended calyces with complete obliteration of sharp angles of calyceal fornices
V. Tortuous elongated serpentine ureters.

Investigations

- Urine microscopy, culture and sensitivity
- Blood urea and serum creatinine
- Intravenous urogram
- Micturating cystourethrogram.

Management

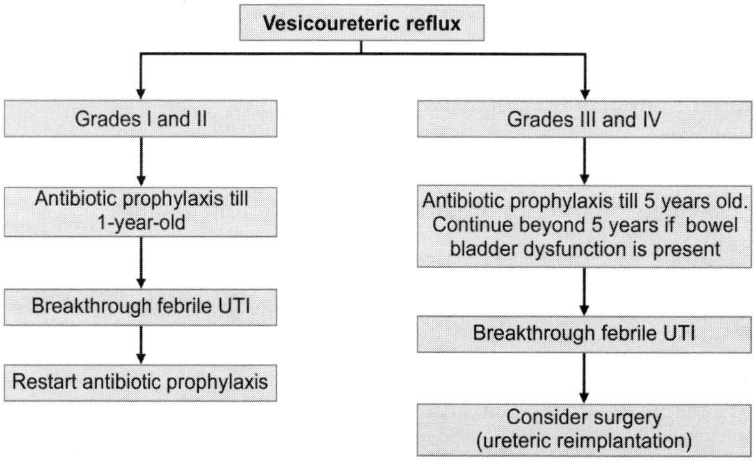

(UTI: Urinary tract infection)

CHAPTER 18

Viva

CASE CHARTS

1. A 10-year-old boy presented with high fever, jaundice, severe myalgia, headache, conjuctival congestion, complete blood count (CBC). There is increase in white blood cell (WBC) count (which predominantly neutrophil).
   a. What is most probable diagnosis?
   b. What is etiological agent?
   c. Give complication.
2. A 2-year-old child is unimmunized. He has fever, cough, coryza since 5 days. On examination, he has maculopapular rash.
   a. Mention most probable diagnosis.
   b. What other pathognomic sign will you look for?
   c. Mention complication.
3. A 1½-years-old child is admitted with cough and fever of 2 days duration. She is lethargic and not feeding. On examination her respiratory rate (RR) is 70/min, cyanosis, lower chest retraction present.
   a. What is your probable diagnosis?
   b. What is Rx?
   c. Name 3 investigations.
4. A 5-year-old Unni fully immunized is admitted with weakness of both lower limbs. No sensory neural symptoms or urinary involvement. No history of trauma.
   a. What is most probable diagnosis?
   b. To whom you report?
   c. Write specification of stool sample collection.
   d. What other investigation you will do?
5. Cerebrospinal fluid (CSF) study in a 5-year-old child with high-grade fever with generalized seizures.
   Pressure—increased, protein—108 mg%, sugar—24 mg%
   Microscopy—cells polymorphs—98%, Lymphocyte—2%
   a. Diagnosis.
   b. Most probable organism.
   c. Drug of choice.
   d. What bedside examination you like to perform before lumbar puncture (LP)?
6. A 4-year-old child admitted with fever, headache, vomiting, CSF, findings are—color clear, tension increased, protein—40 mg%, sugar – 30 mg%, microscopic examination—15 lymphocytes/high-power field (HPF)
   a. What is diagnosis?
   b. What precaution you will take before LP?

7. 8-month-old girl admitted with 1 day history of vomiting, loose watery stools without blood. The mother says baby is thirsty, crying always, urine output decreased.
   a. Discuss the plan of management.
   b. Any 5 relevant clinical signs you look for?
   c. Advice on discharge.
   d. What advice to prevent further episodes?
8. 8-year-old child is brought to casualty with hematuria.
   Urine findings:
   Urine microscopy—plenty of pus cells/hpf
   Urine albumin—++
   a. Write down 5 questions to be asked in history.
   b. What is the most probable diagnosis?
   c. Three common complications.
9. 8-year-old fully immunized boy is admitted with 2 day history of progressive weakness of both lower limb (LL) and difficulty in walking. He gives history of fever and running nose 10 days back. On examination tones of both his LL were reduced with grade 2 power, absent knee and ankle jerks and down going plantars. No sensory impairment or muscle tenderness or signs of meningeal irritation.
   a. Most likely diagnosis.
   b. Three differential diagnosis.
   c. Most dangerous complication.
   d. Specifications of sample to be sent.
   e. Two investigations to confirm the diagnoses.
10. Baby of Mini, born of full-term normal delivery (FTND) weighing 3 kg brought to you with complain of jaundice.
    a. Give 3 questions you will ask mother first.
    b. Name 3 clinical signs you look for.
11. A 4-year-old child brought with multiple ecchymotic patches and purpuric spots.
    a. Write 4 important points you will ask in history.
    b. Name 2 relevant investigations.
    c. Two differential diagnosis.
12. A 3-year-old child gives history of poor vision after sunset. On examination of bulbar conjunctiva shows dry greyish area.
    a. What is nutritional deficiency and eye lesion?
    b. Name 2 other eye signs.
    c. How will you treat the condition?
13. A 12-year-old child was brought with history of difficulty in opening mouth, pain of back and neck muscles. History of wound in left index finger 1 week back.
    a. Most probable diagnosis.
    b. Four essential steps in management.
    c. How will you prevent?
    d. Two complications.
14. A 2 years unimmunized child admitted with weakness and areflexia of 1 week duration.
    a. Define acute flaccid paralysis (AFP)
    b. Step you will take after acute management done.
15. Define kwashiorkor.
    a. Mention 3 complications.
    b. Give the therapeutic diet to be given in initial phase of treatment.
16. A 9-year-old child is admitted with fever, vomiting. She is disoriented and her deep tendon reflexes are brisk. Hemoglobin (Hb) – 12.8 g, total count (TC) – 6500, P – 45%, E – 5%, erythrocyte sedimentation rate (ESR) – 15 mm/1st hour.

Serum bilirubin – 9.6 mg, Direct – 3.6 mg, serum glutamate-pyruvate transaminase (SGPT) – 1176 IU
   a. What is diagnosis?
   b. Write any 2 relevant questions in history.
   c. List 2 investigations.
   d. Management.
17. A 3-year-old child has come with history of poor apetite, poor activity for past few weeks. On examination child is pale, no jaundice, no HSM laboratory investigation given below:
   Hb–7 g%, TC–10500/mm^3, mean corpuscular volume (MCV)–60, mean corpuscular hemoglobin (MCH)–26
   a. What is the first investigation you will do?
   b. Two important points you will ask in history.
   c. Treatment.
18. A 7-year-old child was admitted with fever, cough, not responding to injection CP from outside hospital. RR 20/min, auscultation revealed occasional creps, chest X-ray revealed bilateral disproportionately large non-homogenous opacities.
   a. What is the likely organism?
   b. Other organism causing this.
   c. Drug of choice
19. A 3-week-old child on presented with non-bilious vomiting, since 4 days.
   a. Most likely diagnosis.
   b. Clinical features of child.
   c. Which is the intravenous fluid of choice?
   d. Definitive management.
20. A 2-month-old infant presented with yellowish discolaration of sclera with normal colored urine, pallor.
   a. Most likely diagnosis.
   b. Peripheral smear findings.
   c. Confirmatory test.
   d. Pattern of inheritance.
21. An 11-month-old child presented with epistaxis and gum bleeding. On examination multiple ecchymotic patches are seen. Abdomen within the normal limit (WNL). Bleeding time (BT)-12 minutes, Clotting time (CT)-16 minutes, activated partial thromboplastin time (aPTT)-1 minutes, partial prothromboplastin time (PTT)-12 seconds, platelet-3 lakh mm^3.
   a. What is the likely diagnosis?
   b. Confirmatory test.
   c. Drugs used.
22. A 14-day-old baby of Sangeetha presents with prolonged jaundice delayed passage of meconium, poor cry, floppiness and poor sucking.
   a. Most likely diagnosis.
   b. Radiological investigation you will do.
   c. Important screening test.
   d. Drug used.
23. A 32-week-old preterm of diabetic mother presented with respiratory discomfort. On examination RR-62/min, grunting, cyanosis.
   a. Most likely diagnosis.
   b. What is the bedside test?
   c. Treatment
   d. How will you prevent this?
24. How will you differentiate term and preterm infant?

ANSWERS

1. a. Leptospirosis
   b. Leptospira icterohemorrhagica
   c. Liver failure, renal failure, myocarditis, acute respiratory distress syndrome (ARDS), thrombocytopenia.
2. a. Measles
   b. Koplik's spot
   c. Otitis media, pneumonia, giant-cell pneumonia, croup, meningoencephalitis, subacute sclerosing panencephalitis (SSPE).
   d. Vitamin A, 2 lakh IU (because 2-year-old child).
3. a. Very severe pneumonia
   b. Ampicillin + Gentamicin → Ceftriaxone/Cefotaxime
   c. Chest X-ray, CBC, sputum microscopy.
4. a. Guillain-Barre syndrome (GBS)
   b. District immunization officer.
   c. Two specimen, at least 24 hour apart, collected within 14 days of paralysis onset, each having adequate volume (8–10 g) and sent to World Health Organization (WHO) accredited laboratory in reverse cold chains.
   d. Cerebrospinal fluid (CSF) study, electromyography (EMG).
5. a. Bacterial meningitis
   b. *Neisseria*
   c. Penicillin 4 lakh IU/kg/Day for 7–10 days
   d. Fundoscopy to rule out papilledema.

   CSF Normal Value
   Total protein—20–40 mg/dL
   Glucose—40–60 mg/dL

	Pyogenic	Tuberculous	Viral
Appearance	Turbid	Clear	Clear
On standing	—	Cobweb coagulation	—
Protein	Increased		
Sugar	Decreased	Decreased	Normal
Cells	Predominantly neutrophil	Lymphocyte	Lymphocyte

6. a. TB meningitis
   b. Rule out infection
   Rule out bleeding abnormality
   Rule out increased intracranial pressure (fundoscopy).
7. a. Some dehydration
   b., c., d. } Refer ADD
8. a. History of drug intake (Rifampicin), food intake (Beetroot), oliguria, edema, pyoderma, sore throat.
   b. Acute glomerulonephritis (AGN)
   c. Left ventricular failure (LVF)
   Renal failure
   Hypertensive encephalopathy
9. a. Guillain-Barre syndrome
   b. Polio, traumatic neuritis, transverse myelitis
   c. Respiratory muscle paralysis
   d. Read Q No. 4
   e. CSF study, EMG
10. a. Whether jaundice appeared within 24 hours, it stains nappy.
    Clay colored stool.
    Blood group of baby and mother.
    b. Pallor
    Hepatosplenomegaly (HSM)
    Hypothyroidism

11. a. History of easy fatigability (Aplastic anemia)
    History of recurrent infection, bone pain (leukemia)
    Prior history of viral infection [immune thrombocytopenic purpura (ITP)]
    Drug intake
    Arthralgia, abdominal pain, oliguria [Henoch-Schonlein purpura (HSP)].
    b. Complete blood count (CBC), peripheral smear, bone marrow.
    c. ITP, aplastic anemia.
12. a. Vitamin A deficiency
    Refer chapter—Nutrition
13. a. Tetanus
    b. Neutralize absorbed toxin—TIG 500–1000 IV IM.
    Prevent further toxin production
    Control spasm—diazepam.
    General measurement—hydration, nutrition.
    c. Giving TT vaccination
    d. Respiratory obstruction and convulsion.
14. Read acute flaccid paralysis (AFP)
15. Kwashiorkor—read chapter nutrition [Protein-energy malnutrition (PEM)]
    a. Infection, growth retardation, hypoglycemia
    b. F-75
    Breastfeeding.
16. a. Viral hepatitis with encephalopathy
    b. Similar illness in surrounding
    Food from outside
    History of vaccination
    c. EEG, USG abdomen
    d. Supportive measurement—nutrition, bed rest
    Lactulose
    Treatment of the precipitating factor.
17. a. Peripheral smear
    b. History of pica
    History of worm infestation
    c. $FeSO_4$ (3–6 mg/kg/day) and continue oral Fe 4–6 months after correction of anemia.
18. a. *Mycoplasma pneumoniae*
    b. *Chlamydia, Legionella*
    c. Macrolide (Azithromycin, erythromycin).
19. a. Infantile hypertrophie pyloric stenosis (IHPS)
    b. Abdominal mass, visible gastric peristalisis, succusion splash
    c. Here there is loss of hyponatremia, hypokalemia, hypochloremia with alkalosis (loss of Na, K, Cl, H)
    Treatment: 5% Dextrose, ½ NS, KCl
    d. Ramstedt's pyloromyotomy.
20. a. Hereditary spherocytosis (HS)
    b. Microcytes, spherocytes
    c. Osmotic fragility
    d. Autosomal dominant.
21. a. Von Willebrand disease (vWD)
    b. Ristocetin induced aggregation
    c. Tranexamic acid, epsilon aminocaproic acid (EACA).
22. a. Congenital hypothyroidism
    b. X-ray knee-absence of ossification center in upper tibia and lower femur
    c. TSH >100 μg/mL
    d. L-thyroxine– 10–15 μg/kg/day (ideally lifelong).
23. a. Respiratory distress syndrome (RDS)
    b. Shake test

c. Continuous positive airway pressure, intratracheal surfactant
d. Injection betamethasone 12 mg IM, 2 dose, 24 hour apart.

24. **Clinical assessment of term and preterm**

	Term	Preterm
Hair	Silky hair-individual strands can be made out	Fuzzy hair
Ear	Well-curved pinna, cartilage reaching up to periphery	Flat, soft pinna, cartilage not reaching up to periphery
Breast	Well-formed breast bud (>5 mm)	Poorly formed breast bud
Genitalia	Well pigmented, pendulous scrotal sac with fully descended testes or Labia majora covering clitoris and labia minora	Light pigmentation, not yet descended testes or Prominent labia minora and clitoris
Soles	Deep transverse creases	No deep creases
Popliteal angle	Acute	Obtuse
Scarf sign	Absent	Present
Arm recoil	Recoil	No

ADVICE AND HISTORY TAKING

- **Assessment of a case of diarrhea:**
  - Rapport and consent
  - General appearance of patient
  - Anterior fontanelle
  - Eyes: Sunken/not; tears
  - Tongue, buccal mucosa: Dry/not
  - Skin pinch
  - Edema
  - Pulse, blood pressure (BP)
  - Capillary filling time
  - Ask for urine output frequency
  - If time persists, ask for a glass of water and bring it near the child and assess the thirst.

> **Remember the following things**
> - Stand on right side
> - Always ask name, age, make rapport
> - Ask consent and explain procedure
> - Redress the child
>
> Any marking (with chalk) that you made should be erased before leaving the child

- **Advice on the discharge of a child with diarrhea:**
  - Rapport and consent
  - Explain the condition of disease to the mother
  - Explain to her about preparation of oral rehydration solution (ORS) and the frequency of administration
    - Boil and cool 1L of water (5 glasses)
    - 1 packet of ORS is dissolved in 1L of water
    - 2–3 spoons every 5–10 minutes after every episode of diarrhea
    - Continue breastfeeding and all other home available solutions (kanji, lassi, solution made of sugar and salt)
    - Discourage bottle feeding
    - Next day, new ORS should be used.
  - If there is any complication, take the child to a hospital: Blood in stools, repeated watery stools, marked thirst, drinking poorly, altered sensorium
  - Preventive measures:
    - Drink boiled and cooled water
    - Clean utensils
    - Breastfeeding
    - Immunization
    - Handwashing
    - Discourage bottle feeding
    - Environmental sanitation

  - Do not eat food from outside
  - At last, ask for any doubts.
- **Advice on immunization:**
  - Rapport and consent
  - Ask the age of the child
  - Explain the importance of immunization
  - Why it was not taken?
  - Look for Bacillus Calmette-Guerin (BCG) scar
  - Tell the mother that all are available free of cost
  - Whether other children in the family have been immunized
  - Mention about an optional vaccine
  - It will not cause any harm to the child
  - Not contraindicated in mild illness (fever)
  - Explain the importance of PPI
  - Ask if she has any doubts.
- **Advice on prophylaxis of febrile seizures:**
  - Rapport and consent
  - Explain the condition to the mother
  - During febrile episodes, explain to the mother to decrease the temperature by using: Light clothing, a ventilated room, tepid sponging, tablet paracetamol
  - Clobazam (if on intermittent prophylaxis)
  - Rush to the doctor if temperature does not subside
  - In case of seizures:
    - Keep the child away from danger
    - Do not put anything into the mouth
    - Keep the head tilted to one side
    - Explain about immunization
    - Side effects of diazepam
    - Ask if she has any doubts.
- **A 7-year-old child admitted with seizures, started on antiepileptics (sodium valproate). Advice the mother on discharge.**
  - Rapport and consent
  - Explain the condition to the mother
  - Tell her about the drug administration
  - Never discontinue or miss any drug
  - Inform the doctor if some other drugs are taken
  - Explain the side effects
  - Precautions during an episode of seizures
  - Ask her if she has any doubts.
- **Advice on discharge of a child with nephrotic syndrome:**
  - Rapport and consent
  - Explain the condition to the mother and reassure her
  - Tell her that there are chances for relapse
  - Tell her about the drug administration
  - Side effects of drugs: Moon face
  - Dietary advice: Avoid yolk, fatty food, excess salt
  - Manage infection early
  - Weekly BP monitoring
  - Educate the mother on heat and acetic acid test:
    - Fill 3/4th of a test tube with urine and heat the upper part by tilting it over a flame. Then add 8 drops of vinegar (acetic acid). Hold the test tube in front of a newspaper and try to read through it.
    - Can read small letters clearly: Nil
    - Can read but unclear: 1+
    - Can read only headlines: 2+
    - Cannot read headlines but can see them as a dark area: 3+
    - Cannot see the paper at all : 4+

- If reading comes as 3+ or 4+ for 3 consecutive days, then as her to consult a doctor and report it
- Ask her if she has any doubts.

- **Advice regarding breastfeeding:**
  - Rapport and consent
  - Position: Tummy to tummy; chest to chest; chin to breast; baby to mother and not mother to baby
  - Burping
  - Exclusive breastfeeding up to 6 months
  - Discourage bottle feeds
  - Continue breastfeeding during the disease
  - Breastfeeding up to 2 years
  - Advantage to mother:
    - Reducing chance of postpartum hemorrhage (PPH)
    - Protection against pregnancy
    - Reduces risk of cancer of breast and ovary
    - Emotional bonding
  - Advantage to baby:
    - Nutritional superiority
    - Immunologic superiority
    - Mental growth (IQ)
  - Immunization and advice on weaning
  - Ask her if she has any doubts.
- **Advice on discharge of a child on anti-tubercular treatment (ATT):**
  - Rapport and consent
  - Explain the condition to the mother and reassure
  - Isolation of the child is not needed
  - Tell her about the drug administration
    - 3 drugs—2 months
    - 2 drugs—4 months
    - Rifampicin—on an empty stomach
  - Never discontinue the drug during any other illness
  - Orange discoloration of urine is not a problem
  - Explain about directly observed treatment short (DOTS)
  - Screening of other family members
  - Ask her if she has any doubts.
- **Advice on weaning:**
  - Continue breastfeeding
  - Start weaning at 6 months
  - Weaning food—ragi
  - Start one weaning food at one time
  - Hygiene is very important—clean utensils and handwashing
  - Initially, there may be diarrhea and vomiting; if severe, consult a doctor
  - Immunization
  - Doubts.
- **History taking of a child with febrile seizures:**
  - Rapport and consent
  - Whether it is the first episode or a recurrence
  - Onset (within 24 hours after fever), duration, number of attacks
  - Whether moving all his limbs or local (focal/generalized)
  - Any loss of consciousness
  - Any abnormal behavior in the postictal period
  - Any associated headache, vomiting (increased ICT)
  - Whether seizures in the absence of fever
  - Whether seizures present before 6 months
  - Any stoppage of antiepileptics
  - Any developmental delay
  - Any family history of seizures.

- **Take a case history of diarrhea:**
  - Rapport and consent
  - When the episode began
  - Number of stools passed, frequency, color, consistency, smell, frothy
  - Is it bloody
  - Is there any associated fever, vomiting, abdominal pain
  - Urine output
  - Are eyes sunken or normal
  - Do tears come while crying
  - Thirst of the child
  - History of feeding—bottle feeding, breastfeeding, any history of weaning, food from outside
  - Sensorium, seizures, abdominal distension
  - Contact with similar illness
  - Fully immunized or not
  - Any drugs
  - Source of drinking water, environmental sanitation.
- **Assessment of jaundice in a neonate:**
  - Age of child (pathological/physiological jaundice)
  - Never look in the eyes
  - 1st apply pressure over the tip of the nose and look for yellowish discoloration in the blanched skin
  - Apply pressure over the face, chest, abdomen below umbilicus, overskin, overfoot, palms, soles in that order (Kramer's dermal zone)
  - Urine and stool culture
  - Umbilical sepsis
  - Activity of child
  - Any bleeding
  - Comment on the level of jaundice.

DRUGS—PEDIATRICS

1. **Hydrocortisone**
   Short-acting glucocorticoid
   Uses:
   - Status asthmaticus (25–50 mg/kg/dose IV 6 hourly)
   - Endotoxic shock
   - Adrenal insufficiency.
2. **Aspirin**
   NSAID (acetylsalicylic acid)
   Uses:
   - Anti-inflammatory dose—90–120 mg/kg/day orally 4 hourly in acute rheumatic disease
   - Antipyretic dose—30–60 mg/kg/day orally 4–6 hourly should be avoided in empty stomach

   Side Effects—peptic ulceration, hypersensitivity (Rye's syndrome).
3. **Paracetamol**
   Uses:
   - Analgesic
   - Antipyretic
   - Dose—40–60 mg/kg/day QID
     Or

   5 mg/kg IM (injection).
4. **KCl**
   Used in hypokalemia
   1–2 mEq/kg/day 8th hourly
   Max dose—20 mEq/h.
5. **Ketoconazole**
   Imidazole group of antifungals

PEDIATRICS

Effective in dermatophytes, candidiasis
Dose—3–6 mg/kg/day orally single dose
Side Effects—gynecomastia, thrombocytopenia, photophobia.

6. **Ceftriaxone**
   A 3rd generation cephalosporin
   Widely used in meningitis (high concentration CSF)
   Dose—100–150 mg/kg IV 12th hourly.
7. **Phenytoin**
   Hydantoin class of antiepileptic drug
   Dose—5–10 mg/kg/day
   Uses:
   - Epilepsy
   - 1–2 dose given slow IV
   - Cardiac arrhythmia.

   Side effects:
   - Hirsutism
   - Osteomalacia
   - Fetal hydantoin syndrome
   - Megaloblastic anemia
   - Gum hyperplasia
   - Toxicity, if blood level >20 ng/dL.
8. **Antiretroviral drug**
   Nucleoside reverse transcriptase inhibitor (NRTI)—zidovudine, stavudine, lamivudine
   Non-nucleoside reverse transcriptase inhibitor (NNRTI)—nevirapine, efavirenz
   Protease inhibitor—indinavir, ritonavir.
9. **Atropine sulfate**
   Anticholinergic drug
   0.01 mg/kg/dose SC or IV
   Indicated in supraventricular tachycardia
   Side effects—dry mouth, blurred vision, tachycardia, constipation.
10. **Chloramphenicol**
11. **Cotrimoxazole**
12. **Albendazole refer medicine**
13. **Metoclopramide**
14. **Chlorpheniramine maleate**

    (10–14: Refer medicine)

    0.5 ng/kg/day per orally 8th hourly
    Antihistaminics
    Side effects—hypotension, sedation, urinary retention.
15. **Salbutamol**—bronchodilator
    Short-acting beta agonist
    Bronchodilator and antiasthmatic agent
    Dose—0.1–0.4 ng/kg/dose orally 8th hourly.

INSTRUMENTS

1. **Bone marrow needle**
   - Salah and Klima
   - Salah—with guard

   Indications:
   - Diagnostic—hematological malignancies, immune thrombrcytopenic purpura (ITP), storage disorder, infection like kala-azar, pyrexia of unknown origin (PUO), megaloblastic anemia
   - Therapeutic—intraosseous infusion.

   Contraindication:
   - Infection, bleeding disorder.

PEDIATRICS

Sites: Iliac crest/posterosuperior iliac spine
- Tibia (infants)
- Sternum (Body).

2. **Lumbar puncture needle**
   Site: Between L3 and L4 or L4 and L5
   Indications:
   - Therapeutic—to give drugs, spinal anesthetics.
   - Diagnostic—meningitis, GBS, convulsions, subarachnoid hemorrhage.

   Complication:
   - Infections—trauma, coning

   Contraindications:
   - Bleeding disorder, infection, raised intracranial tension (ICT).
   - Before doing this procedure fundus is examined to rule out papilledema.
3. **Liver biopsy needle**
   - Vim Silverman needle, Menghini needle.

   Indications:
   - Cirrhosis, storage disorder, Wilson's disease, hemochromatosis, malignancies.

   Contraindications:
   - Prolonged prothrombin time (PT), infection at site, thrombocytopenia, biliary obstruction.

   Complications:
   - Infection, bleeding, injury to liver.

   Site:
   - 10th intercostal space (ICS) in midaxillary line (MAL) in the supine position.
4. **Nasogastric tube (Ryle's Tube)**
   - Stomach wash, aspiration of fluid
   - There is metal beads at the end.
5. **Infant feeding tube**
   No metal beads.
   Uses:
   - Gastric lavage
   - To diagnose esophageal atresia, tracheoesophageal fistula
   - To feed a child not taking orally
   - Catheterization
   - Intrarectal diazepam.
6. **Intravenous cannula—venipuncture for infusion of IV fluids, drugs, etc.**
7. **Scalp vein set**
   - Butterfly shaped

   Uses:
   - To withdraw blood
   - To give medication, IV fluids.
8. **A 3 way connector**
   T shaped device containing 2 inlets and 1 outlets
   Uses:
   - Pleural or ascitic fluid
   - Exchange transfusion
   - Hemodialysis.
9. **Endotracheal tube**
   - Curved tube used for intubation
   - Distal end has Murphy's eye (opening in the lateral wall)
   - It can be cuffed or uncuffed
   - Administration of anesthesia
   - Used in unconscious patient with respiratory difficulty
   - To carry out artificial respiration.
10. **Tongue depressor**
    - Examination of throat/oral cavity
    - Oral surgery

- Indirect laryngoscopy
- Spatula test in tetanus.
- Elicitation of gag reflex.

11. Metered close inhaler (**MDI**)
    Contains medicine along with propellent
    Advantages:
    - Rapid onset
    - Very small quantity of drug required
    - Very little medicine reach the systemic circulation so side effect is minimum.

    Disadvantages:
    - Skill is required to coordinate hand mouth movements.
    - Infection like candidiasis.
12. **Spacer:**
    Advantages:
    - Incidence of infection like candidiasis is minimum
    - No need of hand mouth coordination.
13. **Ambulatory mobile breathing unit (Ambu) Bag**
    - In resuscitation for giving intermittent positive pressure ventilation size of bag varies from 250–750 mL for pediatric use
    - It has outlet to which mask is attached, at the other end there are 2 openings (oxygen inlet air inlet)
14. **Biopsy gun**
    To take liver biopsy.
15. **Infusion set (IV set)**
    Uses: Administration of IV fluids, drugs, total parenteral nutrition, etc.
16. **Laryngoscope**
    - It consists of handle and blade
    - Uses:
      - Prior to endotracheal intubation
      - Cord palsy, to detect foreign body.
17. **Thermometer**
    - Used to record body temperature
    - Range—35–420
    - Normal temperature—36.5–37.2°C
    - Two types—(1) axillary, (2) rectal.
18. **Tuberculin syringe**
    It is a 1 cc syringe with white or metal pistol.
    Uses:
    - To administer purified protein derivative (PPD) for Mantoux
    - To administer BCG
    - Insulin injection in diabetes mellitus (DM).
19. **Dry powder inhaler (DPI) (rota haler)**
    - Upper half consists of mouth piece and a slot for capsule, lower half is a kind of reservoir to which upper half can be attached.
    - Advantage—small and portable, no need of hand mouth coordination
    - It cannot be used in children below 5 years.
20. **Hypodermic needle**
21. **Face mask**
    To deliver intermittent positive pressure ventilation by means of Ambu bag.
22. **Fluids**
    - Normal saline (0.9%)
      - Na—154 (mEq/L)
      - Cl—154 mEq/L
      - Osmolarity—308 mosm/L
    - 5% DNS
      - Na—154 (mEq/L)

- Cl—154 (mEq/L)
- Glucose—5 (g/100 mL)
- Ringer lactate
  - Na—130 (mEq/L)
  - Cl—109 (mEq/L)
  - K—4 (mEq/L)
  - HCO_3—28 (mEq/L)
  - Osmolarity—310 (mosm/L)
- Isolyte P (pediatric maintanance solution)
  - Na—25 (mEq/L)
  - Cl—variable
  - K—20 (mEq/L)
  - Glucose—5 (g/100 mL).

X-RAYS

STEPS

1. **Positioning**
   - Distance between medial ends of clavicle from vertebral border must be equal on both sides.
   - Problems:
     - Apparent cardiac displacement, cardiomegaly
     - Hilar prominence.
2. **Soft tissues**
   - Soft tissue swelling—neurofibroma
   - Air—surgical emphysema
   - Muscle shadow
   - Breast shadow—adolescents.
3. **Bony cages**
   - Exposure
   - Normal—intervertebral spaces of first 2–3 vertebrae
   - Over-exposed—all vertebrae are clearly seen
   - Horizontal—emphysema
   - Crowding—collapse.
4. **Trachea**
   - Air column in the trachea casts a black shadow through which vertebral spines are seen in the mid point.
   - Tracheal shift
   - Same side—collapse
   - Opposite—effusion, pneumothorax.
5. **Cardiac border**
6. **Lung fields**
   - Lung zones
   - Upper zone—above anterior ends of 2nd rib.
   - Mid zone—between anterior ends of 2nd to 4th rib.
   - Lower zone—below 4th rib.
   - Inspiratory film—6th rib cut diaphragram anteriorly.
7. **Diaphragm**
8. **Costophrenic and cardiophrenic angles.**

1. **Right upper lobe consolidation**
   - Dense opacity in right upper zone (RUZ)
   - Upper border not clear
   - Lower margin is formed by horizontal fissure
   - No shift of trachea or heart
   - "Silhouette sign" +ve
   - Air bronchogram.

PEDIATRICS

2. **Lower lobe consolidation**
   - Dense opacity in right lower and mid zone
   - Air bronchogram
   - Costophrenic and cardiophrenic angles spared
   - No mediastinal shift
   - Upper border not clear.
3. **Air bronchogram**
   - Intrapulmonary airways have thin walls contain air and surrounded by air in alveoli
   - In consolidation, air in the alveoli is replaced by fluid—air within the bronchi stands out
   - Exclude pleural diseases.
4. **Bronchopneumonia**
   - More patchy alveolar, nodular shadows
   - Not limited by interlobar fissures.
5. **Lobar pneumonia**
   - Dense opacity
   - Limited by fissures.
6. **Collapse**
   - Dense opacity in right upper zone
   - Volume loss—trachea shifted to right
   - Crowding of ribs
   - Interlobar fissure pulled up
   - Hyperlucency on other areas.
7. **Pleural effusion**
   - Tracheal shift to opposite side
   - Cardiac shift to opposite side
   - Homogenous opacity, no air bronchogram
   - Obliteration of costophrenic and cardiophrenic angle
   - Ellis 'S'-shaped curve.
8. **Bilateral effusion-trachea central**

   Differential Diagnosis of Dense Shadow

Consolidation	**Pleural effusion**
Air bronchogram	Homogenous opacity, no air bronchogram
Angles not obliterated	Angles obliterated
Trachea and heart not shifted	Mediastinal shift to opposite side
Upper border indistinct.	Diaphragm not seen clearly
	Ellis 'S'- shaped curve

9. **Pneumothorax (right side)**
   - Increased volume of right hemithorax
   - Hyperlucency on right side
   - Absent lung markings
   - Margin of collapsed lung markings at hilum
   - Mediastinal shift to opposite side.

9A. **Hydropneumothorax**
   - Pleural
   - Elliptical
   - No wall
   - Compressed lung margin.

10. **Lung cavity**
    - Large circular opacity

Differential diagnosis of hyperlucency

Lung markings attenuated, but seen
- Emphysema
- Unilateral or bilateral

Lung markings absent
- Intrapulmonarycavity, i.e. bullae
- Extrapulmonary (collapsed lung markings seen)
- Pneumothorax

+ fluid level
- Hydropneumothorax

Hollow parenchymal lesions
- Lung cavity (abscess)
- Lung cyst
- Pneumatocele
- Bleb/bullae
- Hydatid cyst
- Bronchiectasis
- Cystic adenomatoid lung malformation

- Thick wall
- Fluid level
- No tracheal/heart shift
- Due to necrosis of lung parenchyma with evacuation of necrotic tissue, destruction of alveoli, entry of air.

11. **Air/fluid level**
   - Cavity (lung abscess)
   - Intrapulmonary
   - Round shape
   - Thick wall
   - No compressed lung margin.
12. **Pneumatocele**
   - Seen in staphylococcal pneumonia, *Klebsiella*
   - Breaking down lesion—partial obstruction of small bronchus or bronchiole
   - Thin—ill-defined wall.
13. **Mediastinal mass**
   - Mediastinum—extrapleural space within the thorax lying between the lungs
   - The most common mediastinal mass—thymus
   - Sail sign
   - Lymphoma.
14. **Bronchiectasis**
   - Honeycomb lung—coarse reticular interstitial densities with intervening lucencies that appear as cystic spaces.

Differential diagnosis of fluid level above the hemi diaphragm
- *Inside the lung*
  - Lung abscess
- *Outside the lung*
  - Hydropneumothorax

Ring Shadows and Cavity
- **Thick walled (wall thickness >3 mm)**
  - Lung abscess
- **Thin walled**
  - Bulla
  - Pneumatocele
  - Bronchiectasis
  - Cyst

15. **Miliary mottling**
   - Fine, well-defined, pin point (1–2 mm) shadows uniformly distributed throughout both lung fields
   - Seen in miliary tuberculosis.
16. **Cardiomegaly, pulmonary edema**
   - Cardiothoracic ratio— > 50—**cardiomegaly**
     - Pericardial effusion
     - Myocarditis
     - Cardiomyopathy
     - Critical congenital heart disease (CCHD)—Ebsteins anomaly
     - L-R shunts
     - Multivalvular defects.
   - Left ventricular hypertrophy (LVH)—angle formed between apex and diaphragm is obtuse
   - Right ventricular hypertrophy (RVH)—angle is acute.

16A. **Cardiac border**

17. **Eventeration of diaphragm**
18. **Rickets**
   - Cupping
   - Fraying
   - Splaying
   - Thinning
   - Increased width
   - Green stick fracture.
19. **Hair on end appearance in thalassemia.**

SUGGESTED READING

1. Ghai Essential Pediatrics.
2. Nelson Textbook of Pediatrics.
3. Clinical Pediatrics—Aruchamy Lakshmanaswamy.
4. Practical Aspects of Pediatrics—Dr Mayoor K Chheda.

PEDIATRICS

OBSTETRICS

Practical Examinations	**Marks**
Case 1 (Obstetrics)	25
Case 2 (Gynecology)	25
Case Record	10
Total	60
Viva	
Four Stations	20
(Instruments, Drugs, Partogram, Specimens, Fetal skull, Bony pelvis)	

CHAPTER 19

Clinical Cases

OBSTETRICS—CASE FORMAT

ANTENATAL CASE

- Name:
- Age:
- Address:
- Occupation:
- Blood group (mention if Rh negative)
- She is ____ gravida ____ para with ____ living children with ____ abortion (do not say obstetric score)
- Her last menstrual period (LMP) was on ____, previous 3 cycles regular
- Her estimated date of confinement (EDC) is on ____ and gestational age.

Presenting Complaints

Write what the patient says (if she is not mentioning any complaints, then we can write admitted for safe confinement).

History of Preset Illness

Describe presenting complaints (onset, duration, progression, associated symptoms) (in case of admitted for safe confinement we can avoid this).

History of Present Pregnancy

- **1st trimester (<12 weeks)**
  - She detected to be pregnant ____ weeks after missing her periods by urine pregnancy test (UPT), since then she had regular antenatal check ups
  - Any history of excessive vomiting (admitted/not), bleeding, pain, fever with rash, urinary tract infection (UTI) or radiation exposure, drug intake
  - Mention whether she had taken TT (2 doses), folic acid tablets
  - USG and its interpretation

1st trimester bleeding—causes
- Ectopic pregnancy
- Vesicular mole
- Abortion

- **2nd trimester (13–28 weeks)**
  - Quickening felt at ____ weeks
  - USG taken at ____ months and its interpretations (i.e. whether it is said to be normal/abnormal)
  - Any history of diabetes, hypertension (HTN), bleeding, edema or over distention
  - Folic acid tablets taken
  - Fe and Ca tablets taken.
- **3rd trimester (>28 weeks)**
  - Any history of bleeding, leaking, discharge, pain, edema, HTN, gestational diabetes mellitus (GDM), urinary tract infection

Normally quickening felt
- 16 weeks (in multi)
- 20 weeks (in primi)

Past Obstetric History

- Always start with obstetric score (GPLA)
  Description should be in chronological order.
- First child ____ year back, whether hospital/home delivery, whether normal/cesarean section. Any antenatal complications.
- History of prolonged 2nd stage? If yes, why? History of induction, use of forceps/vacuum.
- Birth weight of baby and any neonatal resuscitation.
- History of prolonged hospital stay.
- Age and condition of child at present.
- Baby breasted up to ____ year (significant when frequent child birth).
  (Describe all the past obstetric history like this, if there is history of abortion, then details of that should be written).

Menstrual History

- Menarche attained ____ age.
- Length of cycle, duration and amount of flow.
- Any history of dysmenorrhea/menorrhagia.
- LMP (always end menstrual history with LMP).
- Previous 3 cycles regular or not.

> Excellent date—previous 3 cycles regular without any contraceptives

Marital History

- Age at marriage, wheather it is a consanguineous.
- Any use of contraceptive/treatment for infertility.
- History of smoking in husband.

Past History

- Any history of diabetes mellitus (DM), HTN, tuberculosis (TB) or jaundice.
- Any history of operative procedures/history of intake of medicine for long-term (antiepileptic drugs).

Family History

- Any history of DM, HTN in family or history of malignancies.
- Any history of repeated abortions.
- Any history of multiple pregnancies.
- Any history of congenital anomalies.

Personal History

- Diet
- Bowel and bladder habit
- Any addictions.

GENERAL EXAMINATIONS

- Built and nourishment, height, weight, body mass index (BMI)
- PICCLE (pallor, icterus, cyanosis, clubbing, lymphadenopathy, edema)
- Skin, hair, nails
- Varicose veins, thyroid swelling
- Breast (never forget to examine)
- Spine.
- Vitals:
  - Pulse
  - Respiratory rate (RR)
  - Blood pressure (BP)
  - Temperature.

> - **Gravida:** Total number of past and present pregnancies regardless of outcome
> - **Para:** Number of past viable pregnancies regardless of number of children whether they are live or dead

OBSTETRICS

Other Systems

- Cardiovascular system (CVS)
- Central nervous system (CNS)
- Gastrointestinal tract (GIT)
- Respiratory.

OBSTETRIC EXAMINATION

Inspection

- Abdomen longitudinally distended/flanks full
- Striae gravidarum, linea nigra
- Umbilicus normal and inverted/everted
- Any scars, dilated veins
  (If there is a scar, then site, length, whether healed by primary or secondary intension)
- Hernial orifice.

Palpation

- After emptying bladder and leg in semi-flexed position
- Fundal height
- Symphysiofundal height
- Abdominal girth.

> **Expected fetal weight** (Johnson's formula)
> Fetal weight (g) = (SFH-12) × 155, if head unengaged
> = (SFH-11) × 155, if head engaged

Fundal Grip

- Broad, soft, irregular, non-ballotable mass felt and corresponding to breech.
- Hard, round, ballotable mass felt and corresponding to head.

Umbilical Grip

- Uniform resistance felt on left side suggestive of back.
- Multiple limb nodules felt, corresponds to limbs.

> Normal FHR—120–160/min

1st Pelvic Grip

- Hard, round, ballotable—cephalic
- Soft, broad, irregular—breech

2nd Pelvic Grip

- Confirm the findings of 1st pelvic grip
- Whether head engaged or not
- Whether head is flexed/deflexed (flexed—sinciput is at a higher level than occiput).

Estimated fetal weight: Adequate on clinical examination and according to Johnson's formula is_____g
Liquor: Adequate on clinical examination.

Auscultation

FHS heard on the left side below the umbilicus (cephalic) or above umbilicus (breech presentation) and FHR is ____/min and FHS is good.

SUMMARY

A____ year old GPLA at gestational age of ____ weeks (with LMP on ___and EDC on___) admitted for____ with history of ___ complications) with previous FTND/LSCS .____ years ago; now regular antenatal check up (mention any significant history of GDM, pregnancy-induced hypertension (PIH), antepartum hemorrhage (APH), blood transfusion). On examination no pallor, edema; PR___, BP___and system___(WNL). On obstetric examination—single live, longitudinal lie, cephalic presentation with left occiput anterior (LOA) with good follicle-stimulating hormone (FHS).

DIAGNOSIS

Age, GPLA, gestational age, single, lie, cephalic, attitude, obstetric complication, medical complication.

NORMAL LABOR

Labor is a process by which the products of conception, after attaining viability are expelled from uterus. Normal labor is the process by which live singleton fetus presenting as vertex, expelled by the natural efforts of mother and pregnancy reached term, there are no complications.

Changes During Pregnancy

- **Chadwick's sign** (Jacquemier's)—bluish discoloration of vagina.
- **Osianders sign**—increased vaginal pulsations, felt through the fornices, also in pelvic inflammatory disease (PID) and in malignancy
- **Hegars sign**—softening and compressibility of lower uterine segment.
- **Goodell sign**—cervix becomes soft
- **Palmer sign**—regular and rhythmic contraction of uterus can be felt at 6–8 weeks.

Schedule of Antenatal Care in India

Booking visit—the first visit that the women makes to the health-care facility.
Booked case—is one who has at least three visits with at least two in the last trimester

- Monthly up to 28 weeks (7 months)
- Two weekly between 28–36 weeks
- Weekly 36 weeks onwards.

Minimum 4 visits
1st—within 12 weeks
2nd—14 to 26 weeks
3rd—28 to 34 weeks
4th—36 to term

MECHANISM OF LABOR

- Engagement
- Descent with increase in flexion
- Internal rotation
- Extension
- Restitution
- External rotation.

STAGES OF LABOR

1. **First stage**—onset of true labor pain to complete cervical dilatation (12 hour—primi and 6 hour—multi).
   - Latent phase: Cervical dilatation up to 3–4 cm
   - Active phase:
     - Acceleration phase
     - Phase of maximum slop
     - Deceleration phase

	True pain	False pain
1. Pain	Lower abdomen and back	Lower abdomen only
2. Frequency and duration of contraction	Regular and gradually increasing	Irregular
3. Relief with enema	No	Yes
4. Show	+	–
5. Cervical changes	+	–

2. **Second stage**—cervical dilatation to delivery of fetus (1–2 hour in primi, ½ to 1 hour in multi).
3. **Third stage**—separation and expulsion of placenta.
   Active management of third stage of labor
   - Prophylactic oxytocics
   - Delivery of placenta by controlled cord traction (modified Brandt Andrews technique)
   - Massaging of uterus.

Moulding—sliding of bone each other, because it is connected by membranes as a result reduction of diameters without damage to brain (But severe moulding is dangerous).

Grading of moulding
Grade I: Obliteration of suture line
Grade II: Reducible overlap
Grade III: Irreducible overlap

ANTEPARTUM HEMORRHAGE

Bleeding from the genital tract after fetal viability and before delivery.

Causes

- Placenta previa
- Abruptio placenta
- Circumvallate placenta
- Vasa previa
- Cervix—erosion, polyp, cancer.

POSTPARTUM HEMORRHAGE

Hemorrhage that requires immediate transfusion (hematocrit drop of 10%).

Causes

- Atonic postpartum hemorrhage (PPH)
- Traumatic PPH
- Retained placenta
- Morbidly adherent placenta
- Coagulopathy
- Uterine inversion.

PUERPERIUM

Period following child birth in which the pelvic organs return to the prepregnant state and physiological changes in pregnancy is reversed (6 weeks following child birth).

MANAGEMENT OF NORMAL LABOR

When patient comes with labor pain

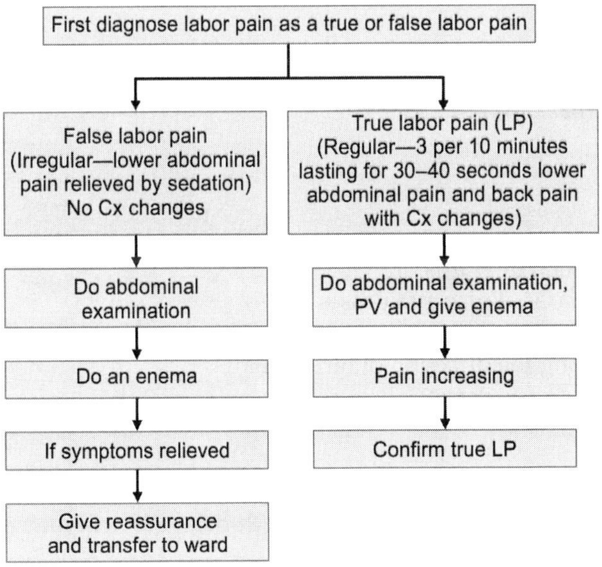

MANAGEMENT IN LABOR ROOM

- Take proper history, look in investigations, if not done prior [URE (urine routine), hemoglobin (Hb), bleeding time (BT), clotting time (CT), random blood sugar (RBS)]
- Check vitals
- Per abdomen (P/A)—lie, presentation, engagement, contractions, fetal heart rate (FHR) [if fetal distress, do cardiotocography (CTG)]
- Do per vaginal (p/v) examination (if in active phase do in every 4th hourly) and assess cervix—position, consistency, effacement, dilation, station of head, membranes intact or not (Bishop score)
- If membranes rupture, asses the liquor status (meconium stained or blood stained)
- Pelvic assessment to rule out cephalopelvic disproportion (CPD)

- If cervix is dilated more than 3 cm transfer to first stage
- Keep the mother in left lateral position (to prevent supine caval syndrome)
- Start IV fluid with 18 G needle with normal saline (meticulous fluid management in heart disease, severe pre-eclampsia), i.e. 75 mL/hr.
- Catheterize bladder if necessary or encourage the mother to pass urine
- Monitor
  - Maternal pulse and BP every ½ hourly
  - Contractions every ½ hourly for 10 minutes
  - FHS every 15 minutes in low risk and continuous CTG monitoring in high-risk
  - Temperature every 4th hourly
  - In pregnancy-induced hypertension (PIH) monitor BP hourly and ask for impending symptoms
  - Monitor progress of labor by setting partogram
- If contractions is not adequate, do artificial rupture of membrane (ARM) if not ruptured [i.e. <1 cm/hr (1 cm right to alert line in partogram)]
- If membrane is already ruptured start IV infusion of P5 (5 units in 500 mL) at an infusion rate of 4 drops/min. or P2.5 in case of multigravida
- If still contractions are not adequate increase infusion rate every half hourly to 8, 12, 16, 20 up to a maximum of 32/min
- If crowning occurs (i.e. full dilatation of Cx), transfer to 2nd stage
- Monitor maternal pulse and BP every 15 minutes and FHS every 5 minutes
- Keep the patient in dorsal position with legs flexed
- Cleanse the vulva and perineum with betadine
- Episiotomy if necessary (only done after crowning has occurred)
- Delivery of head by modified Ritgen maneuver
- Ask assistant to give perineal and para urethral support
- After delivery of head wait for restitution, delivery of anterior shoulder by downward traction and posterior shoulder by upward movement
- Start P20 infusion at a maximum rate or methergin IV 0.2 mg (CI—heart disease, migraine, eclampsia and severe vomiting)
- Clamp the cord
- Wipe the face and eyes, suck the baby's mouth and nose transfer to pediatrician
- Wait for placental separation (look for signs of placental separation)
  Signs of placental separation
  - Gush of fresh blood
  - Lengthening of extravaginal cord
  - Uterus become firm and globular
  - Kustner's sign—cord does not recedes on pushing abdomen upwards
  - Schroeder's sign—uterus rises in the abdomen as the separated placenta passes down
- Vigorous uterine massage and separate placenta by controlled cord traction or modified Brandt-Andrews method (left hand counter traction to uterus and traction along the direction of birth canal)
- Check the placenta for any missing cotyledons. Mop the vulva and cervix
- Place misoprostol per rectally 4 tabletes (one tablete =200 µg)
- Change the glove
- Look for any vulval, vaginal or perineal tear
- Do mucosa suturing—mucosa—continuous, muscle—intermittent, skin—mattress [(with delayed) absorbable sutures—catgut, vicryl]
- Then transfer to IVth stage, i.e. observation room
- Monitor pulse, BP every half hourly for at least 2 hours
- After the uterus has contracted fully (cricket ball consistency), there is no bleeding or pain and she has passed urine, transfer to ward.

MANAGEMENT OF PROLONGED LABOR

- If labor is prolonged in latent phase—give reassurance, hydration, analgesia, ambulation
- If labor is prolonged in active phase/2nd stage
  - Assessment of case—do per vaginal (PV) to rule out CPD, malpresentation
  - Assessment of maternal and fetal condition by monitoring pulse, BP, FHS
  - Give general measure—IV fluid, analgesia, antibiotics

OBSTETRICS

- If CPD or malpresentation do cesarean section (CS)
- If another cause (abnormal uterine contraction)—do ARM if membranes not ruptured start oxytocin P5.

PREREQUISITE FOR VACUUM DELIVERY

- Vertex presentation
- Station +2/below
- No evidence of CPD
- Cervix (Cx) fully dilated (i.e. when narrowing occurs), bladder empty.

Contraindications of vacuum
- Face presentation
- Fetal coagulopathy
- Preterm head

Indications for Vacuum Delivery

- Maternal distress in second stage—anemia, heart disease
- Fetal distress in 2nd stage
- Prolonged 2nd stage
- Deep transverse arrest
- High vacuum for 2nd of a twin
- Vaginal birth after cesarean section (VBAC)
- Medical diseases like PIH.

Modified bishops score

	0	**1**	**2**
Dilatation (cm)	0	1	>2
Effacement (in cm)	2	1	<0.5
Station	–2	–1	0
Position	Posterior	Axial	Anterior
Consistency	Firm	Medium	Soft

DIABETES IN PREGNANCY

Gestational diabetes mellitus: Carbohydrate intolerance of variable severity with onset or first recognition during the present pregnancy.

History Taking

Presenting complaints:
- History of abnormal screening test—glucose challenge test (GCT) and admitted for further evaluation
- Newly detected case of GDM [abnormal glucose tolerance test (GTT) and admitted for management].

History of Present Pregnancy

Preconceptional period:
- Whether known diabetic or not
- If yes, time of detection and duration of disease
- Treatment taken
- Whether diabetes under control when became pregnant.

First trimester:
- In a case of pre GDM, whether oral hypoglycemic drugs changed to insulin.

Second trimester:
- Glucose challenge test—when it was done? result (usually done at 24–28 weeks)
- Glucose tolerance test —when it was done? result
- If GTT abnormal, immediately what treatment was advised? (diet control, exercise, etc.)
- When started on insulin? dosage
- Ask for
  - History of recurrent urinary tract infection (UTI)
  - History suggestive of polyhydramnios.

Third trimester:
- Ask for
  - History of recurrent UTI
  - History suggestive of polyhydramnios.

Past obstetric history: Ask for GDM, abortion, obstructed labor, birth weight >4 kg, over distension.

Family History

History of diabetes.

Past history, dietetic history should be taken in detail

General Examination
- Body mass index (BMI), prepregnant weight

DISCUSSION

Why pregnancy is a diabetogenic state?

Due to estrogen, progesterone, human placental lactogen (HPL), insulinase, plasma cortisol (all changes aimed towards making more glucose available for fetus).

INVESTIGATIONS

- Routine blood
- Urine microscopy for sugar
- GCT, GTT.

Osulliven and Mahan value
- Fasting—90 mg/dL
- 1 hr—165 mg/dL
- 2 hr—145 mg/dL
- 3 hr—125 mg/dL

Glucose Challenge Test

- Irrespective of time of last meal
- 50 gram glucose
- Between 24 and 28 weeks
- Cut off value—140 mg/dL (after 1 hour).

Standard diet of GDM patient (3 meals + 3 snacks):

8.00 am	—	2 idli + sambar
10.00 am	—	1 cup of tea without sugar + 1 plantain
1.00 pm	—	1 spoon of meal + GLV + pulse
4.00 pm	—	coffee + 2–3 biscuits
Night	—	2 chapati + fish curry
At bed	—	milk without sugar, remove supernatant

Glucose Tolerance Test

- Unrestricted or normal diet for previous 3 days and fasting over night
- 75 gram oral glucose.

Risk Factors of GDM

Prepregnancy:
- Age >40 years
- Previous GDM
- Family history of GDM
- PCOD
- Previous big baby (macrosomia)

Pregestational pregnancy:
- Obesity
- Polyhydramnios
- Repeated infections
- Macrosomia

Screening of GDM

*ADA recommendation:
- **At first antenatal visits**
  - FBS >126 mg/dl
  - RBS > 200 mg/dl
  - HbA1C > 6.5%

  If anyone of this is high → overt DM
- **At 24–28 weeks**
  - 75 g oral glucose tolerance test (OGTT)—all women should undergo
  - FBS > 92 mg/dL
  - 1 hr OGTT >180 mg/dL
  - 2 hr OGTT >153 mg/dL

  If one abnormal → GDM.

Management

- **Diet: Medical nutritional therapy (MNT)**

  Goals
  - To prevent postprandial hyperglycemia by splitting main meals
  - Prevent late night hypoglycemia and morning starvation ketosis by bed time snack with complex carbohydrate and protein

  Calorie required
  - Normal weight—30 kcal/kg/day
  - Over weight—24 kcal/kg/day
  - Under weight—40 kcal/kg/day

OBSTETRICS

- **Exercise**—20 minutes daily, upper body exercise.
- **Insulin**
  Mixtard (a mixture of rapid (30%) and intermediate (70%) acting insulin)
  - 2/3rd of dose—morning
  - 1/3rd of dose—at night.

Antepartum Fetal Monitoring

- USG scan [both macrosomia and intrauterine growth restriction (IUGR)]
  - Biometry
  - Amniotic fluid index (AFI)
- Non-stress test (NST)—twice weekly
- Daily fetal movement count
- Cardiff count of 10.

Intrapartum Fetal Monitoring

- Timing of delivery
  - On diet = 40 weeks
  - On insulin, well-controlled = after 38 weeks
  - On insulin, not controlled = 37 weeks
- On receiving at labor room:
  - Do PV—assess Bishop's score
- If not favorable—induce
- Intrapartum glycemic control
  - Morning dose of insulin skipped
  - IV line started with normal saline. A dextrose infusion is piggy backed into a main line on a infusion pump
  - Hourly GRBS
  - If >120 mg/dL start IV infusion of insulin 1–1.5 u/hr
- If RBS >100 mg/dL regular insulin in ringer lactate via a calibrated infusion pump.
- **1st stage**
  - Put on partogram
  - CTG monitoring, RBS, urine ketone body monitoring
- **2nd stage**
  - Shoulder dystocia < should be anticipated >
- **Neonatal care**
  - Good neonatal care facility should be present
  - Early cord clamping to prevent polycythemia
- **Postpartum care**
  - Prophylactic antibiotics
  At 6 weeks postpartum—75 g oral GTT
  - They should be counseled about the risk of future diabetes and lifestyle advise.

Complications

Maternal

- Pre-eclampsia
- Polyhydramnios
- Infection
- Genital trauma
- Puerperal sepsis
- Postpartum hemorrhage (PPH)

Fetal

- Abortion
- Congenital malformation
  - Cardiac anomalies (common)
  - Asymetric septal hypertrophy
  - Caudal regression syndrome (specific)
- Intrauterine device (IUD)
- Macrosomia
- Shoulder dystocia
- Prematurity

Neonatal

- Respiratory distress syndrome (RDS)
- Hypoglycemia
- Polycythemia
- Hyperviscosity syndrome
- Hyperbilirubinemia
- Hypocalcemia
- Erbs or Klumpke's paralysis

PREGNANCY-INDUCED HYPERTENSION (GESTATIONAL HYPERTENSION)

CASE FORMAT

Presenting Complaints

Detected to have high BP.

History of Past Illness

- Onset, duration, drugs, monitoring, controlled or not
- Decreased fetal movements, any impending symptoms.

Past History

HTN, DM, renal disease, heart disease, thrombophilias, connective tissue disorder.

Family History

HTN, severe preeclampsia

GENERAL EXAMINATION

Edema

- Significant pedal edema is seen in 70% normal pregnancies
- Pathological edema is non-dependent or generalized.

Blood Pressure

All rules of BP measurement should be followed:
- Should be measured at the heart level (patient seated in a stool and apparatus is placed on bed)
- Korotkoff phase V or disappearance of sound is used to indicate diastolic BP in pregnancy.

Hypertension in Pregnancy

It is defined as systolic BP >140 mm Hg or diastolic BP >90 mm Hg, at least 2 occasions or rise in systolic BP of 30 mm Hg or rise in diastolic BP of 15 mm Hg at least 6 hours apart or single diastolic BP >110 mm Hg
- Gestational hypertension—hypertension arising 1st time after 20 weeks of gestation in the absence of proteinuria and BP returns to normal within 12 weeks postpartum
- Preeclampsia—gestational hypertension in association with significant proteinuria (300 mg/24 hr)
- Eclampsia—seizures that cannot be attributed to any other cause in a women with preeclampsia
- Chronic HTN—HTN 1st diagnosing before 20 weeks and persisting 12 week postpartum is considered chronic HTN (but not attributable to gestational trophoblastic disease)
- Superimposed preeclampsia—new onset proteinuria in a women with chronic HTN.

Mild Pre-eclampsia

Diastolic BP <110 mm Hg.

Severe Pre-eclampsia

- Diastolic BP >110 mm Hg or more, systolic BP >160 mm Hg
- Proteinuria 5 g in 24 hour or more
- Oliguria/urine output <500 mL/24 hr, <30 mL/hr
- Thrombocytopenia <1 lakh/mm^3
- Headache, visual disturbances, or epigastric pain
- Increased liver enzymes > 50 IU/L
- Increased serum creatinine
- Intrauterine growth restriction (IUGR)
- Pulmonary edema
- Oligohydramnios.

OBSTETRICS

Impending or Imminent Eclampsia

- Headache or flashing lights
- Nausea/vomiting
- Epigastric or right upper quadrant pain
- Brisk tendon reflexes or ankle clonus.

INVESTIGATIONS

PIH Profile

- Complete blood count
  - Increased hematocrit due to contracted vascular volume
  - Thrombocytopenia <1 lakh/dL.
- Bleeding time and clotting time:
  - Prolonged in disseminated intravascular coagulation (DIC).
- Renal function tests:
  - Blood urea normal in pregnancy—15–20 mg/dL
  - Serum creatinine >0.8 mg/dL is significant
  - Serum uric acid raised due to renal tubular dysfunction, placental ischemia leads to increased trophoblastic turnover and increased production of purines
  - It has got prognostic value
- Liver function tests—serum glutamic pyruvic transaminase (SGPT), serum glutamic oxaloacetic transaminase (SGOT), value >70 IU/L is significant. Bilirubin >1.2 mg/dL
- Urine—proteinuria (albumin), pus, cast, red blood cells (RBCs)
- Peripheral smear—features of hemolysis
- LDH >600
- Fundoscopy
- Serum electrolyte.

Prophylaxis

- Low dose aspirin 75 mg—from 12–34 weeks
  In high-risk women—diabetes, hypertension, renal disease, previous severe preeclampsia
- Folic acid—decreases homocysteine level
- Ca supplementation.

Management

- No salt restriction
- No diuretics (worsens IUGR) indicated only in pulmonary edema
- Rest in bed, left lateral position.

Antihypertensive

- Main objective—to reduce cerebral hemorrhage (the disease process is not modified)
- Given when systolic BP >160 mm Hg or MAP >10.5 mm Hg
  - Diastolic BP >100 mm Hg
- Over corrected hypertension leads to IUGR.

Drugs

Drug	*Mechanism of action*	*Dose*	*Side Effect*
• Alpha methyldopa	Central action	250 mg TID > QID 500 mg TID > QID	Postural hypotension Depression, hemolytic anemia
• Nifedipine	Plain/quick action in 6 hours/retard-sustained action in 10–12 hours	10 mg BD/20 mg BD	Postural hypotension, headache, palpitation
• Hydralazine	Peripheral vasodilation	100 mg TID	Headache, flushing, techycardia
• Labetalol	Alpha+beta-blocker	200–400 mg BD	Postural hypotensiom, tremor
*Labetalol is the drug of choice			

Monitoring

Maternal:

After 32 weeks
- Daily BP, urine output
- Weekly PIH profile
- Weekly weight.

Fetal:
- Daily fetal movement count
- Weekly NST

Can go up to 40 weeks, better terminate at 38 weeks.

Preeclampsia

- Watch for impending symptoms
- Twice daily BP
- Daily urine albumin
- Daily urine output
- Twice weekly PIH profile

Fetal
- Daily fetal movement count
- Twice weekly NST
- Weekly BPP
- Once in two week USG (for IUGR, abruption)

In mild preeclampsia, terminate at 37–38 weeks (admit at 34 weeks)

In severe preeclampsia, terminate at 34 weeks.

Mode of delivery:
- If there is no obstetric indications for cesarean section (CS) labor can be induced
- If cervix is favorable with Bishop's score >6, ARM followed by oxytocin
- If unfavorable, PGE2 gel to ripen the cervix.

Indications for CS

- Associated obstetric indications
- Failed induction
- Rapid worsening of maternal condition and delivery is not imminent
- Fetal distress/severe IUGR.

1st Stage

- Limit IV fluid (75 mL/hr) (to prevent pulmonary edema)
- Put partogram
- CTG monitoring
- ½ hour pulse, FHS every 15 minutes
- ½ hourly BP, urine output 4th hourly
- **Control of BP**—diastolic BP should be <110 mm Hg
- Using
  - Oral nifedipine
  - Labetalol IV 2 mg/min infusion or 20 mg IV bolus over 2 min
- Prophylactic magnesium sulfate may be given during labor to prevent eclampsia

Indication for corticosteroid

- In HELLP syndrome
- To accelerate lung maturity
- Betamethasone 12 mg IM 2 doses 12 hour apart.

2nd Stage

- Cut short 2nd stage in severe preeclampsia

Indications for immediate termination:
- Uncontrolled hypertension
- Eclampsia
- Abnormal LFT/RFT/coagulation profile
- HELLP syndrome
- Fetal distress
- Severe IUGR
- Abruption

3rd Stage

- Methergin contraindicated
- Active management of 3rd stage to prevent PPH
- $MgSO_4$ is continued for another 24 hr of delivery/last seizure
- Continue antihypertensive after delivery (methyl dopa avoided to prevent postpartum depression)
- Counsel about—recurrence of PIH in next pregnancy
  - Prophylaxis with low dose aspirin in next pregnancy
- Severe preeclampsia
  - <24 week terminate (refer Medicine)
  - >34 week terminate
  - 24–34 week—place for expectant management
- Aim: Protect mother and fetus from consequences of disease
- Prolong pregnancy to avoid prematurity
- By:
  - Antihypertensive
  - Antenatal corticosteroids—to accelerate lung maturity
  - Close monitoring.

ECLAMPSIA

- May be antepartum, intrapartum or postpartum
- 1/3rd women may experience eclampsia before development of hypertension and proteinuria.

Clinical Features

- Prodromal phase—aura followed by convulsive movements beginning around mouth
- Tonic phase—the entire body becomes rigid. This may last for 15–20 seconds
- Clonic phase—grandmal convulsions occur starting from the facial muscle to involve entire body. Last for about 1 minute.
- Recovery phase—the convulsions slowly subside, and patient passes to stage of variable duration of coma.

Differential Diagnosis

- Epilepsy
- Cerebrovascular accident (CVA)
- Meningitis
- Encephalitis
- Metabolic disturbances

Management

General

- Maintain A, B, C
- Nurse in left lateral position in a cot with railings
- Start IV line—Ringer lactate ideal
- Catheterize the bladder—input output chart
- During fit, mouth gag is placed between teeth
- Oxygen inhalation.

Complications:
- Cerebral hemorrhage
- Hyperpyrexia
- Renal failure
- Pulmonary edema
- Puerperal sepsis
- Aspiration
- Psychosis

Medical

- Drug of choice: magnesium sulphate
- Mechanism of action
  - at neuromuscular junction compete with calcium for entry into the cells,
  - also have central action
- Loading dose—4 g $MgSO_4$ slow IV over 10 minutes in 100 mL saline
  + 4 g deep IM each buttock
- (4 g = 8 mL of 50% $MgSO_4$ diluted with 12 mL sterile water
  or 16 mL of 25% $MgSO_4$ diluted with 4 mL sterile water)
- Maintenance therapy
  - 4 g IM on alternate buttocks every 4 hour
  - Continue till 24 hour postpartum or 24 hour after last seizure; which ever is later.

OBSTETRICS

Monitoring

- Essential because of narrow therapeutic range (therapeutic range 4–8 mEq/L)
- Patellar reflex (lost when $MgSO_4$ = 10 mEq/L)
- Urine output—at least 100 mL in 4 hour, 30 mL/hr (because Mg excreted through kidney).
- Respiratory rate—arrest if level 12 mEq/L
  - In any of this situation skip the next dose:
    - Antidote—10 mL of 10% calcium gluconate is given IV
      In case of respiratory depression → CPR

> - Patellar reflex lost
> - Urine output <30 mL/h
> - Respiratory rate <14/mins

- Absolute contraindications:
  - Myasthenia gravis
  - Recent myocardial infarction (MI)
- Status eclampticus: Thiopentone sodium slow IV.

Obstetric Management

- Immediate termination after controlling seizure
- CS if (1) Convulsions are not controlled, (2) The maternal condition is worsening and delivery is not thought to be possible within 6–8 hours; (3) Failed induction.

HELLP Syndrome

- Hemolysis, elevated liver enzymes, low platelet count
  - Variant of severe preeclampsia
  - Epigastric or right upper quadrant pain, nausea, vomiting
  - Investigations—peripheral smear (p/s), LDH, LFT, platelet count, bilirubin >1.2 mg/dL, decreased hepatoglobulin
  - Treatment—termination of pregnancy
- Supportive—fresh blood/platelet transfusion, high dose steroid therapy
- Differential diagnosis—hepatitis, acute fatty liver of pregnancy, HUS, acute cholestasis of pregnancy

Etiology

i. **Genetic factors:** Family history of preeclampsia
ii. **Obstetric factors** (exposure to chorionic villi for first time or increased chorionic villi).
   Primiparity, past history of PIH, new paternity, multiple pregnancy, hydrops fetalis with large placenta, hydatidiform mole
iii. **Maternal factors:**
   - Chronic hypertension, diabetes, renal disease
   - Antiphospholipid antibodies (APLA), systemic lupus erythematosus (SLE)
   - Insulin resistance
   - Hyperhomocysteinemia.

> **Prediction of preeclampsia:**
> - MAP >90 mm Hg
> - Gant's roll-over test
> - Angiotensin sensitivity test
> - Uterine artery Doppler
> - Persistence of diastolic notch
> - Alpha-fetoprotein (AFP), beta-human chorionic gonadotropin (β-hCG), inhibin A
> - Vascular endothelial growth factor (VEGF)—low level

Complications of Preeclampsia

Maternal

- Eclampsia, cerebral hemorrhage, cortical blindness
- Pulmonary edema, ARDS
- HELLP syndrome, DIC and hemorrhage
- Abruption of placenta
- Renal failure, renal tubular necrosis (RTN)
- Hepatic rupture

Fetal

- Prematurity
- Intrauterine growth restriction (IUGR)
- Perinatal asphyxia
- Intrauterine device (IUD)

OBSTETRICS

MULTIPLE PREGNANCY

PRESENTING COMPLAINTS

- Over-distended abdomen
- Excessive nausea and vomiting.

Over-distended abdomen
Differential diagnosis
- Bladder
- Multiple pregnancy
- Macrosomia
- Molar pregnancy
- Hydramnios
- Ascites
- Tumors

HISTORY OF PRESENT PREGNANCY

Third trimester:
- Respiratory difficulty
- Low backache.

Marital History

Ovulation-induction, assisted reproductive technology (ART)

Family History

History of twin pregnancy in the family

Inspection

Overdistension, shiny skin.

Palpation

- Multiple fetal parts palpable, 3 fetal poles or 2 fetal heads.
  - Fundal height and girth increases

Auscultation

Two fetal heart sound heard by two observers hearing simultaneously at least 10 cm apart, with a difference of 10 beat/min.

DISCUSSION

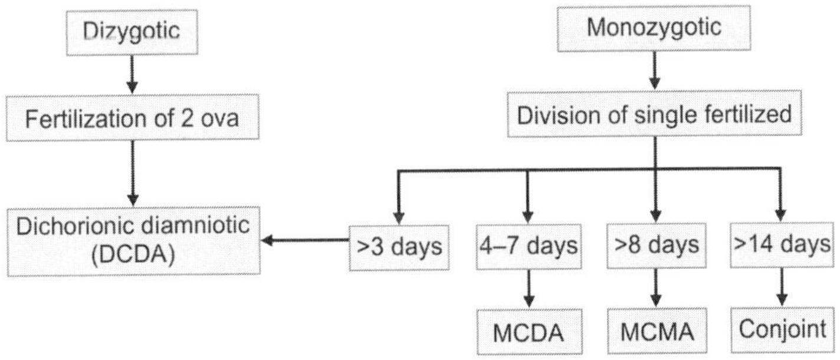

++Zygosity—type of conception
++Chorionicity— type of placentation

Hellin's rule:
Twin 1 in 80
Triplet 1 in 80^2
Quadruple 1 in 80^3

Ultrasound Determination of Chorionicity

- Number of sac
  - Before 10 weeks
  - 2 sac—dichorionic
  - 1 sac—monochorionic
- Placenta—2 placenta—dichorionic
- Sex—discordant sex indicates dichorionicity but concordant sex does not imply monochorionicity
- Intertwin membrane is thicker and more echogenic in dichorionic twin
- Twin peak or lambda sign.

Dichorionic: Chorionic tissue between the 2 layers of intertwine membrane.

MANAGEMENT

- Frequent antenatal visits—monthly USG after 20 weeks

- Admit at 38 weeks—uncomplicated DCDA twin pregnancies
  - Before—complicated pregnancy
- If 1st twin non-vertex—cesarean section

1st stage—Arrange enough blood
- ½ hourly FHS of both twins, uterine contraction
  - Partogram
  - 4th hourly PV
  - Delay ARM

2nd stage
- Necessities before delivery
- Senior obstetrician
- Two neonatal teams
- Anesthetist

Timing of delivery:
DCDA—38 weeks
MC twin—36–37 weeks

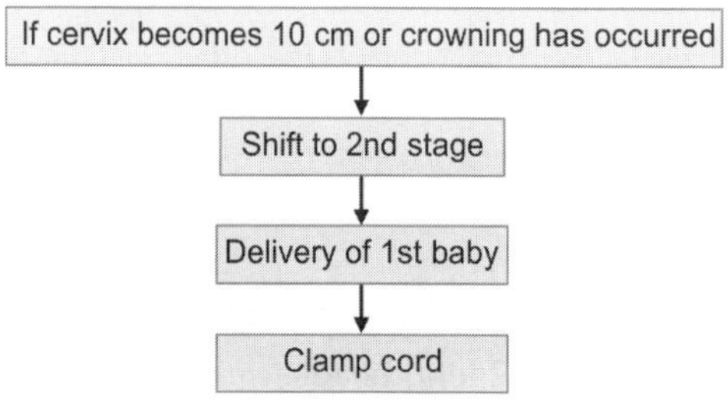

2nd baby should be delivered within 20 minutes

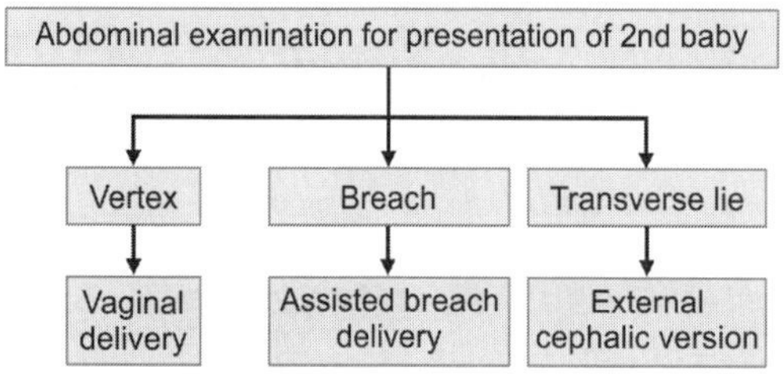

(If fetal distress—high vacuum)

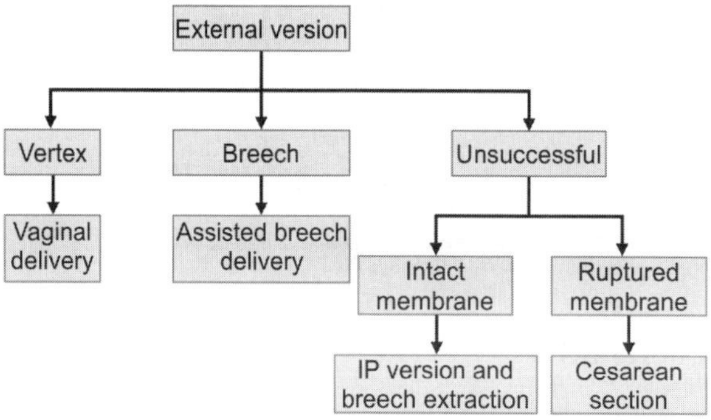

COMPLICATIONS

Maternal Complications

Antepartum:
- Hyperemesis
- Hydramnios
- Preeclampsia
- Pressure symptoms
- Anemia
- Antepartum hemorrhage
- Gestational diabetes mellitus

Intrapartum:
- Dysfunctional labor
- Malpresentation
- Increased chance for casarean section
- Postpartum hemorrhage
- Retained placenta

Fetal Complications

Antepartum:
- Prematurity
- IUGR (concordant, discordant)
- Single fetal demise
- Monochorionic monoamniotic twin
- Twin-twin transfusion syndrome
- Vanishing twin abortion
- Congenital anomalies, e.g. acardiac fetus, conjoint twins

Intrapartum:
- PROM and cord prolapse
- Abruption in the 2nd twin
- Interlocking of twin

Complications specific for monochorionic twins:
- Twin-twin transfusion syndrome
- Monochorionic twinning
- Conjoint twinnig
- Acardiac fetus.

Fetus papyraceous

Seen in vanishing twin syndrome
- Spontaneous cessation of cardiac activity in a previously viable
- When fetus in multiple gestation
- Fetal death occurs after 1st trimester, it results in thin parchment like body—fetus papyraceous

BREECH

MANAGEMENT

At 37 weeks—can try for external cephalic version (ECV).

Why external cephalic version?

a. High perinatal mortality of vaginal breech delivery
b. 1st degree CPD—cannot do vaginal delivery in case of breach presentation (breach is poor dilator of cervix).

External Cephalic Version (ECV)

It is the procedure where by the presentation other than cephalic is converted by external manipulation into cephalic presentation.

Contraindications:
- Multiple pregnancy
- Antepartum hemorrhage
- Uteroplacental insufficiency
- Previous cesarean section
- Contracted pelvis and uterine anomalies

Procedure:

Prerequisite ultrasonography (USG) done by:
- Non-stress test (NST)
- Continuous fetal and maternal monitoring is carried out
- Tocolytics given

Each hand grasp, each fetal pelvis >> The fetal buttocks are gently elevated from maternal pelvis and displaced laterally >> Then the buttocks are gently guided towards fundus while the head is directed to the pelvis >> Take NST >> Monitor 1 hour.

Complications of ECV
1. Fetal distress
2. Preterm labor
3. Abruption
4. Fetomaternal hemorrhage
5. PROM

Assisted Breech Delivery

If ECV fails patient is prepared for assisted breech delivery.

Done for average sized baby, spontaneous onset of labor.

1st stage
- Can induce—inducing may mask the CPD
- Rest in left lateral position
- Nil per oral (NPO)
- In vitro fertilization (IVF)
- Sedation
- Partogram

OBSTETRICS

When climbing perineum, i.e. when the fetal anus is visible at the outlet between contractions >> Shift to 2nd stage >> Do liberal right mediolateral episiotomy (RMLE) >> Breech is delivered up to umbilicus.

Delivery of breech (the mot common position LSA):
- Engagement—bitrochanter diameter (9.5 cm)
- Descent with increase in compaction
- Internal rotation
- Lateral flexion
- Delivery of trunk
- Restitution

Important points:
- Baby's back should always be anterior
- Baby should be held by the femoropelvic grip
- Baby should be wrapped in a warm towel to avoid premature breathing effort due to tactile stimulation

Delivery of shoulder [engaging diameter-bis acromial (12 cm)]
- Lovset's maneuver—once inferior angle of scapula seen, grasped at femeropelvic grip and trunk rotated through 180°.

Delivery of after coming head:

Delivery of head
- Engagement—suboccipitofrontal (10.5 cm)
- Descent with increase in flexion
- Internal rotation
- Flexion

1. **Burns-Marshall maneuver:** When the occiput is seen under the pubic symphysis, steady traction is given on the feet and baby is swung in an arc towards mother's abdomen. By simultaneous suprapubic pressure (Kristellar maneuver) the head is born in flexion.
2. **Mauriceau-Smellie-Veit maneuver:** Here the fetal body rests upon the palm of hand and the left forearm and the index, middle fingers of the same hand are applied over the malar bones to flex the head. Two fingers of right hand are hooked over the fetal neck and grasping the shoulders, downward traction is applied until the suboccipital region appears beneath the symphysis pubis.

INDICATIONS FOR ELECTIVE CESAREAN SECTION

- Complicated breech
- Contracted pelvis
- Large babies
- Hyperextension of fetal head
- Footling or knee presentation
- Several IUGR, previous CS.

Breech Extraction

This is performed when cervix is fully dilated and immediate breech delivery is warranted as in cases of fetal distress, maternal distress or cord prolapse.

The entire body is delivered vaginally by the obstetrician under GA without any effort on the part of patient followed by manual removal of placenta (MROP).

Emergency Cesarean Section Indications

- Cord prolapse
- Failure to progress
- Fetal distress/maternal distress
- Impacted breech

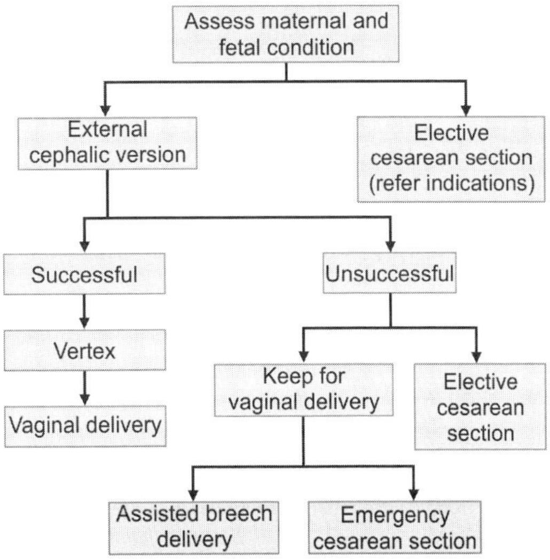

Complications of breech

Fetal
- Soft tissue injury
- Traction of nerve
- Fracture of long bones (femur, humerus)
- Intracerebral hemorrhage
- Hypoxia

Maternal
- Perineal tear
- Increased chance of operative delivery

Complications of assisted breech delivery
- Premature rupture of membranes (PROM)
- Cord prolapse
- Extended arm
- Chin to pubis rotation
- Entrapment of head
- Dysfunctional labor
- Impacted breech
- Nuchal arms

Etiology of breech
- Prematurity (common cause)
- Uterine anomalies
  - Septate/bicornuate
  - Fibroid
- Placental anomalies
  - Placenta previa
- Fetal
  - Anencephaly, hydrocephalus
    - Multiple pregnancy
    - Polyhydramnios
    - Oligohydramnios

Types of breech
- Complete/flexed breech
- Incomplete breech
  - Extended (frank breech)
  - Knee presentation
  - Footling presentation

PREVIOUS CESAREAN SECTION

CASE FORMAT

Presenting Complaints

Write if any like abdominal pain, pain in the area of uterine scar, bleeding per vaginal (PV) or write admitted for safe confinement.

History of Present Pregnancy

As usual.

Past Obstetric History

- Time since last delivery
- Indication for previous cesarean section (CS)

- Emergency or elective
- Any postoperative complications—infection/discharge, cough, etc.
- History of any previous normal delivery.

Other histories as usual.

Abdominal Examination

- Scar—vertical/horizontal, length
- Scar tenderness—palpate just above scar and look any dimpling, give away, pain.

DISCUSSION

Management:

Hospitalization at 38 in LSCS and at 34 weeks in classical CS.

2 options

Elective CS ——— **VBAC trial**

Elective CS:

- If sure about fetal maturity— elective CS at 39 weeks
- Otherwise wait for spontaneous labor and CS performed at onset of labor (to prevent complication of fetal maturity)
- Problems during repeat CS
  - Adhesions, injury to bladder and bowel
  - PPH due to placenta previa/adherent placenta

VBAC trial of labor (TOLAC—trial of labor after cesarean):

- **Successful trial**: Results in vaginal delivery of a live fetus without scar rupture
- **Failed trial**: When emergency CS is required/there is scar rupture.

Selection of Cases

Previous History

- Type of prior uterine incision—lower segment transverse incision
- Prior indication—for non-recurrent indications like breech, fetal distress (favorable) (for recurrent indications like contracted pelvis, previous classical/J shaped—not favorable)
- Prior vaginal delivery—favorable
- Postoperative infection—not favorable
- Interpregnancy interval >6 months.

Present Pregnancy

- Average sized baby
- Vertex presentation
- No CPD
- No medical/obstetric complication

USG

- Presentation
- Assess integrity of scar—if >3.5 mm thickness—decreased risk of rupture
- Placental location—to rule out adherent placenta over scar
- Absence of usual subplacental sonolucent zone
- Estimated fetal weight of baby.

Monitoring

- Arrange cross-matched blood
- Close monitoring of maternal and fetal condition
- Wait for spontaneous of labor
- Put partogram, set IV line,
- Continuous CTG monitoring is ideal.

INDICATIONS FOR EMERGENCY CESAREAN SECTION

a. Unsatisfactory progress of labor
b. Any signs of scar dehiscence

Delivery:

- Cut short 2nd stage—by outlet forceps/vacuum
- Look signs of scar rupture/excessive bleeding—do emergency laparotomy

Signs of scar dehiscence

i. Fetal bradycardia (earliest sign)
ii. Late deceleration on CTG
iii. Meconium staining of amniotic fluid
iv. Vaginal bleeding
v. Persistent maternal tachycardia
vi. Suprapubic discomfort/scar tenderness
vii. Hematuria.

	LSCS scar	Classical scar
Apposition	Better apposition	Difficult to appose
Healing in puerperium	Better as the lower segment is quiescent	Imperfect due to contraction and retraction of upper segment
Timing of rupture	In labor	In pregnancy and labor
Rupture	0.5–2%	4–8%
Placental implantation	May be over scar	Much more likely

Dehiscence: Separation along the line of previous scar and serosa intact.
Rupture: When serosa involved.
Why classical scar more likely to rupture ?
Ans: Refer above box.

INTRAUTERINE GROWTH RESTRICTION

Low birth weight (LBW): Birth weight below 2500 gram
Low birth weight is of two types:
1. Preterm
2. Small for gestational age

Small for gestational age (SGA)—two types:
1. Genetically small fetus
2. IUGR.

Symmetrical	Asymmetrical
1. Uncommon	1. Common
2. Intrinsic fetal pathology	2. Uteroplacental insufficiency
3. All organs equally affected	3. Brain sparing effect
4. Symmetrically small	4. Head larger than abdomen
5. HC/AC, FL/AC normal	5. Increased
6. Ponderal index normal	6. Decreased

ETIOLOGY

Fetal Causes

- Chromosomal abnormality
- Congenital malformations
- Congenital infections—like TORCH infections.

Placental Causes

- Uteroplacental insufficiency
- Thrombophilias—antiphospholipid anibody (APLA) and congenital thrombophilias
- Placental and cord anomalies like minor placental abruption, circumvallate placenta and velamentous insertion of the cord.

Maternal Causes

- Preeclampsia, hypertension, renal disease, diabetes with vasculopathy
- Poor maternal weight gain and under nutrition
- Teratogens like smoking, alcohol, cocaine
- Chronic maternal disease like severe anemia and congenital cyanotic heart disease.

TYPES OF IUGR

- Symmetrical
- Asymmetrical

COMPLICATIONS

Fetal Complications

- Stillbirth
- Fetal distress

Neonatal Complication

- **Metabolic**
  - Hypoglycemia (due to reduced glycogen storage in liver)
  - Hypothermia (due to reduced subcutaneous fat)
  - Hypocalcemia (due to relative hypoparathyroidism)
  - Polycythemia (as chronic hypoxia stimulates erythropoiesis).
- **Complications of hypoxia**
  - Meconium aspiration syndrome
  - Hypoxic-ischemic encephalopathy (HIE)
  - Necrotizing enterocolitis (NEC)
  - Pulmonary hemorrhages
- **Complications related to the cause**
  - Congenital malformations
  - Chromosomal abnormalities
  - Congenital infections.

INVESTIGATIONS

Ultrasonography: Ultrasound biometry/liquor/placental position/to rule out congenital anomaly.

- Ultrasound biometry:
  - Biparietal diameter
  - Head circumference
  - Femoral length
  - Abdominal circumference
  - Estimated fetal weight
  - HC/AC, FL/AC increased in a case of asymmetric IUGR
- AC is the most accurate measure to predict IUGR. AC below 10th centile is taken as the cut-off

Doppler velocimetry:

- Umbilical artery Doppler:
  - In normal pregnancy umbilical and uterine arteries have low resistance, so there will be significant diastolic flow. In IUGR 3 patterns—reduced end-diastolic flow (EDF), absent EDF, reversal of flow. A normal Doppler is reassuring for at least a week and only be repeated weekly to detect compromise.
  - Indices—S/D ratio, resistance index, pulsatility index.
- MCA Doppler—in normal fetus, increased resistance in MCA. In IUGR blood flow preferentially to brain and heart (brain sparing/centralization of flow).
- Venous Doppler—venous flow examined is usually the ductus venosus and the umbilical vein. Reflects function of heart. Reduced/absent flow indicates impaired cardiac function. Umbilical vein pulsations are a terminal sign. (Persistence of diastolic notch in the uterine artery at 20–29 weeks is indicative of increased resistance in the uterine vessels—high-risk of IUGR)

MANAGEMENT

General Management

- Rest, high protein diet, treat associated maternal conditions like anemia, PIH.
- Daily fetal movement count (DFMC)

Group A—clinically IUGR, but normal Doppler and normal AFI
- No risk factor—re-scan monthly
- If risk factor + —re-scan 3 weekly
- If any decrease in AFI—treat as group B
- If no change—terminate at 37 completed weeks.

Group B:
- Normal Doppler, liquor(AFI) reduced at 37 completed weeks consider delivery, if < 37 weeks repeat USG 3 weekly and manage as for group A.

Group C—IUGR with decreased end-diastolic flow repeat Doppler weekly, 2 weekly USG and twice weekly BPP
- Consider termination at 37 completed weeks
- Antenatal steroids if <36 weeks.

Group D—absent or reversed end-diastolic flow
- Antenatal steroids
- Deliver if 34 weeks
- Daily or twice daily CTG, weekly Doppler
- If reversed end-diastolic flow/umbilical vein pulsations deliver at 32 weeks (immediate termination)

Intrapartum Management

- Assess Bishop's score
- If favorable ARM + Oxytocics
- Unfavorable—PGE2 gel.

1st stage:
- Early artificial rupture of membrane
- Continuous monitoring (as there is chance of meconium aspiration)
- Cesarean section—if there is reversal of EDF in the umbilical artery, or abnormal venous Doppler or nonreactive NST.

ANEMIA IN PREGNANCY

PRESENTING COMPLAINTS

- On routine antenatal check up found to have low Hb
- Easy fatigability
- Palpitation, breathlessness
- Edema of limbs.

History of Presenting Complaints

- Easy fatigability—onset, duration, progression
- Dyspnea—onset, duration, progression, aggravating factor, relieving factor
- Edema—site, duration
- Associated symptoms like sweating, syncope

History of Present Pregnancy

- Hyperemesis gravidarum
- Urinary tract infection (UTI)
- Whether taken Fe and folic acid
- Bleeding per vaginum (PV)

Past Obstetric History

It should be explained in details including spacing, Fe tablets taken. History of anemia/blood transfusion in previous pregnancy or postpartum, PPH.

Menstrual History

History of menorrhagia.

Past History

History of worm infestation/anemia/jaundice/blood transfusion

Socioeconomic Status

Family History

History of bleeding disorder.

GENERAL EXAMINATION

Pallor, edema, angular stomatitis, glossitis, cheilosis, jaundice, clubbing, lymph node (LN).

Examination

- Intrauterine growth restriction
- Signs of congestive cardiac failure (CCF)
- Hepatosplenomegaly (HSM)
- Cardiovascular system (CVS)—systolic murmur.

DISCUSSION

According to WHO, pregnancy anemia is defined as Hb level below 11 g/dL.

CLASSIFICATION OF ANEMIA

- Nutritional anemia
  - Iron deficiency
  - Folate deficiency
  - Combined deficiency
  - Protein deficiency.
- Anemia due to blood loss
  - Bleeding during pregnancy
  - Hookworm infestation.
- Hemolytic anemia
  - Hemoglobinopathies
  - Malaria.
- Decreased production of blood
  - Aplastic anemia.

Indian Council of Medical Research (ICMR)
• Mild anemia—10–10.9 g/dL
• Moderate—7–10 g/dL
• Severe—4–7 g/dL
• Very severe—<4 g/dL

ETIOLOGY OF ANEMIA IN PREGNANCY

- Deficient intake and absorption:
  - Inadequate diet
  - Hyperemesis
  - Presence of phosphate and phytate in the diet
  - Achlorhydria and vitamin C deficiency.
- Increased demand:
  - Multiple pregnancy.
- Excessive loss:
  - Repeated pregnancies with inadequate spacing
  - Prior menorrhagia
  - Hookworm infestation
  - Malaria.
- Chronic illness.

COMPLICATIONS OF ANEMIA

- Susceptibility to infections
- Preterm labor
- Inability to withstand PPH
- uerperal sepsis
- Congestive cardiac failure
- Perinatal
  - Intrauterine growth restriction
  - Prematurity
  - Early infantile anemia.

OBSTETRICS

PREVENTION OF ANEMIA

- Routine supplementation of 100 mg of elemental iron and 500 µg folic acid is now recommended daily for all pregnant women in India.
- Deworming—albendazole 400 mg after 1st trimester—single dose
- Dietary modifications.

MANAGEMENT

Investigations

- Hemoglobin (Hb), hematocrit (HCT)—decreases
- PS – microcytic hypochromic
- Red cell indices—decreases
  - Mean corpuscular volume (MCV)
  - Mean corpuscular volume (MCH)
  - Mean corpuscular hemoglobin concentration (MCHC)
- Special tests:
  - Serum iron—decreases
  - Total iron binding capacity (TIBC)—increases
  - % saturation of transferrin—decreases
  - Serum ferritin—decreases
  - Free erythrocyte protoporphyrin —increases
- Investigations to determine etiology
  - PS—malarial parasite
  - Stool examination for occult blood and ova and cyst
  - Renal function test (RFT)—chronic renal disease
  - Test for TB.

TREATMENT

- <30 weeks—oral Fe
- 30–36 weeks—parenteral Fe
- >36 weeks—blood transfusion

a. **Oral iron therapy:**
   - $FeSO_4$—ferrous sulfate thrice daily (one tablet of ferrous sulfate—60 mg of elemental iron)
   - Side effects—nausea, vomiting, abdominal discomfort and constipation.

b. **Parenteral therapy**
   Available preparation—iron dextran, iron sorbitol citrate (not used today), iron sucrose is newer preparation
   Iron needed in mg = (normal Hb – patient's Hb) weight in kg × 2.2 (additional 1000 mg to replenish stores)
   Indications:
   1. Intolerance to oral iron
   2. Non-compliance
   3. Malabsorption syndromes

   IM route
   - Using Z technique and a thick needle
   - Side effects—fever, myalgia, arthralgia.

   IV route
   - Side effects—tachycardia, hypotension, flushing, syncope.

Iron sucrose complex
Available as 2.5 mL, 5 mL vials 1 mL→ 20 mg Fe Given as IV diluted in 100 mL NS on alternate day or twice a week

c. Blood transfusion—diuretic and antihistaminic is given prior to transfusion
   Indications:
   - Severe anemia
   - Immediate correction needed as in intrapartum
   - Hemodynamic instability.

OBSTETRIC MANAGEMENT

1st stage

- Propped up position

- Induce
- Antibiotics—to prevent puerperal sepsis
- O_2—to reduce fetal hypoxia, IVF—75 mL/h.

2nd stage

- Outlet forceps/vacuum
- Active management of third stage
- PPH should be managed promptly
- In the puerperium close monitoring for sepsis, deep vein thrombosis (DVT) and cardiac failure.

CARDIAC DISEASE IN PREGNANCY

PRESENTING COMPLAINTS

- Known case of heart disease (congenital/acquired)
- Dyspnea, orthopnea, paroxysmal nocturnal dyspnoea (PND)
- Chest pain
- Palpitation
- Syncope

NYHA classification
Class 1—No limitation of physical activity
Class 2—Dyspnea on severe exertion
Class 3—Dyspnea on mild exertion
Class 4—Dyspnea at rest

History of Present Illness

If known case of heart disease, describe when detected, treatment, etc.
CVS examination is important

DISCUSSION

- Rheumatic
- Congenital

MANAGEMENT

Pregnancy should be planned in known cases.

Antenatal Care

- On the 1st visit
  - Take pulse rate, BP, examine CVS in detail
  - See a cardiologist
  - Take an echo

In case of **class 3, 4:**

- Admit on 1st visit

In case of **class 1, 2:**

- Follow-up every 2nd week up to 30 weeks, after that weekly.
- Once in month see a cardiologist
- Rest
  - 2 hour rest after lunch
  - 8 hour sleep at night.

Treat anemia

Treatment infection—dental infection, UTI (it may predisposes to IE)

In case of NYHA class 3 and 4—better do MTP at 1st trimester or if they are seen later in pregnancy they should be admitted and should undergo some surgery like closed mitral valvuloplasty or open mitral valvotomy in case of severe MS.

Intrapartum Management

- Admit
  - Class 1–38 weeks
  - Class 2–36 weeks
- Spontaneous onset of labor awaited.

1st stage:

- Left lateral position or propped up position
- Put on a partogram

Infective endocarditis Prophylaxis

- Injection ampicilin 2 g IV stat followed by 500 mg IV 6th hourly
- Injection gentamicin 80 mg IV 12th hourly

OBSTETRICS

- Sedate with morphine/pethidine (decrease pulmonary congestion in active phase of labor)
- Fluid restriction (up to 75 mL/h)
- Infective endocarditis (IE) prophylaxis
- Monitoring
  - With pulse rate (PR), respiratory rate (RR), FHS every 15 minutes, SpO_2
  - BP hourly
  - PV 4th hourly (PR >100, RR >24 = Impending pulmonary edema)
- When there is 5 cm dilatation do ARM (it decreases duration of labor by 1–2 hours)

2nd stage:
- Cut short 2nd stage by forceps (forceps preferred due to lesser maternal effort)
- IV frusemide 40 mg immediately after child is born

3rd stage:
- Avoid ergometrine/methergine
- Active management

Postpartum

- Monitor closely for pulmonary edema
- Look for PPH, infection
- Check for thromboembolism
- Check for new murmur (IE).

Contraception

Barrier contraception and progesterone injection (DMPA, Net-en)

Physiological changes in pregnancy:
- Increase in cardiac output by 40%
- Increase in stroke vol by 10%
- Increase in heart rate by 10% or 15 beats/min
- Increase in blood vol by 40%
- Decrease in peripheral resistance and diastolic BP.

CVS changes in pregnancy (which may mimic heart disease):
- Collapsing pulse due to wide pulse pressure
- Increase in heart rate and ectopic beats
- JVP may be elevated
- Heart size increases
- Apex beat displaced upward and laterally
- S1 may be loud
- ESM may heard over precordium
- Venous hums in neck, Soufflé over breast
- Peripheral edema.

Complications of heart disease:

Maternal	*Fetal*
Congestive cardiac failure	IUGR
Acute pulmonary edema	Asphyxia, stillbirth
Arrhythmias	Prematurity
Subacute bacterial endocarditis	Inheritance of hereditary heart disease
Thromboembolism	

Contraindications for pregnancy (WHO)
- Eisenmenger's syndrome
- Primary pulmonary HTN
- Uncorrected severe coarctation
- Marfan's syndrome with aortic involvement
- Severe mitral stenosis with complication
- Severe symptomatic aortic stenosis

OBSTETRICS

Anticoagulation in Pregnancy

Anticoagulants

Warfarin: Warfarin coagulopathy (chondrodysplasia punctate, nasal hypoplasia, optic atrophy, microcephaly)
Heparin: Does not cross placenta → safe

- Discontinue warfarin at 6 weeks of gestation
- Start heparin
- Restart warfarin at 14 week
- At 34–36 weeks restart heparin—labor should be planned
- Stop heparin 6 hours before labor
- Restart heparin
  - 6 hours after vaginal delivery
  - 12 hours after CS
- Start warfarin after 3 days
- Withdraw heparin if INR is adjusted.

Monitoring

- Heparin—APTT (twice weekly)
- Warfarin—PT-INR (2-3.0)

MOBILE HEAD AT TERM

OCCIPITOPOSTERIOR POSITION

The most common position is right occipitoposterior.

Cause of mobile head at term
O – Occipitoposterior
C – Cephalopelvic disproportion (CPD)
P – Placenta previa
C – Cord around neck
P – Polyhydramnios
D – Distended bladder

ETIOLOGY

- Fetal back on the right side predisposes to this position
- Placenta previa (anterior insertion)
- High assimilation type pelvis (android, anthropoid).

MECHANISM OF LABOR

In occipitoposterior position:

- With well flexed head, it has to rotate 3/8th of a circle, hence labor is prolonged
- If head is deflexed (because the convexity of fetal spine abuts against maternal spine causing extension) and cause larger diameter present at the pelvic inlet (relative disproportion).

ENGAGING DIAMETER

- Suboccipitofrontal in deflexed head
- Occipitofrontal if head is further deflexed.

COURSE OF LABOR

- Normally, the occiput rotates anteriorly (3/8) and baby is born as occipitoanterior
- Posterior rotation—when head is deflexed, sinciput is the leading part, it rotates anteriorly and deliver by face to pubis delivery. Birth is by extreme flexion followed by extreme extension (more common in anthropoid pelvis)
- Failure of rotation
  - The most common in android pelvis (deep transverse arrest)
  - Head is arrested with sagittal suture in transverse diameter at the level of ischial spine.

MANAGEMENT OF DEEP TRANSVERSE ARREST

- Cesarean section
- Vacuum extraction — Not used in modern obstetrics
- Forceps rotation (Kieland's forceps) — Not used in modern obstetrics
- Manual rotation.

OBSTETRICS

CEPHALOPELVIC DISPROPORTION

HISTORY

- History of rickets, osteomalacia, TB, poliomyelitis, fractures
- Previous history of vaginal delivery of average sized baby
- Previous history of instrumental delivery, birth asphyxia, stillbirth.

EXAMINATION

- General Examination—short stature, gait, deformities, spine
- Obstetric examination—mobile head at term.

Pelvic Clinical Pelvimetry

Points to be noted

Inlet	Cavity	Outlet
Sacral promontory	Sacral curvature	Subpubic angle
Diagonal conjugate	Pelvic side walls	Subpubic arch
	Ischial spines	Transverse diameter
	Sacrosciatic notch	

Munrokerr-Muller method: Left hand pushes head downward and backward into pelvis. Right hand, 2 fingers at level of ischial spines and thumb over pubic symphysis (only helpful in active labor)

- If head reaches ischial spine—no CPD
- 1st degree CPD—right hand is flushed with pubis symphysis, head can be pushed down but not reach up to ischial spine
- 2nd degree—head cannot be pushed down, parietal bone over rides pubic symphysis.

Hillis-Muller method: It is done when patient is in labor and during contraction.

In labor at the height of uterine contraction the left hand gives pressure on fundus, 2 finger of right hand are placed at the level of ischial spine when you push. If the head reaches spine, feeling of give is present—no CPD.

INVESTIGATIONS

Radio-pelvimetry (not done usually).

MANAGEMENT

- Elective cesarean section
- Trial of labor

Elective Cesarean Section

- Indication
  - Second degree CPD
  - First degree CPD with one of maternal or fetal complication.

Trial of labor

- Successful trail—birth of healthy baby vaginally with mother in good condition.
- Failed trail—delivery by cesarean section or dead or deeply compromised baby.
- Selection of patient—first degree CPD with no maternal or fetal complication
- Put partogram
- Augmentation of labor
- When to terminate trial of labor:
  - Failure of descend of head
  - Fetal or maternal distress
  - No progress of labor in spite of augmentation.
- Factors which decide outcome of trial of labor:
  - Good uterine contraction
  - Give of the pelvis
  - Moulding of fetal head.

What is mean by CPD?

It is the disparity in relationship between pelvis and fetal head (Never use CPD in breech presentation)
Contracted pelvis—in which any one of the essential diameter are so reduced as to affect mechanism of labor.

ETIOLOGY

- Developmental anomaly
- Vertebral deformity—kyphosis, scoliosis
- Injury or disease of pelvic bones—rickets, osteomalacia, fracture, dislocation of hip.

Complications

Maternal
- Prolonged labor
- Deep transverse arrest
- Increase chance of operative delivery, instrumental delivery
- Postpartum hemorrhage
- Malpresentation
- Premature rupture of membranes

Fetal
- Fetal distress
- Cord prolapse
- Excessive caput

Contracted Pelvis—Types

- Inlet contracted
  - If anteroposterior (AP) diameter <10 cm
  - Transverse <12 cm
  - Diagonal conjugate <11.5 cm
- Cauty contraction: Interspinous diameter <10 cm
- Outlet contraction: Intertuberous diameter <8 cm

BAD OBSTETRIC HISTORY

The term bad obstetric history is applied to a pregnant mother where her present obstetric outcome is likely to be affected adversely by the nature of previous obstetric disaster.

ABORTION

Spontaneous termination of pregnancy before reaching the period of viability (According to WHO it is <22 weeks or fetus weighs less than 500 g).

Types	Clinical picture	Size of uterus	Internal os	Ultrasound
1. Threatened	Slight bleeding	Corresponding	Closed	Live fetus
2. Complete	Bleeding stopped	Smaller	Closed	Uterus empty
3. Incomplete	Bleeding	Smaller	Open	Retained products
4. Inevitable	Bleeding, pain	Equal or less	Open	Dead fetus
5. Missed	Absent/minimal bleeding	Smaller	Closed	Dead fetus

Causes of Abortion

Fetal factors
- Chromosomal abnormalities
- Hydropic degeneration of villi
- Multiple pregnancies.

Maternal factors
- Infections—TORCH
- Maternal disease (HTN, uncontrolled DM)
- Environmental factors (smoking, alcohol, drugs)
- Endocrine factors (thyroid dysfunction, luteal phase defect)
- Immunological factors (APLA)
- Uterine factors (cervical insufficiency, submucous myoma, Asherman's syndrome).

Elderly Primigravida

Women above 35 years.

Grand Multigravida

Women has had 4 or more previous viable birth.

Past Date

Pregnancy crossed EDC—can wait up to 4–5 days

RH ISO (ALLO) IMMUNIZATION IN PREGNANCY

Format

- Ask father's blood group.
- History of previous pregnancy—anti-D given or not, any complication—stillbirth/neonatal death (NND)/ jaundice in neonatal period.

ETIOPATHOGENESIS OF RH ISOIMMUNIZATION

- Sensitization
- Immunization

When the mother is Rh –ve and the father is Rh +ve, the fetus can be Rh +ve and this can cause isoimmunization. Unlike ABO group, where anti-A to anti-B are already present in serum, here there are no naturally occurring antibodies. Hence sensitization must take place for antibodies to be formed.

How does isoimmunization occurs?

Normally fetal red cells carrying Rh antigen do not mix with maternal blood. However, in normal pregnancy there is always some circulating fetal RBC and this stimulate a maternal immune response due to the known self antigen. So produced IgM antibody which are large molecule cannot cross the placenta and hence cannot affect the fetus. IgG is also produced but takes a longer time usually 6 months after a fetomaternal bleed. On subsequent exposure the antigen as in the next pregnancy her previously primed B cells quickly produce IgG, which can be detected.

Factor Determining Maternal Response

- Volume of feto maternal bleed (critical volume 0.1 mL)
- Maternal responsiveness.
- Strength of antigenic stimulus
- ABO compatibility of mother and fetus.

PERINATAL COMPLICATION

- Immune hydrops:
  - This is the most serious form
  - Hemolysis of the fetal red cell results in fetal anemia
  - There is compensatory erythropoiesis in the bone marrow, spleen and liver resulting in hepatosplenomegaly
  - Due to extramedullary erythropoiesis there are immature nucleated erythroblasts in circulation, hence the name erythroblastosis fetalis
  - Severe anemia result in cardiac failure with generalized edema including scalp edema, ascites, pleural and pericardial effusion, hence the name immune hydrops
  - The generalized edema influences the fetal position which is described as 'BUDHA' position with a halo around the head (due to edematous scalp)
- Icterus gravis neonatorum:
  - If the baby is less severely affected it may appear well at birth but become jaundiced within 24 hours. This is because the bilirubin is no longer being cleared by placenta
- Congenital hemolytic anemia:
  - This is the mildest form of the disease, the anemia develops slowly and jaundice is not evident.

MANAGEMENT

All women who are Rh –ve with an Rh +ve partner should have indirect Coombs test (ICT)* at booking visit

↓

If ICT negative

↓

Mother is not immunized

↓

ICT should be repeated at 28th and 34th week in primigravida (should be repeated every month after 28 weeks in multigravida)

↓

If the ICT is persistently negative she can proceed to 40 week.

At delivery early cord clamping and sending blood for Hb, bilirubin and direct Coomb's test is done.

Postpartum Anti-D Prophylaxis

- If the baby is Rh +ve anti-D immunoglobulin must be given within 72 hours
- Anti-D binds to antigen sites on the fetal red cells so that these cells cannot mount an immune response
- Dose – 300 μg of anti-D immunoglobulin will neutralize 15 mL of fetomaternal bleed.

Kleihauer-Betke test

The maternal blood is subjected an acid solution (citric acid phosphate buffer), acid will elute the adult but not the fetal hemoglobin from the red cells, hence fetal red cells appear stained dark red unlike the light colored maternal red cells. The number of fetal red cell in 50 low power field is assessed. If there are 80 fetal red cells in 50 low power field it represents fetomaternal bleed of 4 mL. 100 μg of anti-D will neutralize 4 mL of fetomaternal bleed.

Other indications for anti-D immunoprophylaxis

1st trimester (50 μg)	Later pregnancy (300 μg)
• Miscarriage	• Miscarriage
• Ectopic	• Amniocentesis
• Hydatidiform mole	• Antepartum hemorrhage
• Threatened abortion	• External cephalic version (ECV)
• Medical termination of pregnancy (MTP), CVS	• Routinely at 28 weeks

Indirect Coombs Test

Indirect Coombs test (ICT) is done using the mother's blood and test for incomplete abortion. The mother's serum contains anti Rh-antibodies when treated with Standard Rh +ve red cells, these abortion coat the red cells. This RBC in turn will agglutinate when treated with Coomb's reagent, because now these RBCs are coated with abortion.

Amniocentesis and Amniotic Fluid Bilirubin Evaluation

- This is based upon the fact that when hemolysis occurs, bilirubin is present in the atrial fibrillation (AF). The amount of bilirubin correlates with degree of severity.
- Liley established spectrophotometry as a method of assessing AF bilirubin concentration
- Amniocentesis is done and the bilirubin concentration is measured by spectrophotometry by assessing change in optical density at 450 nm.
- This is plotted on Liley's chart which has 3 zones: Bilirubin concentration at zone 3 > zone 2 > zone 1

Noninvasive Assessment of Early Fetal Anemia

- Liver and spleen enlargement
- Fetal Doppler shows increased vascularity (middle cerebral artery Doppler)
- Sinusoidal pattern with loss of normal baseline variability on CTG.

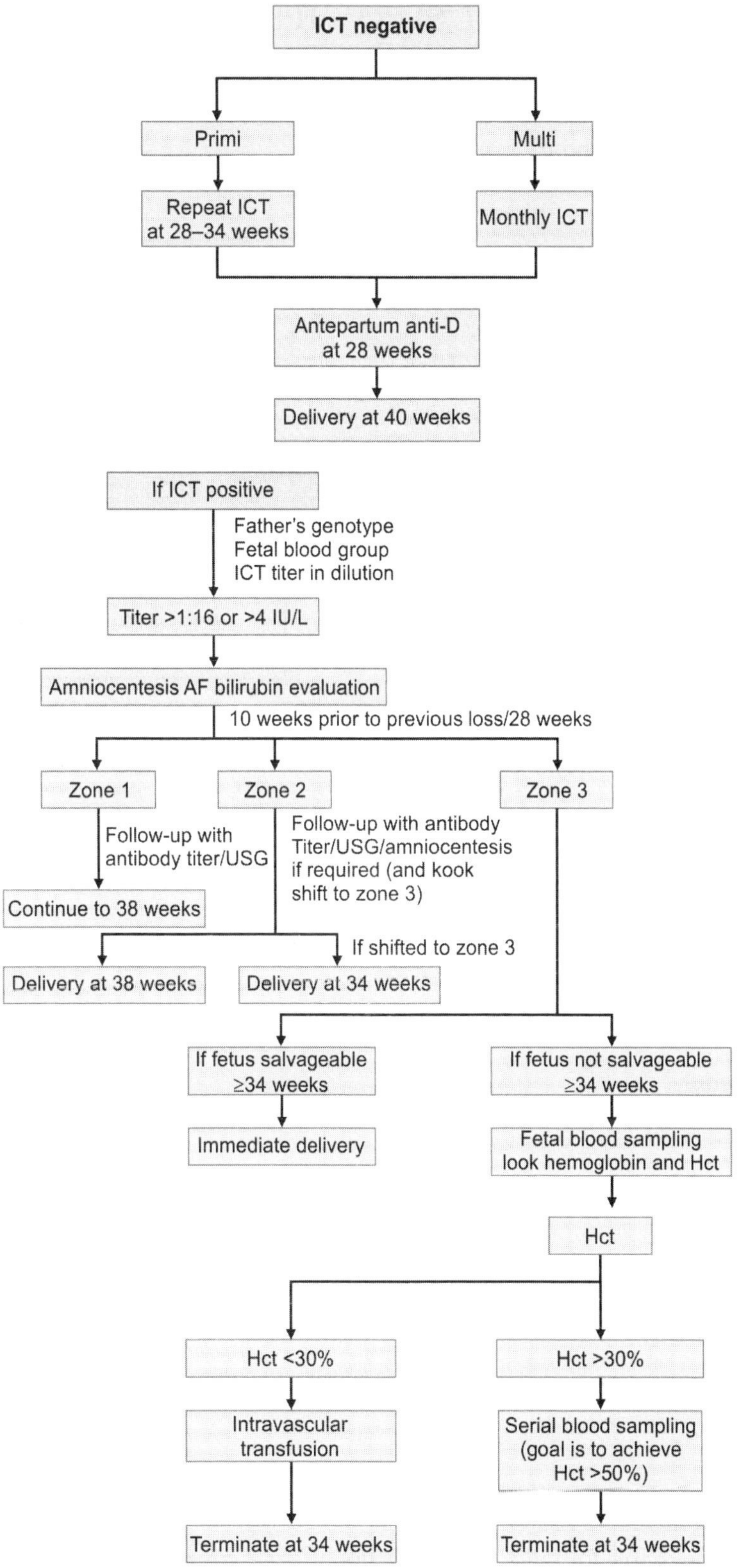

(ICT, Indirect Coombs test, Hct: Hematocrit, USG: Ultrasonography)

FETAL SURVEILLANCE

FETAL MOVEMENT COUNT

Cardiff count-time during which she has felt 10 kicks (ten kick chart) normally at least 10 movements in a 12 hour period (or count up to 3 movements/hour).

NON-STRESS TEST (NST)

Things that is to be looked:
- Fetal heart rate
- Beat to beat variability
- Acceleration
- Deceleration

It may be either reactive or non-reactive.

Reactive NST

Presence of two or more fetal heart rate acceleration during the period of 20 minutes with each acceleration of 12 beats or more per minute and lasting 15 or more second.

Non-reactive NST—causes

- Fetal hypoxia
- Sleep period of fetus
- Gastational age <28 weeks.

- Early deceleration—head compression
- Late deceleration—placental insufficiency
- Variable deceleration—cord compression

BIOPHYSICAL PROFILE

Components:
- Non-stress test
- Amniotic fluid index
- Fetal movement
- Fetal tone
- Fetal breathing

Each having score of 2, max score 10

a. 8–10 normal
b. <4—abnormal
c. 5–7—equivocal

Modified biophysical profile
- Non-stress test
- Amniotic fluid index

Normal value
- AFI— 5–24 cm
- SDP—2–8 cm

Admission Test

Continuous CTG monitoring for 20 minutes on admission to labor ward.

LABOR INDUCTION

BISHOP SCORE

- Cervical dilatation (cm)
- Cervical effacement (cm)
- Status
- Position
- Consistency

Score < 5 is considered unfavorable for induction. Induction may be either medical/mechanical/surgical.

Medical:
- Oxytocin
- Prostaglandin

Mechanical: Foley catheter and extra-amniotic saline infusion (EASI) (220 mL of warm saline introduced).
Surgical: Artificial rupture of membrane using Kochers forceps.
Failed induction: Said to be failed when the women not entered active phase of labor despite induction.

INSTRUMENTAL DELIVERY

FORCEPS

Parts

1. Blade
2. Shank
3. Lock
4. Handle: Wrigley's outlet forceps.

Indication

1. Fetal distress
2. Maternal distress
3. To cut shorten second stage in cardiac disease, preeclampsia, anemia (no maternal effort needed)
4. After coming head in breech.

Prerequisites

1. Vertex presentation
2. Station of the head is known (+2/+3)
3. No CPD
4. Cervix fully dilated
5. Head should be engaged
6. Bladder empty

Complications

1. Maternal
   - Traumatic PPH
   - Injury to vagina, cervix
2. Fetal
   - Intracranial hemorrhage
   - Fracture skull
   - Asphyxia
   - Cephalohematoma.

VACUUM EXTRACTOR

Indications

- Fetal distress
- Maternal distress
- Deep transverse arrest
- Medical disease like preeclampsia

Contraindications for Vacuum
1. Face presentation
2. Preterm head
3. Fetal coagulopathy

Complication—same as that of forceps delivery

Prerequisites

Same as that of forceps delivery.

Application

The center of cup is on flexion point of fetal head (flexing median application, point located on sagittal suture 3 cm in front of posterior fontanelle.

Negative pressure is applied is appliad to create chignon or artificial caput (maximum pressure is 0.8 kg/cm^2).

PRENATAL SCREENING

1. By using USG
   Uses of 1st trimester USG:
   a. Whether pregnancy is intrauterine or extrauterine

b. Dating (+/–3 days)
c. Viability
d. Multiple pregnancy
e. Hydatidiform mole
f. Evaluation of 1st trimester bleeding

11–14 weeks scan:
a. Anencephaly (9–11 weeks)
b. Nuchal translucency (>3 mm, suspect Down syndrome)

18-20 weeks scan (2nd trimester)
a. Targeted anomaly scan
b. Fetal survey (viability, i.e. placentation, liquor status)
c. Fetal biometry
d. Fetal environment

3rd trimester scan
a Fetal growth
b Fetal wellbeing
c Confirmation of presentation, placentation.

2. Triple and quadruple test:
   - Triple test used for screening in Down syndrome (between 15–20 weeks). β-hCG (increases), MS AFP (maternal serum alpha-fetoprotein—decreases) and estriol (decreases)
   - Quadruple test—above mentioned + inhibin A.

PRENATAL DIAGNOSTIC TEST

Karyotyping by:
- Chorionic villi sampling—done between 10–12 weeks (1st trimester)
- Amniocentesis—performed between 15 weeks and 20 weeks
- Cordocentesis—performed at/after 20 weeks.

OPERATIVE PROCEDURES

EPISIOTOMY

Performed when head is crowning the vulva.

Advantages

- Prevent perineal tear
- Easier to repair than ragged tear.

Types

- Midline episiotomy
- Mediolateral episiotomy (common)
- J-shaped episiotomy.

Structures cut:
- Posterior vaginal wall
- Superficial transverse perinei muscle
- Bulbospongiosus
- Deep transverse perinei
- Levator ani
- Fascia overlying muscle
- Subcutaneous tissue
- Skin

Mediolateral Episiotomy

- Vaginal mucosa repaired by continuous suture.
- Muscle repaired by interrupted sutures (suture material—delayed absorbable—catgut or vicryl)
- Skin repaired by mattress sutures.

Complications

- Bleeding, hematoma formation
- Infection
- Fistula formation
- Dyspareunia.

Cesarean Section
Delivery of viable fetus through an incision in the abdominal wall and uterus

OBSTETRICS

PERINEAL TEAR

1°— Laceration involving vaginal mucosa and perineal skin
2°—Involves 1° + facial muscles of perineal body
3°—Involves 2° + anal sphincter
4°—Involves 3° + rectal mucosa

LOWER SEGMENT CESAREAN SECTION

Preparation

- Routine preoperative investigations
- Arrange cross-matched blood
- Tetanus toxoid
- Antibiotic sensitivity
- Written informed consent
- Local area preparation
- Nil per oral after 10 PM
- Enema
- Anxiolytic—alprazolam.

Procedure

- Under spinal anesthesia
- The parts are cleansed with antiseptic solution and draped
- A left lateral tilt will reduce aortocaval compression and the risk of supine hypotension
- Abdominal incision: Pfannensteil incision
- Transverse curvilinear incision just above the pubic hair line, this is deepened through the subcutaneous fat up to the rectus sheath which is incised transversely
- After separating the two recti muscle in the midline the parietal peritoneum is opened.
  - Uterine incision: Once the abdomen is opened dextrorotation corrected
  - A Doyen's retractor is used to visualize LS
  - After identifying the loose peritoneum over LS, it is divided transversely and separated from the bladder by blunt dissection
  - A small incision is made in the LS extended laterally using the scissors or by stretching with the fingers
  - Delivery of the baby—in cephalic presentation the hand is slipped into the uterine cavity and the head is gently levered out of the incision
  - In the breach presentation the feet are first hooked out and the rest of the body is delivered as in the case of vaginal breach delivery
  - In the transverse or oblique lie, the lie is corrected to a longitudinal one before the uterine incision is made.
  - After the delivery of the baby—oxytocin 20 U
  - Closure:
    - Uterus is closed using single layer of No. 1 vicryl
    - Parietal peritoneum—catgut
    - Rectus sheath—PDS, or proline
    - Subcutaneous fat—catgut
    - Skin—vicryl
  - After closure vaginal toilet is done with PGE1, 800 μg is kept PR.

Postoperative Care

- Monitoring of PR, BP, RR, intake output chart, vaginal bleeding, condition of uterus for first 6–8 hours
- IV fluid—on the first days
- Oral fluid started after 6 hours
- Early ambulation and deep breathing exercise started on the next day
- Review after 6–8 weeks.

GYNECOLOGY

CHAPTER 20

Clinical Cases

GYNECOLOGY—CASE FORMAT

Name: Age: Address: Occupation:

Presenting Complaints

(Present in chronological order)

- Bleeding per vaginal (PV)
  - Amount of blood (number of pad she had to use). Any history of passage of clots
  - Associated with pain/discharge/fever
- Discharge PV
  - Whether it is scanty/profuse
  - Color of discharge
  - Whether it is mucoid, frothy (nature)
  - Whether offensive
  - Associated symptoms like pain
- Pain
  - Nature, intensity, onset, location, associated symptoms, relation with menstrual cycle
- Any history of urinary symptoms
  - Burning sensation, retention of urine, urinary incontinence
- Menstrual history
- Marital history
- Obstetric history
- Past history
- Family history
- Personal history.

General Examination

Same as that of obstetric examination.

Other Systems

Abdominal examination

(After evacuation of bladder)

Inspection

- Shape of abdomen
- Umbilicus central and inverted/everted
- All quadrants moving equally with respiration
- Any scar, dilated veins
- Any visible swelling, if yes then shape, size, site of the swelling

Palpation
- Local rise of temperature/tenderness
- Site of swelling, size, whether movable/not lower border palpable/not

Percussion
Auscultation
Perspeculum examination
Summary

FIBROID

ETIOLOGY OF FIBROID

- High estrogen exposure
- Growth factor overexpression—epidermal growth factor (EGF), Insulin-like growth factor (IGF) and transforming growth factor (TGF-β)
- Translocations
- Bcl-2 overexpression.

RISK FACTORS

- Early menarche
- Nulliparity
- Exogenous hormones in oral contraceptive pills (OCP)
- Late menopause.

MECHANISM OF MENORRHAGIA

- Increase in the endometrial surface area
- Increased vascularity
- Endometrial ulceration and hemorrhage over a submucous fibroid
- Interference with normal uterine contractility
- Compression of venous plexus
- Associated endometrial hyperplasia.

Clinical Features

- Menorrhagia
- Abdominal lump
- Pain—causes
  - Red degeneration
  - Expulsion of a submucous fibroid
  - Hemorrhage into fibroid
  - Torsion of pedunculated fibroid
  - Acute retention of urine in cervical fibroid.
- Infertility—causes
  - Cornual myomas can cause tubal occlusion, impaired gamete and embryo transport
  - Distortion of cavity
  - Impaired blood supply leading to atrophy and ulceration of endometrium overlying a submucous fibroid
  - Endometrial hyperplasia
  - Alteration of normal immune response to the implanting fetus
  - Displacement of cervix from vaginal pool of semen.
- Pressure symptoms
  - Cervical fibroid—bladder compression
  - Broad ligament fibroid—compresses ureter and produces hydronephrosis.

Differential Diagnosis

- Ovarian tumor—any age, loss of weight and appetite
- Pelvic inflammatory disease (PID)—tubo-ovarian mass—tender, firm tubo-ovarian abscess—tender, cystic

- Endometriosis tender cystic with reduced mobility
- Chronic ectopic
- Adenomyosis—multiparous, perimenopausal age
- Other surgical causes

Site—midline, firm swelling, all borders except lower border is palpable.
Mass mobile in transverse direction
Bimanual examination: Transmitted mobility, fornices free, uterus not separately palpable.
Perspeculum examination: To visualize vagina and cervix.

Investigations

1. **USG abdomen**
   - Transvaginal and transabdominal USG
   - Seen as hypoechoic area
   - To detect number, size and location of fibroid and also for follow-up
   - Exclude other differential diagnosis.
   - Also to look for hydronephrosis, adenexa, endometrial thickness.
2. **Hysteroscopy**
   - Can see the lesion
   - Remove the submucous fibroid.
3. **Sonosalpingography/hysterosalpingography**
   To detect small submucous fibroid.
4. Magnetic resonance imaging **(MRI)**—to detect sarcomatous changes
5. **Intravenous pyelogram**—in broad ligament fibroid
   Do Pap smear for all women above 30 years.

MANAGEMENT

- Expectant
- Medical
- Surgical
- Conservative
- Uterine artery embolization.

Criteria for Expectant Management

- Absolute certainty of diagnosis (exclusion of ovarian mass)
- Asymptomatic
- No evidence of ureteral compression
- Size: <12–14 weeks
- Willing for follow-up
- Perimenopausal women.

EXPECTANT MANAGEMENT

Medical

Drugs:

- For relief of symptoms and reduction of tumor size
- Nonsteroidal anti-inflammatory drugs **(NSAIDs)**
  - Mefenamic acid 500 mg TDS/QID
  - Decreases bleeding by 40%
- **Antifibrinolytic agents**—tranexamic acid 500 mg TDS
- Ethamsylate
  - 500 mg QID
  - Reduces capillary fragility
- **Progestogens**—medroxyprogesterone acetate 10 mg × 10 days/month or 21 days/month for 3 months
- Gonadotropin-releasing hormone **(GnRH) agonists**
  - Goserelin 3.6 mg or leuprolide 3.75 mg monthly subcutaneous injection
  - Mechanism of action **(MOA)**—Gonadal suppression and hypoestrogenism

Uses of danazol
1. Endometriosis
2. Fibrocystic disease of breast
3. Angioneurotic edema
4. Idiopathic thrombocytopenic purpura (ITP)
5. Hemophilia

GYNECOLOGY

Uses:
1. Large fibroids can be reduced in size
   Abdominal hysterectomy converted to vaginal hysterectomy
   Open procedure—laparoscopic.
2. Anemia can be corrected during waiting period—intraoperative bleeding is less.
3. In women nearing menopause to avoid surgery together.

Drawbacks:
1. Hypoestrogenism—hot flushes, osteoporosis, vaginal dryness
2. Small myomas may be missed
3. The plane of cleavage may be less defined.

Add back therapy—estrogen and progesterone added to prevent side effects of hypoestrogenism
Danazol—antigonadotropin: Side effect—acne, hirsutism, weight gain
Mifepristone—antiprogestin
Mirena intrauterine contraceptive device (IUCD)—to control menorrhagia due to fibroid.

Surgical Management

1. **Hysterectomy**

Types:
i. Simple hysterectomy (type 1): Extra facial, only uterus and cervix removed.
ii. Modified radical hysterectomy (type II): Uterus, cervix, cuff of vagina, parametrial and paracervical tissue medial to ureters are removed
iii. Radical hysterectomy (type III): Parametrium up to pelvic wall removed
iv. Type IV, V: With pelvic exenteration

Abdominal hysterectomy
- Symptomatic fibroids in a woman who has completed family
- Large fibroids (>14 weeks), broad ligament fibroid, cervical fibroid.

Steps:
Incision—Pfannenstiel incision
- Abdomen opened in layers
- The uterus is elevated with surgeon's left hand and a forceps is placed on either sides of cornua to maneuver uterus
- **First pedicle**—tubes, ovarian ligament and round ligament are clamped, cut and ligated (if the ovaries are to be removed the infundibulopelvic ligaments are clamped, cut and ligated).
- Then separate bladder from cervix by opening the uterovesical (UV) fold of peritoneum (this step is essential to avoid damage to ureters while clamping uterine vessel).
- **Second pedicle**—uterine vessels are clamped, cut and ligated.
- **Third pedicle**—includes cardinal and uterosacral ligaments which are cut and ligated.
- Two clamps are placed across the vagina below cervix and uterus is removed.
- Edges of vaginal cut are closed with a locking suture (blanket suture).
- Closure of abdomen—after irrigation with normal saline (NS) the pedicles are closely inspected for hemostasis, ureters are visualized, mops are counted.
- Abdomen is closed in layers.

Complications
- **Immediate**—hemorrhage, injury to ureter, bladder or bowel.
- **Late—**reactionary and secondary hemorrhage, wound infection, pelvic infection, vesicovaginal and uretero-vaginal fistulae, paralytic ileus, deep vein thrombosis (DVT)
- **Sequelae**—vault prolapse, incisional hernia, fistulae

Vaginal hysterectomy—in small fibroids (<14 weeks size).

Laparoscopic hysterectomy
Laparoscopic-assisted vaginal hysterectomy (**LAVH)**—laparoscopic division of structures above uterine artery and remainder of procedure completed vaginally.

2. **Myomectomy**
   - Those who wish to preserve uterus
   - Those who wish for child bearing.

GYNECOLOGY

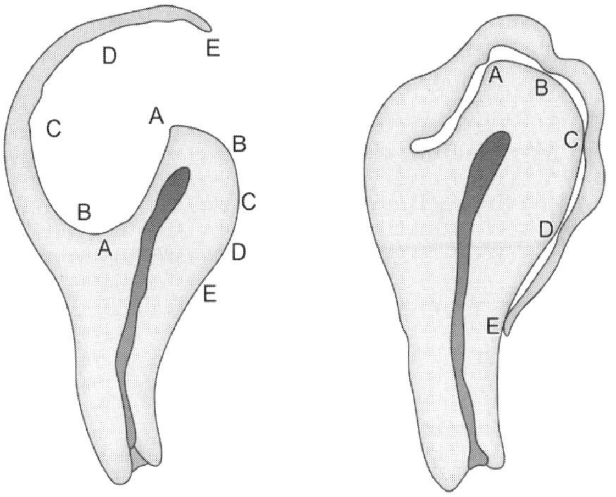

Preopertive counseling
- About risk and complications of myomectomy
- Probability of recurrence 50% in 5 years
- Consent for hysterectomy
- Cross matched blood should be available
- Rule out other causes of infertility.

Incision
- Midline incision—least vascular
- Anterior incision—to prevent adhesions to tubes/ovaries
- Lower incision
- Tunneling incision—for small myoma
- Bonney's hood incision—to remove single posterior fibroid.

After incising myoma, it is enucleated through the cleavage plane of capsule as many myomas as possible must be removed through single incision usually tunneling incision. Myoma screw may help to remove fibroid.

The myometrial defects are closed using 1-0 vicryl without dead space formation to prevent hematoma. Serosa is approximated with 3-0/4-0 vicryl using a baseball stitch.

Methods to limit blood loss
- Timing of surgery—immediate postmenstrual phase
- Hypotensive surgery
- Vasopressin instillation into serosa and myometrium overlying the myoma
- Using tourniquets at internal os to compress the uterine vessels and at the infundibulopelvic ligament to occlude the ovarian vessels
- Bonney's myomectomy clamp to occlude the uterine vessel along with ring forceps to occlude ovarian vessels *release at 20 minutes interval* to prevent accumulation of histamine
- Pretreatment with GnRH agonists
- Plenty of crossmatched blood should be available.

Hysteroscopic myomectomy

Submucous fibroid

Laparoscopic myomectomy
- For pedunculated fibroid and for subserous fibroid not exceeding 10 cm in size and not more than 4 in number
- A morcellator for removal of large fibroid or removal via colpotomy incision.

UTERINE ARTERY EMBOLIZATION (UAE)

For symptomatic women who do not want hysterectomy or myomectomy. It is usually timed for immediate postmenstrual period. Usually, a transfemoral approach is employed. A guide wire is manipulated until it reaches the uterine artery. Embolization is done using polyvinyl alcohol. It is done bilaterally.

Contraindications
- Subserous and pedunculated fibroids
- Infertility
- Pregnancy, infection, coagulopathy.

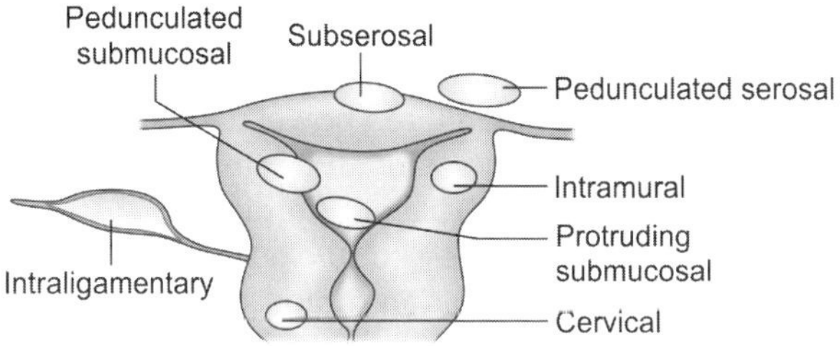

Fibroid types

Complications
- Ischemic pain
- Fever and infection
- Vaginal discharge and bleeding
- Embolism
- Ovarian failure.

Secondary Changes: Degenerations
- Atrophy, calcific degeneration
- Red degeneration (aseptic inflammation, thrombosis, necrosis)—in pregnancy, DCP use, GnRH therapy.

- Sarcomatous changes (only 0.5% of all myomas)
- Hyaline degeneration—most common
- Cystic degeneration
- Fatty degeneration
- Myxomatous degeneration

Other Complications

- Torsion
- Inversion
- Capsular hemorrhage
- Infection
- Associated endometrial carcinoma (3% cases in women >40 years)
- Pseudo-Meigs syndrome
- Polycythemia (due to erythropoietin secretion)
- Leomyosarcoma (0.5%).

Mention adenomyosis as differential diagnosis only when uterus not palpable

ADENOMYOSIS

Islands of endometrium seen in the wall of uterus.

Clinical Features

- Women above 40 years, parous
- Uterus enlarged <14 weeks
- Menorrhagia and progressively increasing dysmenorrhea (congestive type)

Rx-Medical management—NSAID, OCP, GnRH analogue aromatase inhibitor, levonorgestrel intrauterine contraceptive system (LNG-IUS)
Surgical management—Hysterectomy, resection of adenomyoma.

OVARIAN TUMOR

APPROACH

Age: Older (50–60) more chance of malignancy.

History of Present Illness

- Abdominal swelling site—lower abdomen, gradually increasing in size—benign, fast growing—malignant. Abdominal discomfort, dyspepsia, early satiety, abdominal distension
- Pressure symptoms—increased frequency of micturition, urinary retention, constipation, edema of legs, dyspnea (for very large tumor)
- Malignancy characteristics—loss of weight, loss of apetite
- Irregular bleeding/postmenopausal bleeding—feminizing tumor
- Amenorrhea—androgen producing tumor
- Acute pain—torsion/rupture/hemorrhage into cyst/infected dermoid cyst (germ cell tumor in adolescents grow rapidly and cause pain)
- Vomiting—torsion
- Cough, hemoptysis, altered bowel habits—metastasis
- If the patient presents with abdominal mass do not forget to ask the following:
  - Menorrhagia—to rule out fibroid
  - Discharge pv, fever—to rule out PID (forms tubo-ovarian mass)

To rule out metastatic ovarian tumor from gastrointestinal (GI) malignancy, ask bowel habits, malena, etc.

Family History

History of carcinoma (especially breast and ovarian).

General Examination

- Cachexia, supraclavicular lymph node (LNE), breast lump—malignancy
- Pedal edema—pressure effect
- Hirsutism, male pattern baldness—androgen-secreting tumor

Respiratory System

- Pleural effusion signs-Pseudo-Meig's syndrome (ascites + pleural effusion in Brenner, thecoma, granulosa cell tumor and fibroid)
- Meig's syndrome (in fibroma).

PER ABDOMEN

Inspection

Longitudinal distension, visible mass.

Palpation

- Tenderness—torsion, hemorrhage, inflammation
- Describe the mass, e.g. spherical mass of size 6 × 6 cm located in the right iliac fossa, cystic/varying/hard in consistency, smooth/irregular (malignant) surface, well-defined/ill-defined border, all borders palpable, mobile in all direction/fixed (malignant)
  No HSM (may be present in malignancy).

Percussion

- Dull note over the mass.
- Fluid thrill, shifting dullness (present in malignant ascites and sometimes in benign tumors like Brenner and fibroma).

Auscultation

Normal blood sugar (BS)
* Per speculum examination, bimanual pelvic examination (not done).

Diagnosis

For example, ______ year-old P2L2 with benign/malignant ovarian tumor.

Discussion

Risk factors:
- Older age groups
- Nullipara
- Infertility
- Early menarche
- Late menopause
- Endometriosis/PID
- Family history of cancer.

Q. Why do you call it ovarian mass and not uterine?

	Ovarian mass	**Uterine mass**
History		
Menstrual symptoms	Not usually present	Main symptom
Abdominal distension	Main complaint	Not usual
Loss of weight (LOW), LOA	Present if malignant	Not present
Examination		
Site	Towards one side of abdomen	Central
Size	Can reach up to xiphisternum	Smaller usually
Consistency	Cystic (hard if malignant)	Firm
Borders	All borders palpable	Lower not Palpable usually
Mobility	In all directions in benign	Only side to side
Uterus	Normal size separately palpable	Bulky, not separately palpable
Transmitted mobility	Not present	Present

- Bimanual pelvic examination—not done

Q. Why do you tell it is benign?

	Benign	Malignant
History	Slow growing	Fast
	Long-standing	Within months
	No LOW, LOA	Present
General examination	No cachexia	Present
	No supraclavicular lymph node (SCLN)	Present
Per vaginal examination	Smaller, regular surface	Arger, irregular surface
	Cystic consistency	Varying/hard
	Mobile	Fixed
	Unilateral	Bilateral
	No ascites/HSM	May be present

Q. How to differentiate benign and malignant with investigation?

	Benign	Malignant
Ultrasonography (USG)	Thin walled cyst	Thick walled Thin septum Thick septum
	Unilateral	Bilateral
	Anechoic	Heteroechoic
Doppler	———	Increased vascularity, low resistance index (<0.4)
CA-125	——-	Increased

Q. How to proceed with this patient?

1. **Do bimanual pelvic examination**
   - Confirm site, size, etc.
   - Confirm that mass is arising from ovary (refer difference between uterine and ovarian given above)
2. **Do USG**—Transabdominal/transvaginal (TA/TV). TV is better if it is small.
   - USG features; mass, site, ovary separately visible, size, Features of malignancy, Whether contralateral ovary normal?
   - Uterus—whether normal myometrial and endometrial echo? Mass arising from uterus, Endometrial thickness, Liver-metatosis, Free fluid in abdomen, Hydroureteronephrosis.
3. If USG shows features of malignancy, then do CT—Lymph node status, MRI—better for metastasis.
4. Chest X-ray—if symptoms of lung metastasis/pleural effusion.
5. Investigations for fitness for surgery—Hb, blood grouping, liver function tests (LFT), renal function tests (RFT), electrocardiography (ECG).
6. If metastatic ovarian tumor suspected—do barium meal to exclude primary gastrointestinal (GI) carcinoma.
7. Then proceed for treatment.

STAGING

I. Restricted to one/both ovaries
   - I A—One ovary
   - I B—Both ovaries
   - I C—IA/B + surface malignant growth/capsular rupture/malignant ascites/positive washing

II. One/both ovaries with pelvic extension
   - A—Uterus/tubes
   - B—Other pelvic organ
   - C—II A/B + surface malignant growth/capsular rupture/malignant ascites/positive washing.

III. One/both ovary with microscopic implant outside pelvis positive node (inguinal/retroperitoneal), superficial liver metastasis
   - A—Grossly limited to pelvis with microscopic implants in peritoneum
   - B—Peritoneal implants <2 cm
   - C—Peritoneal implants >2 cm/+ve nodes

IV. One/both ovaries with distant metastasis.

If inguinal lymph node involved
- Stage III in ovarian carcinoma
- Stage IV endometrial carcinoma

GYNECOLOGY

TREATMENT OF MALIGNANT OVARIAN TUMORS

Stage I and II (Early stage)

Staging Laparotomy

Steps:

General anesthesia → midline vertical incision → take ascetic fluid/peritoneal wash for astrology → examinations of ovaries and pelvis → systemic exploration of all organs is clockwise fashion → Biopsy from suspicious area and intraperitoneal biopsy → biopsy from diaphragm with Ayre's spatula → Do total abdominal hysterectomy (TAH) + bilateral salpingo-oophorectomy (BSO) → infracolic omentectomy → pelvic and para aortic lymphadenectomy.

Ia and Ib — No need of chemotherapy

Others — adjuvant chemotherapy needed.

Stage III and IV (Advanced stage)

Staging laparotomy

1. Debulking surgery/maximal cytoreductive surgery—to decrease the amount of malignant tissues subjected to chemotherapy and also to relieve symptoms
2. Postoperative adjuvant chemotherapy
3. Neoadjuvant chemotherapy + surgery + postoperative chemotherapy .

CHEMOTHERAPY

- Cisplatin + Paclitaxel or Carboplatin + Paclitaxel.
- Now single agent chemo with cisplatin commonly used.
- Neoadjuvant chemotherapy—in advanced disease. Preoperative chemotherapy to chemically debulk the tumor.

TREATMENT OF BENIGN OVARIAN TUMOR

- Ovarian cystectomy/ovariotomy.
- But if older age and completed family, better do TH with BSO.

WHO CLASSIFICATION OF OVARIAN TUMOR

I. Common epithelial tumor
- Serous
- Mucinous
- Endometrioid
- Clear cell
- Brenner
- Mixed epithelial
- Undifferentiated.

II. Sex cord stromal tumor
- Granulosa—stromal cell tumor
- Theca cell tumor
- Androblastoma
- Gynandroblastoma

III. Lipid cell tumor

IV. Germ cell tumor
- Dysgerminoma
- Endodermal sinus tumor
- Embryonal tumor
- Polyembryoma
- Choriocarcinoma
- Teratoma
- Mixed

V. Gonadoblastoma

VI. Soft tissue tumor

VII. Metastatic tumor

VIII. Tumor-like syndrome

Q. Benign tumors which are solid?
Brenner, thecoma, fibroma

Q. Complications of ovarian tumor.
- Torsion (the most common malignancy causing torsion—dermoid cyst)
- Rupture
- Infection
- Hemorrhage into cyst
- Malignant transformation
- Pseudomyxoma peritonei—spontaneous rupture of mucinous cystadenoma/mucocele of appendix leading to implantation of mucin secreting cells on peritoneum and hence mucinous ascites.

Q. What are the tumor markers used?
- CA 125—epithelial cell tumors
  - >35 U/mL—postmenopausal
  - >200 U/mL—premenopausal
- Carcinoembryonic antigen (CEA), CA 19-9—mucinous cystadenocarcinoma
- Human chorionic gonadotropin (HCG), lactate dehydrogenase (LDH), placental alpha fetoprotein (ALP)—germ cell tumor
- AFP—Endodermal sinus tumor

Tumor maskers
CA 125 – ovarian Ca
CEA – Ca colon
CA 19-9 – pancreatic Ca
PSA – prostate Ca

Q. Screening of ovarian carcinoma.
- Done in high-risk groups, i.e. people with strong family history.
- Six monthly bimanual pelvic examination
- Six monthly TVS
- If needed CA 125, CEA, hCG
- Genetic mapping, polymerase chain reaction (PCR), genetic testing for *BRCA*1, *BRCA*2 genes.
- Doppler— increased vascularity.

Q. What is Krukenberg tumor?
- Metastatic ovarian carcinoma from Ca stomach/large bowel/breast
- Bilateral
- Shape of ovary retained.

DYSFUNCTIONAL UTERINE BLEEDING (DUB)

DEFINITION

Abnormal uterine bleeding without any demonstrable local pathology/systemic disease.
Etiology is purely hormonal—the hypertrophy and hyperplasia of the endometrium are induced by a high titer of estrogen in the circulating blood.

CLASSIFICATION

Anovulatory (80%)	Ovulatory (20%)
1. Metropathia hemorrhagica	1. Idiopathic ovulatory menorrhagia
2. Threshold bleeding	2. Luteal phase defect

Metropathia Hemorrhagica

Failure to develop dominant follicle → No ovulation → No progesterone → unopposed actions of estrogen → endometrial hyperplasia → endometrium out grows its blood supply → bleeding occurs → lack of progesterone cause decreased vasoconstrictors PG production → profuse bleeding occurs.
–characterized by 2–3 months of amenorrhea followed by profuse and prolonged bleeding for 20–30 days.

Threshold Bleeding

Perimenopausal women → insufficient follicular development → continuous action of low level of estrogens → polymenorrhea/polymenorrhagia.

Idiopathic Ovulatory Menorrhagia

Normal progesterone but altered PGE_2 (vasodilator) and PGF_2 (Vasoconstrictor) ratio → bleeding occurs.

GYNECOLOGY

Luteal Phase Defect

Inadequate functioning of corpus lutein → decreased progesterone → decreased PGF2x → premenstrual spotting → bleeding occurs

CAUSES OF MENORRHAGIA

In reproductive age group:

- Pelvic pathology—fibroid, endometriosis, adenomyosis, PID
- Pregnancy related problems—ectopic pregnancy, hydatidiform mole, implantation bleed
- Coagulation and hematological problems—von Willebrand disease (vWD), immune thrombocytopenic purpura (ITP), leukemias
- Medical—hypo/hyperthyroidism, Cushing's disease, liver disease, renal failure
- Intrauterine contraceptive device (IUCD) related bleeding, hormonal contraception.

In perimenopausal age:

- Anovulatory DUB
- Endometrial carcinoma
- Cervical cancer and premalignancy
- Feminizing ovarian tumors
- Other endometrial pathology like fibroids and polyps.

MANAGEMENT OF DUB

1. Perspeculam examination—rule out local pathology
   Bimanual pelvic examination—look size and mobility of uterus
   Any mass—to rule out fibroid, ovarian tumor
2. Routine blood and urine examination—platelet count, LFT, RFT, coagulation profile (if there is clinical suspicion.....etc.
3. Thyroid function test (TFT)—to rule out hypothyroidism
4. Urine pregnancy test (UPT)—to rule out pregnancy
5. Pap smear—to rule out Carcinoma of cervix
6. USG—TAS and TVS—assess size of uterus, uterine cavity and adnexa, measure endometrial thickness
7. Diagnostic curettage—FC in perimenopausal age group and D and C in reproductive age group
8. Hysterosalpingography and saline salpingography.

TREATMENT OF DUB

Endometrial thickness
- Postmenopausal woman—if >4 mm, it should be evaluated
- Premenopausal woman—if >12 mm, should be evaluated

1. Treat anemia
2. Medical therapy—1st line of treatment
   a. Non-hormonal: antifibrinolytics like tranexamic acid, NSAIDs—mefenamic acid, Ethamsylate (reduces capillary fragility)
   b. Hormonal:
      i. Progestogens
         High initial dose of norethisterone 10–30 mg/day—bleeding arrest in 24–48 hours
         ↓
         Continue 5 mg/day for 20 days, withdrawal bleeding occurs within 2–5 days
         Cyclical treatment—5 mg/day for 20 days started on 2nd or 3rd day 3–6 months, and then it is stopped to observe the patient.
         Others: Duphaston (10 mg), MDPA 10 mg—no adverse effect on lipoproteins.
      ii. Mirena/Progestogen impregnated IUCD (LNG-IUS)—effective in controlling menorrhagia. It directly suppresses endometrium with less systemic side effects. Can be left in place for 5 years offering also one time contraception in young women.
      iii. OCPs
      iv. Estrogen only pills
      v. Danazol—200 mg OD for 3–4 cycles. Causes endometrial atrophy. Main problem is androgenic side effects like weight gain, acne, metabolic problems.
      vi. Clomiphene is advocated if pregnancy is desired.
      vii. GnRH analogue last drug when others fail. Depot injection 3.6 mg given monthly for 4–6 months
      viii. Ormeloxifene (Saheli)—60 mg twice weekly for 12 weeks.

OPERATIVE METHODS

1. Curettage: About 30–40% patients will be cured by curettage alone. Also important in diagnosis of genital tract tuberculosis (TB), endometrial carcinoma.
2. Minimally invasive surgery: For example, hysteroscopic endometrial ablation, radiofrequency—induced thermal ablation, cavaterm balloon therapy, uterine tamponade, etc.
3. Hysterectomy: TAH/VH/laparoscopic hysterectomy/LAVH.
   Indicated—if medical/MIS fails or DUB recurs, in older women >40 years
   Not desirous of childbearing and who opt for hysterectomy as a primary procedure.

Notes:

1. Amenorrhea—absence of menstruation. It may be primary or secondary
   Primary refers to failure of onset of menstruation beyond the age of 16 years regardless of development of secondary sexual characters. Secondary amenorrhea refers to failure of occurrence of menstruation for 6 months or longer in women who have previously menstrauted.

Cause:	Primary amenorrhea	Secondary amenorrhea
	Cryptomenorrhea	Polycystic ovary syndrome (PCOS)
	Mullerian agenesis	Asherman's syndrome
		Pituitary hypothalamic dysfunction

2. Menorrhagia—denotes regularly timed episodes of bleeding that are excessive in amount (>80 mL) and/or duration (>8 days).
3. Metrorrhagia—irregularly timed episodes of bleeding superimposed on normal cyclical bleeding.
4. Menometrorrhagia—excessive, prolonged bleeding that occurs at irregularly timed and frequent intervals.
5. Oligomenorrhea—infrequent, irregularly timed episodes of bleeding usually occurring at intervals of >35 days.
6. Polymenorrhea—frequent episodes of menstruation, usually occurring at intervals of 21 days or less.
7. Hypomenorrhea—regularly timed but scanty episodes of bleeding.
8. Dysmenorrhea—painful bleeding.

POSTMENOPAUSAL BLEEDING

FORMAT

Presenting Complaints

Bleeding/spotting per vaginal, postcoital bleeding, vaginal discharge, lower abdominal pain/backache, loss of weight/decreased appetite, fever and constitutional symptoms, bladder and bowel symptoms.

Menstrual History

History of early menarche or late menopause, attained menopause at what age.

Past History

- History of any other malignancies and treatment for same in the form of chemo/radiotherapy, hormone replacement therapy (HRT)/drug therapy, diabetes mellitus (DM), hypertension (HTN).
- Others as usual
- General examination—pallor, hirsutism, obesity.

Abdominal examination—inspection/palpation/percussion/auscultation—usually within normal limits.

DISCUSSION

- Normally 1 year period of amenorrhea after the age of 40 year is considered as menopause.
- Vaginal bleeding occurring any time after 6 months of amenorrhea in a menopausal age group should be considered as postmenopausal bleeding and investigated.
- If a woman over the age of 52 years continues to menstruate, even without amenorrhea, she needs investigations to rule out endometrial hyperplasia and malignancy of the genital tract.

Etiology—endometrial atrophy is the most common cause (60–80%)

Others are, carcinoma endometrial, carcinoma (CA) cervix, atrophic endometrium, endometrial polyp, endometrial hyperplasia, atrophic vaginitis

1. Vulva—trauma, vulvitis, benign and malignant lesions
2. Vagina—senile vaginitis, vaginal tumor, foreign body like pessary
3. Cervix—cervical erosion, cervicitis, cervical malignancy

GYNECOLOGY

4. Uterus—senile endometritis, tubercular endometritis, endometrial hyperplasia, endometrial carcinoma.
5. DUB
6. Fallopian tube malignancy
7. Benign ovarian tumor such as Brenner tumor, granulosa and theca cell tumor; malignant ovarian tumor
8. Others—hypertension, blood dyscrasia.

Management

For per speculum examination

- Bimanual pelvic and per speculum examination

Investigations:

- Blood count and blood smear
- Blood sugar levels
- Cervical cytology for cervical lesion
- USG-(TVS), in postmenopausal women normal endometrium should not exceed 4 mm in thickness. Also to rule out endometrial irregularity and pelvic pathology.
- Fractional curettage (steps described in operative procedure)
- Hysteroscopic inspection and selective biopsy—to improve the predictive value of endometrial study.

Treatment—Treat the cause.

ENDOMETRIAL CARCINOMA

Symptoms—peri- or postmenopausal bleeding, discharge PV, pelvic pain.

Signs

- General examination—obesity, hypertension, lymph nodes (supraclavicular, inguinal)
- Per vaginal examination—usually no positive findings except in advanced cases.

Investigations

1. Fractional curettage—histological study of endocervical scraping before dilating cervix followed by cervical dilatation and curettage from the isthmus, body of uterus and fundus separately, so that extent of lesion can be evaluated.
2. USG—(TVS and TAS), useful in studying endometrial thickness, detecting polyps and associated ovarian tumor or ovarian metastasis.
3. Hysteroscopy and biopsy—for selective biopsy from suspicious areas to reduce chance of missing the lesion.
4. Sonosalpingography
5. CT and MRI—detection of myometrial involvement and nodal enlargement.
6. CA-125: >35 IU/mL, not specific for endometrial cancer.

The International Federation of Gynecology and Obstetrics (FIGO) surgical staging for endometrial carcinoma

Stage		**Finding**
Stage	I	Tumor confined to corpus of uterus
	Ia	No or < half of myometrial invasion
	Ib	Invasion >half of myometrium
Stage	II	Tumor invades the endocervical stroma but does not extend beyond uterus
Stage	III	Local and/or regional tumor spread
	IIIa	Extension to serosa and/or adnexa
	IIIb	Vaginal/parametrial involvement
	$IIIc_1$	Positive pelvic nodes
	$IIIc_2$	Positive para-aortic nodes with or without pelvic nodes
Stage	IV	Tumor involves bladder and/or bowel mucosa and/or distant metastases
	IVa	Invasion of bladder and/or bowel mucosa
	IVb	Distant metastases including intra-abdominal metastases and/or inguinal nodes

Each stage can be G1, 2, 3 which refers to the tumor grade.

Endocervical glandular involvement should be considered as stage I and no longer as stage II

Grading of endometrial carcinoma:

- Grade 1—5% or less shows a solid growth pattern
- Grade 2—6–50% of tumors show solid growth pattern
- Grade 3—>50% show a solid growth pattern.

Management

Stage I

Surgical management:
- TAH with BSO, biopsy or excision of any suspicious lesion.
- Uterus is cut open to assess tumor size, depth of myometrial invasion and cervical involvement.
- Pelvic and para-aortic lymphadenectomy (indications—(i) tumor histology—clear cell, papillary, squamous; (ii) myometrial invasion >1/2; (iii) extension to cervix; (iv) tumor size >2 cm; (v) extrauterine disease.

Postoperative radiotherapy:
Stage 1A, G1, G2 — observations
Stage 1A G3 — vaginal brachytherapy
Stage 1B G1, 2, 3
Stage II
Stage III A, B, C } External pelvic radiation + vaginal brachytherapy
Stage III C2 — Extended field radiation + vaginal brachytherapy
Stage IV — whole abdominal radiation + pelvic radiation + vaginal brachytherapy

Stage II

Radical hysterectomy, BSO, pelvic and para-aortic lymphadenectomy or external pelvic radiation and brachy therapy followed in 6 weeks by TAH and BSO.

Stage III and IV

Debulking surgery; followed by chemoradiation in stage III and palliative treatment in stage IV.
Progestins and chemotherapy:
- In advanced disease and recurrences
- High dose of medroxyprogesterone acetate or megestrol acetate
- Chemotherapy—agents used is doxorubicin, platinum compounds (cisplatin and carboplatin) and paclitaxel (Taxol).

Risk Factors

- Any factor that increases the exposure of endometrium to unopposed or high estrogen level, increases the risk of endometrial carcinoma.
- Endogenous estrogen exposure
- Nulliparity, infertility, early menarche and late menopause, PCOD, functioning ovarian tumors, obesity.
- Exogenous estrogen exposure:
  - Unopposed estrogen therapy as in HRT, tamoxifen for breast cancer.
- Others:
  - Hereditary nonpolyposis colorectal cancer (HNPCC), diabetes, hypertension (obesity, hypertension, diabetes-corpus cancer syndrome)

Epidemiology

Type I
- Estrogen dependent
- Younger age
- Associated with endometrial hyperplasia
- Better differentiated
- Histology—endometroid
- Low grade
- Myometrial invasion minimal
- Good prognosis

Type II
- Estrogen independent
- Older age
- In atrophic endometrium
- Less differentiated
- Papillary serous and clear cell
- High grade
- Deep
- Bad prognosis

Pathological Classification

- Endometroid adenocarcinoma
- Mucinous carcinoma
- Papillary serous carcinoma

- Clear cell carcinoma
- Squamous cell carcinoma.

ENDOMETRIAL HYPERPLASIA

Types—(with in brackets, given are risk of transforming to endometrial carcinoma)

- Simple hyperplasia (1%)—endometrium thickened markedly, glands dilated or cystic with an increased glandular to stromal ratio; but no glandular crowding and cytological atypia—Swiss cheese appearance.
- Complex hyperplasia (3%)—endometrium architecturally complex and there are crowded glands.
- Atypical hyperplasia (simple with atypia—8%; complex with atypia—29%) with cytological atypial.

Management

- If no atypia, progesterone can reverse the hyperplasia. MPA 10–20 mg daily for 10–14 days in a month will suffice.
- Continuous progestins can also be used. Therapy should be continued for at least 6 months.
  - If there is atypia, hysterectomy is the best option.

CARCINOMA CERVIX

Symptoms

- Bleeding per vaginal, discharge per vaginal, pain abdomen and backache, urinary symptoms, bowel symptoms.
- Dyspareunia, postcoital bleeding.

Signs

- General examination—lymphadenopathy (supraclavicular and inguinal), cachexia, pallor, pedal edema.
- Poster anterior—presence of mass or organomegaly, ascites
- Per speculum—cauliflower like growth, barrel shaped carvix, ulcer, vaginal involvement.
- Bimanual examination—friability, induration, bleed on touch, fixity.
- Per rectal examination—induration laterally denoting parametrial spread.
  - Fixed mass indicates that tumor has extended to pelvic side walls.
  - Thick rectovaginal septum.

Classical signs—friability, induration, bleed on touch, fixity.

Investigations

- Deep punch biopsy: If there is obvious lesion or growth, colposcopy and colposcopically directed biopsy along with endocervical curettage. If there is only suspicion (colposcopic findings of invasive carcinoma—abnormal blood vessels, irregular surface contour) (Pap smear is only for screening; not for visible lesion)
- Cone biopsy: If microinvasive carcinoma is suspected.

Other investigations in proven invasive carcinoma

- Barium enema, proctoscopy and sigmoidoscopy—if rectal spread is suspected.
- Cystoscopy, intravenous pyelogram (IVP)
- Chest X-ray
- Skeletal X-ray, if bone spread is suspected.
- CT, MRI: To assess local disease and lymph node involvement.

Staging of Carcinoma Cervix

Stage I	:	**Carcinoma strictly confined to the cervix**
IA	:	Microinvasive carcinoma
IA_1	:	Stromal invasion <3 mm in depth and < 7 mm in horizontal spread
IA_2	:	Stromal invasion 3–5 mm in depth and < 7 mm in horizontal spread
IB	:	Clinically visible lesion
IB_1	:	About 4 cm or less in size
IB_2	:	>4 cm in dimension
Stage II	:	**Cancer spread beyond the cervix, but not to pelvic wall or lower third of vagina.**
IIA	:	Tumor without parametrial invasion.
IIB	:	Tumor with parametrial invasion.

GYNECOLOGY

Stage III : Tumor extends to lateral pelvic wall, involves lower third of vagina and/cause hydronephrosis or nonfunctioning kidney
- IIIA Tumor involves lower third of vagina, no extension to lateral pelvic wall
- IIIB Tumor extends to lateral pelvic wall, and/or involves kidney

Stage IV Tumor spread to pelvic organs or distant metastases
- IVA Tumor involves bladder/rectum or spreads beyond the true pelvis
- IVB Widespread tumor with distant metastases.

Management

IA_1
- Conization with clear margin is considered adequate.
- Hysterectomy in elderly and parous women (who will not comply for long follow-up or in those with diseased uterus)
- Lymphadenectomy not required (LN involvement only 0.5%)
- Lifelong follow-up is necessary.

IA_2
- In old age—modified radical hysterectomy + pelvic lymphadenectomy
  - If node involvement—postoperative radiotherapy
- In young woman desirous of child bearing—conservative treatment—laparoscopic lympadenectomy followed by vaginal trachelectomy (Trachelectomy fertility conserving removal of at least 80% of cervix, upper vagina and cutting the Mackenrodt's ligament on either side)
  - Before conservative treatment—MRI mapping for LN involvement and local extension. If sentinel node/ obturator node –ve, no further lymphadenectomy is required.
  - Contraindication for trachelectomy—lesion >2 cm.

IB_1 and IIA
- Wertheim hysterectomy/or radiotherapy/combined surgery + radiotherapy.

Wertheim's hysterectomy:
- Stage IA with lymph node involvement, tumor size >2 cm, IB and IIA
- It comprises exploratory laparotomy, removal of the entire uterus, both adnexa, pelvic lymph nodes, medial 1/3rd of parametrium on either side and upper 1/3rd of vagina, sparing sacral glands.

IB_2

Radical hysterectomy + pelvic lymphadenopathy

IIB, III, IV

Chemoradiotherapy.

Risk Factors

- Average age 35–45 years.
- Coitus before the age of 18 years.
- Delivery before the age of 20 years.
- Multiple sexual partners.
- Multiparity with poor birth spacing between pregnancies.
- Poor personal hygiene.
- Poor socioeconomic status.
- Smoking, alcohol; women with STD, HIV, HSV2, HPV (16, 18, 31, 33), condyloma.
- Immunosuppressed individuals.
- Combined oral contraceptives (COC) and progestogens use over 8 year period.

CERVICAL INTRAEPITHELIAL NEOPLASIA (CIN)

Refers to histopathological description in which a part or full thickness of the stratified epithelium is replaced by cells showing varying degree of dysplasia, however the basement membrane is intact.

Dysplasias are graded as:
1. Mild dysplasia (CIN-I): Undifferentiated cells are confined to lower 1/3rd of the epithelium.
2. Moderate dysplasia (CIN-II): Undifferentiated cells occupy the lower 50–75% of the epithelial thickness.
3. Severe dysplasia and carcinoma in situ (CIN-III): Entire thickness of the epithelium is replaced by abnormal cells.

Diagnosis

Classification of Pap Smear

Pap class system	Scheme I	Scheme II	Scheme III (Bethesda)
Class I	Negative for malignant cells	Negative	Within normal limits
Class II	Inflammation Squamous atypial kilocytes		Ascus-atypical squamous cells of undetermined significance
Class III	Mild dysplasia	CIN I	Low-grade squamous intraepithelial lesion (LSIL)
Class IV	Moderate dysplasia Severe dysplasia and carcinoma in situ	CIN II	CIN III High grade squamous intraepithelial lesion (HSIL)
Class V	Invasive cancer	Invasive cancer	Invasive cancer

Technique

Patient in dorsal position and insert a Cusco's speculum→longer end of Ayre's spatula is fixed at the external os→rotate through 360° over the portiovaginalis of the cervix→spread on a glass slide and before it dries, is immersed in equal parts of 95% ethyl alcohol and ether and kept for 2 hours to fix it→slide is air dried and then stained with Papanicolaou stain.

Visual inspection with acetic acid (VIA)

- VIA is able to select abnormal areas on the cervix by applying 5% acetic acid.
- Acetic acid dehydrates the abnormal areas containing increased nuclear material and protein which turn acetowhite.

Visual inspection with Lugol's iodine (VILI): or using Schiller's iodine.

- Normal cells containing glycogen take up iodine and turn mahogany brown, and abnormal areas remains unstained because malignant cells are rapidly dividing and devoid of glycogen.

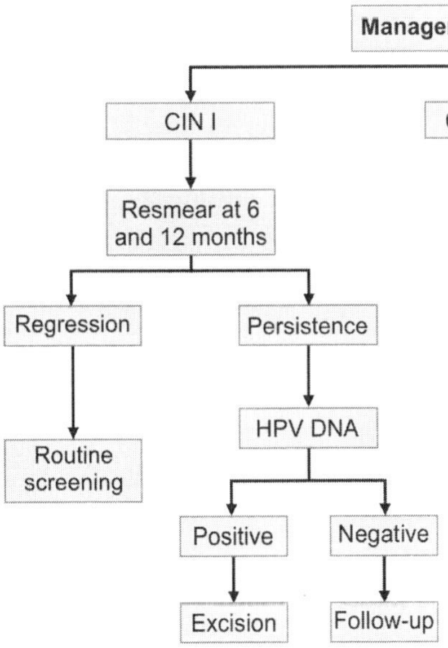

- Ablative procedures
  - Thermoablation
  - Cryotherapy
  - Laser ablatives
- Excisional procedures
  - Loop electrosurgical excision procedure (LEEP)
  - Cold knife conisation
  - Carbon dioxide laser care

PROLAPSE

CASE FORMAT

- Name:
- Age:

Presenting Complaints

Mass descending per vaginum—6 months

Symptoms can be fullness is vagina, mass descending per vaginal, low backache, urinary/bowel symptoms like incomplete emptying, stress incontinence, dysuria, constipation, splinting, vaginal discharge, sexual dissatisfaction.

History of Present Illness

- Patient noticed mass protruding per vaginum 6 months back. It was more towards evening and also straining, coughing. It was reduced in size on lying down position.
- Initially, she was able to reduce it by herself. But for a few days, it is difficult.
- There is increased frequency of micturition and can only empty the bladder by pressing back the swelling.
- No chronic cough, weight lifting, constipation (precipitating factors). Not associated with discharge per vaginum or bleeding per vaginum.

MENSTRUAL HISTORY

Menopause atrophy

MARITAL HISTORY

Obstetric History

- Multiparous
- Home/hospital
- Spacing of deliveries
- Prolonged labor, instrumental delivery, birth weight of baby
- Postnatal exercise.

PAST HISTORY

- Chronic cough
- Constipation
- Mass in abdomen
- Surgery for prolapse/hysterectomy

On Examination

General examination—ligament laxity

Spine examination—nulliparous prolapse (spina bifida)

Abdominal Examination

Mass, free fluid, muscle tone

Local Examination

- Pubic hair clipped
- Labia majora normal, minora atrophic introitus—patulous
- A mass is seen protruding through and leading part is cervix which is hypertrophied. There is no bleeding, ulceration or discharge.

Per Speculum

- Vaginal wall—color, decreased rugosity
- Cystocele and rectocele present ureterocele, enterocoele
- External os is slit-like
- No ulcer, bleeding, discharge.

Palpation

- Tone of levator ani muscle
- Get above swelling (procidentia).

Diagnosis

3rd degree uterovaginal (UV) prolapse
+/- cystocele, urethrocele
+/- rectocele, enterocoele.

Differential Diagnosis

- Cystocele: Anterior vaginal cyst (Gartner's cyst)
- UV prolapse
- Inversion of uterus—A/C, sub A/C, C/C
  - On examination fundus is absent, a dimple is felt
  - Cervix cannot be felt
  - Endometrium is outside
  - Traction on protruding uterine-fundus will cause cervix to move up
- Submucous fibroid polyp: A rim of cervix is felt all around it, no cough impulse
- Congenital elongation of cervix: The fornices are deep.

Increase in distance between external os and bladder sulcus.

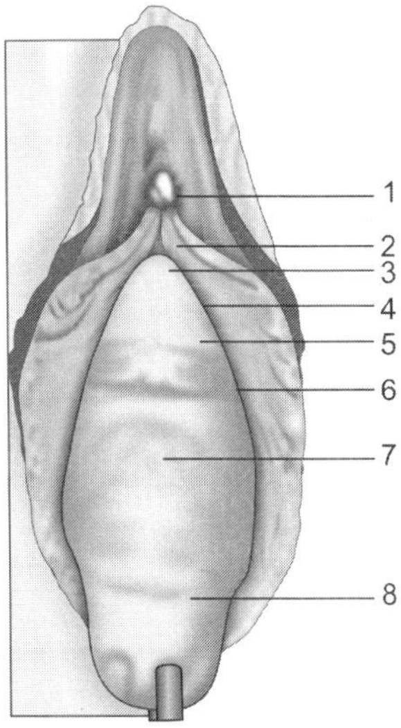

A case of prolapse in which the cervix has been drawn down. (1) Parameatal recess; (2) Hymen; (3) Submeatal sulcus; (4) Paraurethral recess; (5) Oblique vaginal fold; (6) Transverse sulcus of the anterior vaginal wall; (7) Arched rugae of the vaginal wall; (8) Bladder sulcus.

INVESTIGATIONS

Routine

- Hemoglobin (Hb), erythrocyte sedimentation rate (ESR)
- Blood grouping, Rh typing
- Screening
- Liver function tests (LFT), renal function tests (RFT)
- X-ray, electrocardiography (ECG)

Specific

- Pap smear
- USG
  - Uterus—size, fibroid
  - Intra-abdominal mass
  - Rule out inversion
- Urine routine examination, urine C and S
  - To rule out urinary tract infection (UTI)
- Intravenous pyelogram
  - To rule out hydronephrosis.

MANAGEMENT

1. Conservative
2. Surgical

Conservative

- Pelvic floor muscle training by Kegel's exercise (voluntary contraction of pelvic floor muscles)
- Reduce body weight
- Treat cough, constipation (precipitating factor)
- Correct UTI
- Management of decubitus ulcer: Smear for cytology, rest, padding, pessary, estrogen cream.

PESSARIES

Indications

- Pregnancy (especially in first trimester) since the prolapse is usually get corrected thereafter
- Lactation
- Temporary use while clearing infections and decubitus ulcer
- Women who are unfit for surgery.

Types of Pessaries

- Support—for example, Ring pessaries.
- Space filling—Gelhorn and cube pessaries or Smith Hodge

Once the pessary is fit, she is asked to stand and then cough to ensure that pessary is in place. Make sure she is able to pass urine. Regular follow-up is needed.

Complications

Vaginal discharge, vaginal irritation fistulas, ulcerations, forgotten pessary.

Surgery

- Anterior colporrhaphy—for cystocele
- Vaginal hysterectomy—for uterovaginal prolapse
- Posterior colpoperineorrhaphy—rectocele and deficient perineum.

Steps

- Under general anesthesia (GA)/regional anesthesia
- Dorsal lithotomy position
- Parts are cleaned with antiseptic and draped
- Bladder is catheterized with a metal catheter and per vaginal is done to confirm size of uterus.

ANTERIOR COLPORRHAPHY (DIAGNOSIS IN DIAGRAM)

- A sims speculum is introduced and anterior lip of cervix is pulled with a vulsellum forceps. An inverted T shaped incision is made on anterior vaginal wall.
- The horizontal limb of incision is made at the level of bladder sulcus.
- The vertical incision starts from the midpoint of transverse incision to a point just below the external urethral meatus.
- Subepithelial infiltration of adrenaline in saline to define the tissue planes and reduce bleeding.
- Triangular vaginal flaps are separated from bladder throughout its length (the line of cleavage is the vesicovaginal space)
- The pubovesical ligament is cut and bladder is pushed up (rest after VH).

VAGINAL HYSTERECTOMY/WARD MAYO REPAIR (VH+PFR)

- The cervical incision is extended posteriorly and pouch of Douglas (POD) is opened
- The uterus is delivered anteriorly and uterovesical fold of peritoneum incised
  - 1st clamp: Consists of uterosacrals and cardinal ligaments is applied and the pedicle is cut and ligated
  - 2nd clamp: Uterine vessels are clamped, cut and ligated
  - 3rd pedicle containing round ligament, tube and ovarian ligament can be clamped, divided and secured (if oophorectomy has to be performed, infundibulopelvic ligament is clamped and ligated)
- If necessary, McCall's culdoplasty (securing the vaginal vault to uterosacral ligaments) can be done to prevent any future enterocele and vault prolapse. Peritoneum is closed by a purse-string suture.

Complete the Anterior Colporrhaphy

Muscularis and adventitia of the vagina are approximated in midline (bladder buttressing). Then redundant vagina is removed. The bladder is drained with an indwelling Foley's catheter.

POSTERIOR COLPOPERINEORRHAPHY

- A pair of Alley's forceps are placed on either side at lower end of labium minora
- A third one is placed on the posterior vaginal wall in the midline above the bulge of rectocele.
- The first two forceps are joined by a horizontal incision and through this the vaginal mucosa is dissected from underlying prerectal fascia (Denonvillier's) up to the 3rd forceps. A vertical incision is made from the middle of this incision to the apex. Prerectal fascia is then approximated in midline.
- In perineorrhaphy the superficial perineal muscles are plicated in the midline and skin is closed as in the case of an episiotomy.

Complications

- Immediate—hemorrhage, injury to surrounding structures
- Late—reactionary and secondary hemorrhage
  - Pelvic hematoma and pelvic abscess

Fistulae

- Sequel—vault prolapse.

Other Surgeries

Le Forte's Repair/Colpocleisis

- In very elderly women with medical problems
- Here the vaginal epithelium is removed followed by suturing of anterior and posterior walls of denuded vagina **and totally obliterating the vagina.**

Manchester/Fothergill's Operation

- It includes anterior colporrhaphy with amputation of cervix
- Suturing the cut ends of Mackenrodt ligaments in front of the cervix. Covers the raw area on the amputated cervix with vaginal mucosa
- Followed by posterior colpoperineorrhaphy
- For women who have completed family, but wish to retain uterus.
- Complications: (1) Decreased fertility, (2) Cervical incompetence, (3) Cervical stenosis, (4) Recurrence.

Shirodkar's Procedure

- Anterior colporrhaphy
- The uterosacral ligaments divided and stumps of these ligaments are crossed and stitched in front of cervix.

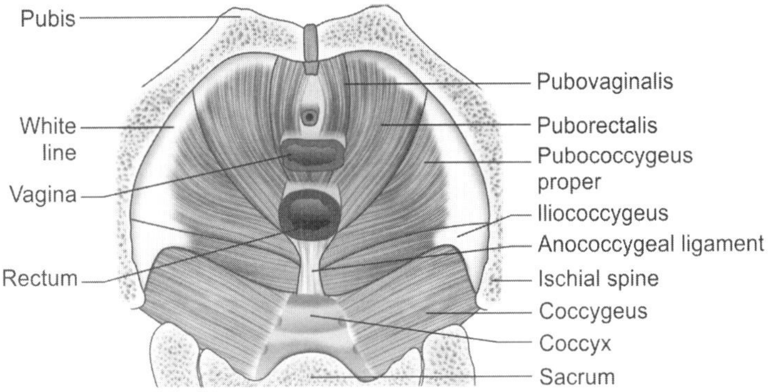

Abdominal Sling Operations

- For young women suffering from 2nd/3rd degree uterine prolapse, who are desirous of retaining their child bearing and menstrual functions.
- **Abdominocervicopexy**
- **Shirodkar's abdominal sling operation**—cervix to sacrum
- **Khanna's abdominal sling operation**—cervix to Anterior superior iliac spine (ASIS)
- **Purandare's sling operation**—cervix to anterior abdominal wall.

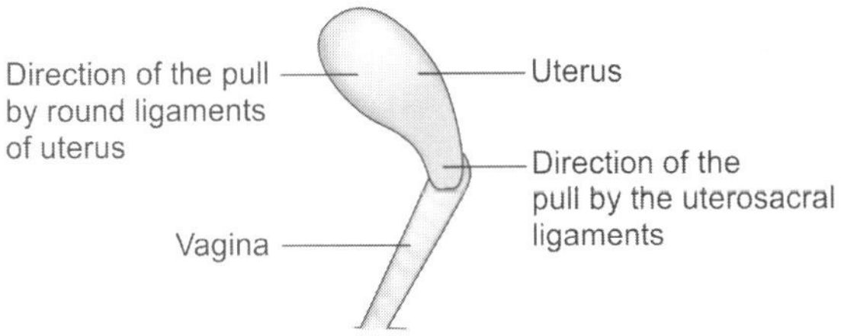

ENTEROCELE

- Vaginal route
  - McCall's Culdoplasty
  - Internal—plicating the uterosacral ligaments
  - External—suture is taken outwards through vaginal vault
- Abdominal—Halban or Moschcowitz procedure—purse string plication of peritoneum of POD

VAULT PROLAPSE

Treatment

- Right transvaginal sacro spinous colpopexy
- Transabdominal sacral colpopexy
- McCall's culdoplasty
- Laparoscopic colpopexy.

Pessary test
The woman is fitted with a ring pessary and checked for stress incontinence. If incontinence is relieved it is likely that surgical correction of prolapse will be beneficial.

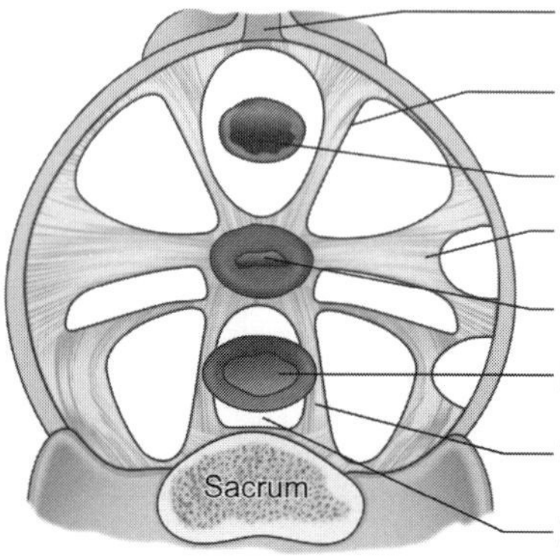

UTERINE SUPPORTS

Primary

- Muscular/active
  - Pelvic diaphragm
  - Perineal body
  - Urogenital diaphragm/Distal urethral sphincter mechanism
- Fibromuscular/mechanical support
  - Uterine axis
  - Pubocervical ligament
  - Transverse cervical ligament of Mackenrodt
  - Uterosacral ligament
  - Round ligament.

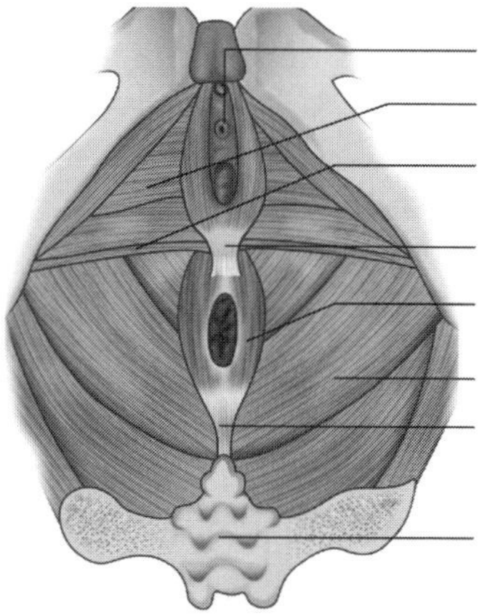

Secondary

- Broad ligament
- Uterovesical fold
- Rectovaginal fold.

DE LANCEY CLASSIFICATION OF SUPPORTS

Level I

- Cervix and upper vagina (suspensory axis) (uterosacral cardinal ligament)
- Defects in this supports leads to apical prolapse (it includes UV prolapse, enterocele, descent of cervix)

Level II—mid vaginal support (attachment axis)

- Anteriorly—pubocervical fascia
- Posteriorly—rectovaginal fascia
  (damage results in paravaginal cystocele/pararectal defects, rectocele).

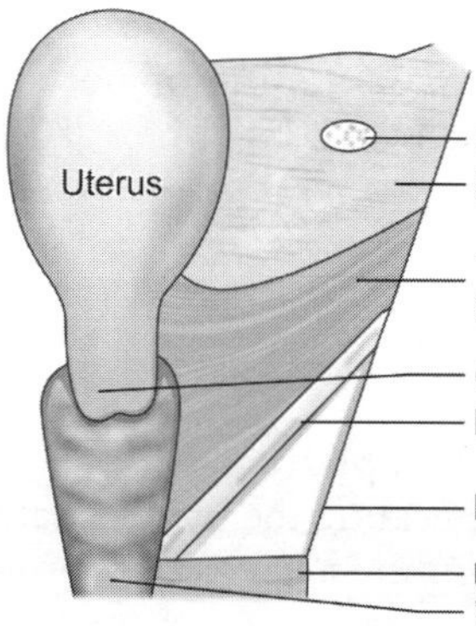

Level III—lower vaginal support (fusion axis)
- Urogenital diaphragm, pubis
- Levator ani
- Perineal body (defects—gaping introitus, deficient perineum, urethrocele).

CLASSIFICATION OF PROLAPSE

1. **Anterior vaginal wall**
   - Upper 2/3rd—cystocele
   - Lower 1/3rd—urethrocele
2. **Posterior vaginal wall**
   - Upper 1/3rd—enterocele
   - Middle 1/3rd—rectocele
3. **Uterine descent**
   - Primary—descent of cervix into vagina (below ischial spine)
   - Secondary—descent of cervix up to introitus
   - Tertiary—descent of cervix outside introitus
   - Procidentia—all of the uterus outside introitus.

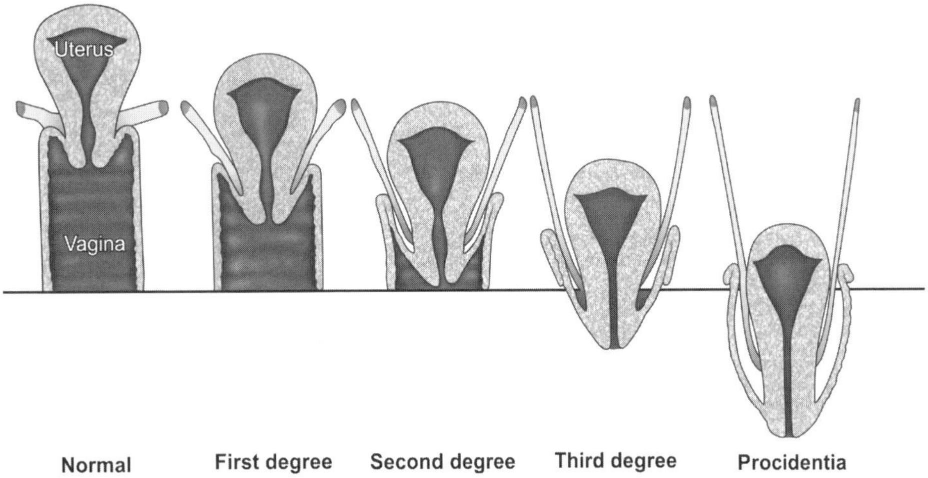

ETIOLOGY OF PROLAPSE

- Atonicity and asthenia of menopause
- Birth injury
- Pudental nerve injury
- Home deliveries
  - Bearing down before full dilatation of cervix
  - No episiotomy
  - Soon resume heavy work
- Hospital deliveries
  - Instrumental
  - Prolonged 2nd stage
- Spina bifida—nulliparous prolapse
- Chronic cough, constipation
- Abdominal mass
- Abdominoperineal resection
- Ligament laxity.

Complications of Prolapse

- Decubitus ulcer
- Cervical malignancy

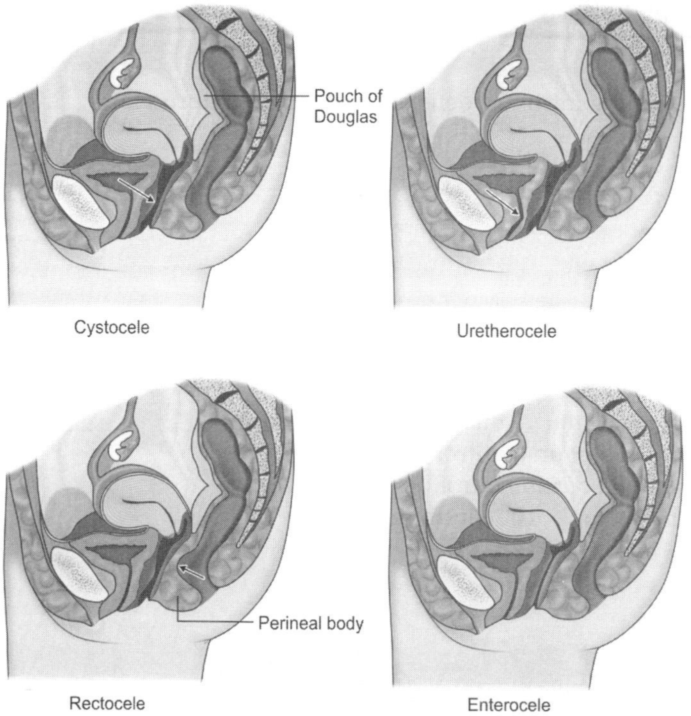

- Ascending infections
- Obstructive uropathy
- Irreducibility
- Gangrene.

Anterior Colporrhaphy

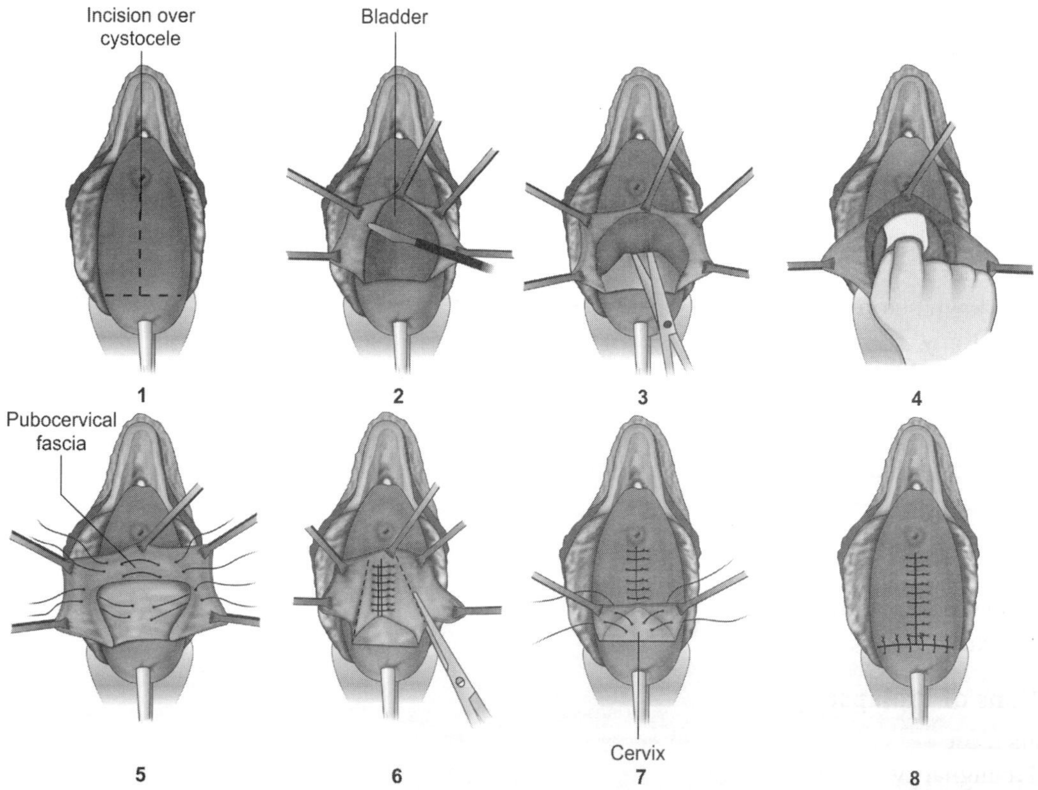

GESTATIONAL TROPHOBLASTIC DISEASE (GTD)

CASE FORMAT

Presenting Complaints

Admitted for 2nd course of chemotherapy.

History of Present Illness

- Detected to be pregnant after 2 week..........
- Regular antenatal care (ANC)
- Bleeding PV/Hyperemesis gravidarum
- USG
- Suction evacuation
- β-hCG follow-up
- Chemotherapy: Why started, single agent/not, how many course, has she tolerated well?

Diagnosis: Persistent trophoblastic disease with—course of chemotherapy. Present β–hCG level is__________.

WHO Classification:

- Benign GTD
  Hydatidiform mole—partial and complete
- Gestational trophoblastic neoplasia (GTN)
  - Nonmetastatic malignant GTD: Persistent GTD, invasive mole, local choriocarcinoma
  - Metastatic GTD: With good prognosis, with bad prognosis.

VESICULAR MOLE

Symptoms

- Amenorrhea of varying duration followed by bleeding
- Passage of vesicles PV
- Hyperemesis.

Signs

- Urethral nodules
- Uterus
  - More than period of amenorrhea 50%
  - Corresponds to period of amenorrhea in 35% or smaller in 20% cases
- No fetal parts felt, no fetal heart rate (FHS)
- Theca lutein cysts
- Early onset preeclampsia
- Thyrotoxicosis.

Investigations

- **Ultrasound**: Snowstorm appearance, theca-lutein cyst in ovaries, partial mole may show fetus
- **Beta-hCG**: Very high.

Differential Diagnosis

- Threatened abortion
- Ectopic pregnancy
- Wrong dates
- Multiple pregnancy
- Tumor complicating pregnancy.

MANAGEMENT

- Suction evacuation and follow-up
- Before procedure
  - Complete blood count (CBC), blood grouping and Rh typing, chest X-ray, LFT, β–hCG
  - Arrange blood
  - PGE1 400 μg is used for 6 hours before procedure to open cervical os

- Do suction evacuation
- Then start oxytocin infusion
- Send the products for histopathology report (HPR)
- Monitor in hospital for 48 hour
  - Watch for bleeding,
  - Post-evacuation β-hCG value, after 48 hours
  - Counseling, advice about contraception.

Risk factors of development of GTN
• Age > 40 years
• Uterus > gestational age
• Theca lutein cyst >6 cm
• Pre-evacuation β–hCG > 1 lakh mIU/mL

Follow-up after suction evacuation
- Clinical follow-up
- Biochemical follow-up
  (History: Bleeding per vaginal, regular periods, contraception, chest symptoms—taken in each visit)
- 2 weekly β-hCG
- Within 8–12 weeks it become normal (<5 IU/mL)
- Examination: Uterine size, thecal cysts, pallor, respiratory system, suburethral nodule.
- Till 3 consecutive values normal
- Then monthly for 6 months
- In 1st visit: Also do Doppler USG—look increased vascularity and myometrial invasion (to rule out persistence)

Contraception:
- Barrier contraception is safest until β-hCG is normal
- Hormonal contraceptive interfere with rate of decline of β-hCG.

Indication for chemotherapy:
- Persistent trophoblastic disease
  - Rising β-hCG values (3 values over 2 weeks)
  - Plateauing of values (4 values over 3 weeks)
  - Failure of β-hCG values to become negative by 8–12 weeks
- HPR of invasive mole
- HPR of choriocarcinoma
- Metastasis in brain, GIT, lung
- Elevated serum, β-hCG 6 months after evacuation.

Chemotherapy:
- Before do CBC, RFT, LFT, chest X-ray
- Drugs: Methotrexate + Folinic acid
- Methotrexate 1 mg/kg—days 1, 3, 5, 7
- Folinic acid 0.1 mg/kg—days 2, 4, 6, 8
- Repeat every 2 weekly
- Until 3 consecutive values of β-hCG normal
- Give 1 more cycle after normalization of β-hCG.
- Then β-hCG follow-up.

Invasive mole	**Choriocarcinoma**
Monthly for 1 year	Monthly for 2 years (lifelong)

- Methotrexate; dihydrofolate reductase inhibitor
- Side effects: Skin reaction, alopecia, stomatitis, gastric hemorrhage, bone marrow suppression, liver dysfunction, renal dysfunction.

Uses of methotrexate
• Choriocarcinoma
• Acute leukemia
• Psoriasis
• Rheumatoid arthritis
• Ectopic pregnancy

High-risk disease: (see below)

Multiple agent chemotherapy (EMACO)

E—Etoposide
M—Methotrexate
A—Actinomycin D
C—Cyclophosphamide
O—Oncovin (vincristine)
EMACO Regimes
Day 1 – EMA
Day 2 – EFA (F—Folinic acid)
Day 8—Co

The cycle is repeated every 2 weeks with serum β-hCG is normal, following which 3 more cycles are given.

GYNECOLOGY

Place for hysterectomy:

- Invasive mole perforating the serosa causing an intraperitoneal bleed
- Drug resistance
- Placental site trophoblastic tumor
- High-risk cases over 40 years, multiparous.

FIGO prognosis scoring system:

	0	1	2	3
Age	<40	>40		
Antecedent pregnancy	H. Mole	Abortion	Term	
Interval (months)	<4	4–6	7–12	>12
Pretreatment hCG	$<10^3$	10^3–10^4	10^4–10^5	$>10^5$
Size of tumor	<3 cm	3–5 cm	>5 cm	
Number of metastosis	–	1–4	5–8	>8
Site of metastasis	Lung	Spleen, kidney	GIT	Brain, liver
Previous chemotherapy			Single drug	2 or more

<4–low risk, 5–8 middle, >8—high-risk

Clinical staging of trophoblastic tumors (FIGO 2000)

- **Stage I**—tumor strictly confined to uterine corpus
- **Stage II**—tumor extends to the adnexa outside uterus but is limited to the genital structures
- **Stage III**—tumor extends to lungs with or without genital involvement
- **Stage IV**—metastasis to other site.

Partial Mole Vs Complete Mole

Partial mole	Complete mole
• 69XXX/69XXY	• 46XX/46 XY
• Embryo present	• Absent
• Fetal RBC present	• Absent
• Theca lutein cyst—uncommon	• Common
• β-hCG slight increase	• Very high
• Complications uncommon	• Common
• Focal hydropic degeneration of villi	• Diffuse
• P57K IP2 immunostaining present	• Negative

Subsequent Pregnancy

- Avoidance of pregnancy for 1 year after chemotherapy
- Early T1—USG
- Placenta should be sent for *HPR*
- Serum β-hCG estimation 6 and 10 weeks after delivery to rule out glucose tolerance test (GTT).

OPERATIVE PROCEDURES

DILATATION AND CURETTAGE

Indications

- Postmenopausal bleeding
- To exclude endometrial cancer
- To complete an incomplete abortion

Procedures

- Consent
- TT should be taken
- Blood sugar to be controlled
- Empty bladder prior to the procedure
- Patient in lithotomy position
- Area prepared and cleaned

- Using Sims speculum, posterior vaginal wall is retracted
- Anterior lip of cervix is held with vulsellum forceps
- Uterine sound is passed to assess the size and position of uterus
- Cervical canal dilated with Hegars dilator
- Using curette, uterus is curetted
- Curetted material sent for HPR
- Review after 3 weeks for report.

Complications
- Perforation
- Bleeding
- Trauma to cervix
- Infection
- Cervical incompetence
- Asherman's syndrome

FRACTIONAL CURETTAGE

In perimenopausal/postmenopausal

Steps:

1, 2, 3, 4, 5, 6, 7, 8, 9—endocervical curettage done

10 11, 12, 13—uterine sound is passed.

COLPOSCOPY

Visualization of cervix under binocular microscope of magnification.

Squamocolumnar junction (SCJ) and transformation zone

- Cervix has two parts:
  1. Ectocervix—lined by squamous epithelium
  2. Endocervix—lined by columnar epithelium.
- The junction of two epithelium is called SCJ.
- If estrogen level is high SCJ moves outward (This is the normal physiological occurring during puberty and pregnancy)
- After menarche squamous metaplasia takes place and new SCJ is formed (SCJ moving inward). This area between original and active SCJ is transformation zone.

Procedure

- Cervix exposed using cuscos speculum
- Wash with normal saline
- Add 2% acetic acid [Visual inspection under acetic acid (VIA)]
  - Acetic acid is a mucolytic agent. It will precipitate protein and abnormal cells appear as acetowhite area.
  - If Lugole's iodine applied, (visual inspection under Lugol's iodine—VILI)
  - Normal epithelial takes mahogany brown color, because in normal epithelial there is mature glycogen.
  - In abnormal epithelial (dysplastic cell) have poor glycogen and appear as pale area.
  - Biopsy is taken from abnormal areas.

VAGINAL HYSTERECTOMY

Described in heading: Prolapse.

ABDOMINAL HYSTERECTOMY

Described in heading: Fibroid.

GYNECOLOGY

CHAPTER 21

Viva

INSTRUMENTS

1. **Sims speculum (Sims double bladed vaginal speculum)**
   Uses:
   - Pap smear
   - Cu T insertion, removal, follow-up
   - Minor OT procedures (dilatation and curettage, fractional curettage cervical biopsy)
   - Major OT procedures—hysterectomy pelvic floor repair

   Advantages:
   - Light weight.
   - Can be moved side to side.
   - Reflects light

   Disadvantage: It is not self-retaining.
2. **Cusco's speculum (Cusco's bivalved self-retaining vaginal speculm)**
   - Bivalved speculum
   - Self-retaining
   - It has the same use as that of sims speculum

   Disadvantages:
   - Cannot reflect light
   - Cannot move the instruments
   - Cannot visualize AP vaginal wall
3. **Vulsellum**
   Curved instrument. Because of this, it cannot obstruct the vision. It is toothed and less traumatic to cervix.
   Uses:
   - To catch the anterior lip of cervix in D and C, vaginal hysterectomy
   - To hold the posterior lip of cervix in culdocentesis, colpotomy.
4. **Uterine sound**
   Long, bend at end, hold like a pen
   - First dilator of cervical canal
   - To know the length of uterus
   - To know the position of uterus
   - To locate IUCD with missing threads by taking X-ray with sound in situ
   - To differentiate between polyp and inversion of uterus

   Complication—perforation
5. **Hegars Dilator**
   - It has blunt end, it is of different size
   - To dilate the cervix
   - Complication—perforation and cervical trauma, cervical incompetence

   If perforation takes place check vitals and if vitals unstable—do laparotomy; if vitals stable—conservative management.

6. **Curette**
   Its one end is blunt and other end is sharp
   a. To curette out the endometrial cavity
   b. To check the completeness of evacuation (gritty feeling)
   Complications:
   a. Perforation
   b. Infection
   c. Uterine synechiae
   d. Incomplete removal

> Blunt curette—Obstetrics (D&E, vesicular mole, retained products)
> Sharp curette—Gynecology (Infertility, check for secretary endometrium)

7. **Punch biopsy forceps**
   To take cervical biopsy
8. **Allis forceps**
   1. To hold the anterior lip of cervix in place of Vulsellum
   2. To hold the peritoneum or rectus fascia
   3. To hold margins of vagina is anterior colporrhaphy of vitamin
9. **Artery forceps**
   To secure bleeding vessels
10. **Wrigley's outlet forceps (Refer Instrumental Delivery)**
11. **Babcock's forceps—nontraumatic**
    To catch tubular structures like fallopian tube during PPS, ureter, vas deferens, bowel, ovarian ligament.
12. **Rubin's cannula**
    To know the patency of the tube—air insufflation test, HSG, manipulate uterus in laparoscopy, hydrotubation
13. **Toothed and nontoothed forceps**
    - Nontoothed forceps—to hold the soft tissue
    - Toothed forceps—skin suturing
    - To hold structures like rectus fascia
14. **Sponge holding forceps**
    - For painting before surgery
    - For holding the cervix to check for injury after delivery—'walking around' the cervix
15. **Mayo scissors**
    Curved scissor for cutting structures
16. **Myoma screw**
    During myomectomy or hysterectomy for fibroid uterus
17. **Leech Wilkinson Cannula**
    During hysterosalpingogram to instill dye
18. **Trocar and cannula**—in laparoscopy
19. **Decapitation hook—RAMSBOTHEM**
    Indications: Neglected shoulder presentation
    Interlocking of twin
20. **CuT**
    - Second generation IUCD
      For example, CuT200, CuT380A (supplied by Govt)(life span of 10 years (paraguard).
    - The no. indicates surface area if Cu on the device in mm^2

    Advantages
    - Postcoital contraceptive
    - Low expulsion rate
    - Better tolerated by nullipara
21. **Doyen abdominal retractor**
    To retract the abdominal wall and bladder in order to visualize the lower segment in LSCS.
22. **Veries needle**—To create pneumoperitoneum.

DRUGS

1. **Oxytocin**
   Uses:
   - Induction of labor

- Second trimester abortion
- Atonic postpartum hemorrhage (PPH)
- Active management of 3rd stage of labor (P5/P10 IM and P20 infusion)

Side effects:

a. Rupture of uterus
b. Neonatal jaundice
c. Water intoxication

2. **Ergometrine**

Uses:

a. Active management of 3rd stage of labor
b. Atonic PPH

Dose: 0.5 mg IV during delivery of anterior shoulder to prevent PPH

Side effects:

a. Hypertension, cardiac ischemia (so contraindicated in heart disease and hypertension)
b. Sometime causes hour glass contraction.

3. **Prostaglandins:**

a. PGE1 (misoprostol)
- For ripening of cervix—25 μg, 4 hours apart, maximum 4 doses (placed in posterior fornix of vagina).
- For the management of PPH 200 μg tablet, 4 tablets kept PR.

b. PGE2 (dinoprostone, cerviprime)—for ripening the cervix 0.5 mg, 6 hours apart intracervically

Side effects:
- Nausea, vomiting, diarrhea
- Fetal distress
- Rupture of uterus
- Contraindicated in asthma.

c. PGF2α

i. 3rd stage of labour
ii. 1st and 2nd trimester MTP
iii. Atonic PPA

4. **Magnesium sulphate**

Pritchards regimen

5. **Methotrexate in ectopic pregnancy, gestational trophoblastic disease (GTD)**
6. **Hormonal contraceptives**

Oral pills
- Combined pills
- Progesterone only pills (mini pills)
- Postcoital pills
- Once a month pill
- Male pill

Depot formulations
- Injectables
- Subcutaneous implants
- Vaginal rings

COMBINED PILLS

- Pills given orally
- Two types:

1. 21 tablet containing strip
2. 28 tablet containing strip (21 OCP+ 7 Fe tabs)

MALA - N - free of cost

0.15 mg levonorgestrel + 0.03 mg ethinylestradiol.

POSTCOITAL PILLS

I Pill:

- Used within 72 hours of unprotected sex
- 1 tab of 0.75 mg within 72 hours + 2nd tab after 12 hours of 1st dose

Mifepristone: 10 mg once within 72 hours

GYNECOLOGY

PARTOGRAM

- It is a graphic record of the events in labor.
- When to start recording?

When the labor is diagnosed:

Regular uterine contractions that bring about demonstrable effacement and dilatation of the cervix.

Admission criteria to labor ward

Painful uterine contractions with any one of the following:

1. Ruptured membranes
2. Bloody show
3. Complete effacement of cervix

Partogram

- Fetal record
- Record of the progress of labor
- Maternal record
- Personal identification
  - Name, age, IP no.: DOA, time of administration
    - Obstetric score
    - Time of rupture of membrane
  - Descend of the head per abdomen—recorded in fifths as the number of finger breadths above the pubic symphysis
  - Cervical dilatation—dilatation in cms of either external or internal os whichever is less
  - Station—cms above and below spines
    - (–5 to +5)
  - Cervical dilatation against time
  - Cervical dilatation is plotted with x-mark.
  - Station with O-mark
  - In about 90% of primigravidae cervix dilates at the rate of 1 cm/hour in active phase
  - Once 3 cm dilatation is reached, labor enters active phase
  - The alert line drawn from 4–10 cm represents the normal rate of cervical dilatation

The Alert Line

- The alert line drawn from 4–10 cm represents the normal rate of cervical dilatation
- If cervical dilatation is more, curve of dilatation is to the left of alert line
- If cervical dilatation moves to the right of alert line, it indicates delay in labor
- Find out the cause and take action.

The Action Line

- Action line is drawn 4 hours to the right of alert line
- Lag of 4 hours unlikely to compromise fetus or the mother
- Giving 4 hours reduce unnecessary intervention

When the Action line is crossed....

- Terminate the labor
- Augment the labor
  - Artificial rupture of membranes (ARM)
  - Oxytocin
  - Hydration
  - Analgesia
- Time limit to terminate labor—6–8 hours of oxytocin

Descend

- **Rate—1.2 cm/hour in Primigravida, 1.5 cm in multipara**

GYNECOLOGY

- **Disorders of descend usually associated with CPD**
- **Time—**Time of examination—0 hour when the patient is admitted to labor room

Moulding – OP/PP (Occipito-parietal or Parieto-parietal)
- + bones close together
- ++ overlapping but reducible
- +++ overlapped not reducible

Caput
- + - mild
- ++ - moderate
- +++ - severe

Liquor
- C – Clear
- M – Meconium (M1, M2, M3)
- B – Blood stained
- A –Absent liquor
- Remarks – Unusual observations

FHS – count – every 15 minutes in 1st stage and after every contraction in 2nd stage

Contractions:
- Shade the number of columns corresponding to the number of contractions in 10 minutes
- Duration is expressed by intensity of shading

Drugs, IVF and medications

Pitocin rate—drops/minute

BP and pulse hourly

Temperature—4th hourly

SPECIMENS

1. **Fibroid**
   - Specimen showing section of uterus with mass showing whorled appearance most probably fibroid
   - Presenting complaints of patient—most probably compressive symptoms like urinary retention, pain, etc. (do not say infertility because in such lady, never do hysterectomy)
   - Read about types, treatment (described in chapter fibroid).
2. **Ovarian cyst**
   - Specimen showing section of uterus with a large cyst which is septate
   - Most probably mucinous cystadenoma ovary
   - Read about classification, treatment of ovarian tumor
3. **Torsion ovarian cyst**
   - Specimen showing section uterus with a large cyst, which is black in color
   - Most probably torsion ovarian cyst
   - Most common ovarian cyst under going torsion—dermoid cyst
   - Treatment—stabilize patient; do detorsion and cystectomy
4. **Vesicular mole**
   - Specimen showing section of uterus which contains vesicles
   - Most probably vesicular mole
   - Read about types, treatment, follow-up
5. **Cervical fibroid**
6. **Wertheim's hysterectomy specimen**
7. **Endometrial carcinoma**
8. **Rupture of uterus**

FETAL SKULL

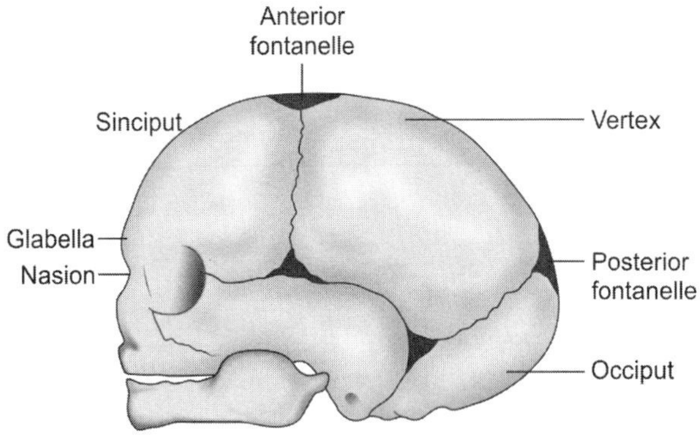

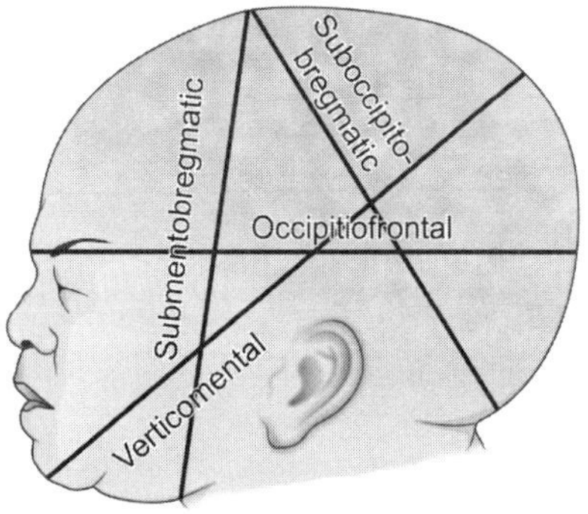

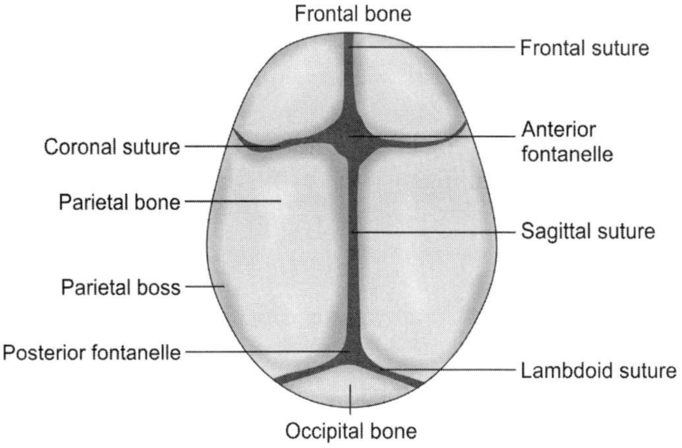

Lie—relationship between long axis of fetal ovoid to long axis of uterine ovoid.
Presentation—part of fetus that lies over pelvic inlet and occupies the lower pole of the uterus.
Presenting part—most dependent part of fetus which is felt first on vaginal examination.
Attitude—relation of fetal parts to each other.
Denominator—arbitrarily chosen point on presenting part of fetus, used to describe position.
Position—relationship of denominator to four quadrants of maternal pelvis.

Presentation	AP diameter	Denominator
1. Vertex head well flexed	Suboccipitobregmatic 9.4 cm	Occiput
2. Vertex head is in attitude of deflexion	Occipitofrontal 11.0 cm	Occiput
3. Brow presentation	Verticomental 13.5 cm (longest diameter of fetal skull)	Sinciput
4. Face presentation	Submentobregmatic 9.4 cm	Chin or mentum
5. Breech presentation		Sacrum
6. Shoulder		Acromian

BONY PELVIS

Pelvic Inlet—boundaries

- Anteriorly—horizontal rami of pubic bone and symphysis pubis
- Posteriorly—sacral promontory and alae
- Laterally—linea terminalis.

1. **Anteroposterior diameter:**
   True/anatomical conjugate—distance between sacral promontory and upper portion of inner surface of pubic symphysis (11 cm).

Obstetric conjugate—distance between sacral promontory and nearest point on the posterior surface of pubic symphysis (10.5 cm) (more important diameter).

Diagonal conjugate—distance between promontory of sacrum to the apex of pubic arch (11.5–12 cm). Normally this conjugate is easily measured and obstetric conjugate is obtained by subtracting 1.5 cm from it.

2. **Transverse diameter**—13.5 cm
3. **Oblique diameter**—12.5 cm.

Mid Pelvis

It extends through lower margin of pubic symphysis, tip of sacrum and ischial spine.

Pelvic Outlet

- Anteriorly—pubic arch
- Posteriorly—tip of coccyx
- Laterally—ischial tuberosity

CLASSIFICATION OF PELVIS

Caldwell and Moloy Classification

1. **Gynecoid pelvis**—normal female pelvis

Inlet	Cavity	Outlet
Transverse diameter more than anteroposterior diameter	Sacrum well curved Side walls parallel Ischial spines not prominent Wide sacrosciatic notch	Subpubic angle 90°

2. **Android pelvis**
   - Male type of pelvis
   - Features are opposite to that of gynecoid type.
   - Deep transverse arrest occurs in android pelvis
3. **Anthropoid pelvis**—Ape like pelvis
   - Face to pubis delivery occurs
   - Inlet is long AP oval with AP diameter longer than transverse.
4. **Platypelloid pelvis**—inlet transvese oval with long transverse and short AP diameter (flat pelvis)
   - Asynclitism occurs in platypelloid pelvis.

SUGGESTED READING

1. Mudaliyar and Menon's Clinical Obstetrics.
2. Textbook of Obstetrics—Sheila Balakrishnan.
3. Shaw's Textbook of Gynaecology.

To study the phenomenon of disease without books is to sail an uncharted sea, while to study books without patients is not to go to sea at all.

—Sir William Osler

Index

INDEX

INDEX

INDEX

INDEX

INDEX